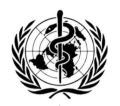

World Health Organization Classification of Tumours

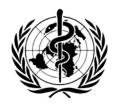

WHO   OMS

International Agency for Research on Cancer (IARC)

4th Edition

WHO Classification of Tumours of Soft Tissue and Bone

Edited by

Christopher D.M. Fletcher

Julia A. Bridge

Pancras C.W. Hogendoorn

Fredrik Mertens

International Agency for Research on Cancer

Lyon, 2013

World Health Organization Classification of Tumours

Series Editors   Fred T. Bosman, MD PhD
Elaine S. Jaffe, MD
Sunil R. Lakhani, MD FRCPath
Hiroko Ohgaki, PhD

WHO Classification of Tumours of Soft Tissue and Bone

Editors   Christopher D.M. Fletcher, MD FRCPath
Julia A. Bridge, MD FACMG
Pancras C.W. Hogendoorn, MD PhD
Fredrik Mertens, MD PhD

Technical Editors   Heidi Mattock, PhD
Rachel Purcell, PhD

Layout   Alberto Machado
Delphine Nicolas

Printed by   Maestro
38330 Saint-Ismier, France

Publisher   International Agency for
Research on Cancer (IARC)
69372 Lyon Cedex 08, France

This volume was produced with support from

Charles Rodolphe Brupbacher Foundation

Institute of Surgical Pathology
University Hospital Zurich

MEDIC Foundation

The WHO Classification of Tumours of Soft Tissue and Bone
presented in this book reflects the views of a Working Group
that convened for a Consensus and Editorial Meeting at the
University of Zurich, Switzerland
18–20 April 2012.

Members of the Working Group are indicated
in the List of Contributors on pages 395–403

Published by the International Agency for Research on Cancer (IARC),
150 cours Albert Thomas, 69372 Lyon Cedex 08, France

Distributed by
WHO Press, World Health Organization, 20 Avenue Appia, 1211 Geneva 27, Switzerland
(Tel: +41 22 791 3264; Fax: +41 22 791 4857; e-mail: bookorders@who.int).

First print run (10000 copies)

Format for bibliographic citations:
Christopher D.M. Fletcher, Julia A. Bridge, Pancras C.W. Hogendoorn, Fredrik Mertens (Eds.):
WHO Classification of Tumours of Soft Tissue and Bone.
IARC: Lyon 2013

IARC Library Cataloguing-in-Publication Data

WHO classification of tumours of soft tissue and bone – 4th edition / edited by Christopher D.M. Fletcher … [et al.]

(World Health Organization classification of tumours)

1. Bone Neoplasms – classification 2. Bone Neoplasms – pathology 3. Neoplasms, Connective and Soft Tissue – classification
4. Neoplasms, Connective and Soft Tissue –pathology
I. Fletcher, Christopher D. M. II. Series

ISBN 978-92-832-2434-1   (NLM Classification: QZ 340)

Contents

WHO Classification of
Tumours of Soft Tissue

WHO classification of tumours of soft tissue[a,b]

ADIPOCYTIC TUMOURS

Benign
Lipoma	8850/0
Lipomatosis	8850/0
Lipomatosis of nerve	8850/0
Lipoblastoma/lipoblastomatosis	8881/0
Angiolipoma	8861/0
Myolipoma	8890/0
Chondroid lipoma	8862/0
Extra-renal angiomyolipoma	8860/0
Extra-adrenal myelolipoma	8870/0
Spindle cell/pleomorphic lipoma	8857/0
Hibernoma	8880/0

Intermediate (locally aggressive)
Atypical lipomatous tumour/	8850/1
well differentiated liposarcoma	8850/3

Malignant
Dedifferentiated liposarcoma	8858/3
Myxoid liposarcoma	8852/3
Pleomorphic liposarcoma	8854/3
Liposarcoma, not otherwise specified	8850/3

FIBROBLASTIC / MYOFIBROBLASTIC TUMOURS

Benign
Nodular fasciitis	8828/0*
Proliferative fasciitis	8828/0*
Proliferative myositis	8828/0*
Myositis ossificans	
Fibro-osseous pseudotumour of digits	
Ischaemic fasciitis	
Elastofibroma	8820/0
Fibrous hamartoma of infancy	
Fibromatosis colli	
Juvenile hyaline fibromatosis	
Inclusion body fibromatosis	
Fibroma of tendon sheath	8813/0
Desmoplastic fibroblastoma	8810/0
Mammary-type myofibroblastoma	8825/0
Calcifying aponeurotic fibroma	8816/0*
Angiomyofibroblastoma	8826/0
Cellular angiofibroma	9160/0
Nuchal-type fibroma	8810/0
Gardner fibroma	8810/0
Calcifying fibrous tumour	8817/0*

Intermediate (locally aggressive)
Palmar/plantar fibromatosis	8813/1*
Desmoid-type fibromatosis	8821/1
Lipofibromatosis	8851/1*
Giant cell fibroblastoma	8834/1

Intermediate (rarely metastasizing)
Dermatofibrosarcoma protuberans	8832/1*
Fibrosarcomatous dermatofibrosarcoma	
protuberans	8832/3*
Pigmented dermatofibrosarcoma protuberans	8833/1*

Solitary fibrous tumour	8815/1*
Solitary fibrous tumour, malignant	8815/3
Inflammatory myofibroblastic tumour	8825/1
Low-grade myofibroblastic sarcoma	8825/3*
Myxoinflammatory fibroblastic sarcoma/	
Atypical myxoinflammatory fibroblastic tumour	8811/1*
Infantile fibrosarcoma	8814/3

Malignant
Adult fibrosarcoma	8810/3
Myxofibrosarcoma	8811/3
Low-grade fibromyxoid sarcoma	8840/3*
Sclerosing epithelioid fibrosarcoma	8840/3*

SO-CALLED FIBROHISTIOCYTIC TUMOURS

Benign
Tenosynovial giant cell tumour	
localized type	9252/0
diffuse type	9252/1*
malignant	9252/3
Deep benign fibrous histiocytoma	8831/0

Intermediate (rarely metastasizing)
Plexiform fibrohistiocytic tumour	8835/1
Giant cell tumour of soft tissues	9251/1

SMOOTH MUSCLE TUMOURS

Benign
Deep leiomyoma	8890/0

Malignant
Leiomyosarcoma (excluding skin)	8890/3

PERICYTIC (PERIVASCULAR) TUMOURS
Glomus tumour (and variants)	8711/0
Glomangiomatosis	8711/1*
Malignant glomus tumour	8711/3
Myopericytoma	8824/0
Myofibroma	8824/0
Myofibromatosis	8824/1
Angioleiomyoma	8894/0

SKELETAL MUSCLE TUMOURS

Benign
Rhabdomyoma	8900/0
Adult type	8904/0
Fetal type	8903/0
Genital type	8905/0

Malignant
Embryonal rhabdomyosarcoma	
(including botryoid, anaplastic)	8910/3
Alveolar rhabdomyosarcoma	
(including solid, anaplastic)	8920/3
Pleomorphic rhabdomyosarcoma	8901/3
Spindle cell/sclerosing rhabdomyosarcoma	8912/3

VASCULAR TUMOURS OF SOFT TISSUE

Benign
Haemangioma	9120/0
Synovial	
Venous	9122/0
Arteriovenous haemangioma/malformation	9123/0
Intramuscular	9132/0
Epithelioid haemangioma	9125/0
Angiomatosis	
Lymphangioma	9170/0

Intermediate (locally aggressive)
Kaposiform haemangioendothelioma	9130/1

Intermediate (rarely metastasizing)
Retiform haemangioendothelioma	9136/1*
Papillary intralymphatic angioendothelioma	9135/1
Composite haemangioendothelioma	9136/1
Pseudomyogenic (epithelioid sarcoma-like) haemangioendothelioma	9136/1
Kaposi sarcoma	9140/3

Malignant
Epithelioid haemangioendothelioma	9133/3
Angiosarcoma of soft tissue	9120/3

CHONDRO-OSSEOUS TUMOURS
Soft tissue chondroma	9220/0
Extraskeletal mesenchymal chondrosarcoma	9240/3
Extraskeletal osteosarcoma	9180/3

GASTROINTESTINAL STROMAL TUMOURS
Benign gastrointestinal stromal tumour	8936/0
Gastrointestinal stromal tumour, uncertain malignant potential	8936/1
Gastrointestinal stromal tumour, malignant	8936/3

NERVE SHEATH TUMOURS

Benign
Schwannoma (including variants)	9560/0
Melanotic schwannoma	9560/1*
Neurofibroma (incl. variants)	9540/0
Plexiform neurofibroma	9550/0
Perineurioma	9571/0
Malignant perineurioma	9571/3
Granular cell tumour	9580/0
Dermal nerve sheath myxoma	9562/0
Solitary circumscribed neuroma	9570/0
Ectopic meningioma	9530/0
Nasal glial heterotopia	
Benign Triton tumour	
Hybrid nerve sheath tumours	9563/0*

Malignant
Malignant peripheral nerve sheath tumour	9540/3
Epithelioid malignant peripheral nerve sheath tumour	9542/3*
Malignant Triton tumour	9561/3
Malignant granular cell tumour	9580/3
Ectomesenchymoma	8921/3

TUMOURS OF UNCERTAIN DIFFERENTIATION

Benign
Acral fibromyxoma	8811/0
Intramuscular myxoma (including cellular variant)	8840/0
Juxta-articular myxoma	8840/0
Deep ("aggressive") angiomyxoma	8841/0*
Pleomorphic hyalinizing angiectatic tumour	8802/1*
Ectopic hamartomatous thymoma	8587/0

Intermediate (locally aggressive)
Haemosiderotic fibrolipomatous tumour	8811/1*

Intermediate (rarely metastasizing)
Atypical fibroxanthoma	8830/1
Angiomatoid fibrous histiocytoma	8836/1
Ossifying fibromyxoid tumour	8842/0
Ossifying fibromyxoid tumour, malignant	8842/3*
Mixed tumour NOS	8940/0
Mixed tumour NOS, malignant	8940/3
Myoepithelioma	8982/0
Myoepithelial carcinoma	8982/3
Phosphaturic mesenchymal tumour, benign	8990/0
Phosphaturic mesenchymal tumour, malignant	8990/3

Malignant
Synovial sarcoma NOS	9040/3
Synovial sarcoma, spindle cell	9041/3
Synovial sarcoma, biphasic	9043/3
Epithelioid sarcoma	8804/3
Alveolar soft-part sarcoma	9581/3
Clear cell sarcoma of soft tissue	9044/3
Extraskeletal myxoid chondrosarcoma	9231/3
Extraskeletal Ewing sarcoma	9364/3
Desmoplastic small round cell tumour	8806/3
Extra-renal rhabdoid tumour	8963/3
Neoplasms with perivascular epithelioid cell differentiation (PEComa)	
PEComa NOS, benign	8714/0*
PEComa NOS, malignant	8714/3*
Intimal sarcoma	9137/3*

UNDIFFERENTIATED/UNCLASSIFIED SARCOMAS
Undifferentiated spindle cell sarcoma	8801/3
Undifferentiated pleomorphic sarcoma	8802/3
Undifferentiated round cell sarcoma	8803/3
Undifferentiated epithelioid sarcoma	8804/3
Undifferentiated sarcoma NOS	8805/3

---

[a] The morphology codes are from the International Classification of Diseases for Oncology (ICD-O) {916A}. Behaviour is coded /0 for benign tumours, /1 for unspecified, borderline or uncertain behaviour, /2 for carcinoma in situ and grade III intraepithelial neoplasia, and /3 for malignant tumours; [b] The classification is modified from the previous WHO histological classification of tumours {870A} taking into account changes in understanding of these lesions. * These new codes were approved by the IARC/WHO Committee for ICD-O in 2012.

TNM classification of soft tissue sarcomas

T – Primary tumour

TX	Primary tumour cannot be assessed
T0	No evidence of primary tumour
T1	Tumour 5 cm or less in greatest dimension
T1a	Superficial tumour*
T1b	Deep tumour*
T2	Tumour more than 5 cm in greatest dimension
T2a	Superficial tumour*
T2b	Deep tumour*

Note: *Superficial tumour is located exclusively above the superficial fascia without invasion of the fascia; deep tumour is located either exclusively beneath the superficial fascia or superficial to the fascia with invasion of or through the fascia. Retroperitoneal, mediastinal, and pelvic sarcomas are classified as deep tumours.

N – Regional lymph nodes

NX	Regional lymph nodes cannot be assessed
N0	No regional lymph-node metastasis
N1	Regional lymph-node metastasis

Note: Regional node involvement is rare and cases in which nodal status is not assessed either clinically or pathologically could be considered N0 instead of NX or pNX.

M – Distant metastasis

M0	No distant metastasis
M1	Distant metastasis

G – Histopathological grading

Translation table for three- and four-grade systems to a two-grade (low grade vs high grade) system.

TNM Two-grade system	Three-grade systems	Four-grade systems
Low grade	Grade I	Grade I
		Grade II
High grade	Grade II	Grade III
	Grade III	Grade IV

Note: If grade cannot be assessed, extraskeletal Ewing and primitive neuroectodermal tumours are classified as high grade. If grade cannot be assessed, classify as low grade.

Stage grouping

Stage IA	T1a, T1b	N0	M0	G1
Stage IB	T2a, T2b	N0	M0	G1
Stage IIA	T1a, T1b	N0	M0	G2, G3
Stage IIB	T2a, T2b	N0	M0	G2
Stage III	T2a, T2b	N0	M0	G3
	Any T	N1	M0	Any G
Stage IV	Any T	Any N	M1	Any G

A help-desk for specific questions about the TNM classification is available at http://www.uicc.org.

References

1. American Joint Committee on Cancer (AJCC) Cancer Staging Manual 7th ed. Edge SB, Byrd DR, Compton CC, Fritz AG, Greene FL, Trotti III H. eds. New York: Springer. 2010
2. Union for International Cancer Control (UICC): TNM classification of malignant tumors 7th ed. Sobin LH, Gospodarowicz MK, Wittekind Ch. eds. Wiley-Blackwell. Oxford. 2010

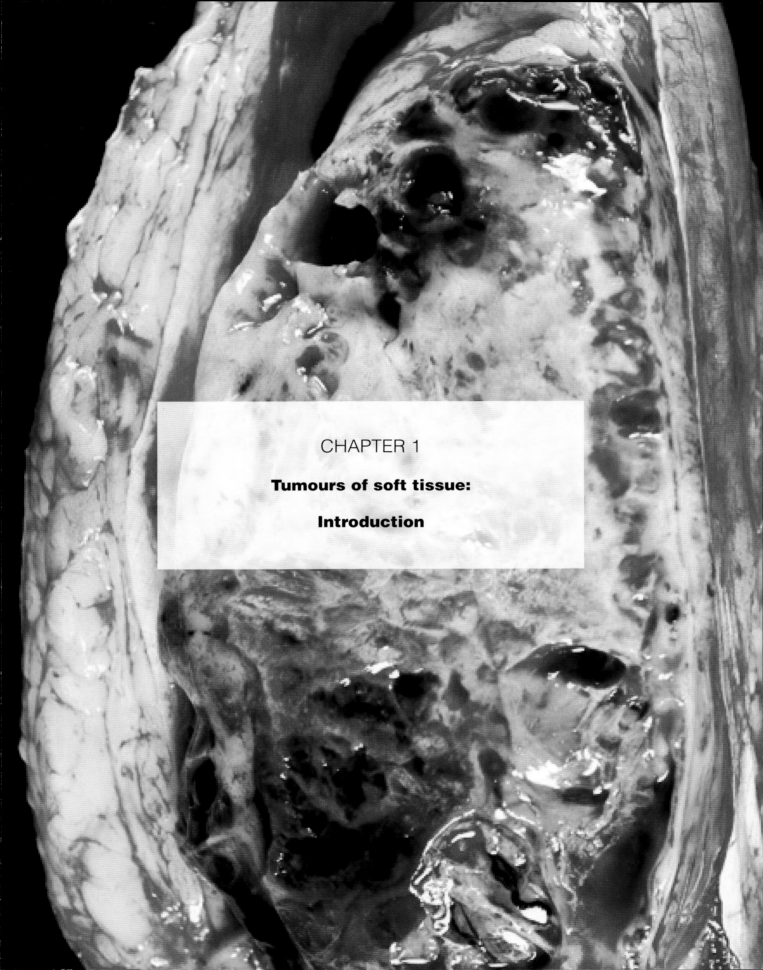

CHAPTER 1

Tumours of soft tissue:

Introduction

Tumours of soft tissue: Introduction

Epidemiology

C.D.M. Fletcher
A. Gronchi

Incidence

Benign mesenchymal tumours outnumber sarcomas by a factor of at least 100. The annual clinical incidence (number of new patients consulting a doctor) of benign tumours of soft tissue has been estimated as up to 3000 per million population {1989}, whereas the annual incidence of soft tissue sarcoma is around 50 per million population {953,1069}, i.e. < 1% of all malignant tumours (but more frequent in children). There are no data to indicate a change in the incidence of sarcoma, nor are there significant geographical differences.

Age and site distribution

At least 30% of the benign tumours of soft tissue are lipomas, 30% are fibrohistiocytic and fibrous tumours, 10% are vascular tumours and 5% are nerve sheath tumours. There is a relationship between the type of tumour, symptoms, location and patient age and sex. Lipomas are painless, rare in the hand, lower leg and foot and very uncommon in children {1989}; angiolipomas are often painful and most common in young men; angioleiomyomas are often painful and common in the lower leg of middle-aged women; half of the vascular tumours occur in patients aged < 20 years {1581,2398}. Of the benign tumours, 99% are superficial and 95% are < 5 cm in diameter {2398}. Soft tissue sarcomas may occur anywhere, but 75% are located in the extremities (most common in thigh) and 10% each in the trunk wall and retroperitoneum. There is a slight male predominance. Of the extremity and trunk-wall tumours, 30% are superficial with a median diameter of 5 cm, while 60% are deep-seated with a median diameter of 9 cm {1069}. Retroperitoneal tumours are often much larger before they become symptomatic.

About 10% of patients have detectable metastases (most common in the lungs) at diagnosis of the primary tumour. Overall, at least one third of patients with soft tissue sarcoma die from tumour-related disease, most of them from lung metastases.

About three quarters of soft tissue sarcomas are histologically classified as undifferentiated pleomorphic sarcoma (previously known as malignant fibrous histiocytoma [MFH]), liposarcoma, leiomyosarcoma, myxofibrosarcoma, synovial sarcoma, or malignant peripheral nerve sheath tumour and three quarters are highly malignant (see *Grading and staging of sarcomas*) {1069}. The distribution of histotypes varies over time and between researchers, probably because of changing definitions of histotypes (as, for example, MFH in the 1990s).

Age-related incidences vary: embryonal rhabdomyosarcoma occurs almost exclusively in children, synovial sarcoma mostly in young adults, whereas undifferentiated pleomorphic sarcoma, liposarcoma, leiomyosarcoma and myxofibrosarcoma dominate in the elderly. Like almost all other malignancies, soft tissue sarcomas become more common with increasing age; median age at diagnosis is 65 years.

Etiology

C.D.M. Fletcher
A. Gronchi

The etiology of most benign and malignant tumours of soft tissue is unknown. In rare cases, genetic and environmental factors, irradiation, viral infections and immunodeficiency have been found to be associated with the development of usually malignant soft tissue tumours. There are also isolated reports of sarcomas arising in scar tissue, at fracture sites and close to surgical implants {1426}. Some angiosarcomas arise in chronic lymphoedema. However, the large majority of soft tissue sarcomas seem to arise de novo, without an apparent causative factor. Some malignant mesenchymal neoplasms occur in the setting of familial cancer syndromes (see below and Chapter 26). Multistage tumorigenesis sequences with gradual accumulation of genetic alterations and increasing histological degree of malignancy have not yet been clearly identified in most tumours of soft tissue.

Chemical carcinogens

Several studies, many of them from Sweden, have reported an increased incidence of soft tissue sarcoma after exposure to phenoxyacetic herbicides, chlorophenols, and their contaminants (dioxin) in agricultural or forestry work {766,1110}. Other studies have not found this association. One explanation for different findings may be the use of herbicides that are contaminated with dioxin at different levels {1790,3046}.

Radiation

The reported incidence of post-irradiation sarcoma ranges from a few cases per thousand to nearly one per hundred. Most incidence estimates are based on patients with breast cancer treated with radiation as adjuvant therapy {1374}. The risk increases with dose; most patients have received 50 Gy or more and the median time between exposure and tumour diagnosis is about 10 years, although there is some evidence that this latent interval is decreasing. More than half of these tumours have been classified as undifferentiated pleomorphic sarcoma, most often being highly malignant. In skin, angiosarcoma is more common. Patients with a germline mutation in the retinoblastoma gene (*RB1*) have a significantly elevated risk of developing post-irradiation sarcoma {1436}, usually osteosarcoma. Similarly, patients with a germline mutation in *TP53* (Li-Fraumeni syndrome) have a significantly high risk of developing post-irradiation sarcoma {1168}, as also do patients with neurofibromatosis type 1 (NF1) {2524}.

Viral infection and immunodeficiency
HHV8 plays a key role in the development of Kaposi sarcoma {253} and the clinical course of the disease is dependent on the immune status of the patient {2923}.

EBV is associated with smooth muscle tumours in patients with immunodeficiency {654}.

Genetic susceptibility
Several types of benign soft tissue tumour have been reported to occur on a familial or inherited basis. However, these reports are rare and comprise an insignificant number of tumours. The most common example is probably hereditary multiple lipoma (or angiolipoma) {2,1003}. Desmoid tumours occur in patients with the Gardner variant of familial adenomatous polyposis (FAP) {1067}. Neurofibromatosis (types 1 and 2) is associated with multiple benign nerve sheath tumours (and sometimes also non-neural tumours).

In up to 5–10% of patients with NF1, malignant peripheral nerve sheath tumours develop, usually in a benign nerve sheath tumour {2956}. Moreover, 5–7% of these patients may develop one or more gastrointestinal stromal tumours (GISTs). Li-Fraumeni syndrome {1184} is a rare autosomal dominant disease caused by germline mutations in the *TP53* tumour suppressor gene, which predispose to the development of sarcoma {1008}. At age 30 years, half of the patients have already developed malignant tumours, of which > 30% are sarcomas of soft tissue or bone. The inherited, or bilateral, form of retinoblastoma, with a germline mutation of the *RB1* gene, may also be associated with development of sarcoma.

Clinical features

S. Singer
A. Gronchi

Clinical features are only occasionally sufficient to distinguish benign from malignant tumours of soft tissue. Most soft tissue sarcomas of the extremities and trunk wall present as painless, incidentally observed tumours that do not influence function or general health, despite their often large volume. The seemingly innocent presentation and the rarity of these sarcomas often lead to misinterpretation as benign conditions. All superficial soft tissue lesions measuring > 5 cm and all deep-seated lesions have a high probability of being a sarcoma and it is therefore recommended that these patients are referred to specialized centres for treatment {396,2019}. Patients with intra-abdominal or retroperitoneal sarcomas often experience nonspecific abdominal discomfort and gastrointestinal symptoms; the diagnosis is usually suspected on finding a soft tissue mass on abdominal imaging.

Biopsy
A biopsy is often appropriate to establish malignancy, assess histological grade and, if possible, determine the histological type and subtype. Most limb masses are best sampled through multiple needle-core biopsies obtained through a single tract, which should be placed so that it can be completely excised during definitive resection. If biopsy is performed with adequate needles and multiple sampling, the accuracy of histological classification,

grading and prognostication is very high. Additional sampling may be required for specific research protocols. When the needle-core approach fails, an alternative for most extremity masses is an incisional biopsy with minimal extension into adjacent tissue planes. Excisional biopsy should be avoided, particularly for lesions > 2 cm, because the contamination of surrounding tissue planes would make definitive re-excision more extensive. Fine-needle aspiration cytology is best performed at centres with specific cytological expertise and the capability for careful clinicoradiological correlation.

For non-extremity tumours, pretreatment biopsy is not required if the tumour appears on imaging to be desmoid, a liposarcoma, or gastrointestinal stromal tumour (GIST) and can be resected with minimal morbidity. However, biopsy (percutaneous CT-guided needle-core biopsy) is recommended under the following circumstances: (i) imaging results may also be suggestive of germ cell tumour, carcinoma or lymphoma; (ii) resection is likely to be incomplete or highly morbid; or (iii) preoperative therapy is an option.

Therapy
Once the histological diagnosis and grade have been established and the work-up for distant metastasis performed, a multidisciplinary team of surgeons, radiation oncologists and medical oncologists

can design the most effective treatment plan for the patient. The plan must balance the goal of minimizing recurrence with the goal of preserving function and quality of life. Surgery remains the principal therapeutic modality in soft tissue sarcoma, while the optimum combination of chemotherapy and radiotherapy is controversial.

Surgery
In principle, surgery should consist of en-bloc removal of the tumour with a cuff of healthy tissue all around. Every attempt should be made to avoid microscopically positive surgical margins, since they are associated with higher risk of local recurrence, distant metastasis and death {1046, 1048,2658,2783,3045}. However, in certain situations a microscopically positive margin may be unavoidable because of the need to preserve critical neurovascular structures. The scope of the excision is generally dictated by the size and histological subtype of the tumour, its anatomical relation to normal structures (e.g. major vessels and neurovascular bundles) and the degree of morbidity and functional loss expected.

Sarcomas of the extremities and trunk wall can often be treated by surgery alone. For subcutaneous or intramuscular high-grade soft tissue sarcoma < 5 cm, or any size of low-grade sarcoma, surgery alone should be considered if the tumour can be excised with a good 1–2 cm cuff of surrounding fat and muscle. If, however, the excision margin is close, or if there is extramuscular involvement, adjuvant radiotherapy should be added. However, irrespective of grade, postoperative radiotherapy is probably used more often than strictly necessary. In fact, a significant subset of subcutaneous and intramuscular sarcomas can be treated by wide-margin excision alone, with a local recurrence rate of only 5–10% {146,353,2250,2399}. Retroperitoneal sarcomas tend to present at a later stage, and because of their large size, their tendency to invade adjacent organs and the difficulty in achieving a clean margin, the survival rate for retroperitoneal sarcomas is much lower than that for extremity soft tissue sarcoma. The most important prognostic factors for survival in retroperitoneal sarcoma are the completeness of the surgical resection, the histological grade and histological type/subtype {562,1601,2562,2563}. Even with an aggressive surgical approach, recurrence is still a significant problem that often leads to unresectable local disease and death. Well-differentiated and dedifferentiated liposarcoma, which account for the majority of retroperitoneal sarcomas, frequently recur locally and multifocally {739,1162,2562}. High-grade leiomyosarcoma, in contrast, is more likely to give rise to liver or lung metastases. The extent of resection of retroperitoneal sarcomas will be affected by proximity of the tumour to important structures. Every effort should be made to achieve a complete resection with negative margins, and adjacent viscera, muscles and fascias should be resected if they are overtly infiltrated. Even if adjacent tissues are not overtly invaded, some have argued that their resection may improve local control and final outcome {268,269,1049,1050}. However, a definitive comparison of aggressive versus more conservative approaches has not been performed.

Some non-metastasizing lesions, such as intramuscular haemangioma, require wide excision comparable to that necessary for a sarcoma; otherwise, local recurrence is very frequent. However, desmoid-type fibromatosis is now most often treated by a conservative approach, avoiding ablative surgery, because of the significant rate of spontaneous growth arrest and occasional spontaneous regressions {849, 2424}.

Adjuvant and neoadjuvant chemotherapy

The value of chemotherapy depends on the specific histological type and the location of the sarcoma. Because of their very high risk of metastasis and sensitivity to chemotherapy, Ewing sarcoma and alveolar/embryonal rhabdomyosarcoma should always be treated with neoadjuvant chemotherapy. For other histological types of high-grade sarcoma, the choice to use chemotherapy depends on the risk of metastasis (governed by size and histology), the sensitivity of the histological type/subtype to neoadjuvant chemotherapy and the patient's age and comorbidities. Many randomized trials of soft tissue sarcoma have shown that chemotherapy improves disease-free survival, with improved local and locoregional control {53,74,297,529}. An improvement in overall survival has been demonstrated in a single randomized trial, which involved an anthracycline (epirubicin) plus ifosfamide, although the trial had relatively short follow-up {918}. This overall survival benefit was confirmed in a recent meta-analysis, with a hazard ratio of 0.77 ($P = 0.01$) {2224}. Given the relatively small benefit, preoperative chemotherapy with an anthracycline and ifosfamide can be justified for large, high-grade tumours in carefully selected patients and for the histological types most likely to respond (e.g. synovial sarcoma, myxoid/round cell liposarcoma, pleomorphic liposarcoma, undifferentiated pleomorphic sarcoma). A recent trial has shown that three cycles of full-dose anthracycline and ifosfamide has equivalent outcomes to five cycles {1047}; the more prolonged treatment may merely increase toxicity.

Agents with activity against particular histological subtypes include gemcitabine and docetaxel for undifferentiated pleomorphic sarcoma and leiomyosarcoma {1709}, trabectedin for myxoid/round cell liposarcoma and leiomyosarcoma {1052}, gemcitabine and taxanes for angiosarcoma {2211,2635} and ifosfamide for myxoid/round cell and pleomorphic liposarcoma {731} and synovial sarcoma {374,730}.

Multimodal protocols

For the multimodal treatment of large, high-grade sarcomas, several sequencing schedules have been developed {2564}:
(i) Neoadjuvant chemotherapy > surgery > postoperative radiotherapy ± adjuvant chemotherapy;
(ii) Neoadjuvant chemotherapy + preoperative radiotherapy > surgery > ± adjuvant chemotherapy;
(iii) Neoadjuvant chemotherapy > preoperative radiotherapy > surgery > ± adjuvant chemotherapy.
An advantage to the first approach, for patients with measurable disease, is the ability to determine at an early stage whether the sarcoma is progressing on chemotherapy and, if so, to avoid further treatment with an agent that appears ineffective.

Imaging of tumours of soft tissue

D. Vanel

The classical criteria explained in the clinical features must be known and used by the radiologist: when deep-seated tumours of soft tissue are encountered on imaging examinations, the patient should ideally be directed to a reference centre, before any aggressive intervention, including biopsy. This initial selection is a crucial responsibility of the radiologist.
Ultrasound is often the first examination used, as it is simple and cheap. It is nevertheless operator-dependent, and nonspecific. Radiographs are useful to rule out a bone tumour invading the soft tissues, detect calcifications and bone erosion, and hence a risk of fracture. MRI is by far superior to CT because of higher contrast. CT is only used to check calcifications seen on radiographs, and sometimes to guide the needle biopsy.
MRI accurately defines tumour size, relationship to muscle compartments, fascial planes (sarcomas are usually, but not always {1947}, in a deep location), and

bone and neurovascular structures in multiple planes. It provides information on haemorrhage, necrosis, oedema, cystic and myxoid degeneration, and fibrosis. The usual sarcoma has a low signal on T1-weighted (T1W) images, and a high heterogeneous signal on T2-weighted (T2W) sequences. It takes up contrast medium heterogeneously. The components lacking uptake after contrast injection are not always necrotic: they can also be a myxoid component of the tumour. This fact must be clearly explained by the radiologist, as myxoid areas may decrease under chemotherapy, while necrosis does not. When the signal is different, the diagnosis capability increases: tumours with a high signal on T1W images contain fat (lipoma or well-differentiated liposarcoma, angioma because of muscle atrophy), blood, or rarely melanin (half of clear cell sarcomas)

{594}. Muscle fibres inside a fat mass usually indicate an intramuscular lipoma, but can rarely also be seen in liposarcomas {678}. Lesions with a low signal on T2W sequences correspond to fibrous tissue (fibrous sarcomas and fibromatosis), or haemosiderin in chronically bleeding masses such as diffuse-type tenosynovial giant cell tumour.

Dynamic MRI after injection of contrast medium is both sensitive and specific for the detection of malignancy {2839}, but not sufficiently to avoid the need for a biopsy. It is the same for MRI diffusion, perfusion and spectroscopy.

MRI aids in guiding biopsy, planning surgery, evaluating response to chemotherapy, restaging, and in the long-term follow-up for local recurrence {2852}. The T2W sequence remains the first indispensable step. The role of a regular MRI

follow-up is very controversial {1517}. Image-guided needle biopsy is the most frequently used technique to perform histological examination. The tract must be chosen with the surgeon who will operate on the patient, to allow easy removal. Tattooing the entrance point is easy and leaves a reliable trace. The radiologist must check the quality of the biopsies with the pathologist, so as to improve technique. Spiral CT is preferable for examining sarcomas of the chest, since air/tissue interface and motion artefacts often degrade MRI quality. CT and MRI are of equivalent value for the imaging of abdominal tumours. A baseline chest CT scan at the time of diagnosis is useful, particularly for sarcomas measuring > 5 cm, for accurate staging of patients. Use of PET is increasing.

Grading and staging of sarcomas

J.-M. Coindre

Grading of sarcomas

Except for some sarcomas, histological typing does not provide sufficient information for predicting the clinical course of disease and, therefore, this must be achieved by grading and staging. While grading is based only on the intrinsic quality of the primary tumour, staging also takes into account tumour extent, and nomograms assess multiple clinical and histological parameters to calculate the probability of recurrence for a given patient {729}.

Grading of sarcomas of soft tissue was first proposed in 1939 by Broders, but the first large-scale effort to use grade and stage in sarcomas was achieved in 1977 by Russell et al. {2395}. This study showed the prominent role of grade for predicting outcome for patients with sarcomas, although the grade used was determined subjectively. In the early 1980s, several grading systems, based on various histological parameters, were reported and proved to correlate with prognosis {513,1990, 2780,2849}. Most grading systems are based on mitotic activity and necrosis. The two most widely used systems are those proposed by the NCI {513} and the FNCLCC {2780}. The FNCLCC system appears to be more precisely defined and potentially more reproducible and, therefore, is the most widely used {658.} In accordance with the College of American

Pathologists (CAP) and the AJCC recommendations, this system is preferred over the NCI system, at least in adults {2387}. Moreover, a comparison of both systems showed greater efficiency of the FNCLCC system in terms of prognostic prediction {1060}. Three independent prognostic factors are used for defining the grade: necrosis, mitotic activity and degree of differentiation. A score is attributed independently

to each parameter and the grade is obtained by adding the three attributed scores {2780}. The weakness of the system lies in the definition of differentiation score, which depends on histological type and subtype.

The main value of grading is to indicate the probability of distant metastasis and overall survival in the whole group of sarcomas considered as a single entity, but

Table 1.1 Definition of histopathological parameters in the FNCLCC grading system

Histological parameter	Definition
Tumour differentiation (see Table 1.2)	• Score 1: Sarcomas closely resembling normal adult mesenchymal tissue and potentially difficult to distinguish from the counterpart benign tumour (e.g. well-differentiated liposarcoma, well-differentiated leiomyosarcoma) • Score 2: Sarcomas for which histological typing is certain (e.g. myxoid liposarcoma, myxofibrosarcoma) • Score 3: Embryonal and undifferentiated sarcomas, synovial sarcomas, sarcomas of doubtful type
Mitotic count (established on the basis of 10 HPF; 1 HPF measures 0.1734 mm^2)	• Score 1: 0–9 mitoses per 10 HPF • Score 2: 10–19 mitoses per 10 HPF • Score 3: > 19 mitoses per 10 HPF
Tumour necrosis	• Score 0: no necrosis • Score 1: < 50% tumour necrosis • Score 2: ≥ 50% tumour necrosis
Histological grade	• Grade 1: total score 2, 3 • Grade 2: total score 4, 5 • Grade 3: total score 6, 7, 8
FNCLCC, Fédération Nationale des Centres de Lutte Contre le Cancer; HPF, high-power field Modified from {494}	

also in undifferentiated pleomorphic sarcomas and synovial sarcomas {500}. On the other hand, it is of poor value for predicting local recurrence, which is mainly related to the quality of surgical margins. Because of the pitfalls and limitations of grading, some rules must be respected: grading is not a substitute for an accurate histological diagnosis; it requires represen-tative and well-processed material that should be obtained before neoadjuvant therapy. Grading is less informative than histological type in dedifferentiated and round cell liposarcomas, rhabdomyosarcoma, Ewing sarcoma, alveolar soft part sarcoma, epithelioid sarcoma, clear cell sarcoma, and it should not be used in tumours that rarely metastasize {494,658}. Several criticisms have been made of histological grading. A universal grading system is not possible for all sarcomas, but it is unrealistic to develop a grading system for every specific histological type of sarcoma and the systems currently used perform correctly for the most frequent sarcoma types and represent an acceptable alternative. The reproducibility of the same grading system among pathologists and of different grading systems for the same tumours is rather poor. Most grading systems are three-grade systems with an intermediate grade that actually corresponds to undetermined prognosis and represents about half of cases. The universal use of needle-core biopsies is another important limitation for grading. Although grading on needle-core biopsies has been reported to show an acceptable degree of accuracy {1196}, determination of grade can be done with certainty for high-grade sarcomas only. Histological grading may be helped by imaging procedures for evaluating necrosis and by a MIB1 score instead of mitotic index {1125}. Despite its limitations, grade remains the most important prognostic factor in most sarcomas, and it is clear that clinicians will continue to expect pathologists to provide a grade for most sarcomas.

Grading can be considered as a morphological translation of molecular events that determine tumour aggressiveness and, therefore, molecular parameters could eventually complement or even replace histological parameters. A molecular grading system based on the expression profile of 67 genes related to chromosome complexity and mitosis management (CINSARC for Complexity INdex in SARComas) has been described on a large series of sarcomas with complex genomic profiles. This molecular grading outperforms histological grading in this category of sarcomas as well as in gastrointestinal stromal tumours (GISTs) {443,1527}.

Staging

Staging of soft tissue sarcomas is based on histological and clinical information. The major staging systems used were developed by UICC and AJCC and are clinically useful and of prognostic value. The TNM system incorporates histological grade as well as tumour size and depth, regional lymph-node involvement and distant metastasis {722}.

Table 1.2 Tumour differentiation score according to histological type in the FNCLCC grading system

Histological type	Differentiation score
Well-differentiated liposarcoma	1
Well-differentiated leiomyosarcoma	1
Malignant neurofibroma	1
Well-differentiated fibrosarcoma	1
Myxoid liposarcoma	2
Conventional leiomyosarcoma	2
Conventional MPNST	2
Conventional fibrosarcoma	2
Myxofibrosarcoma	2
Myxoid chondrosarcoma	2
Conventional angiosarcoma	2
High-grade myxoid (round cell) liposarcoma	3
Pleomorphic liposarcoma	3
Dedifferentiated liposarcoma	3
Rhabdomyosarcoma	3
Poorly differentiated/pleomorphic leiomyosarcoma	3
Poorly differentiated/epithelioid angiosarcoma	3
Poorly differentiated MPNST	3
Malignant Triton tumour	3
Synovial sarcoma	3
Extraskeletal osteosarcoma	3
Extraskeletal Ewing sarcoma	3
Mesenchymal chondrosarcoma	3
Clear cell sarcoma	3
Epithelioid sarcoma	3
Alveolar soft part sarcoma	3
Malignant rhabdoid tumour	3
Undifferentiated (spindle cell and pleomorphic) sarcoma	3

FNCLCC, Fédération Nationale des Centres de Lutte Contre le Cancer; MPNST, malignant peripheral nerve sheath tumour

Modified from {494}

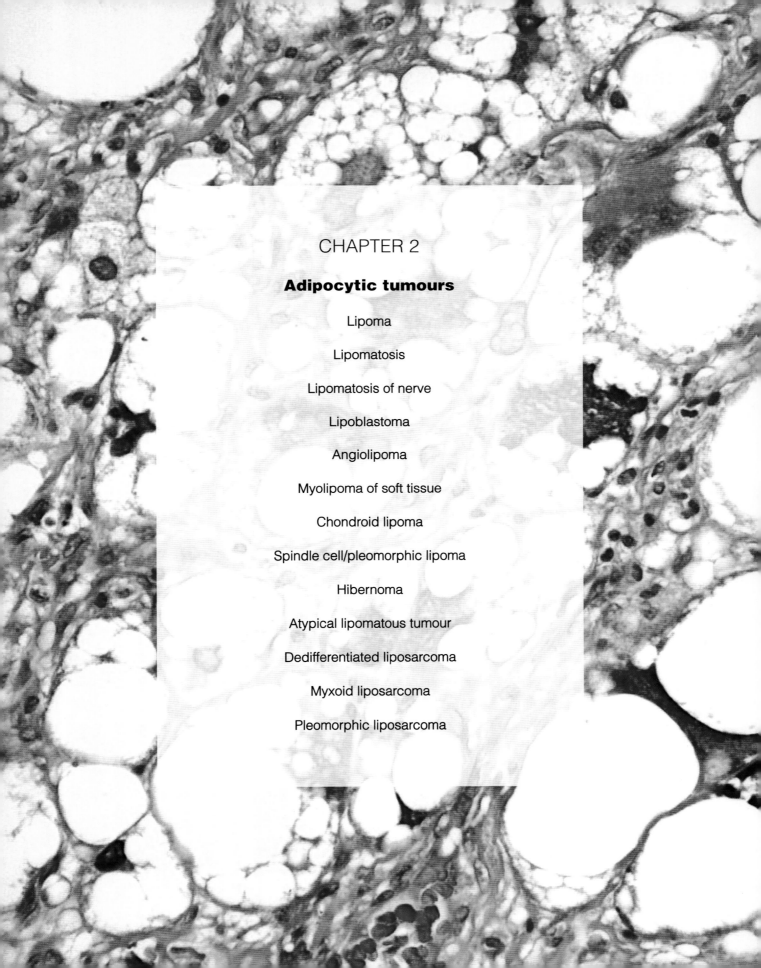

CHAPTER 2

Adipocytic tumours

Lipoma

Lipomatosis

Lipomatosis of nerve

Lipoblastoma

Angiolipoma

Myolipoma of soft tissue

Chondroid lipoma

Spindle cell/pleomorphic lipoma

Hibernoma

Atypical lipomatous tumour

Dedifferentiated liposarcoma

Myxoid liposarcoma

Pleomorphic liposarcoma

Lipoma

G.P. Nielsen
N. Mandahl

Definition
Lipoma is a benign tumour composed of mature white adipocytes.

ICD-O code   8850/0

Epidemiology
Conventional lipoma is the most common mesenchymal neoplasm in adults and is most frequent between age 40 and 60 years {756}. Approximately 5% of patients have multiple lipomas.

Sites of involvement
Conventional lipoma can arise within the subcutaneous tissue or deep soft tissues or on the surfaces of bone (parosteal lipoma) {1385,2355}. Deep-seated lipomas that arise within or between skeletal muscle fibres are called intramuscular or intermuscular lipomas, respectively {868, 1421}. Intramuscular lipoma involves skeletal muscle in a variety of locations, including the trunk, head and neck region, upper and lower extremities {868,1421}. Intermuscular lipoma arises most frequently in the anterior abdominal wall. So-called lipoma arborescens (villous lipomatous proliferation of synovial membrane) is characterized by fatty infiltration of the subsynovial connective tissue {1079,1746}. Retroperitoneal lipomas are very rare and require molecular confirmation {1273,1684}.

Clinical features
Lipoma usually presents as a painless soft tissue mass, although larger tumours can be painful owing to compression of peripheral nerves. Superficial lipomas are generally smaller (5 cm). Patients with lipoma arborescens are usually men complaining of gradual joint swelling {414,1035, 1079,1746,2594}. Imaging studies show a homogeneous soft tissue mass that is isodense to fat. Attenuated fibrous strands can be seen, but are not as prominent as in atypical lipomatous tumours. Intramuscular lipomas are more variably circumscribed.

Macroscopy
Lipomas are well circumscribed and have

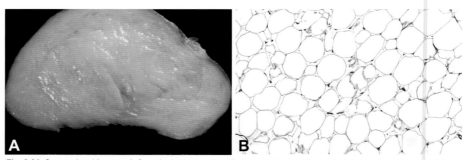
Fig. 2.01 Conventional lipoma. **A** Grossly, the tumour is well-circumscribed and has a homogeneous, yellow cut surface. **B** The mature adipocytes vary only slightly in size and shape and have small eccentric nuclei.

a yellow, greasy, cut surface. Different types are similar in appearance; however, bone formation can be seen in osteolipoma and grey glistening nodules may be seen in chondrolipoma. Intramuscular and intermuscular lipomas do not show any specific gross features except that a portion of skeletal muscle is often attached to the periphery of the tumour.

Histopathology
Conventional lipoma is composed of lobules of mature adipocytes. Lipomas can occasionally have areas of bone formation (osteolipoma), cartilage (chondrolipoma), or abundant fibrous tissue (fibrolipoma). Most lipomas with extensive myxoid change (so-called myxolipomas) are variants of spindle cell lipoma. Intramuscular lipoma may be either well demarcated from the surrounding skeletal muscle or, more often, shows an infiltrative growth pattern with mature adipocytes infiltrating

and encasing pre-existing skeletal muscle fibres that often show evidence of atrophy. Lipoma arborescens shows diffuse fatty infiltration of the subsynovial connective tissue.

Immunophenotype
Lipomas stain for S100 protein, leptin and HMGA2 {699,2119}.

Ultrastructure
The neoplastic cells have a single lipid droplet compressing a peripherally situated nucleus. Pinocytotic vesicles are present and external lamina is seen surrounding the cells {1417}.

Genetics
Cytogenetics
The pattern of aberrations in lipomas is heterogeneous, but three subgroups have been distinguished: (i) aberrations involving 12q13–15 (65% of cases); (ii) loss of

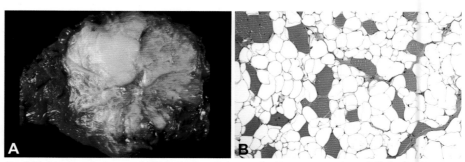
Fig. 2.02 Intramuscular lipoma. **A** This lesion is well-circumscribed in some areas (upper left), but in other areas infiltrates and encases the red skeletal muscle (lower). **B** The lesion is composed of mature adipocytes that infiltrate and encase skeletal muscle fibres.

material from 13q (10%); and (iii) aberrations involving 6p21-23 (5%). Various combinations of these are present in 7% of tumours {160}. Most data come from deep-seated lesions. A fourth subgroup consists of tumours with other aberrations or normal karyotypes. FISH analyses frequently reveal that the aberrations are more complex than appreciated by chromosome-banding patterns. Pseudodiploidy is seen in 87% of the tumours and clonal evolution in 10%. Reported lipomas with ring chromosomes are usually larger and deep-seated {160}, and may actually have been atypical lipomatous tumour.

Two thirds of tumours with abnormal karyotypes show aberrations of 12q13-15. The most common, t(3;12)(q27-28;q13-15), is seen in 20% of tumours. There are many other recurrent recombination partners; those present in 3-8% of tumours include 1p32-34, 2p22-24, 2q35-37, 5q33, 12p11-12, and 12q24. A subset of tumours shows intrachromosomal rearrangements, leading to recombination between 12q13-15 and other segments of chromosome 12. About 13% of lipomas with aberrant karyotypes show loss of material from 13q.

Molecular genetics

The high-mobility group AT-hook 2 (*HMGA2*) gene, localized to 12q14.3, plays an important pathogenetic role in a subset of lipomas {114,2473}. The breakpoints of structural aberrations occur within or outside *HMGA2*, the essential outcome being deregulation of *HMGA2*. Recombination of *HMGA2* with several genes has been reported. The most common chimeric transcript is *HMGA2-LPP* resulting from a t(3;12) {2229}. The fusion gene encodes a novel transcription factor containing the N-terminal AT-hook domain of HMGA2 and C-terminal LIM domains of LPP. Other partner genes include *CXCR7* in 2q37.3 {325,1131}, *EBF1* in 5q33.3 {2053}, *NFIB* in 9p22.3 {1297,2054,2242}, and *LHFP* in 13q13.3 {2230}. The variability of breakpoint localization in many of the fusion partners is in accordance with the idea that truncation of HMGA2 is the critical event.

HMGA2 is rarely expressed in lipomas with 6p21-23 changes and 13q losses, whereas tumours with 12q13-15 re-

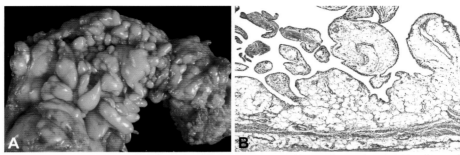

Fig. 2.03 Synovial lipoma (lipoma arborescens). **A** The entire synovium in this resection specimen is bright yellow, and has a nodular or papillary appearance. **B** The subsynovial connective tissue has been replaced by mature adipocytes.

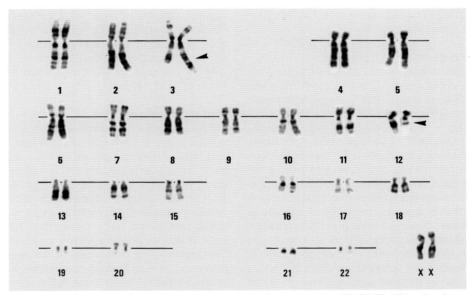

Fig. 2.04 A lipoma karyotype showing the most common structural rearrangement, a t(3;12)(q27;q15) translocation.

arrangement show strong or moderate expression of the full-length gene or a truncated gene (exons 1-3); tumours with t(3;12) express exons 1-3, whereas the majority of tumours with t(5;12) express the entire gene.

Lipomas with loss of 13q material have a minimal deleted region of 3.5 Mb in 13q14, overlapping with one of two deleted regions in spindle cell lipomas {161}. Only the *C13orf1* gene in this region is expressed at significantly lower levels compared with controls and lipomas without 13q deletion.

In tumours with rearrangements of 6p21-23, the breakpoints usually occur adjacent to the coding sequences of *HMGA1* in 6p21, a gene structurally homologous

to *HMGA2* {160,2906}. The most common recombination is with 3q27-28; fusion with *LPP* has not been found.

Some lipomas have gains of *MDM2* {1295,1717}. Rearrangement of 8q11-13 is seen in 2-3% of lipomas; rearrangement of *PLAG1* has been reported in one case {160,299}. These may represent matured lipoblastomas.

Prognostic factors

Lipomas rarely recur. The subclassification of conventional lipoma does not have any prognostic significance except for infiltrating intramuscular lipoma, which has a higher rate of local recurrence {249}.

Lipomatosis

G.P. Nielsen
A.E. Rosenberg

Definition
Lipomatosis is a diffuse overgrowth of mature adipose tissue. It occurs in a variety of clinical settings and can affect different anatomical regions of the body.

Synonyms
In neck: Madelung disease; Launois-Bensaude syndrome

Epidemiology
Diffuse lipomatosis usually occurs in individuals aged < 2 years, but it may also arise in adults {2067}. Pelvic lipomatosis most frequently affects black males ranging in age between 9 and 80 years {1040,1172,1434}. Symmetric lipomatosis develops in middle-aged men of Mediterranean origin. Many patients have a history of liver disease or excessive alcohol consumption. Steroid lipomatosis manifests in patients on hormonal therapy or have increased endogenous production of adrenocortical steroids. Lipodystrophy is frequently seen in HIV-positive patients treated with protease inhibitors, but is also seen in patients receiving other forms of antiretroviral therapy {275,1482}.

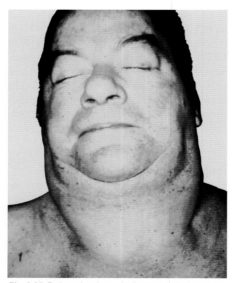

Fig. 2.05 Patient showing typically symmetrical, massive expansion of the neck.

Etiology
The basic mechanism underlying lipomatosis is not well understood. In some cases an autosomal dominant inheritance is suggested {1795}. Point mutations in mitochondrial genes have been implicated in the pathogenesis of symmetric lipomatosis {1440}. The similarity between HIV lipodystrophy and benign symmetric lipomatosis suggests a similar pathogenesis, in that mitochondrial DNA damage may be induced by the drugs used to treat HIV {181,512}.

Sites of involvement
Diffuse lipomatosis may involve the trunk, a large portion of an extremity, the head and neck, abdomen, pelvis or intestinal tract. It may be associated with macrodactyly or gigantism of a digit {1034, 1776,2128}. Symmetric lipomatosis manifests as symmetric deposition of fat in the upper part of the body, particularly the neck. In pelvic lipomatosis there is diffuse overgrowth of fat in the perivesical and perirectal areas. Steroid lipomatosis is characterized by the accumulation of fat in the face, sternal region or the upper middle back (buffalo hump). HIV lipodystrophy typically shows the accumulation of visceral fat, breast adiposity, cervical fat pads, hyperlipidaemia, insulin resistance, and fat wasting in the face and limbs {512,1902}.

Clinical features
In most forms of lipomatosis, the patient presents with massive accumulation of fat in the affected areas that may mimic a neoplasm. Additionally, patients with symmetric lipomatosis can have neuropathy and involvement of the CNS {2013,2253}. Accumulation of fat in the lower neck areas in these patients can also cause laryngeal obstruction, and compression of the vena cava. Patients with pelvic lipomatosis frequently complain of urinary frequency, perineal pain, constipation, and abdominal and back pain. Bowel obstruction and hydronephrosis may even-

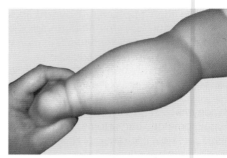

Fig. 2.06 Lipomatosis presenting as diffuse enlargement of the lower leg in an infant.

tually develop. Imaging studies in all forms of lipomatosis show accumulation of fat and are only helpful in determining the extent of its accumulation and excluding other processes.

Macroscopy
The gross appearance of lipomatosis is the same for all the different subtypes. The lesions consist of poorly circumscribed aggregates of soft yellow fat that is identical in appearance to normal fat. The only differences are the site of involvement and the distribution of the fat.

Histopathology
All of the different types of lipomatosis have identical morphological features, consisting of lobules and sheets of mature adipocytes that may infiltrate other structures such as skeletal muscle.

Prognostic factors
All idiopathic forms of lipomatosis have a tendency to recur locally after surgery. The treatment is palliative surgical removal of excess fat. Massive accumulation of fat in the neck region may cause death due to laryngeal obstruction. The fat in steroid lipomatosis regresses after steroid levels have been lowered. Experimental drugs such as recombinant growth hormones have been used to treat HIV lipodystrophy.

Lipomatosis of nerve

G.P. Nielsen

Definition
Lipomatosis of nerve is characterized by expansion of the epineurium by adipose and fibrous tissue. The tissue grows between and around nerve bundles, thereby causing enlargement of the affected nerve.

Synonyms
Fibrolipomatous hamartoma; lipofibroma; fibrolipomatosis; intraneural lipoma of the median nerve; perineural lipoma; median nerve lipoma; macrodystrophia lipomatosa; neural fibrolipoma

Epidemiology
Lipomatosis of nerve is frequently first noted at birth or in early childhood, but patients may not present for treatment until early or mid adulthood. In the largest reported series, the patient age range was 11–39 years. Because the constituent tissues are normal components of the epineurium, some authors have considered this lesion to be a hamartoma {2746}. In some cases it is associated with macrodactyly of the digits innervated by the affected nerve. In one study, associated macrodactyly was present in approximately one third of patients, including five females and two males {2558}. Females are affected more frequently when the condition is accompanied by macrodactyly, while males are more commonly affected when macrodactyly is absent.

Sites of involvement
The median nerve and its digital branches are most commonly affected, followed by the ulnar nerve {224,2558}. The process has also been reported to involve unusual sites such as cranial nerves, brachial plexus and sciatic nerve {202,815,2269}.

Clinical features
Patients present with a gradually enlarging mass in the affected area that may be asymptomatic or associated with motor or sensory deficits. Patients with macrodactyly have symmetric or asymmetric enlargement of the affected finger(s) with enlargement of the involved bones. Imaging studies show fusiform enlargement of the nerve with fatty infiltration {602} and

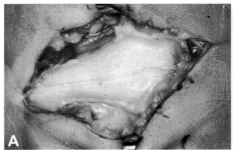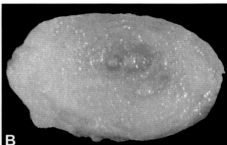

Fig. 2.07 Lipomatosis of nerve. **A** Intraoperative view showing a transition between the normal nerve (left) and the affected area (right). **B** Cross-section reveals nerve bundles entrapped within fibroadipose tissue.

MRI findings are virtually pathognomonic {1736,2980}.

Macroscopy
Grossly there is fusiform enlargement of the nerve by yellow fibrofatty tissue, which is generally confined within the epineurial sheath.

Histopathology
The epineurial and perineurial compartments of the enlarged nerve are infiltrated by mature adipose tissue admixed with fibrous tissue, which dissects between and separates individual nerve bundles {2558}. Concentric perineurial fibrous tissue is a prominent feature. The affected nerve may also show other changes, e.g. perineural septation, microfascicle formation and pseudo-onion-bulb formation mimicking an intraneural perineurioma {2463}. Metaplastic bone formation is rarely present {702}.

Immunophenotype
Immunohistochemistry is not helpful in diagnosing this lesion as all components are seen in normal nerves.

Ultrastructure
The nerve bundles demonstrate onion-bulblike formations with one or two nerve fibres and peripheral perineurial cells {126}.

Prognostic factors
This is a benign lesion with no effective therapy (surgical excision usually causes severe damage of the involved nerve).

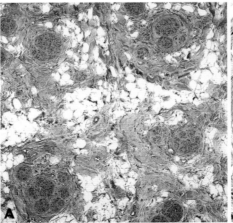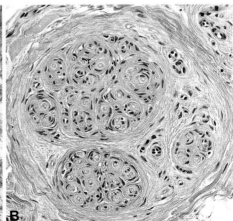

Fig. 2.08 Lipomatosis of nerve. **A** Epineural infiltration of fibroadipose tissue separating nerve bundles. **B** The nerves show pseudo-onion-bulb formation and perineural fibrosis.

Lipoblastoma

C.M. Coffin
N. Mandahl

Definition
Lipoblastoma, a benign neoplasm of embryonal white fat, is a localized or diffuse tumour with a tendency for local recurrence if incompletely excised.

ICD-O code   8881/0

Synonyms
Lipoblastomasis (preferred term, diffuse lipoblastoma); fetal lipoma; fetal fat tumour; fetocellular lipoma; embryonal lipoma; congenital lipomatoid tumour; lipoblastic tumour of childhood {1178}

Epidemiology
Lipoblastoma occurs predominantly in infancy and early childhood, with 90% of cases occurring before age 3 years, although rare cases are seen in adolescents and adults {465,487,604}. There is a slightly higher incidence in males {487, 503,1831,2866}.

Sites of involvement
The trunk and extremities are the most common sites {487}. Lipoblastoma may also arise in the retroperitoneum, pelvis, abdomen, mesentery, mediastinum, head/neck, and solid organs (lung, heart, parotid gland) {672,1353,1369,1756}.

Clinical features
Superficial circumscribed lipoblastoma simulates lipoma. Diffuse lipoblastoma originates in deep soft tissue and is more infiltrative. Since both types recur, the distinction between circumscribed and infiltrative forms is not clinically relevant. Lipoblastoma can compress adjacent structures and interfere with function {487,2238}. MRI reveals a nodular mass with adipose tissue density and non-enhancing cystic change {433,2180,2321}. A subset of patients with lipoblastoma has developmental delays or abnormalities, seizures, congenital malformations, or familial lipomas {487,503,1178}.

Macroscopy
Lipoblastoma is typically 2–5 cm in diameter, although it can exceed 10 cm {465,487, 503}. The soft, lobulated, yellow, white, or tan mass may display myxoid nodules, cystic spaces, or fat nodules separated by fine white fibrous trabeculae on the cut surface.

Histopathology
Lipoblastoma characteristically demonstrates a lobular architecture with sheets of adipocytes separated by fibrovascular septa {265,465,487,503}. Myxoid areas display a plexiform vascular pattern with primitive mesenchymal cells. The fat cells show a spectrum of maturation, ranging from primitive stellate or spindled mesenchymal cells, to multivacuolated or small signet ring lipoblasts, to mature adipocytes. The proportion of these cell types varies from case to case and from lobule to lobule. The fat lobule itself can exhibit a zonal pattern of maturation, with more immature myxoid cells at the periphery and mature adipocytes in the centre, although this pattern is not always maintained. Mast cells are common.

Other histological findings include fibroblastic proliferation with collagen deposition, chondroid metaplasia, extramedullary haematopoiesis, chronic inflammation, and sparse multinucleated or floret cells {487,503,522}. Mitoses are very rare, and abnormal mitoses are absent. A lipomatous or fibrolipomatous pattern is seen as a manifestation of differentiation or maturation, with variable residual lipoblasts in myxoid zones {487, 503,1948}.

Immunophenotype
The adipocytes of lipoblastoma demonstrate reactivity for S100 protein and CD34, and the primitive mesenchymal cells are often reactive for desmin {487}.

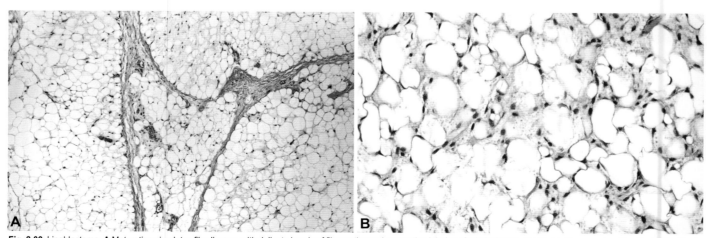

Fig. 2.09 Lipoblastoma. **A** Maturation simulates fibrolipoma, with delicate bands of fibrous tissue demarcating lobules of relatively mature adipose tissue and residual foci of lipoblasts and myxoid change. **B** Lipoblasts range from multivacuolated lipoblasts, to small signet ring cells, to almost mature adipocytes with occasional foci of myxoid material in the background.

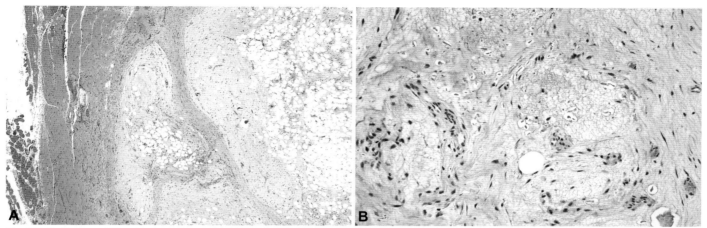

Fig. 2.10 Lipoblastoma. **A** The circumscribed lobulated mass contains a combination of mature adipose tissue, immature myxoid mesenchymal tissue, and lipoblasts in various stages of differentiation. **B** The myxoid area contains bland primitive spindled mesenchymal cells and a delicate lacy network of small blood vessels.

Ultrastructure

Lipoblastoma recapitulates fetal white-fat development, with mitochondria with simple cristae and no dense bodies, cytoplasmic glycogen, pinocytotic vesicles, or basal lamina {265,1174,2866}.

Genetics

The karyotype is pseudo- or hyperdiploid, usually with few structural aberrations {159, 487,981}. Aberrations involving chromosome 8 are found in almost all tumours, with breakpoints clustering to 8q11–13. The most common numerical change is one or more extra copies of chromosome 8 (10–15% of cases), either alone or with rearrangement of 8q11–13. *PLAG1*, a developmentally regulated zinc-finger transcription factor gene in 8q12.1, is the target of the 8q rearrangements {1173,1949}. *PLAG1* has been found to recombine with *HAS2* in 8q24.13 and *COL1A2* in 7q21.3, with a promoter-swapping mechanism that leads to transcriptional up-regulation of *PLAG1* and production of full-length PLAG1 protein. *PLAG1* aberrations can be cytogenetically cryptic {1949}. An alternative mechanism of tumorigenesis is the creation of excess copies of chromosome 8; it is not known whether the extra copies of *PLAG1* are wildtype or not {604,981}. Rearrangement of the *PLAG1* locus as evidenced by FISH is present in variably differentiated cells, indicating that the aberration occurs in a progenitor cell that differentiates {981}. Rearrangement of *HMGA2* has been reported in an isolated case of lipoblastoma, raising the possibility that *PLAG1* and *HMGA2* share a role in lipoblastoma that is similar to that reported in pleomorphic adenoma of the salivary glands {2205}.

Prognostic factors

Lipoblastoma is benign, with an excellent prognosis after excision {465,487,2618, 2866}. The recurrence rate of 13–46% is likely to be attributable to incomplete excision. Re-excision is effective. There is no risk of metastasis or malignant transformation.

Angiolipoma

R. Sciot
N. Mandahl

Definition
A usually subcutaneous nodule consisting of mature fat cells, intermingled with small, thin-walled capillary-type vessels, a number of which contain fibrin thrombi. Some authors believe that these are more appropriately classified as haemangiomas.

ICD-O code   8861/0

Epidemiology
Angiolipomas are relatively common and usually appear in the late teens or early twenties. Angiolipoma is more common in males than in females. Familial incidence has been described (5% of all cases) {2}, with the mode of inheritance being autosomal dominant.

Sites of involvement
The extremities are the most common site of involvement, followed by the trunk (including breast). Intramuscular haemangiomas (formerly known as "infiltrating angiolipoma"), as well as so-called angiolipomas of parenchymal organs or CNS, are different lesions, composed of larger vessels and are more appropriately considered to be haemangiomas {61,120, 966}.

Clinical features
Angiolipomas most frequently present as multiple subcutaneous small nodules, usually tender or painful. There is no correlation between the intensity/occurrence of pain and the degree of vascularity {675}.

Macroscopy
Angiolipomas appear as encapsulated yellowish to reddish nodules.

Histopathology
Angiolipomas typically consist of mature adipocytes and thin-walled capillary-sized vessels, which often contain fibrin thrombi. Vascularity is more prominent in the subcapsular area {675}. Stromal spindle cells

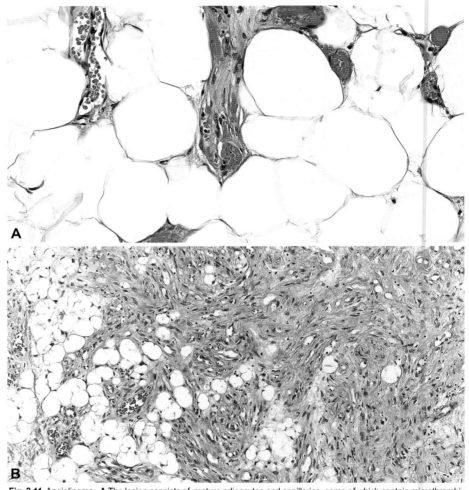

Fig. 2.11 Angiolipoma. **A** The lesion consists of mature adipocytes and capillaries, some of which contain microthrombi. **B** Cellular angiolipoma, in which the vessels predominate.

are variably prominent adjacent to vessels. The relative proportion of adipocytes and vessels varies and some lesions are almost entirely composed of vascular channels. These "cellular" angiolipomas should be distinguished from angiosarcoma and Kaposi sarcoma {1250,1366}.

Genetics
With a single exception, all tumours investigated cytogenetically have had a normal karyotype {2490}. Angiolipomas seem to show aberrant expression of full-length HMGA2, although at levels lower than in lipomas with 12q rearrangements {162}.

Prognostic factors
Angiolipomas are always benign and show no tendency to recur. Malignant transformation does not occur.

Myolipoma of soft tissue

J.M. Meis
L.-G. Kindblom

Definition
Myolipoma of soft tissue is a benign extra-uterine tumour composed of mature adipose tissue and smooth muscle.

ICD-O code   8890/0

Synonym
Extrauterine lipoleiomyoma

Epidemiology
Myolipoma is an extremely rare tumour occurring in adults, predominantly women {1812,1866,2702}. It is not associated with tuberous sclerosis {1866}.

Sites of involvement
Myolipoma is usually a deep-seated mass within the abdominal cavity, retroperitoneum or inguinal region {1812,1866, 2702}. Less commonly it occurs in the subcutis of the trunk wall or extremities {1812}.

Clinical features
Lesions within the abdominal cavity are often found incidentally, whereas those involving the trunk or extremities are palpable {1812}. MRI shows a fatty mass with associated signal-rich areas (corresponding to the smooth-muscle component) that are heterogeneous on T1 post-contrast fat-suppressed images {2862}.

Macroscopy
Deep myolipomas are large, usually 10–25 cm in size. Superficial lesions are smaller. Mature fat intermingles with white-tan fibrous areas that correspond to smooth muscle {1812,1866,2702}.

Histopathology
Thin fascicles of bland smooth muscle traverse mature fat within a relatively well-circumscribed or encapsulated lesion. Smooth muscle varies in amount and may predominate, although fat is clearly an integral component. No atypia or mitotic activity is observed in the smooth-muscle cells and no floret-like cells, lipoblasts or lymphoid aggregates are seen in the lipomatous areas. Prominent thick-walled vessels, as seen in angiomyolipoma, are absent {1812,1866,2702}.

Immunophenotype
Desmin and SMA positivity confirms smooth-muscle differentiation. Expression of estrogen and progesterone receptors has also been reported. Staining for HMB45 is negative {185,1866,2702}.

Genetics
HMGA2 alterations have been reported in extrauterine lipoleiomyoma {1192}.

Prognostic factors
Complete resection is curative.

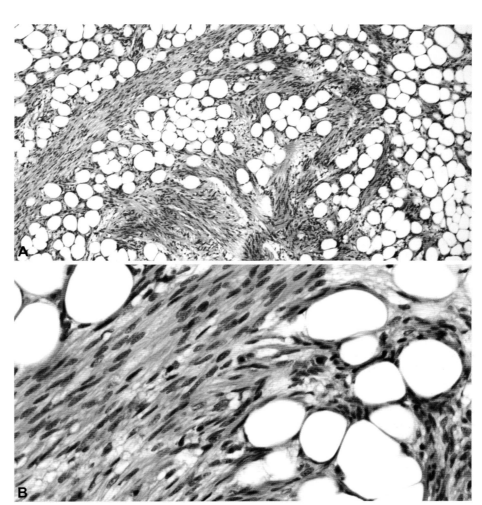

Fig. 2.12 Histological appearance of extrauterine myolipoma of the pelvis. **A** The mature fatty and smooth-muscle components are both integral parts of the tumour. **B** No atypia is seen in either the lipomatous or myoid elements of the lesion.

Chondroid lipoma

L.-G.Kindblom
J.A. Bridge
J.M. Meis

Definition
Chondroid lipoma is a benign adipose-tissue tumour composed of lipoblasts in a myxoid-chondroid matrix that intermingle with mature adipocytes.

ICD-O code   8862/0

Epidemiology
Chondroid lipoma is extremely rare. It most frequently affects women.

Sites of involvement
Tumours are typically deep-seated, involving skeletal muscle, deep fibrous connective tissue, or deep subcutaneous fat. Most occur in the proximal extremities and limb girdles {1815}. Less common sites include distal extremities, trunk, and head and neck, including the oral cavity {930}.

Clinical features
Most patients present with a painless mass of variable duration, with some reporting a recent increase in size {1815}. Imaging studies typically show a heterogeneous fatty and myxoid lesion, deviating from that of lipoma, but otherwise nondistinctive {1648}.

Macroscopy
Chondroid lipomas are well delineated with yellowish cut surfaces suggesting a mature fat component. Tumour size ranges from 2 to 7 cm; those complicated by haemorrhage are usually larger {1815}.

Histopathology
Encapsulation and occasional lobulation may be seen. There are variable proportions of mature adipose tissue intermingled with nests and cords of small round vacuolated cells embedded in a myxoid-chondroid matrix. These tumours may resemble extraskeletal myxoid chondrosarcoma and myxoid liposarcoma. The small cells display a range of lipoblastic differentiation, consisting of undifferentiated bland cells with minimal cytoplasm to small univacuolated and multivacuolated lipoblasts with fat droplets scalloping bland nuclei. Cells with granular, eosinophilic cytoplasm may also be seen. PAS stains accentuate intracytoplasmic glycogen. Toluidine and Alcian blue staining at low pH indicate the presence of chondroitin sulfates. Owing to high vascularity, haemorrhage and fibrosis are common {1423,1815,2037}.

Immunophenotype
Staining for S100 protein is strongly positive in the mature fatty component, weaker in the lipoblastic elements and usually negative in cells without apparent lipoblastic differentiation. Keratins may be detected rarely and EMA is negative {1423}.

Ultrastructure
Ultrastructure confirms the presence of mature fat as well as small embryonal cells with features of lipoblasts, chondroblasts or both. The surrounding matrix consists of a network of thin filaments, thin collagen fibres and abundant proteoglycan particles {1423,2037}.

Genetics
A recurrent t(11;16)(q13;p13) chromosomal translocation has been reported in chondroid lipoma. This results in fusion of the C11orf95 (11q13) and MKL2 (16p13.3) genes {1240}. MKL2, a member of the myocardin/megakaryoblastic leukaemia gene family, encodes a putative DNA-binding domain-containing protein that is functionally implicated in chromatin remodelling and transcriptional coactivation. C11orf95 (chromosome 11 ORF 95) encodes a hypothetical protein of unknown function. Cyclin D1 (CCND1) expression is reportedly strong in chondroid lipoma; however, no abnormalities of the CCND1 locus have been detected by FISH {610}.

Prognostic factors
Surgical excision is usually curative and local recurrences are rare.

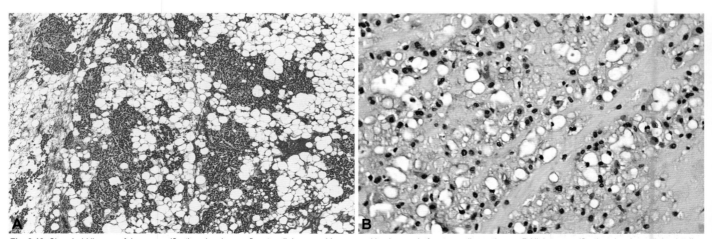

Fig. 2.13 Chondroid lipoma. **A** Low magnification showing confluent, cellular, myxoid areas and background of mature adipose tissue. **B** Higher magnification showing cellular details.

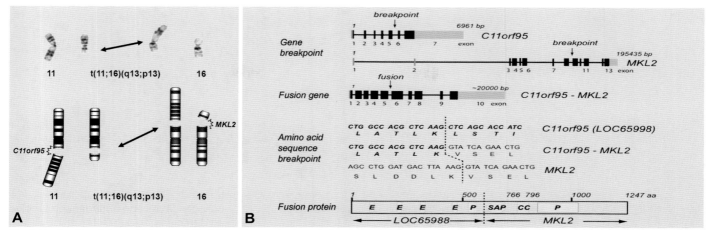

Fig. 2.14 Genetics of chondroid lipoma. **A** Partial karyotype and schematic illustrating the characteristic 11;16 translocation. **B** Schematic of *C11orf95*, *MKL2* and the *C11orf95-MKL2* fusion gene (solid bars represent coding exons; grey boxes are non-translated regions). The amino acid sequence at the breakpoint is shown. The lowest line of the schematic represents the domain structure of the C11orf95-MKL2 fusion protein, with the letters within the bars designating conserved domains (polyglutamic acid regions, E; proline-rich region, P; DNA-binding SAP domain, SAP; and coiled-coiled region, CC).

Spindle cell/pleomorphic lipoma

M.M. Miettinen
N. Mandahl

Definition
Spindle cell/pleomorphic lipomas typically occur in the neck and upper trunk in older males. They are characterized by an admixture of mature fat and bland spindled cells. Additionally, pleomorphic lipoma contains multinucleated giant cells. These lesions represent a morphological continuum.

ICD-O code   8857/0

Synonyms
Spindle cell lipoma; pleomorphic lipoma

Epidemiology
Spindle cell/pleomorphic lipomas typically present in older men with a median age of 55 years, and 10% or fewer of patients are women {65,753,867,2545}. Rarely, patients develop multiple lesions, occasionally on a familial basis {808}.

Sites of involvement
Spindle cell/pleomorphic lipomas are usually subcutaneous and occur predominantly in the posterior neck, back and shoulder. Face, forehead, scalp, buc-cal-perioral area and upper arm are less common sites, and occurrence in the lower extremity is distinctly rare. Dermal examples have a wider anatomical distribution {912}.

Clinical features
The tumour manifests as an asymptomatic, often long-standing subcutaneous mass in most cases.

Macroscopy
Spindle cell/pleomorphic lipoma forms an

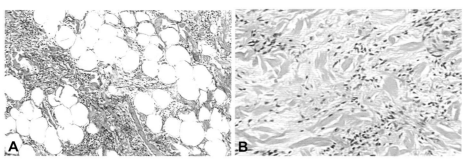

Fig. 2.15 Spindle cell/pleomorphic lipoma. **A** The relative proportions of the adipocytic and spindle cell components are variable. **B** Some lesions are almost devoid of adipocytes and show vague nuclear palisading. Note the typically ropey collagen bundles.

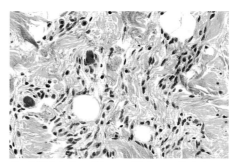

Fig. 2.16 Spindle cell/pleomorphic lipoma. Typical case with bland spindle cells in a background with thick collagen fibres and a small number of adipocytes.

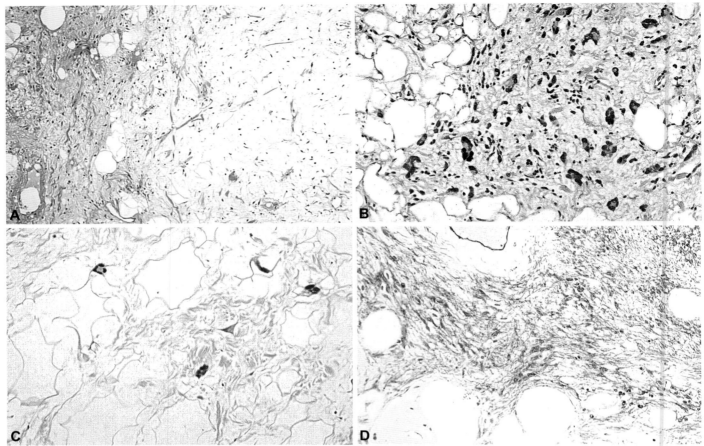

Fig. 2.17 Spindle cell/pleomorphic lipoma. **A** Prominent myxoid change of the stroma is not an uncommon feature. **B** Classical example showing numerous floret-like multinucleate cells. **C** Some spindle cell/pleomorphic lipomas consist almost entirely of mature adipocytes with admixed multinucleated stroma cells, often having floret-like nuclei. **D** Immunopositivity for CD34 is a consistent feature of the spindle-cell component.

oval or discoid yellowish to greyish-white mass depending on the relative extent of the fatty and spindle cell components. The tumour often has a firmer texture than ordinary lipoma, but some examples have a gelatinous texture.

Histopathology

Variants include fat-dominated tumours with scant spindle cells and those with a prominent spindle cell component with only few, if any, fat cells. The spindle cells are bland, mitotically inactive, with short stubby nuclei, surrounded by thick "rope-like" collagen fibres or diffuse sheets of collagen or myxoid matrix. In some cases, nuclear palisading and hyalinized vessels can be seen, as in schwannoma. Matrix can be extensively myxoid. Mast cells are commonly present {65,753,867,2545}. Spindle cell/pleomorphic lipomas with slit-like cleavage spaces have been recognized ("pseudoangiomatoid variant") {1139}. Spindle cell/pleomorphic lipomas

iare characterized by small spindled and rounded cells and multinucleated giant cells. These cells may have radially arranged nuclei in a "floret-like" pattern. Some spindle cell lipomas involve dermis as multinodular lesions with a plexiform architecture. Although fat cells typically lack atypia, some spindle cell/pleomorphic lipomas contain atypical adipocytes and lipo-blasts, showing morphological overlap with atypical lipomatous tumours.

Immunophenotype

The spindle cells are strongly positive for CD34 and may rarely be positive for S100 protein and occasionally for desmin {791,2683,2739}.

Genetics

Spindle cell/pleomorphic have unbalanced karyotypes, mostly hypodiploid, with multiple partial losses {161,543}. Many show monosomy 13, or, more often, partial loss of 13q, always including

13q14. SNP array analyses have revealed two minimal deleted regions in 13q14 {161}. Other frequent losses include chromosome segments 16q22–qter (two thirds of cases), 6q14–21 (one third), 10p (one quarter), 17p (one fifth), and 2q21–qter (one sixth). No recurrent balanced re-arrangement has been identified. No aberrant *HMGA2* expression is detected {162}.

Prognostic factors

Spindle cell /pleomorphic lipomas are benign and conservative local excision is considered sufficient, although local recurrence occurs rarely.

Hibernoma

M.M. Miettinen
J.C. Fanburg-Smith
N. Mandahl

Definition

Hibernoma is a rare, benign, encapsulated, and richly-vascularized adipose tumour composed of variable proportions of brown fat cells admixed with white adipose tissue. Foci of brown fat, sometimes found in cervical, axillary and other locations, should not be classified as hibernoma {931,1165}.

ICD-O code   8880/0

Epidemiology

Based on AFIP data, hibernoma comprises 1.6% of benign lipomatous tumours and approximately 1.1% of all adipocytic tumours. It occurs predominantly in young adults, with a mean age of 38 years: 60% occur in the third and fourth decades of life, only 5% occur in children aged 2–18 years, and 7% in patients aged > 60 years. There are slightly more cases in males than females {931}.

Sites of involvement

The most common site for hibernoma is the thigh, followed by the trunk/chest, upper extremity, and head and neck. Lesions with prominent myxoid and spindle cell morphology tend to be located in the posterior neck and shoulders, similar to spindle cell lipoma {931}. Fewer than 10% of cases occur in the intra-abdominal, retroperitoneal or thoracic cavities {1165}. Intraosseous location has also been reported {1495}.

Clinical features

Hibernoma is a slow-growing, painless, mobile mass, predominantly subcutaneous, but sometimes intramuscular (20%). Larger hibernomas can create local pressure effects and may raise clinical concerns regarding malignancy {931}. MRI reveals non-fat septations and serpentine vascular elements and CT scan shows variable attenuation intermediate between fat and skeletal muscle, as well as contrast enhancement {432,519}.

Macroscopy

The median size in historical series was 9.3 cm (range, 1–24 cm), but hibernomas seen now are usually smaller. Hibernomas are lobular, well-demarcated, and vary from tan-yellow to reddish brown, with a greasy, soft and spongy cut surface {931}.

Histopathology

Hibernomas have a capillary network and vary in the content and appearance of the polygonal brown fat cells and stromal background {931}. Most tumours contain large numbers of brown fat cells with multivacuolation, granular cytoplasm, and a small, central nucleus. The brown fat cells vary from transparent pale cells with larger vacuoles to variably granular, eosinophilic cells; a mixture of pale and eosinophilic cells, while other cases have pure pale brown fat cells. Some hibernomas contain small clusters of brown fat amidst mostly ordinary encapsulated white fat. These multivacuolated cells may resemble lipoblasts. Morphological variations include hibernoma with myxoid stroma or a spindle-cell component, with thick bundles of collagen fibres, scattered mast

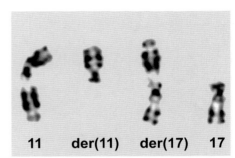

Fig. 2.19 Hibernoma. Partial G-banded karyotype showing a translocation t(11;17)(q13;p13).

cells, and brown fat rather than mature white adipose tissue. Mitoses or cytological atypia are unusual. Such features should not be equated with malignancy, as the biological behaviour of hibernoma is invariably benign. However, scattered normal brown fat cells may be found in an otherwise classic myxoid or well-differentiated liposarcoma.

Immunophenotype

Hibernoma cells are are often positive for S100 protein and negative for CD34. However, CD34 indicates the spindled fibroblastic component in spindle cell hibernoma {931}. Newer markers for hibernoma include UCP1 {1726}.

Ultrastructure

Like brown fat, hibernoma cells contain multiple lipid droplets and numerous large mitochondria {1726}.

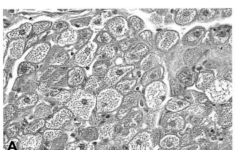
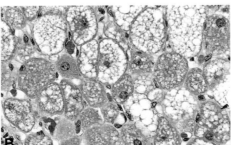
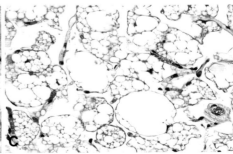

Fig. 2.18 Hibernoma. A The eosinophilic variant is composed mostly of granular-appearing, multivacuolated brown fat cells with prominent nucleoli. B Detail of the eosinophilic variant with granular, multivacuolated brown fat cells and prominent nucleoli. C In the pale-cell variant, the multivacuolated brown fat cells have a pale tinctorial quality.

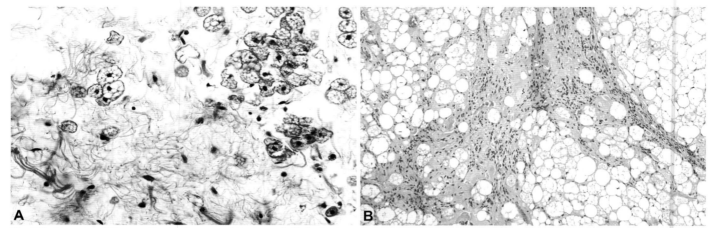

Fig. 2.20 Hibernoma. **A** The myxoid variant has a myxoid background with floating brown fat cells. **B** The spindle cell variant, a hybrid between hibernoma and spindle cell lipoma, shows brown fat cells, mature white fat cells, scattered mast cells and bland spindled cells.

Genetics

Cytogenetically almost all hibernomas have breakpoints in 11q, with a distinctive clustering to 11q13 {162,982,1705,1855}. Many translocation partners are involved, but 9q34 and 14q11 are the only recurrent ones.

FISH analyses have revealed complex re-arrangements with multiple breaks, and that the rearranged chromosome 11, and frequently also the cytogenetically seem-ingly normal homologue, have interstitial deletions in the long arm {982,1705,2072}.

The deletions cluster to a 3 Mb region in 11q13, with a preferential localization to regions covering the tumour suppressor genes *MEN1* and *AIP* {2072}. Combined SNP, MLPA, and FISH analyses of 15 cases disclosed homozygous or hemizy-gous loss of *MEN1* in 10 and 5 cases, re-spectively. The corresponding results for *AIP* were 6 and 8 cases, respectively. Six cases had homozygous deletion of both genes. No mutations of *MEN1* or *AIP* have been detected. Of 132 genes in the 3 Mb region, 13 genes showed significantly

lower expression, including *MEN1*, *EHD1*, *AIP*, and *CDK2AP2* in the homozygously lost regions. *PPARA*, *PPARG*, *PPARGC1A*, and particularly *UCP1* demonstrate high expression in hibernoma compared with lipoma and white adipose tissue. No aber-rant expression of *HMGA2* is detected {162}.

Prognostic factors

Hibernoma is a benign tumour with no significant potential for recurrence after local excision {931}.

Atypical lipomatous tumour

A.P. Dei Tos
F. Pedeutour

Definition

Atypical lipomatous tumour (ALT) is a locally aggressive mesenchymal neoplasm composed either entirely or partly of a mature adipocytic proliferation showing significant variation in cell size and at least focal nuclear atypia in both adipocytes and stromal cells. The presence of scattered hyperchromatic, often multinucleate, stromal cells and a varying number of monovacuolated or multivacuolated lipoblasts (defined by the presence of single or multiple sharply marginated cytoplasmic vacuoles scalloping an enlarged hyperchromatic nucleus) may contribute to the morphological diagnosis. Use of the term "atypical lipomatous tumour" is determined principally by tumour location and resectability.

Terminology in clinical practice

The fact that a well-differentiated liposarcoma shows no potential for metastasis unless it undergoes dedifferentiation led, in the late 1970s, to the introduction of terms such as "atypical lipoma" or "atypical lipomatous tumour" {791} for lesions arising at surgically amenable locations in the limbs and on the trunk. At these sites, complete excision is usually curative and hence the designation "sarcoma" is not warranted. However, the variable, sometimes controversial, application of this new terminology has represented a source of potential diagnostic confusion {782,1419, 2933}. ALT and well-differentiated liposarcoma are synonyms describing lesions that are identical

morphologically and karyotypically (see below), and in terms of biological potential. The choice of terminology is therefore best determined by the degree of reciprocal comprehension between surgeon and pathologist to prevent inappropriate treatment {622}. Most often, the term "well-differentiated liposarcoma" is not appropriate for lesions in somatic soft tissue. However, in sites such as retroperitoneum and mediastinum, it is commonly impossible to obtain a wide excision margin and, in such cases, local recurrence (often repeated and ultimately uncontrolled) is almost inevitable and often leads to death, even in the absence of dedifferentiation and metastasis. Hence, at these sites, retention of the term "well-differentiated liposarcoma" can readily be justified. The same applies for spermatic cord lesions, which often relapse in retroperitoneum.

ICD-O code

Atypical lipomatous tumour   8850/1

Synonyms

Atypical lipoma; well-differentiated liposarcoma; adipocytic liposarcoma; lipoma-like liposarcoma; sclerosing liposarcoma; spindle cell liposarcoma; inflammatory liposarcoma

Epidemiology

ALTs account for about 40–45% of all lipo sarcomas and therefore represent the largest subgroup of aggressive adipocytic

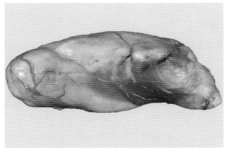

Fig. 2.22 Atypical lipomatous tumour. Surgical specimen showing a well-circumscribed, lobulated mass.

neoplasms. These lesions mostly occur in middle-aged adults with peak incidence in the sixth decade. Convincing examples in childhood are extremely rare, but may be associated with Li-Fraumeni syndrome. Males and females are equally affected, with the obvious exception of those lesions affecting the spermatic cord {758, 860,2930}.

Sites of involvement

ALT occurs most frequently in deep soft tissue of the limbs, especially the thigh, followed by the retroperitoneum, the paratesticular area and the mediastinum {758,859,1076, 2929}. The head and neck region is also affected {2005}. These lesions may also arise in subcutaneous tissue and, very rarely, in skin.

Clinical features

ALT usually presents as a deep-seated, painless enlarging mass that can slowly

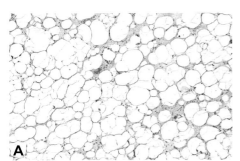
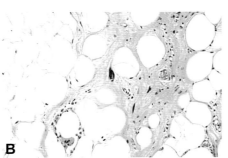
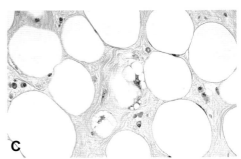

Fig. 2.21 Atypical lipomatous tumour. **A** Marked variation in adipocyte size is one of the most important diagnostic clues. **B** The presence of atypical, hyperchromatic stromal cells represents a common finding. **C** A varying number of lipoblasts can be seen in well-differentiated liposarcoma, but their presence neither makes nor is required for a diagnosis of liposarcoma.

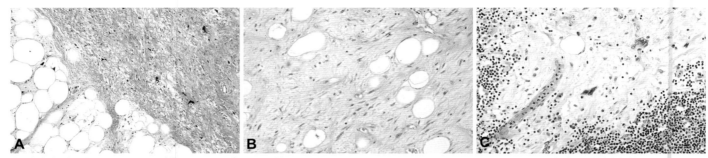

Fig. 2.23 Atypical lipomatous tumour. **A** The presence of scattered bizarre stromal cells exhibiting marked nuclear hyperchromasia set in a fibrillary collagenous background is the most important diagnostic feature of the sclerosing variant. **B** Neural-like spindle cell proliferation in a fibrous and/or myxoid background, associated with an atypical lipomatous component that usually includes lipoblasts, characterize the spindle cell variant. **C** Bizarre, often multinucleate cells in the stroma are an important diagnostic clue in the inflammatory variant. Note the accompanying inflammatory component.

attain a very large size, particularly in the retroperitoneum. Retroperitoneal lesions are often asymptomatic until the tumour has exceeded 20 cm in diameter and may be found by chance.

Macroscopy

ALT consists usually of a large, well-circumscribed, lobulated mass. In the retroperitoneum there may be multiple discontiguous masses. Rarely, an infiltrative growth pattern may be encountered. Colour varies from yellow to white (and firm) depending on the proportion of adipocytic, fibrous and/or myxoid areas. Areas of fat necrosis are common in larger lesions.

Histopathology

ALT can be subdivided morphologically into three main subtypes: adipocytic (lipoma-like), sclerosing, and inflammatory {2924}. The presence of more than one morphological pattern in the same lesion is common, particularly in retroperitoneal tumours.

ALT is composed of a relatively mature adipo-cytic proliferation in which, in contrast to benign lipoma, significant variation in cell size is easily appreciable. Focal adipocytic nuclear atypia as well as hyperchromasia is a consistent finding and scattered hyperchromatic as well as multinucleate stromal cells are often identified. Hyperchromatic stromal cells tend to be more numerous within fibrous septa. A varying number (from many to none) of monovacuolated or multivacuolated lipoblasts may be found. It is important to emphasize that the mere presence of lipoblasts neither makes nor is required for a diagnosis of liposarcoma.

Sclerosing liposarcoma ranks second in frequency among the group of ALTs. This pattern is most often seen in retroperitoneal or para-testicular lesions. The main histological finding is the presence of scattered bizarre stromal cells, exhibiting marked nuclear hyperchromasia and associated with rare multivacuolated lipoblasts, set in an extensive fibrillary collagenous stroma. As the fibrous component may occasionally represent the majority of the neoplasm, lipogenic areas (which are often limited in extent) can easily be overlooked or even missed in a small sample. Extensive sampling of the surgical specimen is therefore mandatory. Inflammatory liposarcoma represents a rare variant, occurring most often in the retroperitoneum, in which a chronic inflammatory infiltrate predominates to the extent that the adipocytic nature of the neoplasm can be obscured. In such instances, the differential diagnosis is mainly with non-adipocytic lesions, such as inflammatory myofibroblastic tumour, Castleman disease and Hodgkin as well as non-Hodgkin lymphomas {95,1481}. The inflammatory infiltrate is usually composed of polyphenotypic lymphoplasmacytic aggregates in which a B-cell phenotype tends to predominate. Cases exist in which a polyclonal T-cell population represents the main inflammatory component. When dealing with cases in which

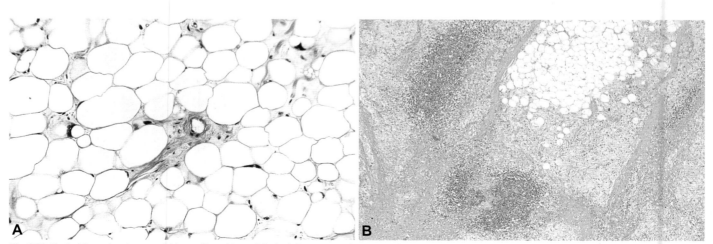

Fig. 2.24 Atypical lipomatous tumour. **A** Lipoma-like subtype. **B** In the inflammatory subtype, the inflammatory infiltrate often predominates and may obscure the adipocytic nature of the neoplasm.

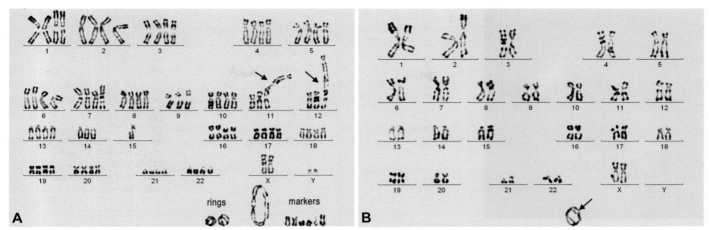

Fig. 2.25 Atypical lipomatous tumour. **A** RHG-banded near-tetraploid karyotype of a well-differentiated liposarcoma: note the random telomeric associations (arrows), three ring chromosomes, including a giant, and a few additional structural anomalies (marker chromosomes). **B** RHG-banded near-diploid karyotype of an atypical lipomatous tumour. The sole chromosomal anomaly is the presence of a supernumerary ring chromosome (arrow).

the adipocytic component is scarce, the presence of bizarre multinucleate stromal cells represents a useful diagnostic clue. Spindle cell liposarcoma {628,1841} is composed morphologically of a fairly bland neural-like spindle-cell proliferation set in a fibrous and/or myxoid background and is associated with an atypical lipomatous component that usually includes lipoblasts. An interesting albeit rare finding in ALT is the presence of heterologous differentiation. In addition to osseous elements {3038}, a well-differentiated smooth or striated muscle component can rarely be seen, but does not of itself imply dedifferentiation {786,2686}.

Immunophenotype

Adipocytic cells usually exhibit S100 protein immunoreactivity that may also highlight lipoblasts {629}. MDM2 and or CDK4 nuclear immunopositivity is present in most cases, in keeping with gene amplification. MDM2 nuclear positivity can often be seen in histiocytes that may be numerous in benign lipomas undergoing fat necrosis. Staining for MDM2 tends to be negative in spindle cell liposarcomas, suggesting that these may be a separate group {1841}.

Genetics

ALT is characterized by supernumerary ring and giant marker chromosomes, typically as the sole change or concomitant with a few other numerical or structural abnormalities {1915,2430}. Metaphase cells are usually near-diploid and occasionally near-tetraploid. Telomeric associations are frequently observed and may give a false

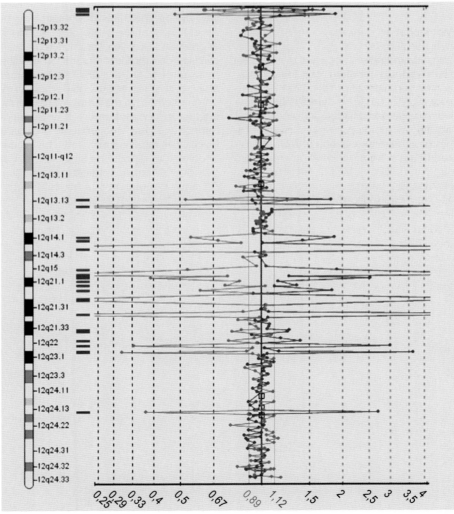

Fig. 2.26 Atypical lipomatous tumour. Quantitative profile of chromosome 12 sequences obtained by array CGH showing characteristic discontinuous high-level amplification of the 12q14–15 region. In this case there is a large degree of amplification, encompassing the 12q13 and 12q23 regions. Amplification of the 12q24.13 and distal 12p13 regions is also present (blue = amplification, red = loss).

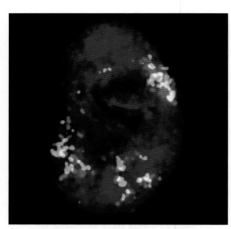

Fig. 2.27 Atypical lipomatous tumour. Interphase FISH using probes for *MDM2* (green signals) and *CDK4* (red signals) showing high-level amplification of both genes. Three clusters of amplified signals are observed in this case, indicating the presence of three ring or large marker chromosomes.

impression of complexity to ALT karyotypes {1723}.

Both supernumerary rings and giant markers invariably contain amplified sequences originating from the 12q14–15 region. *MDM2* (12q15) is consistently amplified and overexpressed in ALT and is considered the main driver gene of the 12q amplicon. Overexpression of MDM2 protein resulting from genomic amplification inactivates TP53; MDM2 targets TP53 degradation toward the proteasome, and inhibits TP53-mediated transactivation.

The *TP53* gene is rarely subject to mutations in ALT/well-differentiated liposarcoma {2245, 2470}. Several other genes located in the 12q14–15 region, including *CDK4* (12q14.1), *HMGA2* (12q14.3), *YEATS4* {156,1293,1294}, *CPM* {765} and *FRS2* {2905} (12q15) are frequently co-amplified with *MDM2*. The amplicons are discontinuous and variable in size. Of note, *CDK4* is not amplified in approximately 15% of ALT; these cases are mostly lipoma-like low-grade tumours of peripheral location {1293}. Quantitative detection of *MDM2* by FISH {2567}, PCR {1230}, array CGH {2720}, or indirectly by immunohistochemistry {41,624,2567,3058} serves to distinguish ALT from benign adipose tumours.

The rings and giant marker chromosomes of ALT are very complex genomic structures. In addition to 12q14–15 amplified sequences, they always contain co-amplification of at least one other genomic segment {2206}. The chromosomal origin of these co-amplified regions varies. The most frequent is 1q21–25 {1484}. Another striking feature of ALT supernumerary chromosomes is that they consistently contain a "neocentromere" {1298}. Neocentromeres are functional, as indicated by positive labelling with anti-CENPC antibodies that bind to the kinetochore, but they do not contain α-satellite sequences. Although generation of a neocentromere is a very rare event in tumour cells, it is a specific hallmark of ALT ring and marker chromosomes. In support of the evolving concept that spindle cell liposarcoma may represent a distinctive entity among the ALT family of tumours, monosomy of chromosome 7 but not 12q amplification has been identified in two cases {1296}.

Prognostic factors

The most important prognostic factor is anatomical location. Lesions located in surgically amenable soft tissue do not recur after complete (preferably wide) excision with a clear margin. Tumours occurring in deep anatomical sites such as retroperitoneum, spermatic cord or mediastinum tend to recur repeatedly to the extent that they may cause death as a result of uncontrolled local effects, or they may dedifferentiate and metastasize. Preliminary data indicate that, in retroperitoneum, multivisceral resections may increase relapse-free survival {268}. The ultimate risk of dedifferentiation varies according to site and lesional duration and is probably > 20% in the retroperitoneum but < 2% in the limbs. Overall mortality ranges from essentially 0% for ALT of the extremities to > 80% for well-differentiated liposarcomas occurring in the retroperitoneum, if the patients are followed up for 10–20 years. Median time to death ranges from 6 to 11 years {1670,2933}.

Dedifferentiated liposarcoma

A.P. Dei Tos
A. Marino-Enriquez
F. Pedeutour
S. Rossi

Definition

An atypical lipomatous tumour (ALT)/well-differentiated liposarcoma showing progression, either in the primary or in a recurrence, to (usually non-lipogenic) sarcoma of variable histological grade. In most cases there is substantial amplification of *MDM2*. A well-differentiated component may not be identifiable. Rarely, the high-grade component may be lipogenic.

ICD-O code   8858/3

Epidemiology

Dedifferentiated liposarcoma (DDLPS) is a common form of liposarcoma, accounting for most pleomorphic sarcomas in the retroperitoneum. Dedifferentiation occurs in up to 10% of well-differentiated liposarcomas, although the risk is higher for deep-seated (particularly retroperitoneal) lesions and significantly lower in the limbs. This is likely to represent a time-dependent more than a site-dependent phenomenon. DDLPS affects the same patient population as liposarcoma and is equally frequent in males and females. About 90% of cases arise de novo, while 10% develop in recurrences {860, 2930}.

Sites of involvement

Retroperitoneum is the most common location, outnumbering somatic soft tissue by at least 5 : 1. Other locations include the spermatic cord and, more rarely, the head and neck and trunk. Occurrence in subcutaneous tissue is extremely rare {860,2930}.

Clinical features

DDLPS usually presents as a large painless mass, which may be found by chance (particularly in the retroperitoneum). In the limbs, the history of a longstanding mass exhibiting recent increase in size often indicates dedifferentiation. Radiological imaging shows coexistence of both fatty and non-fatty solid components which, in the retroperitoneum, may be discontiguous.

Macroscopy

DDLPS usually consists of large multinodular yellow masses containing discrete, solid, often tan-grey non-lipomatous (dedifferentiated) areas. Dedifferentiated areas often show necrosis. The transition between the lipomatous and the dedifferentiated areas may sometimes be gradual.

Histopathology

The histological hallmark of DDLPS is transition from ALT/well-differentiated liposarcoma to non-lipogenic sarcoma, which, in most cases, is of high grade. The extent of dedifferentiation is variable, but is usually evident to the naked eye. The prognostic significance of microscopic foci of dedifferentation is uncertain. Transition is usually abrupt; however, in some cases this can be more gradual and, exceptionally, low-grade and high-grade areas appear to be intermingled.

Dedifferentiated areas exhibit a variable histological picture, but most frequently

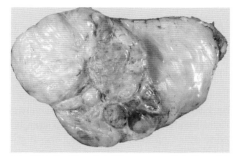

Fig. 2.29 Dedifferentiated liposarcoma. Note the solid, fleshy areas with haemorrhage, indicating the presence of a high-grade component in this otherwise well-differentiated retroperitoneal liposarcoma.

resemble undifferentiated pleomorphic sarcoma or intermediate- to high-grade myxofibrosarcoma {1787,2933}. Although dedifferentiation was originally defined by high-grade morphology {778}, cases with low-grade dedifferentiation have increasingly been recognized {739,1162}. Low-grade dedifferentiation is characterized most often by the presence of uniform fibroblastic spindle cells with mild nuclear atypia, often organized in a fascicular pattern and exhibiting cellularity intermediate between well-differentiated sclerosing liposarcoma and usual high-grade areas.

Low-grade DDLPS should not be confused with well-differentiated spindle cell liposarcoma: the latter contains atypical adipocytes or lipoblasts, while dedifferentiated areas, both low- and high-grade, are generally non-lipogenic. Low-grade DDLPS is virtually indistinguishable from cellular well-differentiated liposarcoma {786}.

DDLPS may exhibit heterologous differentiation in about 5–10% of cases; this does not affect clinical outcome. Most often the line of heterologous differentiation is myogenic or osteo-/chondrosarcomatous, but angiosarcomatous elements have also been reported. A peculiar "neural-like" or "meningothelial-like" whorling pattern of dedifferentiation has been described, which is often associated with ossification {812,2009}. Local recurrences of DDLPS may be entirely well differentiated {1787, 2933}. Occasionally, the high-grade

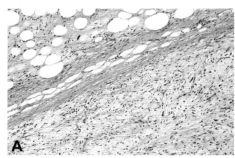 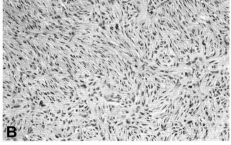

Fig. 2.28 Dedifferentiated liposarcoma. **A** Abrupt transition between well-differentiated liposarcoma and a high-grade non-lipogenic area is seen. **B** The morphology of the dedifferentiated component usually overlaps with undifferentiated sarcoma.

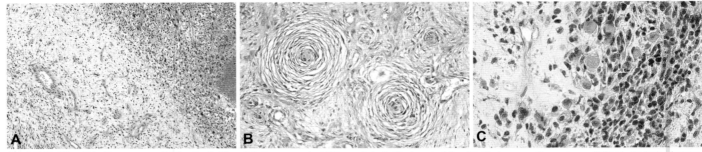

Fig. 2.30 Dedifferentiated liposarcoma. **A** Often the dedifferentiated component exhibits morphological features indistinguishable from myxofibrosarcoma. **B** Rarely, the lesion features a peculiar whorling growth pattern reminiscent of neural or meningothelial structures. **C** Approximately 5% of cases exhibit heterologous differentiation, most often myogenic. This example shows rhabdomyosarcomatous differentiation.

component may exhibit overt lipoblastic differentiation, either in the form of isolated lipoblasts scattered throughout the high-grade component, or as sheets of atypical pleomorphic adipocytic cells resulting in areas morphologically indistinguishable from pleomorphic liposarcoma. This phenomenon has been referred to as "homologous lipoblastic differentiation" or "pleomorphic liposarcoma-like features" {264,1162, 1733}.

Immunophenotype

The main role of immunohistochemistry is in the recognition of divergent differentiation and exclusion of other tumour types. Diffuse nuclear expression of MDM2 and/or CDK4 is almost invariable {2567}, and allows separation of "homologous" DDLPS from pleomorphic liposarcoma, which has a considerably worse prognosis {1733}.

Genetics

Like ALT/well-differentiated liposarcoma, DDLPS most often has ring or giant marker chromosomes wherein *MDM2* (12q15) is consistently amplified and over-expressed, representing the main driver

gene of the 12q amplicon {264,623, 862,983,1820,1852,2245, 2568}. A peculiarity of DDLPS may be the presence of multiple abnormal clones, with one or more containing supernumerary rings or giant marker chromosomes {1820, 1852, 2430}.

CGH and FISH analyses have revealed amplification of the 12q13–21 region associated with coamplification of other regions, as also observed in ALT/well-differentiated liposarcoma {1820,2245,2568, 2699}. However, in contrast to pure ALT/well-differentiated liposarcoma, DDLPS is characterized by coamplifications involving mainly 1p32 and 6q23 {446}, which include *JUN* {1732} and its activating kinase *ASK1* {445} as target genes, respectively, suggesting that the c-Jun pathway may be implicated in progression from ALT/well-differentiated liposarcoma to DDLPS. In this scenario, ASK1 triggers a phosphorylation cascade that activates the c-Jun N-terminal kinase JNK, which then phosphorylates and stabilizes c-Jun, ultimately blocking adipogenesis by interfering with C/EBPb {1732}. However, since Jun protein is frequently expressed in the well-differentiated component of DDLPS

{2591} and *JUN* amplification {2591} and 1p32 region copy-number gain {446} have also been reported in the well-differentiated component of DDLPS, it is possible that the activation of the c-Jun pathway per se may not always be sufficient to inhibit adipocytic differentiation {2591}. Although the role of c-Jun in the dedifferentiation process is still debated, its oncogenic role in liposarcoma has been demonstrated in cellular and xenograft models {1732,2591}.

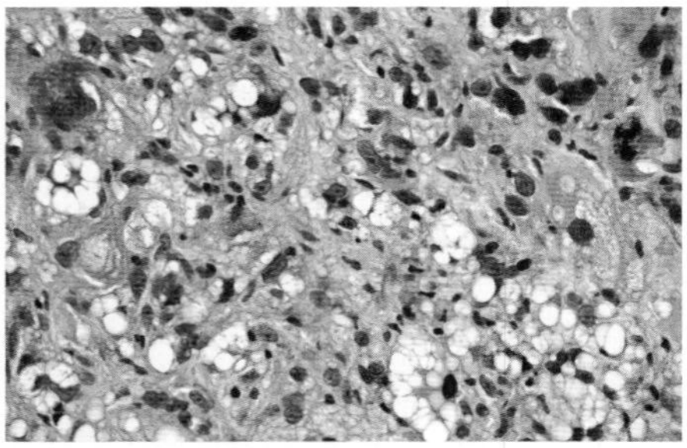

Prognostic factors

DDLPS is characterized by local recurrence in at least 40% of cases. However, almost all retroperitoneal examples seem to recur locally if patients are followed for 10–20 years. Distant metastases are observed in 15–20% of cases, with an overall mortality of 28–30% at 5-year follow-up {1162, 1787,2933}, although this figure is undoubtedly much higher at 10–20 years. The most important prognostic factor is anatomical location, with retroperitoneal lesions exhibiting the worst clinical behaviour. The extent or morphological pattern of dedifferentiated areas does not predict outcome. DDLPS, despite its high-grade morphology, exhibits a less aggressive clinical course than other types of high-grade pleomorphic sarcoma, and an accelerated clinical course is observed in only a minority of patients. However, the basis for this difference is unknown {1162, 1787,2933}. Relative absence of complex karyotypic aberrations as well as rarity of *TP53* gene aberrations (unlike in other high-grade pleomorphic sarcomas) may at least partly explain the discrepancy between morphology and clinical outcome {510,623}. Multivisceral resections appear to increase relapse-free survival {268}

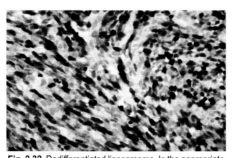

Fig. 2.31 Homologous dedifferentiated liposarcoma. Rarely, the high-grade component of dedifferentiated liposarcoma can be lipogenic, mimicking pleomorphic liposarcoma.

Fig. 2.32 Dedifferentiated liposarcoma. In the appropriate morphological context, diffuse and intense nuclear immunoreactivity for MDM2 represents a useful clue favouring the diagnosis of dedifferentiated liposarcoma.

Myxoid liposarcoma

C.R. Antonescu
M. Ladanyi

Definition

A malignant tumour composed of uniform round to oval-shaped primitive non-lipogenic cells and a variable number of small signet-ring cell lipoblasts in a prominent myxoid stroma with a characteristic branching vascular pattern. These tumours usually show either *FUS-DDIT3* or *EWSR1-DDIT3* rearrangement. Included in this category are more cellular lesions formerly known as round cell liposarcoma.

ICD-O code   8852/3

Synonym

Round cell liposarcoma

Epidemiology

Myxoid liposarcoma (MLS) accounts for 15–20% of liposarcomas and represents about 5% of all soft tissue sarcomas in adults. MLS is a disease of young adults. Peak incidence is in the fourth and fifth decades of life and, although rare, it is the commonest form of liposarcoma in children and adolescents {1247}. MLS is equally common in males and females.

Sites of involvement

MLS occurs more commonly in the deep soft tissues of the extremities, and in more than two thirds of cases develops within the musculature of the thigh. MLS rarely arises primarily in the retroperitoneum or subcutaneous tissue.

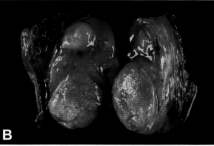

Fig. 2.33 Myxoid liposarcoma. **A** Grossly, this low-grade tumour has a distinctive gelatinous haemorrhagic appearance. **B** Gross appearance of a high-grade lesion showing solid fleshy areas.

Clinical features

MLS typically occurs as a large painless mass within the deep soft tissue of the limbs. One third of patients develop distant metastases, this being dependent on the histological grade of the primary tumour. In contrast to other types of liposarcoma or myxoid sarcomas of the extremities, MLS tends to metastasize to unusual locations in soft tissue (such as retroperitoneum, opposite extremity, axilla, etc) or bone (particularly spine), even before spreading to the lungs.

In a significant number of cases, MLS patients present with synchronous or metachronous multifocal disease {77}. This unusual clinical manifestation is caused by haematogenous metastasis to other sites, involving tumour cells seemingly incompetent to seed the lungs.

Macroscopy

Grossly, MLSs are well-circumscribed, multinodular intramuscular tumours, showing glistening, gelatinous cut surface in predominantly low-grade myxoid tumours. In contrast, higher-grade areas have instead a fleshy tan appearance. Gross evidence of tumour necrosis is uncommon.

Histopathology

At low power, MLS has a nodular growth pattern, with enhanced cellularity at the periphery of the lobules. There is a mixture of uniform round to oval-shaped non-lipogenic cells and small signet ring lipoblasts in a prominent myxoid stroma, rich in a delicate, arborizing, "chicken-wire" capillary vasculature. Frequently, the extracellular mucin forms large confluent pools, creating a microcystic lymphangioma-like or so-called "pulmonary oedema" growth pattern. Typically, MLS lacks nuclear pleomorphism, giant tumour cells, prominent areas of spindling or significant mitotic activity.

A subset of MLS shows histological progression to hypercellular or round cell

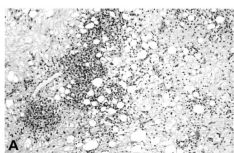
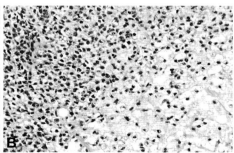
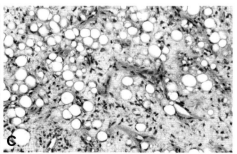

Fig. 2.34 Histological spectrum of myxoid liposarcoma (MLS). **A** Low-power view of a low-grade MLS showing focal areas of increased cellularity. **B** High-power view of a transitional area, showing increased cellularity. Tumour cells are not closely packed, retaining a small amount of intercellular myxoid stroma. **C** Uniform round to oval-shaped primitive nonlipogenic mesenchymal cells and a variable number of small lipoblasts in a prominent myxoid stroma.

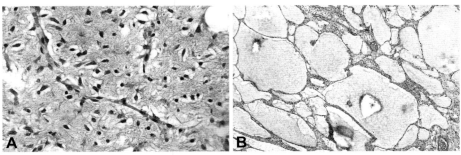

Fig. 2.35 Low-grade myxoid liposarcoma. **A** Delicate arborizing vasculature. **B** Characteristic "pulmonary oedema" growth pattern attributable to pools of stromal mucin.

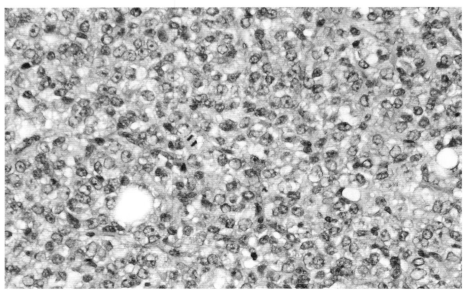

Fig. 2.36 High-grade myxoid liposarcoma characterized by solid sheets of back-to-back primitive round cells with a high nuclear to cytoplasmic ratio, and no intervening myxoid stroma.

morphology, which is associated with a significantly poorer prognosis. The higher-grade ("round cell") areas are characterized by solid sheets of back-to-back primitive round cells with a high nuclear to cytoplasmic ratio, with no intervening myxoid stroma. The cytomorphology of the round cell component may resemble that of the relatively small cells seen in the myxoid areas or may less often consist of larger rounded cells with variable amounts of eosinophilic cytoplasm. These two morphological patterns show no difference with regard to patient prognosis. The presence of gradual transition from myxoid to hypercellular/round cell areas provides strong support that myxoid and round cell liposarcoma represent a histological continuum of MLS. This concept is also supported by the presence of the identical translocation in both histological types (see below). So-called transitional areas are defined as ar-

eas of increased cellularity, not reaching the level of round cell component and still retaining small amount of intercellular myxoid stroma. The appearance of MLS in fine-needle aspirate cytology is also well described {1439}.

Immunophenotype
In most cases, immunohistochemical studies are not needed for establishing a diagnosis of MLS. In tumours with predominantly high-grade morphology, immunostains are performed to exclude other round-cell malignancies, since S100 protein is variably positive in the high-grade component.

Ultrastructure
Ultrastructurally, the undifferentiated cells are typically devoid of lipid droplets and show rich arrays of vimentin-type intermediate filaments. Lipoblasts in variable

stages of adipocytic maturation can be identified, containing either relatively few small lipid droplets or large confluent lipid vacuoles that displace the nucleus at the periphery. Flocculent mucoid stromal material coating the cells and extracellular spaces is common.

Genetics
MLS is characterized by the recurrent translocation t(12;16)(q13;p11) {2628, 2804} that results in *FUS-DDIT3* gene fusion, present in > 95% of cases {530, 2219,2284}. In the remaining cases, a variant t(12;22)(q13;q12) is present in which *DDIT3* (also known as *CHOP*) fuses instead with *EWSR1*, a gene that is highly related to *FUS* {2156}. There are at least 11 different isoforms of the *FUS-DDIT3* fusion transcript and four known forms of the *EWSR1-DDIT3* fusion transcript. In the most common variants, a portion of the amino terminus of *FUS* is fused to the entire coding region of *DDIT3*. Three major recurrent fusion transcript types have been reported in which exon 2 of *DDIT3* is fused in frame with either *FUS* exon 5 (type I, accounting for two thirds of cases), exon 7 (type II), or exon 8 (type III) {83,1445, 2157}. The monoclonal origin of synchronous/metachronous multifocal MLS has been confirmed by *FUS-DDIT3* genomic rearrangement structures in tumours from different sites {77}. The presence of the *FUS-DDIT3* fusion is highly sensitive and specific for MLS and is absent in other morphological mimics, including predominantly myxoid well-differentiated/dedifferentiated liposarcoma of the retroperitoneum and in myxofibrosarcoma {78}. No convincing genetic evidence has been presented to date to support the concept of a mixed-type liposarcoma composed of MLS and dedifferentiated liposarcoma. *RET*, *IGF1R* and *IGF2* are highly expressed in MLS and promote cell survival through both the PI3K/Akt and Ras-Raf-ERK/MAPK pathways {439,2021}. Activating *PIK3CA* mutations were recently demonstrated in 14–18% of cases, in either the helical (E542K and E545K) or kinase (H1047L and H1047R) domains {156, 636}. Mutations were more frequent in round cell tumours and were associated with shortened disease-specific survival. Homozygous loss of *PTEN*, an alternative mechanism for PI3K/Akt activation, was found in an additional subset of patients, mutually exclusive with *PIK3CA* mutation.

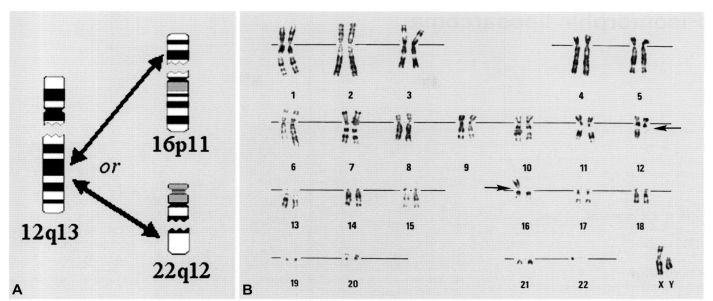

Fig. 2.37 Myxoid liposarcoma. **A** Schematic illustration of the breakpoints involved in the specific translocations reported for myxoid liposarcoma, t(12;16)(q13;p11) and t(12;22)(q13;q12). **B** Karyotype showing the translocation t(12;16)(q13;p11) in a myxoid liposarcoma. Arrowheads indicate breakpoints.

Prognostic factors

High histological grade (often defined as > 5% round cell component), presence of necrosis, and *TP53* and *CDKN2A* alterations are predictors of unfavourable outcome in localized MLS {83,1099,1946, 2094}. The prognostic significance of more limited hypercellularity (transitional areas) is less certain. Low-grade MLS is associated with a metastatic risk of < 10%. The different isoforms of the *FUS-DDIT3* fusion transcripts are not associated with differences in histological grade or clinical outcome {83,260}.

Pleomorphic liposarcoma

J.-M.Coindre
F. Pedeutour

Definition

A pleomorphic, high-grade sarcoma containing a variable number of pleomorphic lipoblasts and with a complex genomic profile. No areas of atypical lipomatous tumour/well-differentiated liposarcoma or other line of differentiation are present.

ICD-O code   8854/3

Epidemiology

Pleomorphic liposarcoma is the rarest subtype of liposarcoma, accounting for about 5% of all liposarcomas {128}. Most cases occur in adults in later life, with peak incidence in the seventh decade and a slightly higher incidence in males than females {695,955,1213,1877,2118}.

Sites of involvement

Pleomorphic liposarcoma occurs on the extremities in two thirds of cases (lower > upper limbs), while the trunk wall, retroperitoneum and spermatic cord are less frequently affected {695,955,1213,1877}. Rare sites of involvement include mediastinum, heart, pleura, breast, scalp, colon and orbit {354,955,1213}. Most cases arise in deep soft tissue, but about 25% develop in subcutaneous fat {955,1213}, with purely dermal cases being very rare {627,695,955,1213}.

Clinical features

Most patients complain of a rapidly growing painless mass, usually with a short preoperative duration (median, 3–6 months); a subset of patients report pain, while some patients have symptoms related to tumour location {955,1213}.

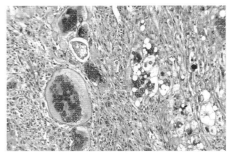

Fig. 2.39 Pleomorphic liposarcoma. A notable feature is the presence of extremely large cells.

Macroscopy

Most tumours are large with a median size of 8–10 cm {955,1213}. They are well-demarcated but non-encapsulated, or ill-defined and infiltrative and sometimes multinodular. On sectioning, most tumours are white to yellow. Myxoid changes as well as foci of necrosis are quite often observed.

Histopathology

Histologically, most cases have infiltrative margins and all tumours contain a varying proportion of pleomorphic lipoblasts in a background of a high-grade, usually pleomorphic, sarcoma. The presence of lipoblasts is necessary for the diagnosis, but their number varies considerably between cases and between areas twithin the same tumour, emphasizing the importance of

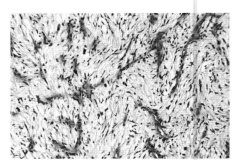

Fig. 2.40 Pleomorphic liposarcoma with areas resembling myxofibrosarcoma.

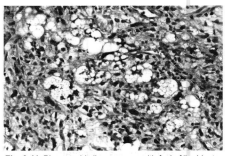

Fig. 2.41 Pleomorphic liposarcoma with foci of lipoblasts.

adequate sampling. In most cases, the non-lipogenic component resembles undifferentiated pleomorphic sarcoma with spindle and multinucleate giant cells arranged in short fascicles, with some notable features: presence of extremely large tumour cells often showing clear or vacuolated cytoplasm, and the presence of extracellular and occasionally intracellular eosinophilic hyaline droplets. Almost half

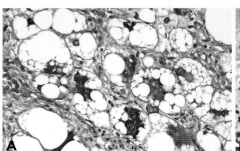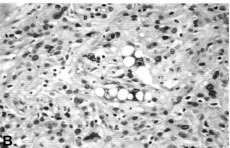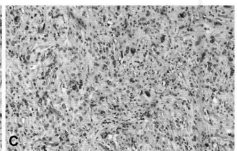

Fig. 2.38 Pleomorphic liposarcoma. **A** This lesion is characterized by the presence of pleomorphic lipoblasts that contain enlarged and hyperchromatic nuclei scalloped by cytoplasmic vacuoles. **B** In about one third of cases, lipoblasts are sparse and represent < 10% of the tumour surface. **C** The dominant pattern of the non-lipogenic pattern resembled that of an undifferentiated pleomorphic sarcoma (previously known as pleomorphic malignant fibrous histiocytoma).

of cases contain at least focal areas similar to intermediate- to high-grade myxofibrosarcoma associated with pleomorphic lipoblasts. This myxofibrosarcoma-like component is predominant in some cases. Epithelioid morphology is seen in about one quarter of cases with areas resembling poorly differentiated carcinoma, renal clear cell carcinoma, adrenocortical carcinoma or melanoma {955,1213, 1877}. A haemangiopericytoma-like vascular pattern, and areas resembling round cell, well-differentiated or spindle cell liposarcomas may be seen. All these patterns may be associated or predominant. An unusual subset of pleomorphic liposarcoma with myxoid morphology is recognized in the mediastinum of children {32}. The mitotic rate is variable, but with a median of 19–25 mitoses per 10 HPF. Necrosis is present in more than half of cases.

Immunophenotype
Staining for S100 protein is positive in lipoblasts in fewer than half of cases. SMA and CD34 are at least focally positive in almost half of cases, while pankeratin, EMA, desmin and HMGA2 may also be positive {699,955,1213}. Staining for MDM2 and CDK4 is typically negative {239}.

Ultrastructure
Pleomorphic lipoblasts contain abundant and coalescent lipid droplets and numerous cytoplasmic organelles.

Genetics
The cytogenetic profile of pleomorphic liposarcoma more closely resembles those of other pleomorphic sarcomas than those of well-differentiated/dedifferentiated liposarc-

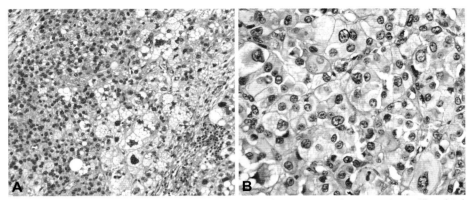

Fig. 2.42 Pleomorphic liposarcoma. Epithelioid morphology is present in some cases and may suggest an undifferentiated carcinoma (**A**) or even a renal clear cell carcinoma (**B**).

omas or myxoid/round cell liposarcomas {1852}. Metaphase cells show high chromosomal counts and complex structural rearrangements. This complexity is represented by unidentifiable marker chromosomes, non-clonal aberrations, polyploidy and intercellular heterogeneity. No pathognomonic structural rearrangement, such as recurrent translocation or consistent presence of supernumerary ring chromosomes, has been identified.
Studies using aCGH have shown complex profiles with numerous chromosomal imbalances {917,1274,2337,2468,2733}. Gains are more frequent than losses. The most frequently gained regions are 1p21, 1q21–22, 5p13–15, 7q22 and 20q13, while the most frequent losses involve 11q22, 12p13, 13q14 (including the *RB1* locus) and 15q21. Deletions affecting chromosome 17, as well as mutations of *TP53* and *NF1,* have also been reported {156,2470,2733}, in contrast to other types of liposarcoma. In addition, the presence

of amplification of 13q material has been correlated with a worse prognosis {2468} and it has been noted that the genomic profiles of pleomorphic liposarcoma and myxofibrosarcoma are similar {156,1274}. No consistent amplification or overexpression of the 12q14–15 region has been detected in pleomorphic liposarcoma {917,2565}. Hence, absence of *MDM2/ HMGA2/CDK4* amplification can help distinguish pleomorphic liposarcoma from dedifferentiated liposarcoma.

Prognostic factors
Pleomorphic liposarcomas are aggressive sarcomas exhibiting local recurrence and with metastatic rates of 30–50% and overall 5-year survival of about 60%. Metastases occur mostly in the lungs and pleura. Central location, tumour depth, size and mitotic index have been associated with a worse prognosis {955,1213}.

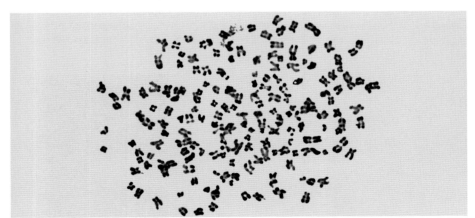

Fig. 2.43 Metaphase cell (RHG banding) from a pleomorphic liposarcoma showing > 170 chromosomes and a few structural alterations. Large ring or giant marker chromosomes are not observed.

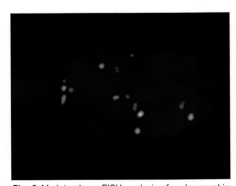

Fig. 2.44 Interphase FISH analysis of a pleomorphic liposarcoma with probes for the *MDM2* (red signal) and *CDK4* (green signal) genes indicating polysomy 12 (more than two signals for each probe) rather than amplification where more than ten signals grouped in clusters would be seen.

CHAPTER 3

Fibroblastic/myofibroblastic tumours

Nodular fasciitis

Proliferative fasciitis and proliferative myositis

Myositis ossificans and fibro-osseous pseudotumour of digits

Ischaemic fasciitis

Elastofibroma

Fibrous hamartoma of infancy

Fibromatosis colli

Juvenile hyaline fibromatosis

Inclusion body fibromatosis

Fibroma of tendon sheath

Desmoplastic fibroblastoma

Mammary-type myofibroblastoma

Calcifying aponeurotic fibroma

Angiomyofibroblastoma

Cellular angiofibroma

Nuchal-type fibroma

Gardner fibroma

Calcifying fibrous tumour

Palmar/plantar fibromatosis

Desmoid-type fibromatosis

Lipofibromatosis

Giant cell fibroblastoma

Dermatofibrosarcoma protuberans

Extrapleural solitary fibrous tumour

Inflammatory myofibroblastic tumour

Low-grade myofibroblastic sarcoma

Myxoinflammatory fibroblastic sarcoma

Infantile fibrosarcoma

Adult fibrosarcoma

Myxofibrosarcoma

Low-grade fibromyxoid sarcoma

Sclerosing epithelioid fibrosarcoma

Nodular fasciitis

A. Lazar
H.L. Evans
A.M. Oliveira

Definition

Nodular fasciitis is a self-limiting fibrous neoplasm that usually occurs in subcutaneous tissue. It is composed of plump but uniform fibroblastic/myofibroblastic cells and typically displays a loose or tissue culture-like growth pattern.

ICD-O code   8828/0

Synonym

Pseudosarcomatous fasciitis

Epidemiology

Nodular fasciitis is comparatively common {45,200,1255,1463,1821,2539,2610}. It occurs in all age groups but more often in young adults. Intravascular fasciitis {2194,2268} and cranial fasciitis {1565} are rare. Intravascular fasciitis is found mostly in persons aged < 30 years, while cranial fasciitis develops predominantly in infants aged < 2 years. Nodular fasciitis and intravascular fasciitis occur equally frequently in males and females, but cranial fasciitis is more common in boys.

Etiology

Some patients with nodular fasciitis report trauma to the site of the lesion, but most do not. Birth trauma may be a factor in the genesis of cranial fasciitis.

Sites of involvement

Nodular fasciitis typically develops from the surface of fascia and extends into subcutis, although occasional cases are intramuscular. Dermal localization is very rare {598}. Any part of the body can be involved, but the upper extremity, trunk, and head and neck are most frequently affected. Intravascular fasciitis is usually subcutaneous. It occurs in small to medium-sized vessels, predominantly veins but occasionally arteries. Cranial fasciitis typically involves the outer table of the skull and contiguous soft tissue of the scalp, and may extend downward through the inner table into the meninges.

Clinical features

Nodular fasciitis typically grows rapidly

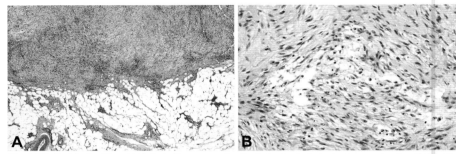

Fig. 3.001 Nodular fasciitis. **A** This typical low-power view illustrates the typical subcutaneous location. **B** This high-power view demonstrates the typical plump, but regular fibroblasts/myofibroblasts with discohesive areas.

and has a preoperative duration in most cases of not more than 2–3 months. Soreness or tenderness may be present. It usually measures 2 cm or less and almost always < 5 cm. Intravascular fasciitis may enlarge more slowly, but is also normally not more than 2 cm in size. Cranial fasciitis expands quickly, like nodular fasciitis, and may become somewhat larger than the usual example of the latter. When the skull is involved, X-ray imaging shows a lytic defect, often with a sclerotic rim. In

contrast, nodular fasciitis presents as a nondistinctive soft-tissue mass on imaging studies.

Macroscopy

Grossly, nodular fasciitis may appear circumscribed or infiltrative, but is not encapsulated. The cut surface varies from myxoid to fibrous, and occasionally there is central cystic change. Intravascular fasciitis ranges from nodular to plexiform, the latter contour resulting when there is

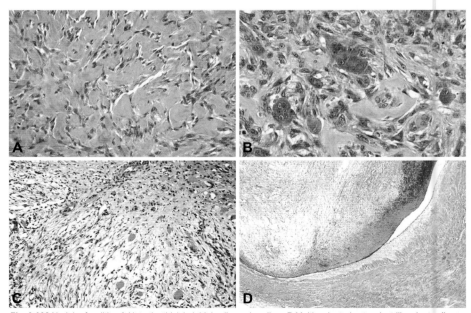

Fig. 3.002 Nodular fasciitis. **A** Note the thick keloidal collagen bundles. **B** Multinucleated osteoclast-like giant cells are sometimes present. **C** Intramuscular variant. There is a loose and torn appearance, but greater fibrosis than usual in one area (upper right). **D** Intravascular fasciitis. The intravascular location is demonstrated at scanning magnification.

extensive intravascular growth. Cranial fasciitis is typically circumscribed and rubbery to firm, and may be focally myxoid or cystic in its centre.

Histopathology

Nodular fasciitis is composed of plump but regular spindle-shaped fibroblasts (or myofibroblasts) lacking nuclear hyperchromasia and pleomorphism. Mitotic figures may be plentiful, but not atypical forms. The lesion may be highly cellular, but typically it is at least partly discohesive and myxoid, with a torn, feathery, or tissue culture-like character. In more cellular areas, there is often growth in S- or C-shaped fascicles, or sometimes in a storiform pattern. There is normally little collagen, but this may be increased focally, and keloidal collagen bundles may be present and occasionally prominent. Extravasated erythrocytes, lymphocytes and osteoclast-like giant cells are frequently identified. The lesional border is typically, at least focally, infiltrative, although it may be well delineated; peripheral extension is often seen between fat cells in the subcutis and between muscle cells in intramuscular locations. Small vessels are numerous, resulting in a resemblance to granulation tissue.

Intravascular fasciitis and cranial fasciitis are similar to nodular fasciitis histologically, although the former often displays a greater number of osteoclast-like giant cells. Intravascular fasciitis ranges from predominantly extravascular, with only a minor intravascular component, to predominantly intravascular. Osseous metaplasia is occasionally seen in nodular fasciitis (fasciitis ossificans) {572,1512} and cranial fasciitis.

Immunophenotype

Stains for SMA and MSA are usually strongly and diffusely positive, but desmin

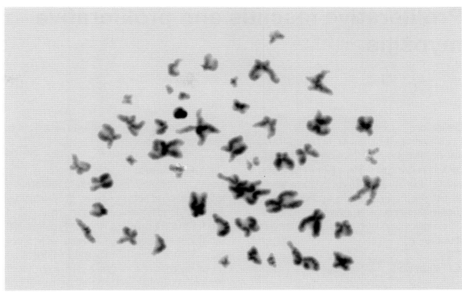

Fig. 3.003 Nodular fasciitis. FISH of metaphase showing rearrangement of the *USP6* locus on chromosome 17 (separation of green and orange signals). This chromosomal translocation is difficult to identify using traditional cytogenetic methods since both genes are located in light bands at the terminal end of the chromosomes. *USP6* rearrangements are found in > 90% of cases of nodular fasciitis.

positivity is rare {1938}. CD68 staining is present in the osteoclast-like giant cells and occasionally in spindle cells. Staining for keratin and S100 protein is typically negative.

Genetics

The identification of the *MYH9-USP6* gene fusion as a recurrent event in nodular fasciitis has firmly established its previously disputed clonal neoplastic nature {241,681,764,1457,2448,2865,2918}. *MYH9* (22q13) encodes non-muscular myosin heavy chain 9 and is involved in cell-shape maintenance, cell motility, adhesion, differentiation and development. USP6 (17p13) is a deubiquitinating protease involved in cell trafficking, protein degradation, signalling and inflammation {2115}. The *MYH9-USP6* fusion causes transcriptional upregulation of the entire coding sequence of *USP6* driven by the active *MYH9* promoter in a classic promoter-swapping mechanism {764}. Whether this translocation is featured in the less common intravascular and cranial fasciitis is uncertain. Structurally similar *USP6* fusion genes are found in aneurysmal bone cyst {2117,2121}, which shares some common histological features with nodular fasciitis. As an example of a consistently self-limited and regressing lesion with a recurrent fusion gene, the term "transient neoplasia" has been suggested {764}.

Prognostic factors

Recurrence of nodular fasciitis after excision is rare, but is occasionally observed after incomplete excision during the active growth phase.

Proliferative fasciitis and proliferative myositis

A. Lazar
J.A. Bridge
H.L. Evans

Definition
Proliferative fasciitis is a mass-forming subcutaneous proliferation characterized by large ganglion-like cells in addition to plump fibroblastic/myofibroblastic cells similar to those seen in nodular fasciitis. Proliferative myositis has the same cellular composition but occurs within skeletal muscle.

ICD-O code   8828/0

Epidemiology
Proliferative fasciitis and proliferative myositis are much less common than nodular fasciitis. Both occur predominantly in middle-aged or older adults {466,752,1401}, i.e. an older age group than nodular fasciitis. A rare variant of proliferative fasciitis is described in children {1814}.

Etiology
There is sometimes a history of trauma to the site of proliferative fasciitis and myositis, but usually there is not.

Sites of involvement
Proliferative fasciitis develops most frequently in the upper extremity, particularly the forearm, followed by the lower extremity and trunk. Proliferative myositis arises predominantly in the trunk, shoulder girdle, and upper arm and less often in the thigh. By definition, proliferative fasciitis is subcutaneous and proliferative myositis is intramuscular.

Clinical features
Both proliferative fasciitis and proliferative myositis characteristically grow rapidly and are usually excised within 2 months of the time they are first noted. Proliferative fasciitis almost always measures < 5 cm and is most often < 3 cm. Proliferative myositis may be slightly larger, but not greatly so. Either lesion may be painful or tender, but this is more common with proliferative fasciitis. The imaging characteristics of proliferative myositis may be suggestive of the diagnosis; those for proliferative fasciitis are less well studied {2149,3033}.

Macroscopy
Proliferative fasciitis typically forms a poorly circumscribed mass in the subcutaneous tissue and may extend horizontally along fascia. The rare childhood variant is often better circumscribed. Proliferative myositis is also poorly marginated and replaces a variable proportion of the involved muscle.

Histopathology
Both proliferative fasciitis and myositis contain plump fibroblastic/myofibroblastic spindle cells similar to those seen in nodular fasciitis, but also demonstrate large cells with rounded nuclei, prominent nucleoli, and abundant amphophilic to basophilic cytoplasm {466}. These cells are often described as ganglion-like. They usually have one nucleus but may have two or three. They may be evenly or patchily distributed. Mitotic figures are found in both the spindle cells and ganglion-like cells and may be relatively numerous, but are not atypical. The stroma varies from myxoid to collagenous, and the lesional borders are typically infiltrative or even ill defined. Proliferative fasciitis may grow laterally along fascial planes, while proliferative myositis extends between individual muscle fibres, creating the characteristic "checkerboard" pattern. The childhood variant of proliferative fasciitis normally has better delineated borders than the adult form, greater cellularity, dominance of ganglion-like cells and more mitoses. Focal necrosis and acute inflammation may also be present. Proliferative myositis may contain metaplastic bone, demonstrating kinship to myositis ossificans.

Immunophenotype
The immunohistochemical profile of proliferative fasciitis/myositis is similar to that of nodular fasciitis, usually staining positive for SMA and MSA and negative for desmin {732,1676}. The ganglion-like cells are often negative for actins.

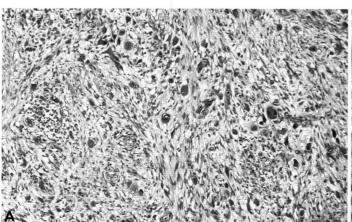
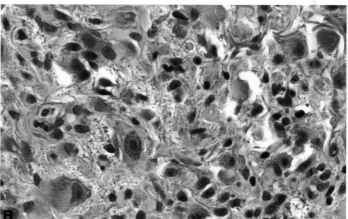

Fig. 3.004 Proliferative fasciitis. **A** Ganglion-like cells are admixed with spindle cells and lymphocytes in a loose myxoid matrix. **B** Ganglion-like cells at higher power.

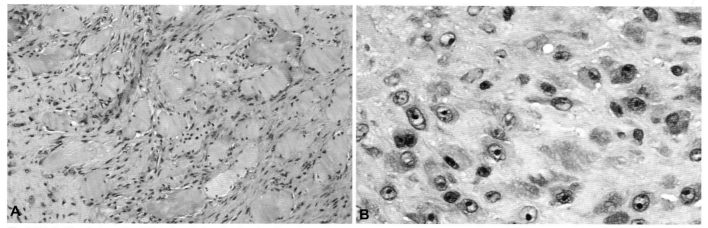

Fig. 3.005 Proliferative myositis. **A** Note the spindle cells. Ganglion-like cells sporting amphophilic cytoplasm are admixed. **B** Details of the cytological features of the ganglion-like cells with prominent nucleoli.

Ultrastructure

As with nodular fasciitis, the ultrastructural features of proliferative fasciitis and myositis are those of fibroblasts and myofibroblasts {732,1676}. The ganglion-like cells demonstrate abundant, dilated rough endoplasmic reticulum and lack neuronal characteristics.

Genetics

Trisomy of chromosome 2 has been detected as the sole abnormality in one case each of proliferative fasciitis and prolifer-

ative myositis {633,2105}. The significance of these findings, however, is not entirely clear as nonrandom trisomy 2 has also been documented in vitro in senescent lymphocytes from elderly patients {350}. Thus the possibility that trisomy 2 in these cases of proliferative fasciitis and proliferative myositis represents an acquired age-related anomaly cannot be entirely excluded.

A second case of proliferative myositis lacking trisomy 2 has demonstrated a t(6;14)(q23;q32) translocation {1785}.

Prognostic factors

Both proliferative fasciitis and proliferative myositis recur only rarely after conservative local excision and do not metastasize.

Myositis ossificans and fibro-osseous pseudotumour of digits

A.E. Rosenberg
A.M. Oliveira

Definition
Myositis ossificans (MO) and fibro-osseous pseudotumour of digits (FP) are localized, self-limiting lesions that are composed of reactive hypercellular fibrous tissue and bone. Rapid growth of these lesions, which frequently arouses clinical suspicion, in conjunction with hypercellularity and mitotic activity makes them classic pseudosarcomas.

Synonyms
Pseudomalignant osseous tumour of soft tissue; myositis ossificans circumscripta; myositis ossificans traumatica

Epidemiology
MO and FP have a broad age distribution ranging from infancy to late adulthood (14 months to 95 years); however, they usually occur during young adulthood (mean age, 32 years) {474,608,1874,2081,2370, 2678}. Males are affected more frequently than females (sex ratio, 3 : 2); however, females are more commonly affected by FP. Patients with MO are typically physically active.

Etiology
Injury to soft tissue is the initiating event in most instances and a history of trauma is documented in 60–75% of cases {474, 2081,2678}. Repetitive small mechanical injuries, ischaemia or inflammation have been implicated in atraumatic cases.

Sites of involvement
MO can develop anywhere in the body, including the extremities, trunk, and head

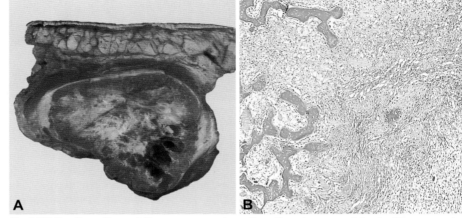

Fig. 3.007 Myositis ossificans. **A** Gross appearance of myositis ossificans in a young adult male. **B** Low-power view showing typical zonation with fasciitis-like features (centre right), immature osteoid (centre) and bone formation at the periphery.

and neck {474,608,2081,2370,2678}. The common locations are susceptible to trauma, such as the elbow, thigh, buttock, and shoulder {1195,1769}. MO-like lesions have also been reported in the mesentery {3053}. The process often develops within skeletal muscle; similar lesions that occur in the subcutis, tendons or fascia are known as panniculitis ossificans and fasciitis ossificans, respectively.

FP usually affects the subcutaneous tissues of the proximal phalanx of the fingers and less frequently the toes {430,1945, 1998}.

Clinical features
The clinical and radiographical findings for MO parallel the stage of development of the lesion. In the early phase (1–2 weeks), the involved area is swollen and painful. Similarly, in FP the digit is painful and there is a localized fusiform swelling. Plain X-rays and CT scans of MO may demonstrate soft-tissue fullness and oedema, while MRI reveals signal heterogeneity and high-signal intensity on T2-weighted images {1476,2807}. Flocculent dense calcifications become evident in the periphery of the mass 2–6 weeks after the onset of symptoms, and eventually produce a lacy pattern of bone deposition that sharply demarcates the periphery of the lesion in an eggshell-like fashion. In FP, the lesional calcification has a more random distribution. Over time, MO and FP become hard and well demarcated.

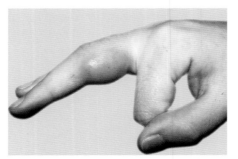

Fig. 3.006 Fibro-osseous pseudotumour of digits presenting as a red and swollen mass.

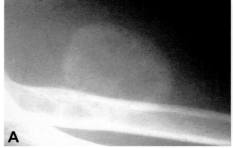

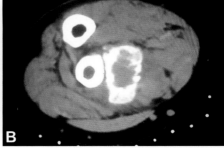

Fig. 3.008 Myositis ossificans. **A** Plain X-ray. **B** Cross-sectional CT of a forearm lesion of approximately 6 weeks duration with a well-circumscribed, ossified periphery and a more lucent centre.

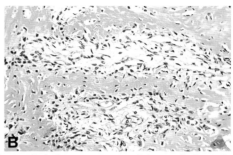

Fig. 3.009 Myositis ossificans. **A** The centre is composed of randomly arranged plump fibroblasts in a myxoid stroma. **B** The periphery of the fibroblastic component merges with the region containing trabeculae of woven bone. **C** Woven bone is prominently rimmed by osteoblasts.

Macroscopy

MO is well delineated, ovoid, with a glistening soft tan haemorrhagic centre and a firm, grey-white gritty periphery. The lesion ranges in size from 2 to 12 cm, but most are 5 cm in size. FO is usually smaller and less well-demarcated.

Histopathology

MO is characterized by a zonal proliferation of fibroblasts and bone-forming elements that progress through various stages over time {474,608,2081,2370,2678}. In the early stages, MO is most cellular, bearing a resemblance to nodular fasciitis, and is composed of proliferating fibroblasts that are oriented randomly or in short intersecting fascicles. The fibroblasts have eosinophilic cytoplasm and nuclei that are vesicular or finely granular and contain nucleoli. Normal mitoses may be numerous. The stroma is richly vascular, myxoid and contains fibrin, extravasated erythrocytes, scattered lymphocytes and osteoclast-like giant cells and injured myocytes. Peripherally, the fibroblastic component merges with ill-defined trabeculae and sheets of unmineralized woven bone that are rimmed by prominent osteoblasts and harbour large osteocytes. In FP, the bone is randomly distributed throughout the lesion. In some cases of MO, nodules of cellular hyaline cartilage with foci of enchondral ossification are present. The most peripheral portions of MO are composed of well-formed bony trabeculae and cortical-appearing bone, which initially has a woven architecture but eventually is remodelled into lamellar bone. As the central area undergoes ossification, the mass becomes composed of cortical and cancellous bone with fatty or haematopoietic marrow. In some cases of MO, the zonal pattern is not well developed.

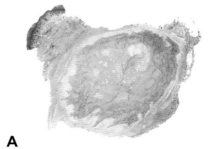

Fig. 3.010 Fibro-osseous pseudotumour of digits. **A** In this case, the lesion presents as a well-circumscribed mass in subcutis. **B** Reactive woven bone lined by osteoblasts is present throughout the lesion.

Immunophenotype

The fibroblasts and myofibroblasts may express actin, SMA and desmin.

Ultrastructure

The spindle cells have the features of fibroblasts and myofibroblasts, including dilated rough endoplasmic reticulum and aggregates of cytoplasmic filaments occasionally associated with dense bodies {2259}. The osteoblasts contain mitochondria and abundant rough endoplasmic reticulum.

Genetics

The molecular genetics of MO and FP are unknown. The finding of *USP6* rearrangements in some putative cases of MO with classic radiological and histological features, but a more protracted clinical course suggests that they may be better classified as aneurysmal bone cyst of soft tissue {2674}.

Prognostic factors

The treatment of MO and FP usually consists of simple excision. Prognosis is excellent as recurrence is exceptional and malignant transformation into osteosarcoma is very rare {1460}.

Ischaemic fasciitis

B. Liegl-Atzwanger

Definition
Ischaemic fasciitis is a distinctive reactive pseudosarcomatous fibroblastic/myofibroblastic proliferation, sometimes associated with physical immobility.

Synonym
Atypical decubital fibroplasia

Epidemiology
Ischaemic fasciitis affects mainly elderly patients, with a peak incidence between the seventh and ninth decades of life. Males are affected slightly more frequently than females {1614,1939,2220}.

Etiology
Ischaemia caused by constant pressure or trauma to a predisposed region (e.g. a bony prominence) may contribute to the pathogenesis in some patients {1939, 2220}.

Sites of involvement
Ischaemic fasciitis is frequently located around the limb girdles, sacral region and greater trochanter; however, the chest wall and back may also be affected. While this lesion usually develops in the deep subcutis, infiltration of the deep dermis, tendinous tissue and skeletal muscle can occur {1614}.

Clinical features
This lesion occurs as a painless mass with a median size of 4.7 cm. An association with patients' immobility or debilitation may occur but is inconsistent {1614}.

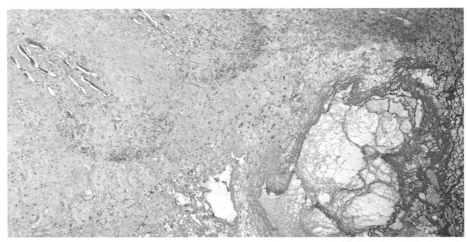

Fig. 3.011 Ischaemic fasciitis showing a distinct zonal appearance with a central area of fibrinoid degeneration/necrosis with pseudocystic changes, surrounded by a granulation tissue-like vascular proliferation.

Macroscopy
Ischaemic fasciitis presents as a white fibrous to tan-yellow lesion with central necrosis or occasional cystic change.

Histopathology
The histological hallmark of ischaemic fasciitis is a distinct zonal appearance. The central part of the lesion is characterized by a hypocellular area of fibrinoid degeneration/necrosis with or without pseudocystic degeneration or infarcted fat. The central area is surrounded by a granulation tissue-like vascular proliferation mixed with fibroblasts and myofibroblasts, partly with ganglion cell-like appearance similar to proliferative fasciitis.

Fibrosis/fibrohyalinosis or myxoid stromal change, hyalinosis of vessel walls, vessels with fibrin thrombi, an inflammatory infiltrate and commonly extravasated erythrocytes can often be seen.

Immunophenotype
Immunohistochemical expression of SMA and desmin can be observed in lesional cells, indicating the fibroblastic/myofibroblastic nature of this lesion {1614}.

Prognostic factors
Patients are usually cured by local excision even if incomplete. Recurrences may rarely develop in immobilized patients, due to persistence of the underlying cause.

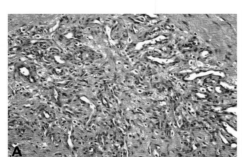
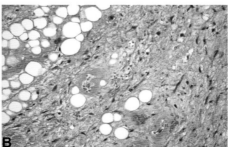
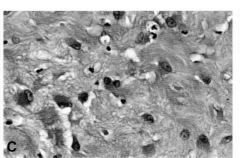

Fig. 3.012 Ischaemic fasciitis (IF). **A** Vascular proliferation with endothelial cells showing reactive hyperchromatic nuclei (no endothelial multilayering) jumbled up with a reactive fibroblastic/myofibroblastic proliferation. **B** IF with myxoid stroma changes, infarcted fat, hyalinosis of vessel walls and a reactive fibroblastic/myofibroblastic component with extravasated erythrocytes. **C** Polygonal-shaped fibroblasts showing enlarged nuclei, prominent nucleoli and amphophilic cytoplasm, similar to ganglion-like cells in proliferative fasciitis.

Elastofibroma

M. Hisaoka
J. Nishio

Definition
A benign, ill-defined proliferation of elastofibrous tissue characterized by an excessive number of abnormal elastic fibres.

ICD-O code   8820/0

Synonyms
Elastofibroma dorsi

Epidemiology
Elastofibroma occurs almost exclusively in the elderly, with a peak incidence between the seventh and eighth decades of life. There is a striking predominance in females {1992}. Although elastofibroma was previously considered to be rare, its exact prevalence remains unknown. Incidental lesions were detected by CT in 2% of adults aged > 60 years and in 16% of autopsies in adults aged > 55 years {302, 1321}.

Etiology
Elastofibroma has an unknown etiology, but may be induced by a response to repeated trauma or friction between the lower scapula and the thoracic wall {1322}. Elastotic degeneration of collagen or abnormal elastotic fibrinogenesis may underlie its pathogenesis {921,1497, 2648}.

In contrast, recurrent chromosomal alterations and a nonrandom inactivation of the X-chromosome-linked human androgen receptor gene described in some cases imply a clonal fibrous proliferation {1186}. Approximately one third of the patients in Okinawa had a family history of elastofibroma, suggesting a familial predisposition {1992}.

Sites of involvement
Elastofibroma mostly arises in the deep soft tissue between the lower scapula and the thoracic wall. However, it may rarely occur in extrascapular locations, such as other parts of the thoracic wall, extremities, limb girdles, and the gastrointestinal tract or other viscera. Although it is usually identified as a unilateral or solitary mass, bilateral or multiple elastofibromas have been reported.

Clinical features
The lesion presents as a slowly growing mass and rarely causes pain, stiffness, scapular snapping and impingement-like features. CT and MRI show a poorly defined, heterogeneous soft-tissue mass with attenuation similar to that of skeletal muscle interlaced with fatty strands {2018}.

Macroscopy
Elastofibroma is poorly defined and rubbery, and it appears as grey or whitish fibrous tissue with variably intervening streaks of yellow fatty tissue. The diameter of the lesion ranges from 2 to 15 cm.

Histopathology
Elastofibroma is composed predominantly of fibrocollagenous tissue containing prominent abnormal elastic fibres and

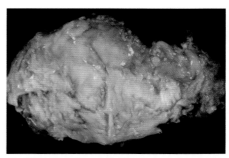

Fig. 3.013 Elastofibroma. An ill-defined mass comprising an admixture of grey-white fibrous tissue and intervening yellow fat.

dispersed, bland-appearing fibroblasts with a variable amount of mature adipose tissue. Myxoid change is common. The elastic fibres are typically thick or coarse, deeply eosinophilic and fragmented into linearly arranged globular or serrated disc-like structures, simulating beads on a string, which are highlighted using elastic stains.

Immunophenotype
The abnormal elastic fibres are positively reactive with antibodies against elastin or its precursor, tropoelastin {1186,1497}. The spindle cells are usually positive for CD34, but not for SMA or desmin {1186, 3017}.

Ultrastructure
The abnormal elastic fibres contain electron-lucent central cores surrounded by electron-dense fibrillar or granular substance, showing an irregular radial

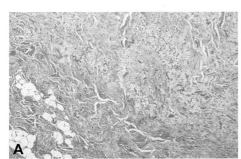
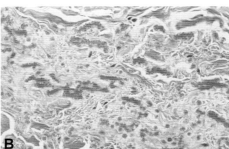
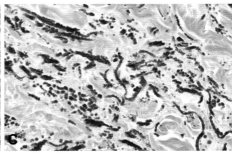

Fig. 3.014 Elastofibroma. **A** Hypocellular fibrocollagenous tissue with mature fatty tissue. **B** Thick or coarse, deeply eosinophilic elastic fibres arranged in beaded strings or globules. **C** Elastic van Gieson staining highlights the abnormal elastic fibres.

appearance {189,921,1497}. The constituent spindle cells have features of fibroblasts, but myofibroblastic cells are essentially absent {1497,3017}. The spindle cells exhibit intimate cell-to-matrix association or contain intracytoplasmic non-membrane-bound dense granular bodies with an intensity similar to that of extracellular elastin, suggesting elastogenesis {3017}.

Genetics
Elastofibroma exhibits chromosomal instability, manifested as both clonal and non-clonal structural changes {165,1784, 2854}. Aberrations of the short arm of chromosome 1 are particularly prominent. Metaphase- and array-based CGH studies have shown recurrent gain of Xq12–22 and loss of 1p, 13q, 19p, and 22q {1164, 2065}. In addition, deletion of *CASR* (3q21), *GSTP1* (11q13), *BRCA2* (13q12)

and gains of *APC* (5q21) and *PAH* (12q23) have been detected by MLPA in two cases of elastofibroma {1164}. No mutation of the *ABCC6* gene has been identified {1999}.

Prognostic factors
Elastofibroma is a benign lesion, which is cured by simple excision. Local recurrence is very rare. No cases of malignant transformation have been reported.

Fibrous hamartoma of infancy

C.M. Coffin

Definition
Fibrous hamartoma of infancy is a poorly circumscribed superficial soft-tissue mass with a characteristic organoid pattern of three histological components: intersecting fascicles of dense fibrocollagenous tissue, loosely textured areas of immature basophilic or myxoid round or primitive mesenchymal cells, and mature adipose tissue.

Synonym
Subdermal fibromatous tumour of infancy

Epidemiology
Fibrous hamartoma of infancy is very rare. Nearly all cases are diagnosed by age 2 years and 20% are congenital {664,727, 749,2607}. Males are affected predominantly {2150,2256,2607}.

Sites of involvement
The tumour most often involves the axillary and inguinal regions, upper arms, and trunk, and external genitalia {749,2150,2256, 2607}. It occasionally arises in the head, hands, or feet {760,1319,1323,1914}.

Clinical features
This solitary dermal and subcutaneous mass grows slowly or rapidly, without pain. The overlying skin may display eccrine changes {1055} or hypertrichosis {3036}. Rare cases have been associated with tuberous sclerosis {1098} or Williams syndrome {2765}.

Macroscopy
The soft, poorly demarcated mass has a lumpy texture and a white or yellow cut surface; margins are difficult to discern. Most are 3–5 cm in diameter, although very large tumours have been reported {664,1789}.

Histopathology
Fibrous hamartoma of infancy has a characteristic organoid architectural pattern with three components: fibrous tissue, adipose tissue, and immature mesenchymal tissue {749,2256,2607}. Well-defined

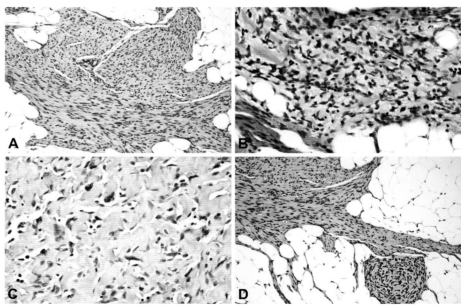

Fig. 3.015 Fibrous hamartoma of infancy. **A** The mature fibrous tissue component consists of interlacing fascicles of bland spindle cells with eosinophilic cytoplasm and collagenized background. **B** The immature component has a myxoid appearance with spindled, irregular, and round cells. **C** Pseudoangiectoid , scar-like, or neural-type pattern with dense collagen separated by clefts lined by spindled and irregular cells and a sparse mononuclear infiltrate. **D** The triphasic organoid pattern with mature adipose tissue, interlacing bundles of fibroblastic spindle cells, and immature basophilic mesenchymal tissue is characteristic.

intersecting fascicles of mature fibrous tissue with narrow straight or wavy nuclei are embedded in a collagenized stroma. The adipose tissue is mature and may form a major proportion of the lesion. The immature mesenchymal tissue is basophilic or myxoid and consists of sheets or bundles of primitive spindle, stellate, or ovoid cells which may surround small veins. Mitotic figures are rare. In some cases, a dominant area with disorderly randomly oriented fibroblasts in a collagenized vascular background or with abundant collagen and pseudoangioectoid spaces lined by angulated, occasionally multilobulated cells simulates a vascular, myxoid, or fibrohistiocytic neoplasm {749}. A sparse inflammatory infiltrate of mast cells, lymphocytes, and eosinophils may be present. This area may occupy the majority of the lesion and the characteristic triphasic organoid components are usually visible at the periphery.

Immunophenotype
The fibroblastic areas express SMA, while the primitive mesenchymal component does not {869,1045,1872,2256}. The mature adipose tissue is reactive for S100 protein. Desmin is usually not expressed, although it may occasionally be present in the fibroblastic areas {1045}. The sclerotic zone with angiectoid spaces expresses CD34.

Ultrastructure
The spindle-cell component displays fibroblastic and myofibroblastic features, and the primitive mesenchymal component contains slender cytoplasmic processes with few intracytoplasmic organelles {1045,1872}.

Genetics
Cytogenetic abnormalities have been described in rare examples, but no recurrent aberration has been detected {1529,2377,2730}.

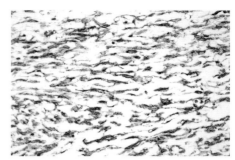
Fig. 3.016 Fibrous hamartoma of infancy. The pseudoangiectoid areas show diffuse cytoplasmic immunoreactivity for CD34.

Prognostic factors
Local excision is effective treatment {386}. Some 15% of cases recur, probably due to incomplete resection, and are cured by re-excision {664,749,1920,2607}.

Fibromatosis colli

J.X. O'Connell

Definition
A benign site-specific "tumour" that occurs in the distal sternocleidomastoid muscle of infants. The mass results in fusiform thickening of the muscle and cervico-facial asymmetry due to its shortening (torticollis) {238,1572}.

Synonyms
Congenital muscular torticollis; sternocleidomastoid tumour of infancy; pseudotumour of infancy

Epidemiology
Fibromatosis colli is uncommon. It occurs in approximately 0.4% of live births {1503}. Incidence is slightly greater in males {1665}. Most affected infants are diagnosed before age 6 months {238,1665}. There is a clear association with other musculoskeletal developmental abnormalities

that are associated with abnormal intra-uterine positioning, including forefoot anomalies and congenital hip dislocation {238,1503,2442}.

Etiology
It is most likely that fibromatosis colli represents a cellular scar-like reaction to injury of the sternocleidomastoid muscle acquired in the last trimester of intrauterine growth, or at the time of delivery {238,1503,2442}.

Sites of involvement
Fibromatosis colli affects the lower one third of the sternocleidomastoid muscle.

Clinical features
The affected infants present with a smooth fusiform swelling of the distal sternocleidomastoid muscle {238,1503,2442}. This

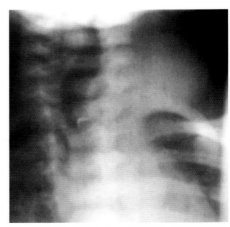
Fig. 3.017 Fibromatosis colli. Plain X-ray showing a soft-tissue mass in the region of the sternocleidomastoid muscle.

usually measures < 5.0 cm in length. The muscle is expanded, although rarely measures > 2.0 cm. Typically the infants

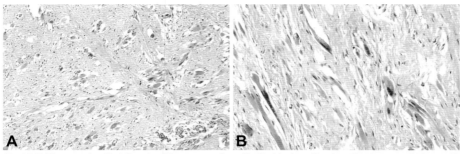

Fig. 3.018 Fibromatosis colli. **A** Note the diffuse pattern of scar-like fibroblastic proliferation within the sternocleidomastoid muscle. **B** The entrapped skeletal muscle fibres commonly show both degenerative and reactive sarcolemmal nuclei.

exhibit facial tilt due to the shortening of the affected muscle {238,1503,1572, 2442}. Ultrasound investigation demonstrates a uniform isoechoic mass confined to the muscle {524}. MRI also allows precise localization and characterization of the mass {1984,2179}.

Macroscopy
The lesion appears as a tan, gritty mass confined to the muscle.

Histopathology
Like many presumed reactive proliferations, the microscopic appearance of fibromatosis colli varies depending on the time at which it is examined. If biopsy is considered necessary, the favoured means of investigation of these masses is fine-needle aspiration cytology {1492,1503}. This demonstrates cellular specimens with aggregates of uniform plump spindle cells embedded in myxoid to collagenous ground substance {1492,1503}. Multinucleate skeletal myocytes may be admixed.

These aspiration specimens correspond to the cellular proliferative phase of the process. Surgical specimens, which are obtained only from a minority of patients at the time of tenotomy for persistent torticollis, usually demonstrate less cellular collagen-rich tissue that resembles scar or conventional fibromatosis {238,1572,2442}.

Immunophenotype
There is positive staining for vimentin and muscle actins. Nuclear β-catenin is not expressed {378,2756}.

Prognostic factors
The treatment involves passive stretching and physiotherapy {238,1665}. The vast majority of children will have complete resolution of the mass and demonstrate normal cervico-facial posture and movement with this approach {238,1665}. Surgical intervention, principally tenotomy, is required in < 10% of patients {1665}.
The deformity is greater in those infants who are diagnosed and treated when aged > 1 year.

Juvenile hyaline fibromatosis

J.X. O'Connell

Definition
Juvenile hyaline fibromatosis is a rare autosomal recessive disorder that typically presents in infancy {1632}. It is characterized by the accumulation of extracellular "hyaline material" within skin, somatic soft tissues and the skeleton, resulting in tumour-like masses {1360,1402}. The hyaline material is produced by fibroblasts. The clinical manifestations vary depending on the number, location and rate of "growth" of the masses {1360,1402,1716}. Infantile systemic hyalinosis is a clinically related disorder that presents earlier, is more severe and is typically fatal within 2 years. It is caused by similar genetic mutations as juvenile hyaline fibromatosis {694,1100}. While juvenile hyaline fibromatosis and

infantile systemic hyalinosis were originally considered to be separate and distinct conditions, the allelic nature of the diseases and the existence of patients with overlapping features of each disorder has resulted in the concept that the classical disorders are better considered as two ends of a pathogenetic spectrum {73,694,1100,2068}.

Synonyms
Molluscum fibrosum; mesenchymal dysplasia

Epidemiology
Juvenile hyaline fibromatosis is an extremely rare disorder {1360,1402,1716}. It typically presents in infancy {1360,1402, 1716,2975}. Incidence is similar in males

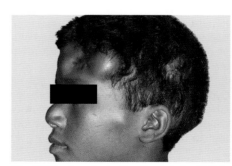

Fig. 3.019 Juvenile hyaline fibromatosis. Multiple subcutaneous nodules on the scalp and face are the most consistent finding.

and females, and affected infants are often the progeny of consanguinous parents {1360,1402,1716,2975}.

Etiology

Juvenile hyaline fibromatosis and infantile systemic hyalinosis are caused by inactivating mutations in the *ANTXR2* gene encoding capillary morphogenesis protein 2, located on the long arm of chromosome 4. This gene encodes a transmembrane protein that functions as a receptor for anthrax toxin and binds extracellular matrix proteins laminin and collagen IV {694,1100}. Inheritance is autosomal recessive. Mutation and dysfunction of this gene is likely to result in dysregulation of basement membrane matrix homeostasis, which leads to the accumulation of hyaline material at the affected tissue sites {694}. Biochemically, the hyaline deposits in juvenile hyaline fibromatosis have significantly less hyaluronic acid and increased amounts of dermatan sulfate and chondroitin sulfate {2808}.

Sites of involvement

The tumour-like masses of hyaline material develop in the skin (particularly the face and neck resulting in papules and nodules), gums (producing "gingival hyperplasia"), periarticular soft tissues (resulting in joint contractures) and bones (especially the skull, long bones and phalanges) {1360,1384,1402,1716,2975}.

Clinical features

The clinical phenotype of affected children varies {1716}. Patients present with skin papules affecting the face and neck, in particular, around the ears. Perianal skin papules may resemble genital warts. Periarticular deposits of the hyaline material result in joint contractures, particularly involving the knees and elbows {1360,1384, 1402,1716,2975}. Imaging studies reveal generalized osteoporosis and discrete lytic lesions in the affected bones {1360, 1402,1918}. Most often there is progressive increase in the number and size of superficial and deep nodules with resulting deformity and dysfunction. Survival into adulthood may occur {1384,1402}.
Infantile systemic hyalinosis results in visceral as well as somatic soft-tissue deposits. Involvement of the gastrointestinal tract characteristically causes severe diarrhoea and recurrent infections.

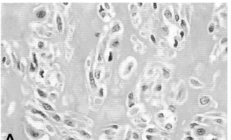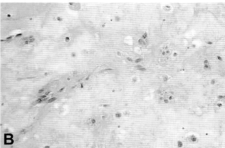

Fig. 3.020 Juvenile hyaline fibromatosis. **A** Cellular focus of a nodule. Note the clustered arrangement of the fibroblasts and the extracellular amorphous material. **B** An older, less cellular, nodule that is dominated by the hyaline material.

Macroscopy

The nodules have a solid uniform appearance.

Histopathology

The individual nodules obliterate the normal tissues in which they are found. They are composed of an admixture of plump fibroblastic cells associated with extracellular uniform hyaline material that is non-fibrillar and eosinophilic on H&E.
In younger patients or "newer" lesions, the nodules are relatively more cellular {1770,1918}. The constituent fibroblasts have clear cytoplasm and may exhibit a vague fascicular arrangement. Nuclear atypia or necrosis is not seen. Older lesions are less cellular and the fibroblasts may appear compressed by the extracellular material. PAS staining is strongly positive and diastase-resistant.

Immunophenotype

Staining for muscle actins and S100 protein is negative {9,2511}.

Ultrastructure

The lesional cells are fibroblasts and demonstrate numerous cystically dilated membrane-bound vesicles. These contain granular and filamentous material similar to the extracellular ground substance. Continuity between the vesicles and the extracellular space may be evident {1360, 1716,1918,2975}.

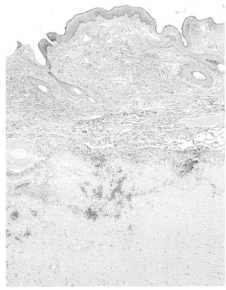

Fig. 3.021 Juvenile hyaline fibromatosis. Low-power view of a typically well-circumscribed hypocellular nodule in deep dermis/subcutis.

Genetics

See Etiology.

Prognostic factors

The "tumour masses" are treated by surgical excision depending on their location. Local recurrence rates are high {1360}. The prognosis is determined by the number, size and location of the nodules and the degree of the patient's functional impairment.

Inclusion body fibromatosis

W.B. Laskin

Definition
A benign, predominantly myofibroblastic tumour, sometimes multicentric, with potential for local recurrence. Its name reflects its characteristic eosinophilic paranuclear inclusions.

Synonyms
Infantile digital fibroma/fibromatosis; recurring digital fibrous tumour of childhood

Epidemiology
The classic (infantile digital) subtype comprises 0.1% of soft tissue tumours {46} and 2% of paediatric fibroblastic tumours {482}. It is usually detected during the first year of life, with about 30% of cases presenting at birth {174,464}. This tumour occurs equally in males and females. Rare (non-classic) examples occur in adults and/or at extra-digital sites {1554}.

Etiology
No established etiology exists. Rare cases follow antecedent trauma or toxin ingestion {1554,2016}. A histogenetic relationship with digital fibromas of the X-chromosome-linked syndrome digitocutaneous dysplasia is uncertain {703,1212}.

Sites of involvement
The classic variant typically involves the dorsal or dorsolateral aspect of the distal or middle portion of the second, third, and fourth digits (while typically sparing the first digit), and less often, the hand or foot

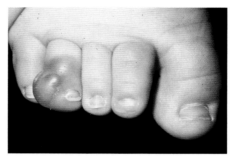

Fig. 3.022 Inclusion body fibromatosis. A single protuberant nodule with an erythematous surface on the lateral aspect of the distal toe.*

{174,464,1554}. Extra-digital cases were reported on the leg, arm, and breast {1554}.

Clinical features
The classic variant presents as an asymptomatic, dome-shaped or polypoid cutaneous nodule, typically no larger than 2 cm {174,464,1554}. Synchronous and/or metachronous lesions sometimes affecting different digits occur {46,174,2400}, but simultaneous involvement of both fingers and toes is rare {174}. Non-classic lesions present as solitary masses or nodules {1554}.

Macroscopy
Tumours are firm or rubbery, ill-defined protuberant or polypoid dermal nodules. The cut surface is fibrous, off-white to grey in colour.

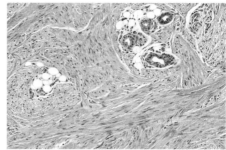

Fig. 3.023 Inclusion body fibromatosis showing characteristic growth patterns, with spindled cells in short fascicles and whorls surrounding adnexa.*

Histopathology
Spindle cells with lightly eosinophilic cytoplasm and an elongated, cytologically bland nucleus proliferate in whorls, interlacing short fascicles, or storiform arrays within a variably collagenous dermis. Cells characteristically grow perpendicular to the epidermis and surround adnexa {46,464}. The process occasionally involves deeper tissues {46,1554}. A variable number of cells harbour a 1.5–24 μm, rounded, pale pink paranuclear inclusion that often indents the nucleus {464,2330} and is highlighted by trichrome (red), phosphotungstic acid-haematoxylin (dark purple), and Movat (pink) stains {1554}.

Immunophenotype
Classic examples express muscle actins (often in a peripheral "tram-track" pattern), calponin, and desmin, and in a few cases,

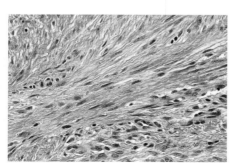

Fig. 3.024 Inclusion body fibromatosis. High-power view demonstrates spindled cells with elongated, cytologically bland nuclei and rounded, pink, intracytoplasmic inclusions, some indenting the nucleus.

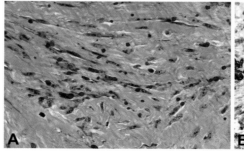

Fig. 3.025 Inclusion body fibromatosis. **A** Gomori's trichrome staining highlights intracytoplasmic inclusions (red).* **B** Immunostaining for SMA demonstrates a peripheral ("tram-track") pattern of expression.

*Am J Surg Pathol 2009;33(1):1–13. Copyright © (2009), with permission from Wolters Kluwer Health.

nuclear β-catenin, myosin, and caldesmon {1554,1935,1970}. Non-classic tumours express actin, but desmin only focally {1554}. Inclusions mark with actin after pre-treatment with potassium hydroxide {1969} and occasionally with caldesmon {1554}.

Ultrastructure
Most tumour cells exhibit myofibroblastic features, including actin-rich bundles of myofilaments with dense bodies. The dense, non-membrane-bound inclusion has loosely aggregated microfilaments at its periphery that are in continuity with the myofilamentous aggregates {220,1141, 1970}.

Prognostic factors
The recurrence rate for the classic subtype is between 61% and 75% {464, 1554}. Recent studies suggest that complete (wide) excision results in considerably lower recurrence rates {799,2338,2707}. Tumours have been known to spontaneously regress {2029}. Approximately 25% of non-classic tumours recur {1554}.

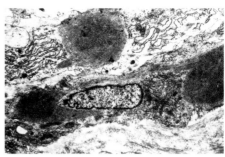

Fig. 3.026 Ultrastructure of inclusion body fibromatosis. Myofilamentous bundles at the periphery of a tumour cell merge with a dense intracytoplasmic inclusion.

Fibroma of tendon sheath

R. Sciot
P. Dal Cin

Definition
A benign fibroblastic nodular neoplasm, usually attached to a tendon (sheath).

ICD-O code   8813/0

Synonyms
Tenosynovial fibroma

Epidemiology
Fibroma of tendon sheath is uncommon and typically occurs in patients aged between 20 and 50 years {469,2274}.

Sites of involvement
The lesion typically occurs on the finger tendons. The thumb, index, and middle fingers are most frequently involved. Intra-articular locations (knee, elbow, wrist) have been described rarely {472,620, 1498,2183}.

Clinical features
The tumour presents as a firm, small (usually ≤ 3 cm) and slowly growing nodule.

Macroscopy
Fibroma of tendon sheath has a circumscribed, lobular fibrous appearance, reminiscent of a tenosynovial giant cell tumour of localized type, except that it lacks pigmentation.

Histopathology
The lesion is well circumscribed, lobulated, and contains bland fibroblastic/myofibroblastic spindle cells in a collagenous background {469}. There is generally no atypia. The cellularity is usually low, but can be variable and is often higher at the edge, sometimes resembling nodular fasciitis. There are characteristic elongated ("slit-like") thin-walled vessels or clefts. Degenerative features such as myxoid/cystic changes, chondroid or osseous metaplasia or bizarre pleomorphic cells can be seen.

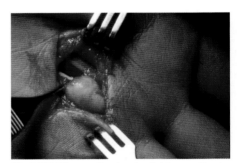

Fig. 3.027 Fibroma of tendon sheath. Intra-operative picture showing the smooth nodular surface and attachment to a tendon.

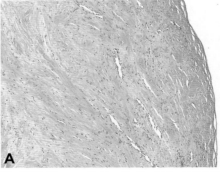
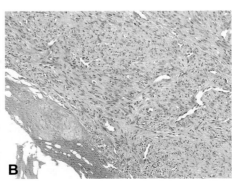

Fig. 3.028 Fibroma of tendon sheath. **A** Low-power view showing the highly sclerotic and poorly cellular aspect. Note the small vessels and clefts. **B** Some cases can show increased cellularity, which is most obvious at the edge.

Immunophenotype
Positive staining for SMA is often seen, at least focally.

Ultrastructure
The tumour cells show (myo)fibroblastic features.

Genetics
A clonal chromosomal abnormality, t(2;11)(q31–32;q12), has been described in one case {558}. Notably, an apparently identical translocation has been also observed in three cases of desmoplastic fibroblastoma {196,2059,2496}.

Prognostic factors
Fibroma of tendon sheath is benign, but can recur in approximately 20% of cases if marginally or incompletely excised.

Desmoplastic fibroblastoma

M.M. Miettinen
J.A. Bridge
J.F. Fetsch

Definition
A benign, paucicellular, soft-tissue tumour with abundant collagenous or myxocollagenous matrix, low vascularity, and scattered, bland, stellate-shaped and spindled fibroblastic cells.

ICD-O code   8810/0

Synonym
Collagenous fibroma

Epidemiology
This relatively uncommon tumour has a 2 : 1 male predominance and is usually diagnosed in the fifth to seventh decades of life (70% of cases). It only rarely occurs in children and adolescents {1879}.

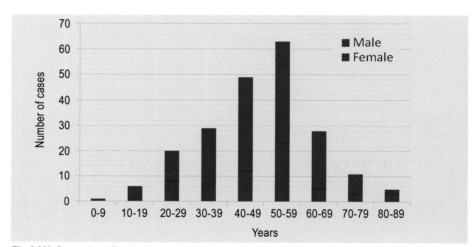

Fig. 3.029 Desmoplastic fibroblastoma: age distribution among 212 patients.

Sites of involvement
The most common sites are the upper arm, shoulder, lower limb, back, forearm, hands and feet.

Clinical features
The tumour typically presents as an asymptomatic, slowly growing subcutaneous mass, but fascial and skeletal-muscle involvement is fairly common {784, 1124,1879,2038}.

Macroscopy
Desmoplastic fibroblastomas are usually relatively small, often measuring 1–4 cm in greatest dimension, but examples of > 10 cm and as large as 20 cm have occurred. Grossly, the lesions appear well circumscribed and form oval, fusiform, or discoid masses. Some examples have an externally lobulated, cobblestone-like surface. The tumours have a firm, cartilage-like consistency, and on cut section, they have a homogeneous pearl-grey colour.

Histopathology
Although often well demarcated grossly, most tumours microscopically infiltrate into subcutaneous fat, and approximately 25% extend into skeletal muscle. Rare examples

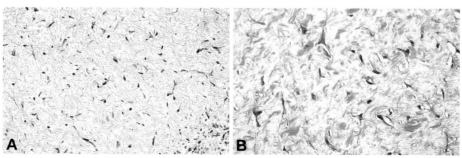

Fig. 3.030 Desmoplastic fibroblastoma. **A, B** The tumour is paucicellular and composed of uniform, often stellate-shaped fibroblasts.

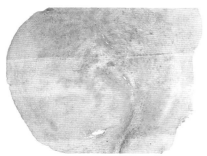

Fig. 3.031 Desmoplastic fibroblastoma. The lesion has a smooth, rounded contour.

are purely intramuscular. The lesions have abundant collagenous or myxocollagenous matrix with low vascularity. Cellularity ranges from low to moderate, and the neoplastic cells tend to be uniformly distributed within the extracellular matrix. The lesional cells are stellate-shaped, bipolar and spindled, and they have uniform, bland nuclei with distinct small nucleoli. Mitotic figures are uncommon. Rare examples have focal intravascular growth.

Immunophenotype
The tumour cells may be focally positive for SMA. Rarely, a few cells with keratin (AE1/AE3) expression may be present. The neoplastic cells are negative for desmin, EMA, S100 protein and CD34 {1879}.

Genetics
Cytogenetic abnormalities of chromosomal band 11q12 are characteristic of desmoplastic fibroblastoma, with the presence of an identical t(2;11)(q31;q12) translocation or three-way variant thereof featured in a subset of these lesions {196, 2059,2420}. A 2;11 translocation with slightly distal breakpoints (2q35 and 11q13) has been reported in one desmoplastic fibroblastoma {2059}.
On the basis of global gene-expression profiling and quantitative real-time PCR, deregulated expression of FOSL1 has been proposed as the functional outcome of 11q12 rearrangements in desmoplastic fibroblastoma {1685}.

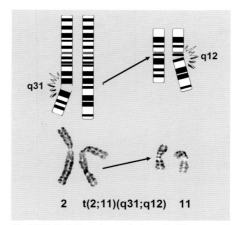

Fig. 3.032 Partial karyotype and schematic of the recurrent t(2;11)(q31;q12) translocation in desmoplastic fibroblastoma.

Prognostic factors
The behaviour of this tumour is benign, and none of the published clinicopathological series have documented any recurrences.

Mammary-type myofibroblastoma

M. McMenamin
M. Debiec-Rychter

Definition
A benign mesenchymal neoplasm, composed of spindle-shaped cells with features of myofibroblasts, embedded in a stroma that contains coarse bands of hyalinized collagen and conspicuous mast cells, admixed with a variable amount of adipose tissue. It is histologically identical to myofibroblastoma of breast and is part of a spectrum of lesions that includes spindle cell lipoma and cellular angiofibroma.

ICD-O code   8825/0

Epidemiology
Lesions have arisen in adults with a wide age range of 35–85 years (median, 56 years) and equal sex distribution {110, 674,1237,1696,1699,1801,1974,2498, 2916,3063}.

Etiology
It has been postulated that tumours may be related to the patient's hormonal status, in that lesions are relatively common in older men and postmenopausal women {1698}. Occasional cases tested (including one male) showed at least focal positivity for estrogen receptor {110,2498, 2916}. The apparently higher frequency of tumours originating along a putative "milk line" might suggest the possible existence of hormonally responsive mesenchymal

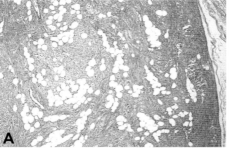
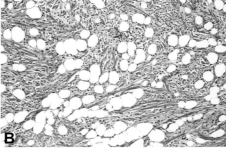

Fig. 3.033 Mammary-type myofibroblastoma. **A** Sharply circumscribed margin. **B** Fasicles of spindle cells separated by coarse bands of intersecting hyalinized collagen. Note the admixed adipose tissue.

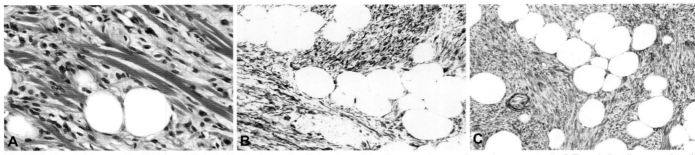

Fig. 3.034 Mammary-type myofibroblastoma. **A** Note the bland spindle cells with tapering nuclei, collagenous stroma and conspicuous mast cells. **B** The spindle cells are consistently immunopositive for desmin. **C** In most cases, the spindle cells are also immunopositive for CD34.

tissue, although rare cases in distal extremities argue against this.

Sites of involvement
The most common locations are the inguinal/groin, paratesticular and vulvovaginal areas. Other reported sites include perianal, buttock, abdominal wall, back, neck and popliteal fossa. Incidence appears to be higher along the putative anatomical "milk line" that extends from axilla to medial groin. Lesions arise most commonly in subcutaneous tissue; however, one case arose deep to the abdominal muscle wall.

Clinical features
Tumours generally present as painless masses or incidental lesions, but some are painful. Lesions may be present for years before clinical presentation. Radiological features are not specific.

Macroscopy
Size ranges from 0.8 to 13 cm (median, 5.5 cm). The tumours are generally well circumscribed, mobile and firm. The colour can be variable (white, yellow, pink, tan or brown). The cut surface may be whorled or nodular. Soft areas of "mucoid" appearance reflecting myxoid change were present in one case.

Histopathology
Tumours are unencapsulated, but well circumscribed. The spindle cells resemble myofibroblasts and are characterized by oval to tapered nuclei with finely dispersed chromatin, small nucleoli, eosinophilic to amphophilic cytoplasm and poorly defined cytoplasmic borders. The spindle cells are generally arranged in variably sized, usually quite long fascicles. The stroma has broad bands of coarse hyalinized collagen and usually scattered mast cells. Tumours can vary from being cellular to being paucicellular and hyalinized. There is generally an admixture of adipose tissue that can vary from only rare adipocytes to a prominent fatty component. Rare cases lack adipose tissue.

Epithelioid change of the lesional cells and focal nuclear atypia with enlarged nuclei and multinucleation have been described {1801}. Such morphological variation is also well recognized in breast myofibroblastomas {1698}.

The blood vessels in myofibroblastoma are generally not conspicuous, being small, often focally hyalinized and commonly having a perivascular lymphocytic infiltrate in contrast to the prominent medium to large vessels with markedly hyalinized walls that are characteristic of cellular angiofibroma or the large branching "haemangiopericytoma-like" blood vessels that are seen in lipomatous haemangiopericytoma, two potential morphological mimics.

Mitotic figures range from 0 to 6 per 10 HPF.

Immunophenotype
As is characteristic of the breast counterpart, the typical immunophenotype of extramammary myofibroblastoma is diffuse coexpression of desmin and CD34 in the spindle cells. Rare cases are negative for CD34. Expression of SMA is present in a third of cases.

Genetics
Partial monosomy 13q has been detected in two mammary myofibroblastomas, as well as partial monosomy 16q in one of these {2201}. Similar rearrangements of 13q and 16q are characteristic of spindle cell lipoma {560}. Interphase FISH analysis using *RB1* and *FOXO1* probes of two extramammmary myofibroblastomas revealed loss of 13q14 sequences {1237, 1696}. A similar FISH study of cellular angiofibroma also demonstrated loss at 13q14 {877,1696}. The latter entity shares morphological and immunophenotypical features with (extra)mammary-type myofibroblastoma and spindle cell lipoma, further supporting a pathogenetic link between these entities.

Prognostic factors
All tumours have followed a benign course after marginal local excision, with a follow-up of up to 6 years.

Calcifying aponeurotic fibroma

S.E. Kilpatrick

Definition
Calcifying aponeurotic fibroma is a rare tumour, usually of childhood and adolescence, which is usually found on the hands or feet and has a tendency for local recurrence.

ICD-O code   8816/0

Synonyms
Juvenile aponeurotic fibroma; aponeurotic fibroma

Epidemiology
Calcifying aponeurotic fibroma is an extraordinarily rare lesion. Although these tumours occur over a wide age range, the vast majority present in childhood and adolescence {47}. There is a slight male predominance.

Sites of involvement
The most common sites of involvement are the palmar surface of the hands and, less commonly, the plantar surface of the feet, wrist, digits, and ankles. The proximal extremities and trunk are rarely involved {839,1391}.

Clinical features
Patients present with small, slowly growing and ill-defined soft-tissue masses, generally not tender. Plain-film X-rays may reveal calcifications.

Macroscopy
Resected specimens usually reveal small (1–3 cm), ill-defined, grey-white to gritty lesions that infiltrate adjacent soft tissues and are often associated with tendons and aponeuroses. Rare cases are much larger.

Histopathology
Calcifying aponeurotic fibroma is a biphasic lesion that displays a moderately cellular and infiltrative, fibromatosis-like component and nodules of calcification accompanied by more rounded, epithelioid cells, often radiating from the centre of the calcifications and forming linear arrays {47}. Individual cells of both components typically appear uniform, lack significant cytological atypia, and show only scattered, infrequent

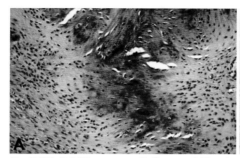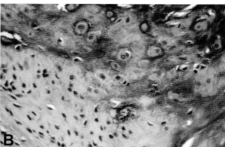

Fig. 3.035 Calcifying aponeurotic fibroma. **A** The classic areas of calcification are immediately surrounded by hyalinization. **B** This view shows early chondroid differentiation, displaying rounded tumour cells within lacunae.

mitotic figures. The background stroma, especially in the calcified areas, ranges from hyalinized to focally chondroid. Cartilaginous differentiation in the calcified area is more common in older children and adults, while lesions seen in infants may lack calcifications altogether. Multinucleate osteoclast-type giant cells are frequently present.

Immunophenotype
Most cases express SMA, but appear negative for desmin, supporting a fibroblastic/myofibroblastic phenotype. EMA and S100 protein are sometimes expressed by the lesional cells, but nuclear expression of β-catenin is absent {378}.

Ultrastructure
The ultrastructural findings reflect the fibroblastic/myofibroblastic (and minor chondrocytic) nature of these neoplasms.

Prognostic factors
Not surprisingly, the infiltrative nature of calcifying aponeurotic fibroma translates to a high rate of local recurrence, up to 50%, which may occur many years after the initial excision {839,1987}. The risk of local recurrence seems to be higher in young children. Recurrences are not generally destructive.

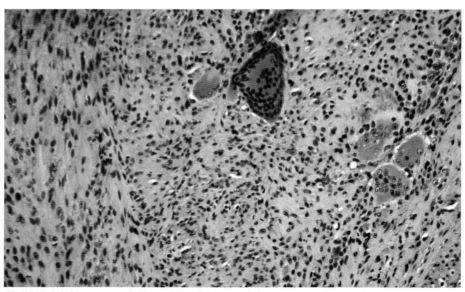

Fig. 3.036 Calcifying aponeurotic fibroma. The cellular, non-calcified component with osteoclast-type giant cells.

Angiomyofibroblastoma

C.D.M. Fletcher

Definition
A benign, well-circumscribed myofibroblastic neoplasm, usually arising in the pelviperineal region, especially the vulva, and apparently composed of stromal cells distinctive to this anatomical region.

ICD-O code   8826/0

Epidemiology
Angiomyofibroblastoma is uncommon, with an incidence comparable to that of aggressive angiomyxoma. These tumours arise predominantly in females, principally in adults between menarche and menopause {870,1189,1552,2042}. About 10% of patients are postmenopausal. Convincing examples have not been described before puberty. Rare cases occur in males {870,2089}.

Sites of involvement
Virtually all cases arise in pelviperineal subcutaneous tissue, with the majority arising in the vulva. About 10–15% of cases are located in the vagina. Lesions in men occur in the scrotum or paratesticular soft tissue.

Clinical features
Most cases present as a slowly enlarging, painless, circumscribed mass. The most frequent preoperative diagnosis is Bartholin's gland "cyst".

Macroscopy
These lesions are well-circumscribed but not encapsulated, with a tan/pink cut surface and a soft consistency. Necrosis is not seen. Most cases measure < 5 cm in maximum diameter, although rare examples measuring up to 10 cm have been reported.

Histopathology
Tumours are generally well demarcated by a thin fibrous pseudocapsule and, at low power, show varying cellularity with prominent vessels throughout. Vessels are mostly small, thin-walled and ectatic and are set in an abundant loose, oedematous stroma. The tumour cells are round to

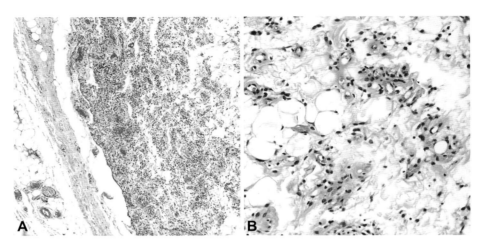

Fig. 3.037 Angiomyofibroblastoma. **A** A typically well-demarcated tumour. **B** This tumour is more cellular and vascular than aggressive angiomyxoma. Note the adipocytic component.

spindle-shaped with eosinophilic cytoplasm and are typically concentrated around vessels. Mitoses are rare. Binucleate and multinucleate tumour cells are common. Some cases show very plasmacytoid or epithelioid cytomorphology and

rare examples show degenerative ("ancient") nuclear hyperchromasia and atypia. About 10% of cases have a variably prominent well-differentiated adipocytic component. In postmenopausal patients, the stroma is often less oedematous and

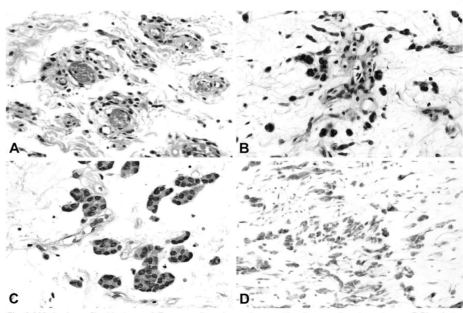

Fig. 3.038 Angiomyofibroblastoma. **A** Tumour cells and vessels are set in a loose oedematous stroma. **B** Binucleate and multinucleate cells are frequent and may have a plasmacytoid appearance. **C** In this example, the tumour cells are focally clustered with an epithelioid appearance. **D** Immunopositivity for desmin is a typical feature in most cases.

more fibrous, and there may be hyalinization of vessel walls. Rare cases show morphological overlap with aggressive angiomyxoma {1027}.

Immunophenotype
The majority of cases show strong and diffuse positive staining for desmin, while, at most, there is usually only focal positivity for SMA or pan muscle actin {870,2042, 2089}. Desmin staining may be reduced or absent in postmenopausal cases. Tumour cells are consistently positive for estrogen and progesterone receptors {1552,2089}, occasionally positive for CD34 and negative for S100 protein, keratin and fast myosin.

Ultrastructure
Tumour cells show fibroblastic or myofibroblastic features by electron microscopy {870,2042}.

Genetics
Angiomyofibroblastomas lack rearrangements of *HMGA2* and *HMGA1* {1806}.

Prognostic factors
Angiomyofibroblastoma is entirely benign and recurrence appears to be exceedingly rare, even after marginal local excision.

Cellular angiofibroma

C.D.M. Fletcher
U. Flucke
Y. Iwasa

Definition
Cellular angiofibroma is a benign, cellular and richly vascularized fibroblastic neoplasm that usually arises in the superficial soft tissues of the vulva or inguinoscrotal regions. The tumour is closely related to spindle cell lipoma and mammary-type myofibroblastoma.

ICD-O code   9160/0

Synonym
Male angiomyofibroblastoma-like tumour {1551}

Epidemiology
Cellular angiofibroma is a rare neoplasm arising in adults. Females and males are roughly equally affected, with a peak incidence in the fifth decade of life in females and seventh decade in males {877,1301, 1551,2077}.

Etiology
The immunohistochemical expression of estrogen and progesterone receptors in both sexes {1301,1551,1781} suggests that these hormones may have a role in the pathogenesis of this tumour.

Sites of involvement
Although these tumours typically arise in the superficial soft tissues of the vulvovaginal region and the inguinoscrotal or paratesticular region, rare examples have been described in the retroperitoneum, midtrunk {1301}, iliac spine {1363}, oral mucosa {792}, knee and upper eyelid {877}.

Clinical features
Patients usually present with a slowly growing painless mass. The most frequent preoperative diagnosis is (Bartholin) cyst {877,1301,2077}. In males, the mass may be associated with a hernia or hydrocoele {1301,1551}

Macroscopy
The tumour varies in size, from 0.6 to 25 cm. Those in women are generally smaller (median, 2.8 cm) than those in men (median, 7.0 cm). The tumours appear as round, oval, or lobulated well-circumscribed nodules. The consistency of the

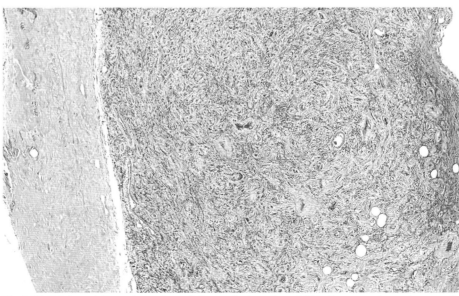

Fig. 3.039 Cellular angiofibroma is usually a well-circumscribed neoplasm. A thick, fibrous pseudocapsule surrounds this example.

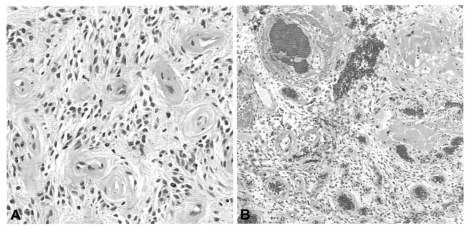

Fig. 3.040 Cellular angiofibroma. **A** The vascular component consists primarily of numerous small to medium-sized open vessels with hyaline walls. **B** Regressive and degenerative changes include organizing intraluminal thrombi, intramural inflammation, extravasated erythrocytes, and haemosiderin deposits.

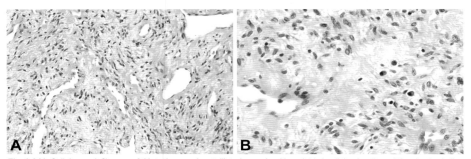

Fig. 3.041 Cellular angiofibroma. **A** Note the prominent dilated vessels with variably hyalinized walls and the short spindle-cell fascicles. **B** The spindle-cell cytomorphology is reminiscent of spindle cell lipoma. Note also the stromal mast cells.

lesion varies from soft to rubbery and the cut surface is solid with a grey-pink to yellow-brown colour {1301,1551}. Foci of haemorrhage or necrosis are exceptional {1301}.

Histopathology

These tumours are generally well circumscribed. Poorly marginated, more infiltrative tumours occur rarely, in men. Tumours are composed of uniform, short spindle-shaped cells, in an oedematous to fibrous stroma containing short bundles of delicate collagen fibres and numerous small to medium-sized thick-walled vessels with rounded, irregularly ectatic or branching lumina. Vessel walls may show hyaline fibrosis. The spindle cell component is usually moderately to highly cellular and randomly distributed throughout the lesion, occasionally with a fascicular arrangement or nuclear palisading. Spindle cells have short, oval to fusiform nuclei with inconspicuous nucleoli and scanty amounts of palely eosinophilic cytoplasm with ill-defined borders. Mitoses are generally sparse, but can be more frequent (up to 10 per 10 HPF) in some cases. The stroma consists primarily of wispy collagen, with occasional short bundles of densely eosinophilic collagen fibres. Variable stromal oedema, hyalinization or myxoid change is often seen, especially in males. Perivascular lymphoid aggregates are often present. Mast cells are frequent. Small aggregates or individual adipocytes are observed in close to 50% of cases. Degenerative changes of slight nuclear enlargement and hyperchromasia, intravascular thrombi, and cystic change are seen in some cases {1301,1551, 1781,2077}.

Morphological sarcomatous transformation has been described rarely, mostly in the vulva {434,877,1363}. Abrupt transition from cellular angiofibroma to a discrete sarcomatous nodule composed of multivacuolated lipoblasts, or pleomorphic and hyperchromatic spindle cells showing morphological features either of pleomorphic liposarcoma, atypical lipomatous tumour, or pleomorphic spindle cell sarcoma has been reported. Other rare cases show severely atypical cells scattered in conventional cellular angiofibroma. No necrosis or haemorrhage is observed. Mitoses in sarcomatous areas are fewer than 3 per 10 HPF, but one case with atypical mitoses has been reported {434,877}.

Immunophenotype

CD34 expression has been documented in 30–60% of tumours. Variable expression of SMA and desmin is identified in a minority of cases. Staining for S100 protein and keratin is negative. Estrogen and progesterone receptors are expressed in many cases {1301,1551,1781}. Tumour cells in sarcomatous areas show multifocal or diffuse expression of p16, while tumour cells in usual cellular angiofibroma are negative {434}.

Genetics

A single cytogenetically investigated case showed loss of chromosomes 13 and 16, suggesting a genetic link with spindle cell lipoma and mammary-type myofibroblastoma {560,1091,1695,2201}. This relationship is also supported by interphase FISH showing deletion of the *RB1* and *FOXO1* loci on chromosome 13q14 {877,1091,1695}.

Prognostic factors

Local recurrence is very infrequent {1301, 1551,1781}. The rare cases with atypia or sarcomatous transformation have not developed recurrence or metastasis {434, 877,1363}.

Nuchal-type fibroma

M. Michal

Definition
Nuchal-type fibroma (NTF) is a rare tumour-like lesion representing accumulation of collagen.

ICD-O code   8810/0

Synonyms
Nuchal fibroma; collagenosis nuchae

Epidemiology
NTF is significantly more common in men, with peak incidence during the third to fifth decades of life.

Sites of involvement
NTF typically affects the posterior neck region, but can also occur elsewhere. Most of the extranuchal tumours are located on the upper back, but other locations such as the face, extremities, can be encountered {755,2627}. Because these extranuchal lesions are histologically indistinguishable from the nuchal cases, the designation "nuchal-type fibroma" was proposed to encompass all histologically similar lesions, irrespective of location {1869}.

Clinical features
There is an interesting relationship between NTF and diabetes mellitus {7}. Up to 44% of patients with NTF in one series also had diabetes mellitus {1869}. Histologically, NTF and diabetic scleredema, which is another tumour-like change in fibrous tissues in patients with diabetes mellitus type 2, are identical. As in NTF, the sites prone to be affected by diabetic scleroedema are the skin and underlying soft tissues of the posterior neck, upper back, and shoulders {493,855}.

Macroscopy
The mean greatest dimension is slightly

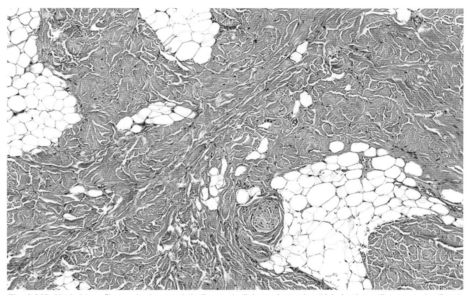

Fig. 3.042 Nuchal-type fibroma is characteristically paucicellular and contains thick, haphazardly arranged collagen fibres with entrapment of adipose tissue and peripheral nerve.

more than 3 cm {1869}. NTF has a hard consistency and white colour.

Histopathology
NTF is an unencapsulated, poorly circumscribed, paucicellular lesion composed of thick, haphazardly arranged collagen fibres. Centrally, the collagen bundles intersect and form a vaguely lobular architecture. Compared with normal tissue from the nuchal area, NTFs show similarly thick collagen fibres. However, in NTF there is an expansion of collagenized dermis with encasement of adnexa, effacement of the subcutis with entrapment of adipocytes, and, in many cases, extension into underlying skeletal muscle. A delicate network of elastic fibres is observed between the collagen fibres. Thus, NTFs appear to represent a localized accentuation of the poorly cellular, collage-

nous connective tissue that normally resides in these sites. Scant numbers of lymphocytes are present in occasional cases. Many NTFs contain a localized proliferation of nerve twigs, similar to those seen in traumatic neuromas {145} and, in rare cases, there can be also perineurial fibrosis. These changes probably represent the result of repetitive minor trauma or a response by small nerves to the local accumulation of collagen.

Immunophenotype
Immunohistochemically, the lesions are CD34-positive {1634} and give negative results with antibodies to actins and desmin {1869}.

Prognostic factors
NTFs often recur, but they do not metastasize.

Gardner fibroma

C.M. Coffin

Definition
Gardner fibroma is a benign plaque-like proliferation of thick, haphazardly arranged collagen bundles with interspersed fibroblasts and is associated with Gardner-type familial adenomatous polyposis (FAP).

ICD-O code   8810/0

Synonyms
Soft fibroma; desmoid precursor lesion

Epidemiology
Gardner fibroma mainly affects children in the first decade of life, although the age range extends through the fourth decade, with no difference between males and females {484,2914}.

Etiology
More than 80% of cases are associated with Gardner-type FAP, *APC* mutation, or familial desmoids {484,1599,2914}. Gardner fibroma is a sentinel event for FAP.

Sites of involvement
Sites include superficial and deep soft tissues of the paraspinal region, back, chest wall, abdomen, head/neck, and extremities {484,2240,2914}. Mesenteric Gardner fibroma in FAP has been reported as "desmoid precursor lesion" {475}.

Clinical features
The ill-defined mass is usually asymptomatic {484,2914}.

Macroscopy
Gardner fibroma ranges from 1 to 10 cm. The poorly circumscribed mass is firm and rubbery, with a tan surface and scattered yellow areas {484,2914}.

Histopathology
The uniform hypocellular proliferation contains haphazardly arranged, coarse collagen fibres with cracks, bland spindle cells, and sparse mast cells {484,2914}. It entraps fat, nerves, and muscle fibres.

Immunophenotype
Gardner fibroma is reactive for CD34 and non-reactive for SMA, MSA and desmin {484,2914}. Focal nuclear reactivity for β-catenin is common {378,484}.

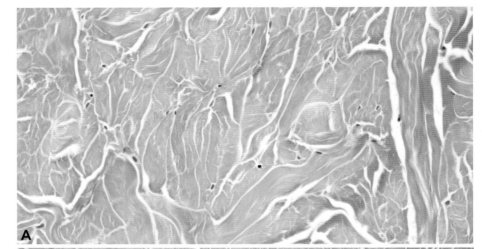

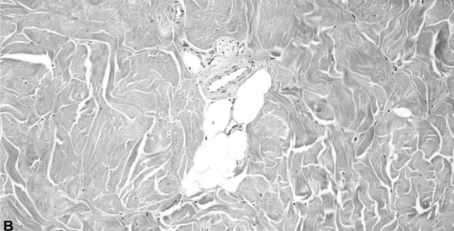

Fig. 3.043 Gardner fibroma. **A** Small bland spindle cells are dispersed in cracks between collagen fibres. **B** Entrapped mature adipose tissue and benign nerve fibres are frequently seen in Gardner fibroma.

Prognostic factors
Some 50% of patients with Gardner fibroma develop a desmoid-type fibromatosis at the same site, spontaneously or after surgery. Gardner fibroma should be considered in young patients with putative nuchal-type fibroma {2913}. Diagnosis of Gardner fibroma in a child should prompt screening of the family for FAP.

Calcifying fibrous tumour

A.F. Nascimento

Definition
Calcifying fibrous tumour (CFT) is a rare benign lesion characterized by a hypocellular fibroblastic proliferation with associated chronic inflammation and variably prominent calcification.

ICD-O code   8817/0

Synonyms
Childhood fibrous tumour with psammoma bodies {2373}; calcifying fibrous pseudotumour

Epidemiology
CFT affects people of a wide age range, with tumours of somatic tissues often occurring in children (median age, 3 years), while visceral tumours arise more frequently in adults (median age, 43 years). Males and females are equally affected {15,841,1177,2006,2556}.

Etiology
This lesion has been described following trauma {2247,3050} and in association with Castleman disease {570}. Rare cases are familial {437}. A putative relationship with inflammatory myofibroblastic tumour {2255,2841} and IgG4-related sclerosing disease has not been substantiated, and ALK staining is negative {15,1177,1499, 2006,2556}.

Sites of involvement
CFT is anatomically ubiquitous, having been described in superficial and deep somatic soft tissues, such as upper and lower extremities, neck, scrotum, back and abdominal wall, as well as in intracavitary and visceral locations, such as gastrointestinal tract, mesentery, mediastinum, omentum, peritoneum and pleura {15,841,1177,2006,2247,2556}.

Clinical features
CFT often presents as a painless mass in extremities. Visceral lesions are usually found incidentally, but occasionally may lead to mass-like effects in the affected organ. Some patients develop multiple lesions.

Macroscopy
CFT is an unencapsulated, well-circumscribed firm mass, ranging in size from 0.5 to 25 cm. The cut surface is tan-white and homogeneous with variable degrees of grittiness.

Histopathology
CFT is a circumscribed lesion with peripheral entrapment of native structures such as adipose tissue, small nerves and vessels. The tumour is characterized by a hypocellular hyalinized collagenous stroma and variably prominent chronic

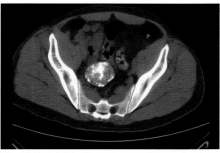

Fig. 3.044 Calcifying fibrous tumour. CT scan showing a calcified intra-abdominal mass.

inflammation and calcifications. Stromal cells are bland, elongated with fine chromatin, inconspicuous nucleoli and scant pale cytoplasm. The inflammatory component is composed of scattered small lymphocytes and plasma cells and/or the formation of follicles with germinal centres. Calcifications are dystrophic or psammomatous in appearance.

Immunophenotype
Lesional cells show positivity for CD34, and may rarely be positive for SMA and desmin.

Prognostic factors
Local recurrences occur in a subset of patients, and occasionally the tumour may recur repeatedly; however, there is no potential for metastasis {841,2006}.

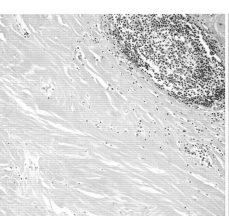 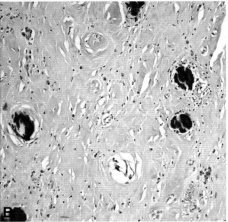

Fig. 3.045 Calcifying fibrous tumour. **A** Note the hypocellularity of the tumour and a follicle on the upper part. **B** Calcifications may be psammomatous or dystrophic.

Palmar/plantar fibromatosis

J.R. Goldblum
J.A. Fletcher

Definition
Palmar/plantar fibromatoses are fibroblastic proliferations that arise in the palmar or plantar soft tissues and are characterized by infiltrative growth. They have a tendency toward local recurrence but do not metastasize.

ICD-O code   8813/1

Synonyms
Palmar fibromatosis: Dupuytren disease; Dupuytren contracture
Plantar fibromatosis: Ledderhose disease

Epidemiology
Palmar fibromatosis affects adults, with a rapid increase in incidence with advancing age. Patients aged < 30 years are seldom affected. It is three to four times more common in men and is most frequent in northern Europe and in those parts of the world settled by northern Europeans {170}. Plantar lesions, although still most common in adults, have a noticeable incidence in children and adolescents {836}. Plantar lesions also arise more commonly in males, but the difference between the sexes is not as great as for palmar lesions. Both forms of fibromatosis have been linked with numerous disease processes, including other forms of fibromatosis, diabetes mellitus and alcoholism {348}. Approximately 5–20% of palmar fibromatoses are associated with plantar lesions, and up to 4% also have penile fibromatosis (Peyronie disease) {344}.

Etiology
The pathogenesis of both plantar and palmar fibromatosis is multifactorial and includes a genetic component, as many patients have a significant family history of this disease {611}. Trauma is also likely to play an important role, but other factors are probably involved given the coexistence of these fibromatoses with a myriad of seemingly unrelated disorders, some of which were documented in biased populations such as mental institutions in the past.

Sites of involvement
Palmar lesions occur on the volar aspect of the hand, and almost 50% are bilateral. Rare lesions occur on the dorsal aspect {2825}. Plantar lesions arise within the plantar aponeurosis usually in non-weight-bearing areas. Cases arising in children tend to occur in the anteromedial portion of the heel pad {836}.

Clinical features
For palmar lesions, the initial manifestation is that of an isolated firm palmar nodule that is usually asymptomatic, but ultimately results in cord-like indurations or bands between multiple nodules and adjacent fingers. This leads to puckering of the overlying skin and flexion contractures, principally affecting the fourth and fifth digits. Plantar lesions present as a firm subcutaneous nodule or thickening that adheres to the skin and is frequently associated with mild pain after long standing or walking. Plantar lesions rarely result in contraction of the toes.

Macroscopy
Both lesions consist of small nodules or an ill-defined conglomerate of nodular masses intimately associated with aponeurosis and subcutaneous fat. On cut section, both have a grey-yellow or white surface, although the colour depends on the collagen content of the lesion.

Histopathology
The proliferative phase is characterized by a cellular proliferation of plump, immature-appearing spindled cells that vary little in size and shape, have normochromatic nuclei and small pinpoint nucleoli. Plantar lesions are quite consistently hypercellular. Mitotic figures are usually infrequent but may be focally prominent. Cells are intimately associated with moderate amounts of stromal collagen and elongated blood vessels. Older lesions are considerably less cellular and are

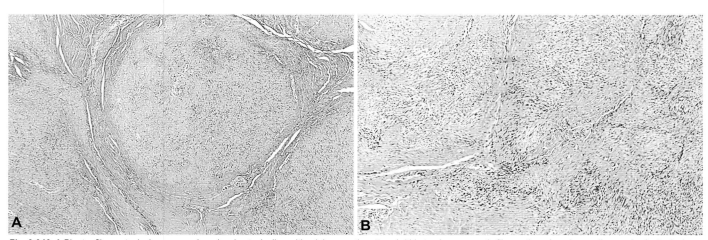

Fig. 3.046 A Plantar fibromatosis: low-power view showing typically multinodular growth pattern (within tendoaponeurotic fibrous tissue), as is usually seen in plantar lesions. **B** Palmar fibromatosis: in the early (proliferative) phase, palmar fascial or aponeurotic tissue is expanded by hypercellular spindle cell nodules.

often more densely collagenized. Occasional cases of plantar fibromatosis contain notable multinucleate giant cells.

Immunophenotype

The cells stain variably for MSA and SMA, depending upon the extent of myofibroblastic differentiation. At least 50% may show nuclear immunopositivity for β-catenin {378}, in the absence of a mutation {1935}.

Genetics

Standard karyotypic analysis reveals clonal chromosomal aberrations in approximately 10% of cases arising in palmar locations {553}. Fewer plantar cases of superficial fibromatosis have been reported {306}; however, simple numerical changes appear to predominate in both palmar and plantar locations, particularly gains of chromosomes 7 or 8 as demonstrated cytogenetically and by FISH. A reciprocal translocation t(2;7)(p13;p13) has been identified in one case of plantar fibromatosis {2449}.

Prognostic factors

Risk of local recurrence is most closely related to the extent of surgical excision. Dermofasciectomy followed by skin grafting

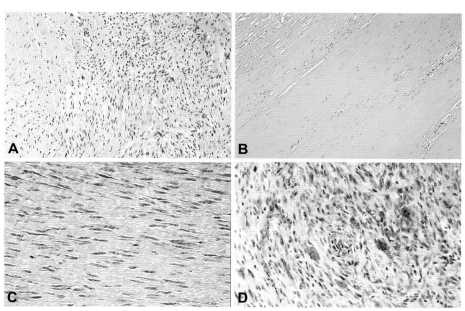

Fig. 3.047 A Early (proliferative) lesion of palmar fibromatosis showing bland fibroblastic/myofibroblastic cells. **B** Late lesions of palmar fibromatosis associated with contracture consist largely of densely hyalinized hypocellular collageneous tissue. **C** High-power view of cytologically bland cells in a palmar fibromatosis. In this example, the cells are widely separated by collagen. **D** Plantar fibromatosis: the lesion may contain scattered osteoclastic giant cells.

is associated with the lowest rate of local recurrence {169}. For plantar lesions, there is an increased risk of local recurrence in cases with multiple nodules, in patients with bilateral lesions, those with a positive family history and those who develop a postoperative neuroma {597}.

Desmoid-type fibromatosis

J.R. Goldblum
J.A. Fletcher

Definition
Desmoid-type fibromatosis is a locally aggressive (myo)fibroblastic neoplasm that usually arises in deep soft tissues and is characterized by infiltrative growth and a tendency toward local recurrence, but lacks metastatic potential.

ICD-O code
Desmoid-type fibromatosis   8821/1
Abdominal (mesenteric)
    fibromatosis   8822/1

Synonyms
Aggressive fibromatosis; musculoaponeurotic fibromatosis; desmoid tumour

Epidemiology
Deep fibromatoses are rarer than their superficial counterparts. In the paediatric population, these lesions occur with equal frequency in male and females, and most are extra-abdominal. Patients between puberty and age 40 years tend to be female; in these patients, the abdominal wall is the favoured site of involvement. Later in adulthood, these tumours are equally distributed between abdominal and extra-abdominal locations and occur equally in men and women {2322}.

Etiology
The pathogenesis is multifactorial and includes genetic, endocrine and physical factors. Features suggesting an underlying genetic basis include the existence of familial cases and the presence of these lesions, particularly mesenteric fibromatoses,

in patients with Gardner-type familial adenomatous polyposis (FAP) {774}. Like their superficial counterparts, trauma (most often surgery) is also likely to be a contributory factor.

Sites of involvement
Extra-abdominal fibromatoses may be located at virtually any anatomical site, although the principal sites of involvement are the shoulder, chest wall and back, thigh and head and neck region. Abdominal tumours arise from musculoaponeurotic structures of the abdominal wall, especially the rectus and internal oblique muscles and their fascial coverings. Intra-abdominal fibromatoses arise in the mesentery or pelvis.

Clinical features
Extra-abdominal fibromatoses typically arise as a deep-seated, firm, poorly circumscribed mass that grows insidiously and causes little or no pain. Some patients develop multifocal lesions. Although rare, some lesions cause decreased joint mobility or neurological symptoms. Abdominal wall lesions usually arise in young, gravid or parous women during gestation or, more frequently, during the first year after childbirth. Pelvic fibromatoses arise as a slowly growing palpable pelvic mass that is usually asymptomatic and is often mistaken for an ovarian neoplasm. Mesenteric lesions may be sporadic or arise in patients with Gardner-type FAP. Most patients present with an asymptomatic abdominal mass, but some have mild abdominal pain or, even less frequently, present with gastrointestinal

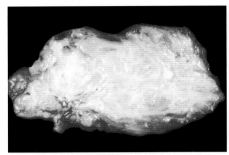

Fig. 3.048 Extra-abdominal desmoid fibromatosis. Note the whorled fibrous cut surface and poorly defined margins with surrounding skeletal muscle.

bleeding or acute abdomen secondary to bowel perforation.

Macroscopy
These lesions are firm and cut with a gritty sensation. On gross section, the cut surface reveals a glistening white, coarsely trabeculated surface resembling scar tissue. Lesions in the abdomen may appear well circumscribed. Some have a grossly myxoid appearance. Most tumours measure 5–10 cm at the time of excision.

Histopathology
The lesions are typically poorly circumscribed with infiltration of the surrounding soft-tissue structures. All are characterized by a proliferation of elongated, slender, spindle-shaped cells of uniform appearance, set in a collagenous stroma containing variably prominent blood vessels, sometimes with perivascular oedema. The cells lack nuclear hyperchromasia or

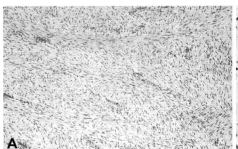
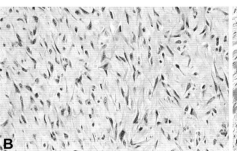
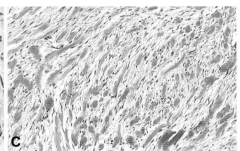

Fig. 3.049 Extra-abdominal desmoid fibromatosis. **A** Note the whorled fibrous cut surface and poorly defined margins to surrounding skeletal muscle. **B** Cellular proliferation of bland spindled cells arranged into ill-defined long fascicles. **C** Cells are spindled or stellate in shape and have bland nuclear features.

cytological atypia and have small pale-staining nuclei with one to three minute nucleoli. Cells are usually arranged in long sweeping bundles. As with superficial fibromatoses, the mitotic rate is variable. Keloid-like collagen or extensive hyalinization may be present and in some lesions, particularly those arising in the mesentery or pelvis, extensive myxoid change may be found. Isolated cases are associated with coexisting Gardner fibroma.

Immunophenotype
The cells stain variably for MSA and SMA, and are typically negative for desmin, h-caldesmon and S100 protein. Approximately 70–75% of tumours show nuclear positivity for β-catenin, more often in cases associated with FAP than in sporadic lesions {378,2027}.

Ultrastructure
Most of the cells have features of fibroblasts, although a proportion has myofibroblastic features.

Genetics
Desmoid-type fibromatosis may harbour cell subpopulations with trisomies for chromosomes 8 and/or 20 {322,611,872}. These numerical chromosomal aberrations are found in no more than 30% of the fibromatosis cells, and it is unlikely they play a crucial role at the inception of the tumours. Some clinical series suggest a relationship between trisomy and more advanced disease, but there is no consensus that any of these aberrations are of prognostic significance {89,1857,2423}. Tumours arising in the setting of Gardner-type FAP harbour inactivating mutations of the *APC* gene {1919}. Up to 85% of sporadic lesions harbour mutations in the gene encoding β-catenin (*CTNNB1*) {1574,2423}. Both *CTNNB1* and *APC* mutations result in the intranuclear accumulation of β-catenin protein {1936}. The prognostic significance of these mutations is uncertain {676,1574}.

Prognostic factors
Local recurrence is common, but is nowadays recognized to be inconsistently related to adequacy of surgical excision {1847}. Attempts to achieve tumour-free resection margins may result in significant morbidity. Despite the lack of metastatic potential, rare desmoid tumours prove fatal owing to local effects of growth, especially in the head and neck region.

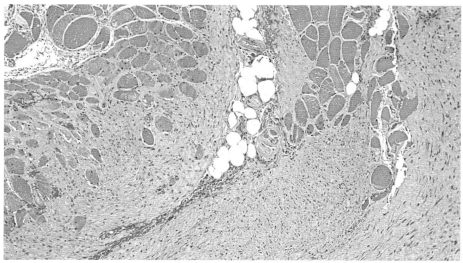

Fig. 3.050 Desmoid fibromatosis. Note the irregular infiltration into adjacent skeletal muscle and adipose tissue.

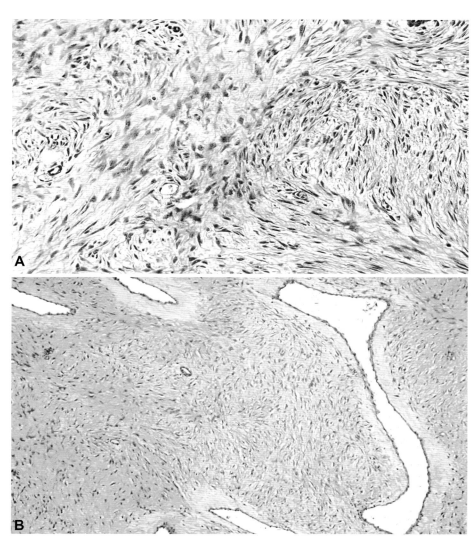

Fig. 3.051 Mesenteric desmoid fibromatosis. **A** Mesenteric fibromatosis with extensive myxoid change. **B** Ectatic blood vessels with perivascular hyalinization in a mesenteric fibromatosis.

Lipofibromatosis

M.M. Miettinen
J.F. Fetsch
E. Zambrano

Definition
A benign paediatric tumour with abundant, usually mature, adipose tissue admixed with a spindle cell (fibromatosis-like) component, often concentrated in septal and perimysial locations.

ICD-O code
8851/1

Synonym
Infantile/juvenile fibromatosis variant (non-desmoid type)

Epidemiology
This is a very rare childhood tumour and two thirds of patients are male.

Sites of involvement
Almost half of the reported examples have involved the hand or foot. About 17% of cases have affected the head and neck or a truncal location {122,1355}.

Clinical features
Patients have ranged in age from newborn to 14 years. Approximately 20% of cases are congenital. The process typically forms an ill-defined, slowly growing, painless mass, located in the subcutis or deep soft tissue of an extremity {122,619,840,1030, 1355,1399,2441,2443,2742}.

Macroscopy
The tumours are usually 1–5 cm in size {840}, but some are larger and rare examples have involved an entire extremity {1030,2742}. The process has a grossly fatty appearance and is yellowish or

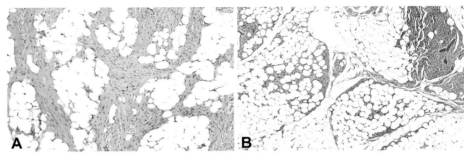

Fig. 3.052 Lipofibromatosis. **A** There is an even admixture of fibroblastic and adipocytic components. **B** The relative proportion of the two components is variable and the spindle cell areas may form delicate trabeculae.

whitish tan and poorly marginated. Close inspection may reveal fibrous streaks within the fat.

Histopathology
All contain abundant adipose tissue that usually accounts for > 50% of the tumour {840}. The fat cells are usually mature and lack atypia. However, in newborn patients, the fat lobules may have an immature appearance with myxoid matrix. In addition, there is a spindled fibroblastic element that characteristically forms fascicles concentrated in septal regions and along the perimysial surface of skeletal muscle. The fibroblastic element has only mild atypia and a low mitotic rate. This element does not exhibit the diffuse sheet-like and destructive growth pattern of desmoid-type fibromatosis. Small collections of univacuolated cells may be evident at the interface between the fibroblastic component and the mature fat. In rare instances, melanin-laden cells have been documented

amongst the fibroblastic population {122,840}.

Immunophenotype
The fibroblasts show variable immunoreactivity for CD34 and SMA {840,1355}. Focal staining for S100 protein, MSA and, rarely, EMA may occur. There is no reactivity for desmin or keratins and no nuclear expression of β-catenin {378, 2756}. The uncommon pigmented cells express melanocytic markers {122,840}.

Genetics
A t(4;9;6)(q21;q22;q2?4) was present in one case {1399}.

Prognostic factors
This tumour has a high rate of local recurrence {840}, but has no metastatic potential. Congenital onset, male sex, acral location, mitotic activity in the fibroblastic component and incomplete excision may be risk factors for recurrence {840}.

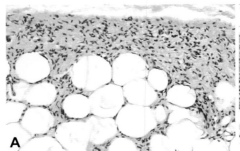
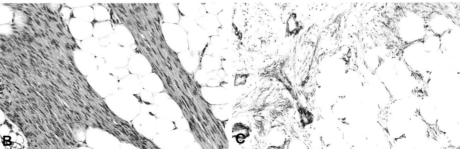

Fig. 3.053 Lipofibromatosis. **A** The spindle-cell component is bland and may have a rather primitive fibroblastic appearance. **B** Fascicular growth of the fibroblastic element. **C** Focally positive immunostaining for SMA, consistent with fibroblastic/myofibroblastic differentiation.

Giant cell fibroblastoma

J.-M. Coindre
F. Pedeutour

Definition
Giant cell fibroblastoma (GCF) is a locally aggressive histological variant of dermatofibrosarcoma protuberans (DFSP) that primarily affects children and is characterized by the presence of multinucleated giant cells and pseudovascular spaces.

ICD-O code 8834/1

Epidemiology
GCF is a rare tumour which affects predominantly children with a median age of 6 years. Occasional cases have been reported in adults. About two thirds of patients are male {1331,2546}.

Sites of involvement
Most cases occur in the trunk wall, groin and axillary area, but cases have also been reported in extremities, head and neck {717,1331,2546,2744}. Like DFSP, all cases develop in superficial soft tissues, specifically dermis and subcutaneous fat.

Clinical features
Most patients complain of a slow-growing painless cutaneous mass that is, in almost half of cases, protuberant and sometime polypoid {1331,2546}.

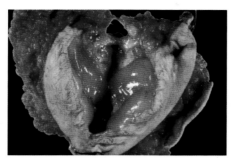
Fig. 3.054 Giant cell fibroblastoma is characterized grossly by a mucoid cutaneous and subcutaneous mass.

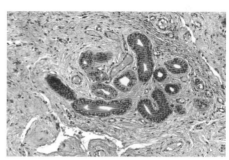
Fig. 3.055 Giant cell fibroblastoma. A characteristic feature is the entrapment of cutaneous adnexal structures.

Macroscopy
Grossly, GCF consists of grey to yellow mucoid mass that is ill-defined and infiltrative. It measures from 1 to 8 cm with a mean of 3–4 cm {1331,2546}.

Histopathology
GCF is a subcutaneous tumour that infiltrates the deep dermis and, rarely, the superficial skeletal muscle. Almost all cases infiltrate the subcutaneous fat in honeycomb or parallel growth patterns with adnexal sparing. Areas of pure GCF show variable cellularity, but are mostly hypocellular with a myxoid or collagenous stroma and are composed of wavy bland spindle cells and scattered giant cells. These giant cells are characteristic of GCF and most show several nuclei either conglomerated towards the centre of the cell

or arranged peripherally in a wreath or floret pattern. Irregularly branching pseudovascular spaces are characteristic, but are not seen in all cases. These spaces are lined by a discontinuous row of spindle and multinucleate cells identical to those seen in the surrounding stroma. Mitotic activity is low and there is no necrosis. Tumours with areas of conventional DFSP in primary or recurrent lesions are seen in about 15% of cases; the extent of DFSP is variable {1331,2744}.

Rare cases may contain pigmented cells (Bednar tumour), myoid whorls or fibrosarcomatous areas {1331}.

Immunophenotype
Spindle and giant cells are positive for CD34 but negative for SMA, desmin, and S100 protein {1331,2744}.

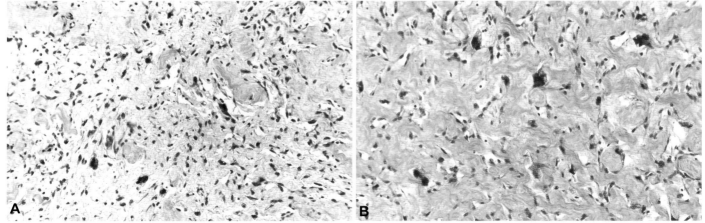
Fig. 3.056 Giant cell fibroblastoma areas are mostly hypocellular with a myxoid (**A**) or collagenous (**B**) stroma and are composed of spindle cells and scattered giant cells.

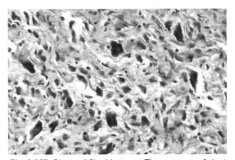

Fig. 3.057 Giant cell fibroblastoma. The presence of giant cells is characteristic; these cells usually show several small and regular nuclei.

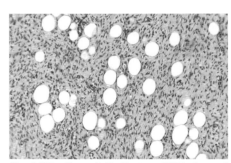
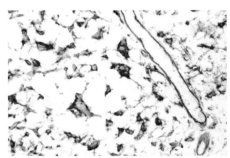

Fig. 3.058 Giant cell fibroblastoma. **A** Irregular branching pseudovascular spaces are characteristic, but are not seen in all cases. **B** These spaces are lined by spindle cells and multinucleate cells.

Genetics

GCF and DFSP share chromosomal and molecular features, consisting of re-arrangements of chromosomes 17 and 22 and formation of a chimeric gene that fuses the α1 type 1 collagen preprotein gene (*COL1A1*; 17q21) with the platelet-derived growth factor β-chain gene (*PDGFB*; 22q13) {2560}. Only a few cases of GCF have been analysed by conventional cytogenetics {2431,2569}. Two cases of GCF were characterized by the presence of an unbalanced translocation t(17;22)(q21.3;q13) similar to that observed in DFSP. In two other cases of GCF, a balanced t(17;22) was reported {521,559}. A balanced t(17;22) has not been reported in classical DFSP. At the molecular level, GCF is indistinguishable from DFSP; the breakpoint in *COL1A1* is variable between patients (from exon 6 up to exon 49), while the breakpoint in *PDGFB* is consistently located in intron 1 {2569}. There is no evidence for the correlation of a specific breakpoint within *COL1A1* related to GCF in comparison with classical DFSP or other DFSP-related tumours {969}.

Prognostic factors

GCF recurs locally in about half of cases, but metastases have not been reported {2546}.

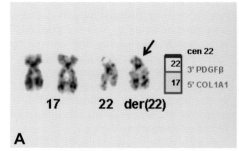

Fig. 3.059 Giant cell fibroblastoma (GCF). Areas of dermatofibrosarcoma protuberans are seen in about 15% of cases, either admixed with GCF or as a recurrent tumour.

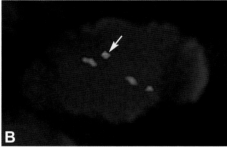

Fig. 3.060 Giant cell fibroblastoma. Spindle cells and giant cells are immunopositive for CD34.

Fig. 3.061 Giant cell fibroblastoma. **A** Partial G-banded karyotype showing an unbalanced t(17;22) translocation. The abnormal chromosome 22 derived from the translocation der(22)t(17;22)(q21.3;q13.1) is indicated by an arrow. The schematic representation shows the structure of the abnormal chromosome containing the *COL1A1-PDGFB* fusion gene. **B** Interphase FISH analysis. The arrow indicates the *COL1A1-PDGFB* fusion gene (juxtaposition of red and green signals) observed in addition to two normal *COL1A1* (green signals) and *PDGFB* (red signals) alleles, respectively.

Dermatofibrosarcoma protuberans

T. Mentzel
F. Pedeutour
A. Lazar
J.-M. Coindre

Definition

Dermatofibrosarcoma protuberans (DFSP) is a superficial, low-grade, locally aggressive fibroblastic neoplasm carrying a COL1A1-PDGFB fusion gene. Higher-grade fibrosarcomatous progression is shown in 10–15% of cases.

ICD-O code

Dermatofibrosarcoma protuberans	8832/1
Fibrosarcomatous dermatofibrosarcoma protuberans	8832/3
Pigmented dermatofibrosarcoma protuberans	8833/1

Epidemiology

DFSP usually presents in young to middle-aged adult patients, with a slight male predominance. However, a significant number of cases are seen in children (including congenital presentations) {1286, 2744}, and in the elderly. Although it represents a rare neoplasm (< 1 per 100 000 people each year), DFSP is one of the most common dermal sarcomas.

Etiology

Most of these tumours occur sporadically. A high incidence of DFSP with unique features, such as multicentricity and occurrence at early age, has been shown in children affected with adenosine deaminase-deficient severe combined immunodeficiency (ADA-SCID) {1403}, possibly because of the known DNA-repair defect associated with this condition.

Sites of involvement

These neoplasms occur most commonly on the trunk and the proximal extremities, followed by the head and neck region; rarely regions, such as the genital area {1580}.

Clinical features

DFSP typically presents as a nodular or multinodular cutaneous mass, often with a history of slow but persistent growth. Early lesions may show plaque-like growth with peripheral red discoloration and clinically resemble morphea. These neoplasms may show rapid enlargement due to progression to fibrosarcomatous DFSP.

Macroscopy

DFSPs are indurated plaques with one or multiple nodules. Multiple protuberant tumours are often seen in recurrent lesions. These ill-defined and infiltrative neoplasms have firm, grey-white cut surfaces with occasional gelatinous areas, whereas areas of tumour necrosis are only rarely observed.

Histopathology

DFSP is characterized by diffuse infiltration of the dermis and subcutis. The neoplastic cells grow along the fibrous septa of the subcutaneous tissue and interdigitate with fat lobules, resulting in a typical honeycomb appearance. The epidermis is usually uninvolved and tumour cells encase skin appendages without destroying them. DFSP is composed of cytologically uniform spindled tumour cells containing plump or elongated wavy nuclei arranged in a predominantly storiform, whorled or cartwheel growth pattern. Cytological atypia is minimal and mitotic activity is usually low. The collagenous stroma contains small blood vessels. The superficial portion of the neoplasm may be less cellular and thus cause considerable challenges in the differential diagnosis on small, superficial biopsies. Rarely, DFSP may present as a subcutaneous mass

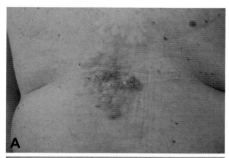
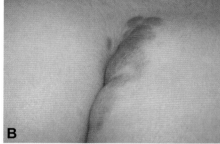

Fig. 3.062 Dermatofibrosarcoma protuberans (DFSP). **A** Clinically, DFSP is characterized by an exophytic, multinodular growth. **B** A boy aged 7 years presented with a 2-year history of a slowly increasing, gluteal lesion.

with infiltration of deep soft tissues {137}. Rare cases may show prominent vessels {2719} or granular cell change.

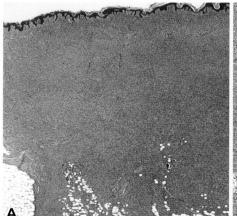
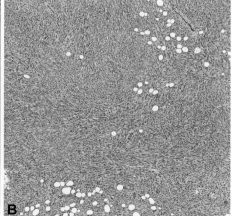

Fig. 3.063 A Dermatofibrosarcoma protuberans (DFSP): there is a diffuse infiltration of subcutaneous fat by neoplastic cells that grow along preexisting fibrous septa. **B** Fibrosarcomatous DFSP: a transition to cellular, fascicular areas with increased atypia is seen.

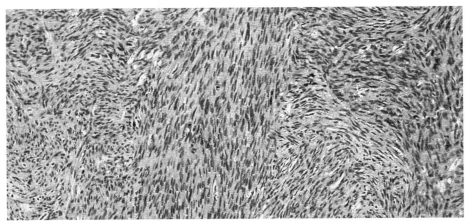

Fig. 3.064 Fibrosarcomatous dermatofibrosarcoma protuberans. Increased cytological atypia and increased mitotic activity are seen in fibrosarcomatous areas.

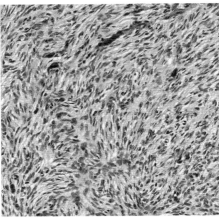

Fig. 3.065 Pigmented dermatofibrosarcoma protuberans (Bednar tumour). Higher-power view reveals elongated pigmented cells and fibroblastic tumour cells arranged in a storiform growth pattern.

Pigmented DFSP (also known as Bednar tumour)
Some cases of DFSP may contain a variable number of pigmented, dendritic melanocytic cells.

Myxoid DFSP
Rarely, DFSP may show prominent myxoid stroma with a more nodular growth and numerous vessels with slightly fibrotic vessel walls, often producing a more variable architecture, which may mimic other myxoid mesenchymal neoplasms {1843,2319}.

DFSP with myoid differentiation
In addition to a myointimal, non-neoplastic proliferation in entrapped vessels, bundles and nests of spindled, myofibroblastic tumour cells are rarely observed {360}, more often in the fibrosarcomatous variant.

Plaque-like DFSP
In rare cases, DFSP may show a flat, plaque-like growth resembling benign plaque-like CD34-positive dermal fibroma {581,1511}.

Fibrosarcomatous DFSP
Fibrosarcomatous DFSP represents morphological progression to a usually fascicular pattern with acquisition of metastatic potential. Fibrosarcomatous changes occur de novo or more rarely in local recurrences and either abrupt or more gradual transformation can be encountered. The fibrosarcomatous component often shows a nodular, rather well-circumscribed growth and is composed of cellular spindle cell fascicles with a "herringbone" appearance. The neoplastic cells in fibrosarcomatous areas are characterized by increased atypia and proliferative activity {293,1001,1642,1829}. Very rarely, transformation to pleomorphic sarcomatous areas has been reported {2687}

Immunophenotype
Tumour cells stain positively for CD34, and may show aberrant, weak expression of EMA {2941,3052}. Importantly, fibrosarcomatous DFSP may show loss of CD34 expression in about half of the cases {1829}, whereas increased expression of TP53 is often noted. Tumour cells in myoid nodules and bundles stain positively for SMA. Staining for desmin, S100 protein, and keratins is negative {525}.

Genetics
DFSP is cytogenetically characterized by the presence of supernumerary ring chromosomes {2431,2569}. These ring chromosomes usually contain the centromere of chromosome 22 and comprise interspersed sequences from chromosomes 17 and 22 {2207}. Secondary chromosomal aberrations, such as trisomy 5 and trisomy 8, are also often observed {2431,2569}. Rather than ring chromosomes, unbalanced t(17;22)(q21.3;q13.1)

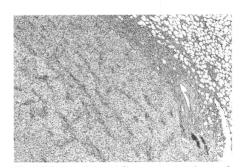

Fig. 3.066 Myxoid dermatofibrosarcoma protuberans. A diffusely infiltrating myxoid neoplasm is seen. Note the numerous blood vessels with slightly fibrosed vessel walls.

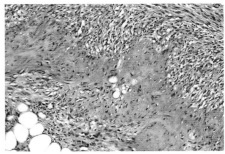

Fig. 3.067 A case of dermatofibrosarcoma protuberans. with focal myoid differentiation, showing focal proliferation of eosinophilic spindled cells set in hyalinized stroma.

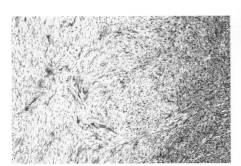

Fig. 3.068 Fibrosarcomatous dermatofibrosarcoma protuberans. A reduction or loss of expression of CD34 is seen in about half of cases.

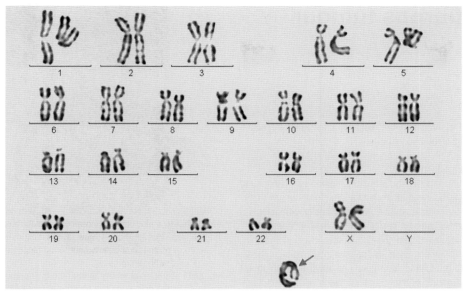

Fig.3.069 Representative RHG-banded karyotype of a dermatofibrosarcoma protuberans in an adult. The arrow indicates the supernumerary ring chromosome.

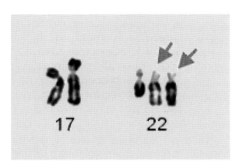

Fig. 3.070 Representative RHG-banded karyotype of a paediatric case of dermatofibrosarcoma protuberans. The arrows indicate the two abnormal chromosomes 22 derived from a t(17;22)(q21.3;q13.1).

translocations are present in most paediatric cases and more rarely in adult cases {2431,2569}. Balanced t(17;22) translocations have been described in giant cell fibroblastoma, but not in DFSP. Therefore, most DFSP cells harbour not only a structural rearrangement but also a gain of 17q21.3–17qter and 22q10–q31 sequences {1379,1633}.

Both ring and der(22)t(17;22) chromosomes contain a chimeric gene that fuses the α1 type I collagen preprotein gene (*COL1A1*; 17q21) with the platelet-derived growth factor β-chain gene (*PDGFB*; 22q13) {2560}. The breakpoint in *COL1A1* is highly variable: the chimeric gene is composed of at least the first 6 exons up to exon 49 of *COL1A1* and of a consistent fragment retaining all but exon 1 of the *PDGFB* gene. The fusion gene *COL1A1*-

PDGFB can be detected by multiplex RT-PCR or preferably by FISH in DFSP as well as in related tumours, such as giant cell fibroblastoma {1642,2426}. No correlation has been established between the various locations of the breakpoint within *COL1A1* and the different clinical and histological variants of DFSP and related tumours {969,1643}. The *COL1A1-PDGFB* fusion gene encodes a fusion protein that is proteolytically processed to normal PDGFB ligand. Because tumour cells contain the PDGFB receptor on their cell surfaces, autocrine stimulation of neoplastic cells drives tumorigenesis. This molecular pathway provides a rationale for targeted therapeutics with tyrosine kinase inhibitors capable of interfering with the phosphorylation and activation of PDGFRB for unresectable or metatstatic DFSP.

Prognostic factors

DFSP is characterized by locally aggressive growth and an increased number of often repeated local recurrences unless widely excised. The rate of local recurrence varies from 20% to 50% and is strongly related to the lack of wide tumour-free margins (a 2–3 cm cuff of surrounding tumour-free tissue should be achieved) {1001,1824}. In striking contrast, ordinary DFSP almost never metastasizes, and metastases usually occur only after multiple local recurrences. Cases of fibrosarcomatous DFSP show a similar rate of local recurrence compared with ordinary DFSP; however, distant metastases were detected in 13% of all analysed cases {293,1642,2887}.

Extrapleural solitary fibrous tumour

C.D.M. Fletcher
J.A. Bridge
J.-C. Lee

Definition

A ubiquitous mesenchymal tumour of fibroblastic type, which shows a prominent haemangiopericytoma-like branching vascular pattern. In the past, most cases were termed "haemangiopericytomas."

ICD-O code

Solitary fibrous tumour	8815/1
Malignant solitary fibrous tumour	8815/3

Synonyms

Haemangiopericytoma (obsolete); giant cell angiofibroma

Fat-forming variant: lipomatous haemangiopericytoma

Epidemiology

Extrapleural solitary fibrous tumours (SFTs) are uncommon mesenchymal neoplasms that are anatomically ubiquitous and occur most often in middle-aged adults aged 20–70 years, with cases in children and adolescents being rare. Males and females are affected equally, except in the case of the fat-forming SFT variant, which tends to slightly predominate in males (male to female ratio, 3 : 2).

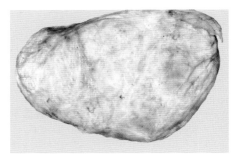

Fig. 3.071 Extrapleural solitary fibrous tumour. Grossly, the lesion is well delineated and shows a multinodular whitish appearance on cut section.

Sites of involvement

SFTs may be found at any location; 40% are found in subcutaneous tissue, while others arise in deep soft tissue of extremities or in the head and neck region (especially the orbit), thoracic wall, mediastinum, pericardium, retroperitoneum, and abdominal cavity. Other locations described include meninges, spinal cord, salivary gland, lung, thyroid, liver, the gastrointestinal tract, adrenal, kidney, urinary bladder, prostate, spermatic cord, testis, bone, and skin {336,933,1119,1121,1827, 2039,2088,2684}.

The fat-forming variant of SFT often affects the deep soft tissues of a wide variety of anatomical locations, including the lower extremity (especially the thigh), trunk, abdominopelvic regions (especially retroperitoneum), and head and neck.

Clinical features

Most tumours present as well-delineated, slowly growing, painless masses. Large tumours may give rise to compression symptoms, especially in the nasal cavity, orbit and meninges. Malignant tumours are often locally infiltrative {924,925, 1121,2830}. Rarely, large tumours may be the source of paraneoplastic syndromes such as hypoglycaemia due to the production of IGF2 {2645}.

Macroscopy

Most SFTs are well circumscribed, often partially encapsulated masses, measuring between 1 and 25 cm (median, 5–8 cm;

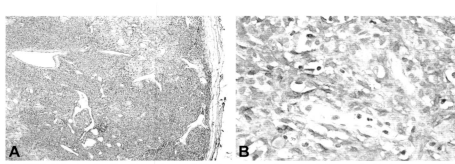

Fig. 3.072 Extrapleural solitary fibrous tumour. A The tumour presents as a well-circumscribed but nonencapsulated mass. B There is strong immunoreactivity of the tumour cells for CD99, but this is not specific.

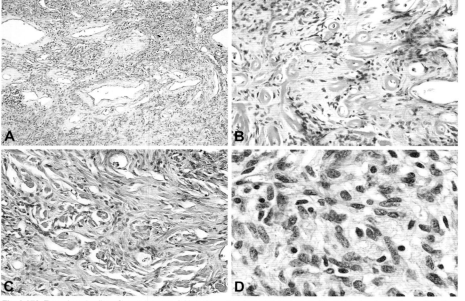

Fig. 3.073 Extrapleural solitary fibrous tumour. A Note the patternless architecture. B Stromal and perivascular hyalinization are common. C Keloidal-type deposition of collagen is frequent. D Typically bland spindle cells with rather vesicular nuclei.

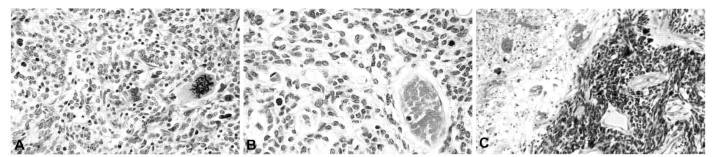

Fig. 3.074 Malignant extrapleural solitary fibrous tumour. **A** Hypercellularity and marked cytological atypia. Note the atypical mitosis. **B** Moderately cellular area with brisk mitotic activity. **C** Hypercellularity, marked cytological atypia, and areas of tumour necrosis (left).

generally smaller in the head and neck region). On section, they frequently have a multinodular, whitish and firm appearance; myxoid and haemorrhagic changes are infrequent {924,1121,1827,2039,2684, 2830}. Tumour necrosis and infiltrative margins (about 10% of cases) are mostly observed in locally aggressive or malignant tumours {925,1121,2830}.

Histopathology

Typical SFTs show a patternless architecture characterized by a combination of hypocellular and hypercellular areas separated by thick bands of hyalinized, sometimes keloidal, collagen and thin-walled branching haemangiopericytoma-like vessels. There may also be perivascular hyalinization. Tumour cells are ovoid to spindle-shaped with limited pale cytoplasm having indistinct borders and dispersed chromatin within vesicular nuclei. Rarely, epithelioid or rhabdoid cells can be found focally. Myxoid change, areas of fibrosis and interstitial mast cells are commonly observed. Mitoses are generally scarce, rarely exceeding 3 mitoses per 10 HPF. Some SFTs may contain giant multinucleate stromal cells and pseudo-vascular spaces {416,1121,2088}, being formerly known as "giant cell angiofibroma". Malignant SFTs are usually hypercellular lesions, showing increased mitoses (> 4 mitoses per 10 HPF), variable cytological atypia, tumour necrosis, and/or infiltrative margins {925,1121, 2830}, of which mitoses seem to be most prognostic {998}. Rare cases show abrupt transition from conventional benign-appearing SFT to high-grade sarcoma, likely representing a form of dedifferentiation {1963}. Lesions may show cytological atypia in the absence of mitoses or necrosis.

Fat-forming SFT is an uncommon, usually slowly growing, mesenchymal neoplasm closely resembling typical or cellular SFT with, in addition, a variably prominent adipocytic component {883,1061,2034}.

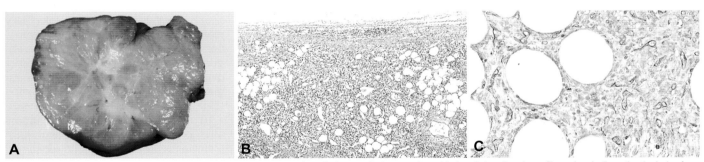

Fig. 3.075 Fat-forming solitary fibrous tumour (SFT). **A** Gross appearance of a well-circumscribed retroperitoneal lesion. Cut section shows fibrous bands dissecting the lesion from centre to periphery. **B** Like extrapleural solitary fibrous tumour, fat-forming SFTs are well-delineated, often encapsulated masses. **C** The tumour cells show immunoreactivity for CD34.

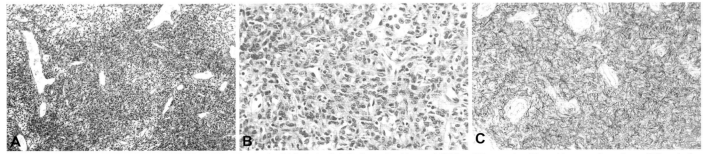

Fig. 3.076 Cellular solitary fibrous tumour (SFT). **A** Note the evenly distributed cellularity (in contrast to usual SFT) and the prominent branching vascular pattern. **B** Even in the more solid areas, tumour cells are arranged around numerous thin-walled vessels. Tumour cells are small with monomorphic nuclei and eosinophilic cytoplasm. **C** Diffuse positivity for CD34 is evident. A lesion such as this would have been labelled "haemangiopericytoma" in the past.

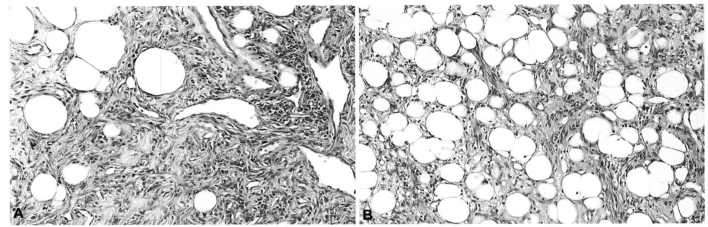

Fig. 3.077 Fat-forming solitary fibrous tumour (SFT). **A** Many such lesions show features of solitary fibrous tumour in addition to containing numerous mature adipocytes. Note haemangiopericytoma-like branching vessels. **B** An intimate admixture of bland spindle cells and mature adipocytes.

Morphologically, it is a well-demarcated neoplasm consisting of a varying combination of patternless cellular areas, prominent haemangiopericytoma-like vessels, variably collagenized extracellular matrix, and admixed mature adipocytes, which range from being singly scattered to being the predominant component. A small subset of fat-forming SFTs show malignant histological features (as seen in "classical" malignant SFTs); of note, lipoblasts and/or atypical lipomatous tumour-like areas can be found in these malignant tumours, closely mimicking liposarcoma {141,1061,1585}.

Immunophenotype
Tumour cells are characteristically immunoreactive for CD34 (90–95% of cases) {336,1827,2039,2684,2830}; 20–35% of cases are variably positive for EMA and SMA. Focal and limited reactivity for S100 protein, keratins and/or desmin has also occasionally been reported {924,2830}. Fat-forming SFT has a similar immunophenotype {1061,1585}.

Genetics
SFTs are karyotypically diverse, with aberrations detected primarily in tumours > 10 cm in diameter. Recurrently involved breakpoints are few, although structural rearrangements of 2p21, 4q13, 6p11, 9p22–23, 9q22, 9q31–32, 12q15, and 12q24 have each been identified in more than one SFT {2691,2768}. With respect to imbalances, gain of chromosomes 5, 8, and 21 and loss of 13 or 13q are most prominent {1741,1899,1963}. *TP53* mutations are rare, although TP53 overexpression has been observed in the high-grade component of benign-appearing SFTs exhibiting an abrupt transition to nondistinctive high-grade sarcoma {1951,1963}. Mutation testing of various genes encoding proteins with potential for targeted therapy has been negative, with the exception of rare isolated cases exhibiting missense gain-of-function mutations involving the enzymatic tyrosine kinase domain of *PDGFRA* {1078,2465,2634}. *IGF2* loss of imprinting corresponds with IGF2 overexpression in some SFTs {1078}.

Prognostic factors
Although most cases are benign, the behaviour of SFT can be unpredictable. About 10% behave aggressively, and local or distant recurrence can occur many years after primary resection {924,1121, 1281,2830}. Although there is no strict correlation between morphology and behaviour, malignant histology (especially high mitotic counts) remains the best indicator of poor outcome {520,998}; most (but not all) histologically benign SFTs prove to be non-recurring and non-metastasizing lesions, and most histologically malignant tumours behave aggressively. Lesions located in the mediastinum, abdomen, pelvis, retroperitoneum, and/or meninges also tend to behave more aggressively than those in the limbs {520,924,925,1121,2830}. Tumour size > 10 cm and positive surgical margins also predict poorer prognosis {998}. Metastases are most frequently observed in lungs, bone and liver {2830}. The behaviour of SFT with atypia alone is unpredictable.

Inflammatory myofibroblastic tumour

C.M. Coffin
J.A. Fletcher

Definition
Inflammatory myofibroblastic tumour (IMT) is a distinctive neoplasm composed of myofibroblastic and fibroblastic spindle cells accompanied by an inflammatory infiltrate of plasma cells, lymphocytes, and/or eosinophils. It occurs primarily in soft tissue and viscera of children and young adults.

ICD-O code   8825/1

Synonyms
Plasma cell granuloma; inflammatory myofibrohistiocytic proliferation; omental-mesenteric myxoid hamartoma; inflammatory pseudotumour; inflammatory fibrosarcoma; inflammatory myofibroblastic sarcoma {485,991,1734,1811}

Epidemiology
IMT primarily affects children and young adults, although the age range extends throughout adulthood {483,489,991}. The mean age at diagnosis is 10 years (median, 9 years) and IMT is most frequent in the first three decades of life. There is a slight female predominance.

Sites of involvement
IMT occurs throughout the body, most frequently in the mesentery, omentum, retroperitoneum, pelvis, and abdominal soft tissue in 73% of cases, followed by the lung, mediastinum, and head and neck {489, 991,1375,2290}. Unusual locations include somatic soft tissue, gastrointestinal tract, uterus, bladder, pancreas, and CNS {40,1198,2800}. Pseudosarcomatous myofibroblastic proliferations in the genitourinary tract can be difficult to distinguish from IMT {1112, 1183}.

Clinical features
The site of origin determines the symptoms {489,991,1375,2940}. Abdominal tumours may cause gastrointestinal obstruction {2249}. Pulmonary IMT is sometimes associated with chest pain and dyspnoea {2235}. Up to one third of patients have a clinical syndrome, possibly cytokine-mediated, of fever, malaise, weight loss, and laboratory abnormalities including microcytic hypochromic anaemia, thrombocytosis, polyclonal hyperglobulinaemia, elevated erythrocyte sedimentation rate, and elevated C-reactive protein {462,489,2609,2718}. When the mass is excised, the syndrome disappears, and its reappearance heralds recurrence.
Imaging studies reveal a lobulated heterogeneous solid mass with or without calcification {1375}.
IMT is clinically and pathologically distinct from IgG4-related sclerosing disease {2401,3015}.

Macroscopy
IMT is a nodular, circumscribed or multinodular mass with a tan, whorled, fleshy, or myxoid cut surface and variable haemorrhage, necrosis, and calcification {483, 489,991}. The diameter of the lesion ranges from 1 to > 20 cm. Some IMTs display a

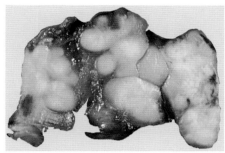

Fig. 3.078 Inflammatory myofibroblastic tumour presenting as a circumscribed, multinodular mass with a variegated cut surface.

zonal appearance with a central scar and softer red periphery. Multinodular tumours are generally restricted to the same anatomical region and may be contiguous or separate.

Histopathology
The spindled, fibroblastic-myofibroblastic, and inflammatory cells form three basic histological patterns {483,489,991}. Loosely arranged plump or spindled myofibroblasts in an oedematous myxoid background with abundant blood vessels and an infiltrate of plasma cells, lymphocytes, and eosinophils stimulate granulation tissue, or a reactive process. A second pattern is characterized by a compact fascicular spindle cell proliferation with variable myxoid and collagenized regions and the distinctive inflammatory infiltrate with diffuse inflammation or small aggregates of plasma cells, eosinophils,

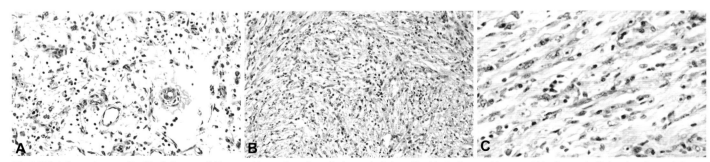

Fig. 3.079 Inflammatory myofibroblastic tumour. **A** The myxoid vascular pattern displays spindled myofibroblasts dispersed in a myxoid background with lymphocytes and plasma cells. **B** Interlacing bundles of spindle cells intermingled with plasma cells and lymphocytes are characteristic of the cellular phase. **C** Spindled and plump polygonal ganglion-like myofibroblasts with prominent nucleoli are dispersed in a collagenized background with intermingled lymphoplasmacytic inflammation.

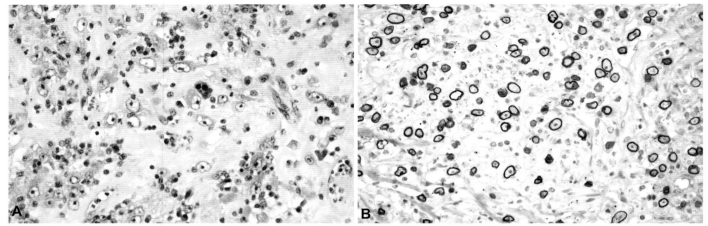

Fig. 3.080 Inflammatory myofibroblastic tumours (IMT) with *ALK-RANBP2* rearrangement. **A** Plump polygonal and epithelioid tumour cells with prominent nucleoli intermingled with lymphoplasmacytic inflammation. **B** Distinctive paranuclear membranous and occasional dot-like cytoplasmic immunoreactivity for ALK is seen.

and lymphocytes. Infrequently, the spindle cells surround blood vessels or bulge into vascular spaces. Ganglion-like myofibroblasts with vesicular nuclei, eosinophilic nucleoli, and abundant amphophilic cytoplasm are typical. The third pattern consists of a scar-like proliferation of plate-like collagen with lower cellularity and a relatively sparse inflammatory infiltrate of plasma cells and eosinophils. Dystrophic calcifications and osseous metaplasia are occasionally seen. Necrosis is uncommon. Mitotic activity varies but is generally low. Rare cases progress to frankly sarcomatous morphology in recurrences.

An IMT variant with plump round epithelioid or histiocytoid tumour cells is associated with *RANBP2-ALK* gene rearrangement and seems to portend more aggressive clinical behaviour {438,1734}.

Immunophenotype

IMT displays variable staining for SMA, MSA, and desmin. Focal keratin immunoreactivity is seen in approximately one third of cases. Focal reactivity for CD68 occurs in histiocytic-appearing cells. Cytoplasmic reactivity for ALK protein is detectable in 50–60% of cases and correlates well with the presence of a rearrangement of the *ALK* gene {411,417,488, 507,991}. A nuclear membrane pattern of ALK staining may be associated with the *RANBP2* fusion partner and a granular cytoplasmic pattern with the CLTC fusion partner {1683,1734}. Development of more sensitive immunohistochemical techniques for the detection of ALK protein may improve detection of ALK protein in IMTs {2705}.

Genetics

IMT are heterogeneous genetically, as is hardly surprising given the varied clinicopathological entities that have been grouped in this category. IMT in children and young adults contain clonal cytogenetic rearrangements involving chromosome band 2p23 that fuse the 3' kinase region of the *ALK* gene with various partner genes, including *TPM3*, *TPM4*, *CLTC*, and *RANBP2*, and *ATIC*, among others in a growing list, in 50–70% of cases {317, 1036,1570,2671}. In contrast, such rearrangements are uncommon in IMT diagnosed in adults aged > 40 years {417, 1570}. Notably, certain *ALK* gene fusions can be found in both IMT and anaplastic large cell lymphoma, and ALK-positive

B-cell lymphoma {951,2273}. IMT with *ALK* genomic rearrangement features activation and overexpression of the ALK C-terminal kinase regions, which is restricted to the neoplastic myofibroblastic component {317,488,507,1036,1570}. Therefore, immunohistochemical detection of the ALK C-terminal end is undoubtedly the most efficient method for identifying ALK oncoproteins in IMT {488, 507}. In questionable cases, diagnosis by *ALK* split-apart FISH may be useful.

Prognostic factors

Approximately 25% of extrapulmonary IMTs recur in a fashion that is related to anatomical site, resectability, and multinodularity {31,489,991}. Metastasis occurs in < 2% of cases. Metastasis may be associated with specific *ALK* fusion partners such as *RANBP2* and round cell morphology {1734}. ALK-negative IMTs may have a higher likelihood of metastasis {613}. Distant metastases are rare and involve the lungs, brain, liver and bone. Tumour size, cellularity, and histological features are not reliable prognostic indicators, although aneuploidy may indicate aggressiveness {246,483,1253}.

Low-grade myofibroblastic sarcoma

T. Mentzel

Definition
Low-grade myofibroblastic sarcoma represents a distinct atypical myofibroblastic tumour, often having fibromatosis-like features, which tends to arise in the head and neck region and that rarely metastasizes.

ICD-O code   8825/3

Synonym
Myofibrosarcoma

Epidemiology
Given the lack of well-defined diagnostic criteria, myofibroblastic sarcomas in general are probably more common than currently believed, and include a variety of clinicopathological forms. Low-grade myofibroblastic sarcoma represents a distinct entity that occurs predominantly in adults with a slight male predominance; children are more rarely affected {1836,1934,2584}.

Sites of involvement
Low-grade myofibroblastic sarcoma shows a wide anatomical distribution; however, extremities and the head and neck region, especially the tongue and oral cavity, seem to be preferred locations, while the skin and gastrointestinal tract are rarely affected {18,1836,1934}. These neoplasms arise predominantly in subcutaneous and deeper soft tissue, while dermal presentation is very uncommon {424}. Rare cases involving salivary gland and nasal cavity/paranasal sinus have been reported {244,1459}.

Clinical features
Most patients complain about a painless swelling or an enlarging mass. Pain or related symptoms have been more rarely reported. Clinically, local recurrences are common, but metastases only rarely occur and often after a prolonged time interval {1836}. Radiologically, these lesions have a destructive growth pattern.

Macroscopy
Grossly, most cases are described as a firm mass with pale, fibrous cut surfaces and usually ill-defined margins {1836}; a

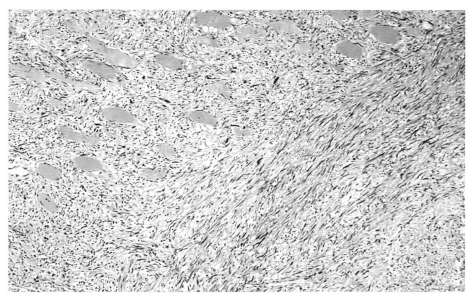

Fig. 3.081 Low-grade myofibroblastic sarcoma, deep-seated, presenting as a diffusely infiltrative spindle cell tumour with a fascicular arrangement of neoplastic cells.

minority are well circumscribed with pushing margins {1934}.

Histopathology
Histologically, most low-grade myofibroblastic sarcomas are characterized by a diffusely infiltrative growth pattern and, in deeply located neoplasms, tumour cells often grow between individual skeletal muscle fibres. Most cases are composed of spindle cells arranged in cellular fascicles or a storiform growth pattern. Neoplastic cells have ill-defined palely eosinophilic cytoplasm and fusiform nuclei that are either elongated and wavy with evenly distributed chromatin, or plumper, more rounded and vesicular with indentations and small nucleoli. More rarely, hypocellular neoplasms with a more prominent collageneous (sometimes hyalinized) matrix have been described. Importantly, neoplastic cells show at least focally moderate nuclear atypia with enlarged, hyperchromatic and irregular nuclei and slightly

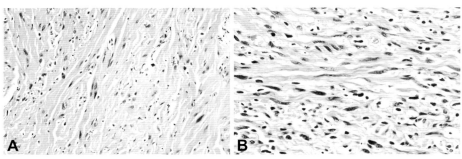

Fig. 3.082 Low-grade myofibroblastic sarcoma. **A** This hypocellular example is composed of atypical spindled neoplastic cells set in a prominent collagenous matrix. **B** Fusiform tumour cells containing ill-defined, pale, eosinophilic cytoplasm and spindle-shaped nuclei that are either vesicular with small nucleoli and indentations or elongated and wavy, resembling neural differentiation.

increased proliferative activity. These neoplasms may contain numerous thin-walled capillaries.

Immunophenotype

Neoplastic cells in low-grade myofibroblastic sarcoma show variable positivity for actin and/or desmin. In addition, there may be staining for calponin, and focal expression of CD34 has been reported, while staining for S100 protein, epithelial markers, nuclear β-catenin, and h-caldesmon is typically negative {219,1836, 2280}.

Ultrastructure

In contrast to smooth muscle cells, the neoplastic cells in low-grade myofibroblastic sarcoma have indented and clefted nuclei, variable amounts of rough endoplasmic reticulum, and are surrounded by a discontinous basal lamina. Unlike fibroblasts, randomly oriented intermediate filaments and thin filaments with focal densities and subplasmalemmal attachment plaques, a discontinous basal lamina and often micropinocytic vesicles are noted, and in some cases fibronexus junctions have been found {1836,2908}.

Genetics

Genetic aberrations have been described in only a few cases. Preliminary reports are of karyotypes with a moderate number of chromosomal aberrations, substantially less complex than the karyotypes seen in most high-grade myofibroblastic sarcomas, but nevertheless quite different from fibromatosis {864}.

Prognostic factors

Metastasis is very rare in low-grade myofibroblastic sarcoma.

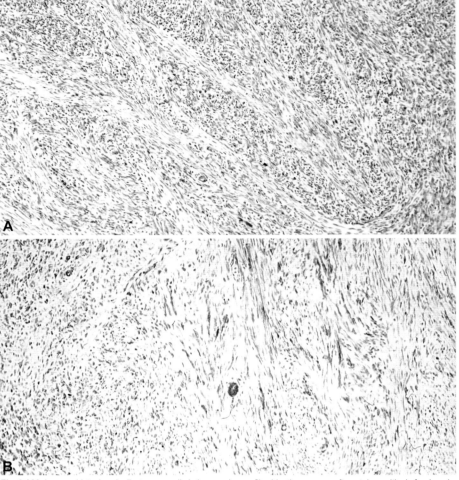

Fig. 3.083 Immunohistochemically, tumour cells in low-grade myofibroblastic sarcoma often stain positively for desmin (**A**) and SMA (**B**).

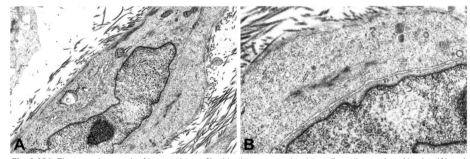

Fig. 3.084 Electron micrograph of low-grade myofibroblastic sarcoma showing a discontinuous basal lamina (**A**) and thin filaments with focal densities, subplasmalemmal attachment plaques, and micropinocytic vesicles (**B**).

Myxoinflammatory fibroblastic sarcoma

J.M. Meis
L.-G. Kindblom
F. Mertens

Definition

Myxoinflammatory fibroblastic sarcoma (MIFS) is a locally aggressive fibroblastic neoplasm, occuring primarily in the distal extremities, and characterized by epithelioid fibroblasts with macronucleoli interspersed with a prominent mixed inflammatory infiltrate and a variable myxoid matrix.

ICD-O code   8811/1

Synonyms

Atypical myxoinflammatory fibroblastic tumour; Acral myxoinflammatory fibroblastic sarc-oma {1817}; inflammatory myxohyaline tumour of the distal extremities with virocyte/Reed-Sternberg-like cells {1937}; inflammatory myxoid tumour of the soft parts with bizarre giant cells {1867}.

Epidemiology

MIFS occurs in middle-age and is equally frequent in males and females {1538,1817, 1937}. Cases in children are rare.

Sites of involvement

The overwhelming majority of MIFS occur in the distal extremities, with 80% in the hands (predominantly fingers) {720,1538, 1817,1937}. More proximally situated cases are rare {1354}.

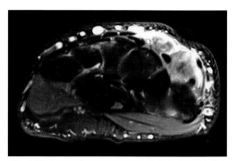

Fig. 3.085 Myxoinflammatory fibroblastic sarcoma of the dorsal radial aspect of the left wrist. MRI shows a 3.7 x 3.6 x 1.8 cm mass, which has a heterogeneously increased signal on axial proton density-weighted fat-suppression images. The tumour is encasing the extensor tendons and the radial artery with a small extension between the carpal bones.

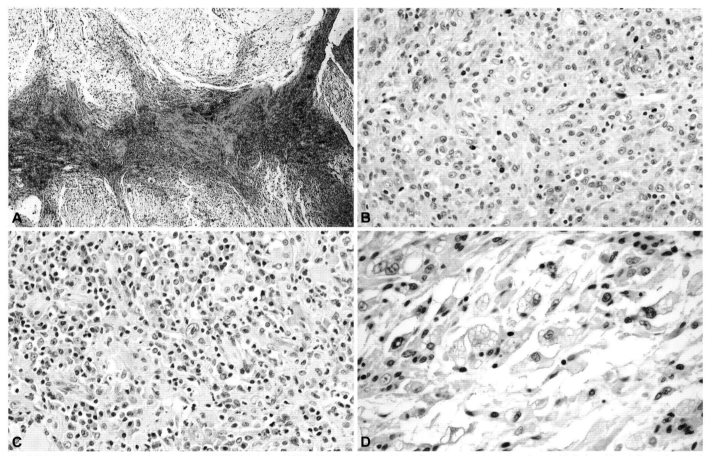

Fig. 3.086 Myxoinflammatory fibroblastic sarcoma (MIFS). A Lobulated MIFS with alternating myxoid and fibrous zones and prominent haemosiderin deposition similar to pigmented villonodular synovitis. B Relatively uniform population of cells in another MIFS, with features overlapping with a tenosynovitis. C Tumour cells are more apparent. D Early cytoplasmic vacuolization in blander appearing cells.

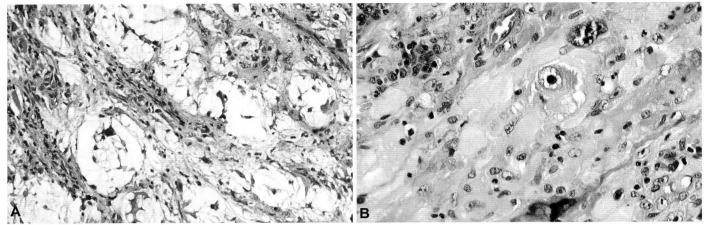

Fig. 3.087 Myxoinflammatory fibroblastic sarcoma. **A** Vacuolated cells. **B** "Virocyte"-like cells are commonly seen.

Clinical features

Most patients present with a slowly growing mass that is judged clinically to be a benign condition, such as tenosynovitis or a ganglion cyst. Thus incomplete excision and local recurrences, sometimes multiple, are not uncommon. Metastases to regional lymph nodes may occur, although this is relatively rare (< 3% of reported cases) {1817,2412}.

Macroscopy

Most lesions have a multinodular appearance with fibrous and myxoid zones. Tumour size is usually < 5 cm, although some may be larger {1817}.

Histopathology

Involvement of tenosynovial structures is typical {2001}, with extension into the subcutis and rarely into bone. MIFS shows a prominent mixed inflammatory infiltrate, haemosiderin deposition, macrophages, Touton-type giant cells and a mononuclear cell background with varying degrees of nuclear atypia. The latter component ranges from relatively bland to bizarre epithelioid cells with inclusion-like nucleoli, sometimes resembling virocytes or Reed-Sternberg cells. When a myxoid matrix is prominent, the cytoplasm of the bizarre cells becomes vacuolated, resulting in a bubbly lipoblast-like appearance. The tumour periphery often reveals insidious extensions of scattered tumour cells within inflammatory zones, rendering complete excision difficult.

Immunophenotype

There is variable positivity for CD68, CD34 and SMA {1817}. Focal staining for keratin may be seen. Importantly, lymphoid markers such as CD30 are negative {1937}.

Genetics

Most cytogenetically abnormal MIFS cases share a near-diploid chromosome count, a balanced or unbalanced t(1;10)(p22–31;q24–25) and loss of material from chromosome arm 3p {1084, 1534}. However, some cases have displayed near-triploid clones or other structural rearrangements {1084,1272,1729}. The breakpoints in the t(1;10) map to the *TGFBR3* gene in 1p22 and to, or near, the *MGEA5* locus in 10q24; the functional outcome seems to be transcriptional upregulation of the *FGF8* gene, located close to *MGEA5* on chromosome 10 {1084}. The 3p rearrangements are associated with amplification and overexpression of genes, including *VGLL3*, in 3p11–12 {87,1084}. The same t(1;10) and amplification of 3p are seen in haemosiderotic fibrolipomatous tumour and tumours with mixed morphology {87,736}.

Prognostic factors

The rate of local recurrence ranges from 20% to 70% {1817,1937}; the discrepancy may reflect differences in referral patterns. Repeated local recurrences with proximal extension eventuating in amputation have been reported in up to one third of cases. {1817,2001,2412} Regional lymph-node metastases and local bone invasion occasionally occur {1817,2412}. Distant metastasis seems exceedingly rare. There are no reported histological criteria or immunohistochemical stains that predict aggressive behaviour.

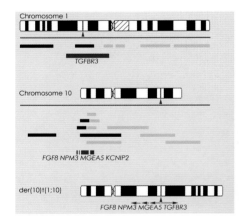

Fig. 3.088 Schematic illustration of the breakpoints in the t(1;10), resulting in upregulation of FGF8, that is characteristic of myxoinflammatory fibroblastic sarcoma. Black and grey horizontal bars represent BAC clones; the genes located in or near the breakpoints are indicated {1084}.

Infantile fibrosarcoma

C.M. Coffin
P.H. Sorensen

Definition

Infantile fibrosarcoma (IFS) simulates classic adult fibrosarcoma histologically, but has a distinctive *ETV6-NTRK3* gene fusion. It occurs in infants and rarely metastasizes. The renal counterpart is cellular congenital mesoblastic nephroma (CMN).

ICD-O code   8814/3

Synonyms

Congenital fibrosarcoma; congenital-infantile fibrosarcoma; juvenile fibrosarcoma; medullary fibromatosis of infancy; congenital fibrosarcoma-like fibromatosis; desmoplastic fibrosarcoma of infancy {486,2662}

Epidemiology

Nearly all cases of IFS occur in the first year of life, 36–80% are congenital {467, 482,486,1302,2662}. There is a slight male predominance.

Sites of involvement

The superficial and deep soft tissues of distal extremities are the origin in nearly two thirds of cases {150,256,467,2641}. The trunk and head/neck are other major sites; rare cases occur at visceral locations {337,1455,2348,2536}.

Clinical features

IFS presents as a solitary rapidly enlarging mass, sometimes grotesque in proportion to the child's size {256,467,486,2662}. The diameter can exceed 30 cm. The overlying skin is erythematous and ulcerated. Intratumoral haemorrhage may cause anaemia {2458}. Imaging reveals a heterogeneously enhancing soft-tissue mass and variable osseous erosion {150,728}. IFS may be diagnosed antenatally {516, 713,1279}.

Macroscopy

The poorly circumscribed lobulated mass infiltrates soft tissue {467,486,2371,2662}. Compression of adjacent tissue creates a pseudocapsule, but actual margins are irregular. The cut surface is fleshy and tan with variable areas of myxoid or cystic change, haemorrhage, necrosis, and yellow or red discoloration.

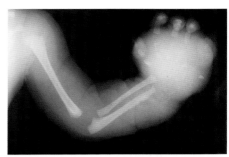

Fig. 3.089 X-ray of a large infantile fibrosarcoma of the hand.

Histopathology

This is a densely cellular neoplasm composed of intersecting fascicles of primitive round, ovoid, and spindle cells with a focal herringbone pattern, or more commonly

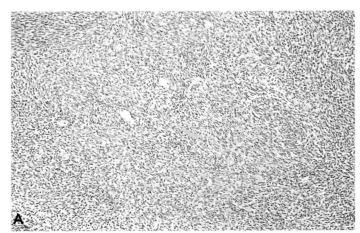
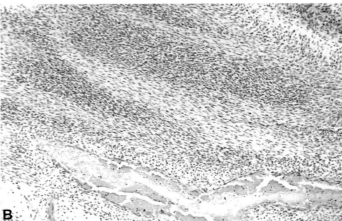

Fig. 3.090 Infantile fibrosarcoma (IFS). **A** IFS of the knee presenting as a large mass with purple discoloration and focal cutaneous ulceration. **B** IFS in soft tissue, displaying a fleshy, tan-white cut surface with focal haemorrhage, necrosis, and myxoid change.

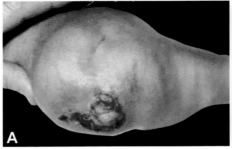
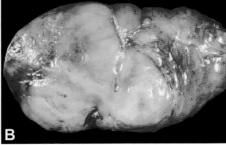

Fig. 3.091 Infantile fibrosarcoma. **A** Poorly formed fascicular growth pattern. **B** A herringbone pattern is present with variable deposition of collagen.

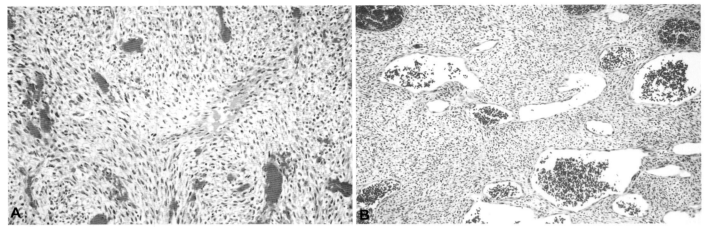

Fig. 3.092 Infantile fibrosarcoma (IFS). **A** Short interlacing fascicles, congested blood vessels, and zonal necrosis. **B** Dilated, irregularly branching blood vessels in IFS.

forming interlacing cords, sinuous bands, or sheets {467,486,2662}. Zonal necrosis and haemorrhage may be associated with dystrophic calcification. The cells show little pleomorphism. Mitotic activity may be prominent. Histological variations include collagenization, chronic inflammation, focal extramedullary haematopoiesis, a focally prominent haemangiopericytoma-like vascular pattern, fibrin thrombi, myxoid foci, or a predominantly round or ovoid immature cellular proliferation with minimal collagen {486, 542, 2294}. Infiltrative growth results in entrapment of adipose tissue, skeletal muscle and other structures. Composite tumours with overlapping features of infantile myofibroma and infantile fibrosarcoma are occasionally encountered {29, 2858}. Chemotherapy causes fibrosis with fibrovascular proliferation {2394}.

Immunophenotype
The immunohistochemical features are nonspecific {486,1453,2529}.

Genetics
IFS is characterized by a chromosomal translocation, t(12;15)(p13;q25), which fuses exons 1–5 of the 12p13 *ETV6* (*TEL*) gene to exons 13–18 of the 15q25 neurotrophin-3 receptor gene, *NTRK3* (*TRKC*) and generates fusion transcripts encoding the ETV6-NTRK3 chimeric tyrosine kinase {1444}. ETV6-NTRK3 is a potent oncoprotein that constitutively activates signal transduction cascades of the NTRK3 tyrosine kinase, namely Ras-Erk and PI3K-Akt pathways {2763}. This fusion is present in the majority of IFS. *ETV6-NTRK3* fusions are absent in infantile myofibromatosis and adult-type fibrosarcoma {278,2529}. Identical *ETV6-NTRK3* fusions are expressed in CMN {1443,2386}. Tumours lacking karyotypically evident (12;15) translocations may still harbour these fusions {1444,2386,2641}. FISH and RT-PCR are useful for diagnosis {12,96, 97}. Immunostaining for NTRK3 is not reliable for the detection of the fusion {278,705}. Trisomy of chromosomes 8, 11, 17, and 20

is characteristic of IFS and CMN {201,552, 2475}. *ETV6-NTRK3* fusions have also been reported in myeloid leukaemias {901,1473, 1639}, secretory breast carcinoma {2764}, and mammary-type secretory carcinoma of skin and salivary gland {822,2577}.

Prognostic factors
IFS has a relatively favourable outcome, with mortality of < 5% and a recurrence rate of 5–50% {467,486,2129,2611}. Metastasis is rare in recent series {406,486,516,2427}. No definitive prognostic factors are known. Haemorrhage and involvement of vital structures by locally aggressive tumours may cause death {713}. Spontaneous regression and non-recurrence of incompletely excised IFS have been reported {406,1500,1515, 1649,1692,1774,2611}.

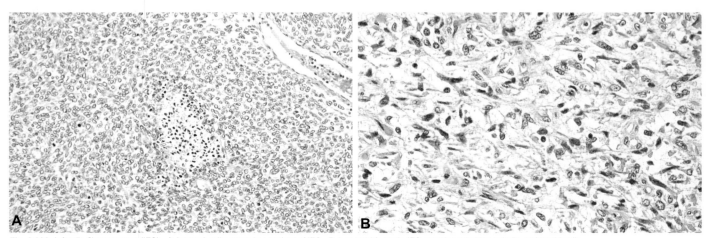

Fig. 3.093 Infantile fibrosarcoma (IFS). **A** A round-cell pattern is a variant of IFS. **B** A myxoid focus in IFS contains primitive spindle and ovoid cells.

Adult fibrosarcoma

A.L. Folpe

Definition
Adult fibrosarcoma is a malignant neoplasm composed of fibroblasts with variable collagen production and, in classical cases, a "herringbone" architecture. It is a diagnosis of exclusion.

ICD-O code   8810/3

Epidemiology
Adult fibrosarcoma was once considered to be the most common soft tissue sarcoma in adults {1862}. However, incidence has declined dramatically over the past seven decades, with recent data showing it to account for only 3.6% of sarcomas arising from soft tissues {2770}. A recent review from a single institution showed strictly defined adult fibrosarcoma to account for < 1% of adult soft tissue sarcomas {139}. Adult fibrosarcoma is most common in middle-aged and older adults (median age, 50 years), but may rarely occur in children. Historically, no difference between the sexes has been noted, although this tumour may be slightly more common in males {139}.

Etiology
There are no specific predisposing factors. Some tumours arise in the field of previous therapeutic irradiation, and rarely in association with implanted foreign material {139}.

Sites of involvement
Fibrosarcomas most often involve the deep soft tissues of the extremities, trunk, head and neck. Those in skin and subcutis are more likely to represent fibrosarcomatous change in dermatofibrosarcoma protuberans. The veracity of the diagnosis for cases reported as "fibrosarcoma" in visceral organs is questionable. Retroperitoneal fibrosarcoma is very rare, and is likely to represent low-grade dedifferentiated liposarcoma in most instances.

Clinical features
Fibrosarcoma presents as a mass with or without pain.

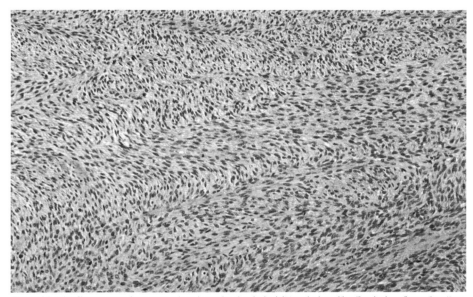

Fig. 3.094 Adult fibrosarcoma. Low-power view shows the classical adult-type lesion with a "herringbone" growth pattern.

Macroscopy
The typical fibrosarcoma is a circumscribed, firm, white or tan mass. Haemorrhage and necrosis can be seen in high-grade tumours.

Histopathology
Fibrosarcomas are composed of relatively monomorphic spindled cells, showing no more than a moderate degree of pleomorphism. Tumours showing a greater degree of pleomorphism are better classified as undifferentiated pleomorphic sarcoma. The tumour cells are characteristically arranged in long, sweeping fascicles in a herringbone pattern. Storiform areas can occasionally be present. The cells have tapered, darkly staining nuclei with variably prominent nucleoli and scanty cytoplasm. Mitotic activity is almost always present but variable. The stroma has variable collagen, from a delicate intercellular network to paucicellular areas with diffuse or "keloid-like" sclerosis or hyalinization. Some fibrosarcomas may contain relatively bland zones mimicking fibromatosis.

Immunophenotype
Fibrosarcomas occasionally show limited expression of SMA, representing myofibroblastic differentiation. CD34-positive tumours showing fibrosarcoma morphology probably represent fibrosarcoma arising in dermatofibrosarcoma protuberans or fibrosarcoma-like progression in solitary fibrous tumour.

Ultrastructure
Fibrosarcoma is composed of fibroblasts with prominent rough endoplasmic reticulum and absence of myofilaments, external lamina or intercellular junctions. An occasional cell has peripheral filament bundles suggestive of myofibroblastic differentiation, but tumours in which this is a prominent feature should be classified as myofibrosarcomas.

Genetics
Adult fibrosarcoma has been reported to show multiple numerical and structural chromosomal abnormalities, without involvement of a specific locus {556,1624, 2834}.

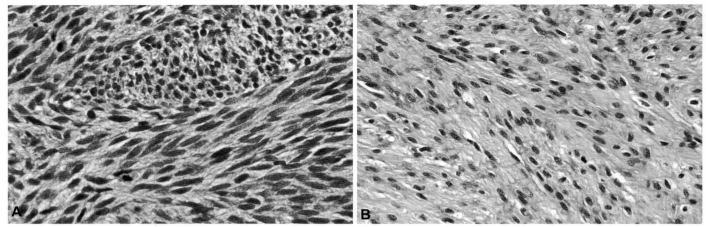

Fig. 3.095 Adult fibrosarcoma. **A** High-grade fibrosarcoma consisting of monomorphic spindled cells with brisk mitotic activity. **B** Low-grade fibrosarcoma showing lower cellularity, increased stromal collagen, and a lesser degree of nuclear atypicality.

Prognostic factors

In the recent series of strictly defined adult fibrosarcomas reported by Bahrami and coworkers, > 80% of tumours were high grade (FNCLCC grade 2 or 3), with one of the four low-grade lesions progressing to high-grade sarcoma in a local recurrence {139}. These fibrosarcomas were aggressive, with multiple local recurrences, lymph-node and parenchymal metastases, and overall survival of < 70% at 2 years, and < 55% at 5 years. Owing to the relatively small number of fibrosarcomas in the Bahrami et al. series, no correlation could be made between clinicopathological variables (including grade) and outcome. In the older literature, behaviour has been related to grade, tumour size and depth. The probability of local recurrence relates to completeness of excision, with historically reported recurrence rates of 12–79% {2271,2497}. Fibrosarcomas metastasize to lungs and bone, especially the axial skeleton, and rarely to lymph nodes. Widely variable rates of metastasis and survival have been reported in older series of fibrosarcomas, probably reflecting diagnostic heterogeneity.

Myxofibrosarcoma

T. Mentzel
P.C.W. Hogendoorn
H.-Y. Huang

Definition
Myxofibrosarcoma comprises a spectrum of malignant fibroblastic neoplasms with variably prominent myxoid stroma, cellular pleomorphism and a distinctive curvilinear vascular pattern.

ICD-O code
8811/3

Synonym
Myxoid malignant fibrous histiocytoma

Epidemiology
Myxofibrosarcoma is one of the most common sarcomas in elderly patients, with a slight predominance in males. Although the overall age range is wide, these neoplasms mainly affect patients in the sixth to eighth decades of life, whereas they are exceptionally rare under the age of 20 years {1834,1849,2926}.

Sites of involvement
Most of these tumours arise in the limbs, including the limb girdles (lower > upper extremities), but they are seen only rarely on

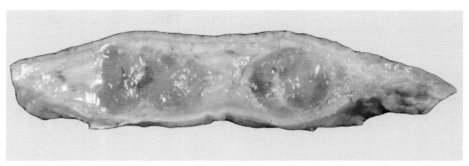

Fig. 3.096 Superficially located, low-grade myxofibrosarcoma with multinodular growth pattern and gelatinous, myxoid cut surface.

the trunk, in the head and neck area, and on the hands and feet {1243,1834,1849,2434, 2926}. Origin in the retroperitoneum and in the abdominal cavity is extremely uncommon, and most lesions with myxofibrosarcoma-like features in these locations represent dedifferentiated liposarcomas {78, 1190,1820}. Notably, about half of cases develop in dermal/subcutaneous tissues, with the remainder occurring in the underlying fascia and skeletal muscle {2434}.

Clinical features
Most patients present with a slowly enlarging and painless mass. Local, often repeated recurrences, unrelated to histological grade, occur in up to 50–60% of cases. In addition to pulmonary and osseous metastases, lymph-node metastases are seen in a small but significant number of cases {1243,1834,1849,2434, 2926}.

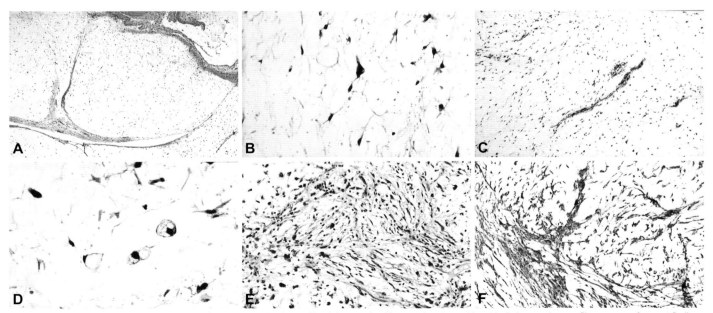

Fig. 3.097 Myxofibrosarcoma. **A** Low-grade myxofibrosarcoma showing multinodular growth with a prominent myxoid matrix. In low-grade myxofibrosarcoma, frequent findings include: **B** Atypical fibroblastic cells with enlarged and hyperchromatic nuclei on a background of low cellularity; **C** Elongated, curvilinear blood vessels; and **D** Pseudolipoblasts. **E**, **F** Intermediate-grade myxofibrosarcomas retain a myxoid stroma and characteristic vascular pattern, but are more cellular and pleomorphic than low-grade lesions.

Macroscopy

Superficially located neoplasms typically consist of multiple, variably gelatinous or firmer nodules, whereas deep-seated neoplasms often form a single mass with an infiltrative margin. In high-grade lesions, areas of tumour necrosis are often found.

Histopathology

Myxofibrosarcoma shows a broad spectrum of cellularity, pleomorphism, and proliferative activity; however, all cases share distinct morphological features, particularly multinodular growth with incomplete fibrous septa, and a myxoid stroma. Subcutaneous examples of myxofibrosarcoma commonly have very infiltrative margins, often extending beyond what is detected clinically. The type of glycosaminoglycan content may correlate with histological grade {2967}.

The low-grade end of the morphological spectrum is characterized by hypocellular neoplasms composed of only a few, non-cohesive, plump spindled or stellate tumour cells with ill-defined, slightly eosinophilic cytoplasm and atypical, enlarged, hyperchromatic nuclei. Mitotic figures are infrequent in low-grade lesions. A characteristic finding is the presence of prominent elongated, curvilinear, thin-walled blood vessels with perivascular condensation of tumour cells and/or inflammatory cells (mainly lymphocytes and plasma cells). Frequently, so-called pseudolipoblasts (vacuolated neoplastic fibroblastic cells with cytoplasmic acid mucin) are noted.

In contrast, high-grade neoplasms are composed partly of solid sheets and cellular fascicles of spindled and pleomorphic tumour cells with numerous, often atypical mitoses, areas of haemorrhage and necrosis. In many cases, bizarre, multinucleated giant cells with abundant eosinophilic cytoplasm (resembling myoid cells) and irregular shaped nuclei are noted. However, high-grade lesions also focally show features of a lower-grade neoplasm with a prominent myxoid matrix and numerous elongated capillaries.

The intermediate-grade lesions are more cellular and pleomorphic than purely low-grade neoplasms, but lack well-developed solid areas, pronounced cellular pleomorphism and necrosis.

The rare epithelioid variant is composed predominantly of atypical epithelioid tumour cells with abundant eosinophilic cytoplasm and round vesicular nuclei arranged in small clusters in the myxoid areas or forming sheets in the hypercellular areas, mimicking

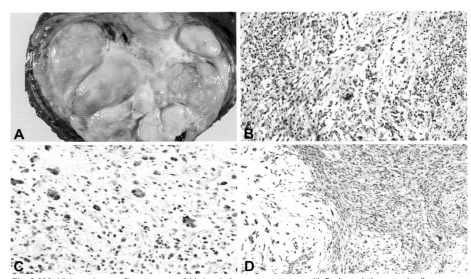

Fig. 3.098 High-grade myxofibrosarcoma. **A** Variegated gross appearance with fleshy, gelatinous and yellow-orange areas of necrosis. **B** This example shows features of a high-grade unclassified pleomorphic sarcoma. **C** The lesion also shows frequent multinucleated giant cells with abundant eosinophilic cytoplasm. **D** Focally, areas of lower-grade myxofibrosarcoma with a prominent myxoid matrix are usually present in high-grade myxofibrosarcoma.

metastatic carcinoma, melanoma or malignant myoepithelioma of soft tissues. These morphological features are seen mainly in high-grade neoplasms {2002}.

Immunophenotype

In a minority of cases, some spindled or larger eosinophilic tumour cells express MSA and/or SMA, suggestive of focal myofibroblastic differentiation; staining for desmin and histiocyte-specific markers is negative {1834}.

Genetics

Karyotypes tend to be highly complex, with extensive intratumoral heterogeneity and chromosome numbers in the triploid or tetraploid range in most cases, including even grade 1 neoplasms {1720, 1926,2132, 2561,2965}. Progression in grade is accompanied by an increase in cytogenetic aberrations {2965}. No specific aberration has emerged. There is a diverse pattern of NF1 aberrations, including point mutations and deletions, in 10% of analysed myxofibrosarcomas {156}. Local recurrences may show more complex cytogenetic aberrations than the primary neoplasms, suggesting tumour progression {2965}. In contrast to intramuscular myxoma, no activating mutations of the GNAS gene are seen in myxofibrosarcoma {2966}.

Prognostic factors

Metastases and tumour-associated mortality are closely related to tumour grade {2926}. Although none of the low-grade neoplasms metastasize, intermediate- and high-grade neoplasms may develop metastases in about 20–35% of cases. A local recurrence within 12 months increases tumour-associated mortality {1834,1849}, and better local control may translate into final survival benefits {2434}. Proliferative activity, the percentage of aneuploid cells, and tumour vascularity are associated with the histological tumour grade, but no clear relationship to clinical outcome has been found {1830,1834}, whereas tumour size, morphological grade, and margins are statistically significant predictors of survival of affected patients {2434}. Importantly, low-grade lesions may become higher grade in subsequent recurrences and hence acquire metastatic potential. The overall 5-year survival rate is 60–70%.

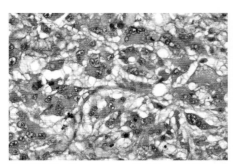

Fig.3.099 Myxofibrosarcoma, epithelioid variant. Enlarged epithelioid tumour cells contain abundant eosinophilic cytoplasm, vesicular nuclei with prominent nucleoli, and easily identified mitoses set in a prominent myxoid stroma.

Low-grade fibromyxoid sarcoma

A.L. Folpe
J.L. Hornick
F. Mertens

Definition
Low-grade fibromyxoid sarcoma is a distinctive malignant fibroblastic neoplasm, characterized by admixed heavily collagenized and myxoid zones, deceptively bland spindled cells with a whorling growth pattern and arcades of curvilinear blood vessels. These tumours consistently have either a *FUS-CREB3L2* or a *FUS-CREB3L1* gene fusion.

ICD-O code   8840/3

Synonyms
Hyalinizing spindle cell tumour with giant rosettes

Epidemiology
Low-grade fibromyxoid sarcomas are rare, with approximately 350 reported cases {237,781,783,787,888,1059,1536, 1851,2323}; however, it is likely that many cases go unrecognized. These tumours occur equally frequently in men and women and typically affect young adults. However, patients of any age may be affected and up to 20% of cases occur in patients aged < 18 years {237,888,1059,1316}.

Sites of involvement
Low-grade fibromyxoid sarcomas typically arise in the proximal extremities or trunk, but may occur at unusual locations {787,1059,1316,1567}. The overwhelming

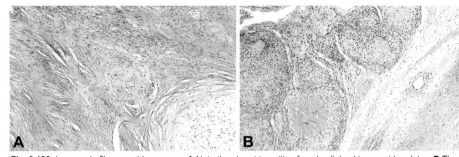

Fig. 3.100 Low-grade fibromyxoid sarcoma. **A** Note the abrupt transition from hyalinized to myxoid nodules. **B** There are numerous giant collagen rosettes.

majority occur in a subfascial location; rare superficial tumours appear to be more common in children {237}.

Clinical features
Up to 15% of patients report a prebiopsy duration of > 5 years. The tumour presents as a painless mass.

Macroscopy
Grossly, low-grade fibromyxoid sarcomas are well-circumscribed, fibrous, and often focally mucoid. The tumour ranges in size from 1 cm to > 20 cm in greatest dimension (median size, 5 cm).

Histopathology
Classical low-grade fibromyxoid sarcoma shows an admixture of heavily collagenized, hypocellular zones and more cellular

myxoid nodules. Short fascicular and characteristic whorling growth patterns are seen. The tumour vasculature consists of arcades of small vessels, and arteriole-sized vessels with perivascular sclerosis. The tumour cells are very bland, with only scattered hyperchromatic cells. Mitotic figures are scarce. Approximately 10% of cases show areas with increased cellularity, nuclear atypia, pleomorphism, or epithelioid morphology {696,888,1059}. Occasional cases show areas indistinguishable from sclerosing epithelioid fibrosarcoma {696,787,1059,2323}. Rarely tumours recur with an undifferentiated round cell appearance or with osteoblastic differentiation {787}. Approximately 30% of otherwise typical cases show the focal presence of collagen rosettes, consisting of a central core of hyalinized collagen

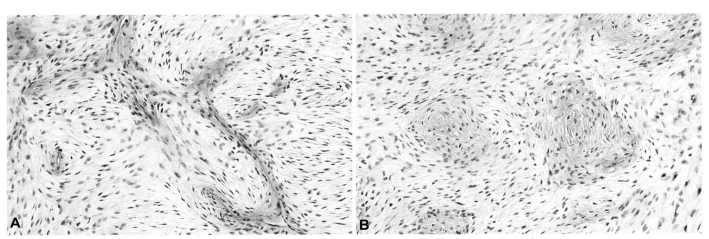

Fig. 3.101 Low-grade fibromyxoid sarcoma. **A** Arcades of small blood vessels are present. **B** Early formation of collagen rosettes can be seen.

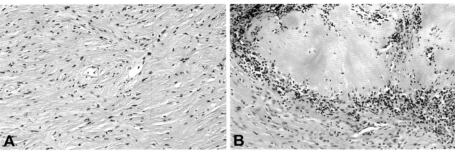

Fig. 3.102 Low-grade fibromyxoid sarcoma. **A** The lesion consists of very bland spindle cells embedded in a densely collagenous background. **B** In cases with giant collagen "rosettes," the tumour cells are arranged in cuffs around nodules of hyaline collagen.

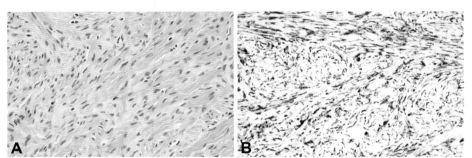

Fig. 3.103 Low-grade fibromyxoid sarcoma. **A** Genetically confirmed low-grade fibromyxoid sarcoma. **B** There is immunoexpression of MUC4.

surrounded by a cuff of epithelioid fibroblasts. In the subset of low-grade fibromyxoid sarcomas in which these collagen rosettes are particularly prominent and well-formed, the term "hyalinizing spindle cell tumour with giant rosettes" was formerly applied {888,1536}. The immunohistochemical features, genetic features, and behaviour of tumours with and without giant collagen rosettes are identical {787,888}.

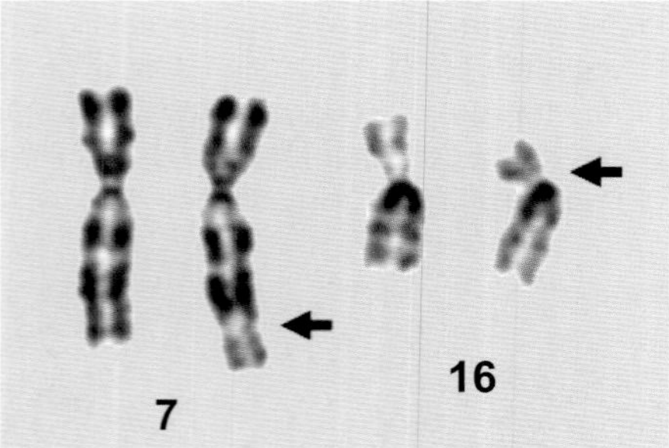

Immunophenotype
EMA is at least focally positive in up to 80% of cases {696,1059}. MUC4, an epithelial glycoprotein, is expressed by low-grade fibromyxoid sarcoma and is highly sensitive and specific among fibroblastic tumours {696}. Myofibroblastic differentiation, as reflected by focal expression of SMA, may be seen on occasion {237,696, 888,1059}.

Genetics
The cytogenetic hallmark of these tumours is the t(7;16)(q33;p11), which is present, often as the sole change, in approximately two thirds of cases. Another 25% of cases

Fig. 3.104 Partial karyogram for a low-grade fibromyxoid sarcoma showing the characteristic t(7;16)(q33;p11) resulting in a *FUS-CREB3L2* fusion gene. Arrows indicate breakpoints.

show a supernumerary ring chromosome {182,1864,2316,2660}. Both aberrations result in fusion of the 5' part of the *FUS* gene in 16p11 with the 3' part of the *CREB3L2* gene in 7q33 {1851,2162, 2660}. A rare variant t(11;16)(p11;p11) results in a *FUS-CREB3L1* fusion {1851}. Molecular genetic studies have identified the *FUS-CREB3L2* and *FUS-CREB3L1* fusion genes in 76–96% and 4–6%, respectively, of cases {1059,1765,1851, 2367}. Low-grade fibromyxoid sarcomas arising in atypical locations and those with giant rosettes or foci resembling sclerosing epithelioid fibrosarcoma also display t(7;16)/*FUS-CREB3L2* {1059,1567,2162, 2195,2316}. The chimeric FUS-CREB3L2 protein functions as an aberrant transcription factor, causing deregulated expression of wildtype CREB3L2 target genes {1927}.

Prognostic factors
Although low-grade fibromyxoid sarcoma shows low rates of recurrence and metastasis in the first 5 years after excision of the primary tumour (approximately 10% and 5%, respectively), rates are much higher with long-term follow-up {237,781, 783,787,888,1012,1059}. A recent series from a referral centre with prolonged follow-up showed recurrences, metastases, and death from disease in 64%, 45%, and 42% of patients, respectively {787}. Metastases occurred up to 45 years after primary excision (median, 5 years), and the median interval to tumour-related death was 15 years {787}. The most common metastatic sites are the lungs and pleura. Histological features do not correlate with clinical behaviour {787,888}, although the rare tumours that progress with an undifferentiated round cell morphology pursue an aggressive course {787}.

Sclerosing epithelioid fibrosarcoma

L.-G. Kindblom
F. Mertens
J.-M. Coindre
J.L. Hornick
J.M. Meis

Definition
Sclerosing epithelioid fibrosarcoma (SEF) is a rare, distinctive malignant fibroblastic neoplasm characterized by epithelioid fibroblasts arranged in distinct cords and nests in a densely sclerotic, hyalinized stroma. A subset of SEF appears to be related to low-grade fibromyxoid sarcoma.

ICD-O code   8840/3

Epidemiology
SEF occurs primarily in middle-aged and elderly patients. There is no clear difference in incidence between males and females {1819}.

Sites of involvement
SEF is a deep-seated tumour, most commonly affecting the lower extremity or limb girdle, followed by the upper extremity, shoulder region, trunk, and head and neck areas {82,878,1819}. Rare cases occur in the pelvis, retroperitoneum, viscera or bone {113,1054,2907}.

Clinical features
Most patients present with a mass of variable duration; one third have a history of recent enlargement and pain {1819}. Imaging studies are helpful for preoperative evaluation of tumour extent {459}.

Macroscopy
SEF is typically well circumscribed, lobular or multinodular and involves deep musculature with frequent periosteal attachment. Occasional erosion of underlying bone occurs. The cut surface is predominantly firm and white. Areas of calcification are often seen. Most tumours are < 10 cm in size, although some of > 20 cm have been reported {82,1819}.

Histopathology
At low magnification, SEF appears well delineated, but lacks encapsulation and frequently shows areas with infiltration of muscle, fascia or periosteum. Peripheral tumour nodules surrounded by clefts, suggestive of angiolymphatic invasion are often seen. The hallmark of SEF is the prominent hyalinized, sclerotic collagen matrix that is associated with small epithelioid bland cells arranged in distinct cords, nests and clusters. Occasionally, tumour cells are arranged in a pseudoalveolar or acinar-like pattern. SEF may have rare foci with more prominent pleomorphism, focal necrosis and readily identifiable mitoses, although most have a very low mitotic rate. Paucicellular, myxoid or sclerotic, fibroma-like zones are common. Chondro-osseous foci and calcifications may also be seen. Some SEF contain relatively small areas of more conventional low-grade fibrosarcoma or minor areas closely resembling low-grade fibromyxoid sarcoma, with transition to higher-grade fibrosarcoma, particularly in recurrent tumours {82,794,878, 1819}.

Immunophenotype
Up to 70% of SEF cases are MUC4-positive {696}. Focal positivity for EMA and S100 protein may be seen. Staining for keratins, CD34, SMA, and desmin is typically negative {680,878,1819}.

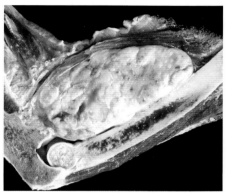

Fig.3.105 Deep, large sclerosing epithelioid fibrosarcoma of the upper arm.

Ultrastructure
Despite the distinct epithelioid features seen under light microscope, the tumour cells of SEF have the ultrastructural features of fibroblasts, with prominent Golgi zones, well-developed rough endoplasmic reticulum and perinuclear whorls of intermediate filaments. The extracellular matrix may be indistinguishable from osteoid {680,794,1819}.

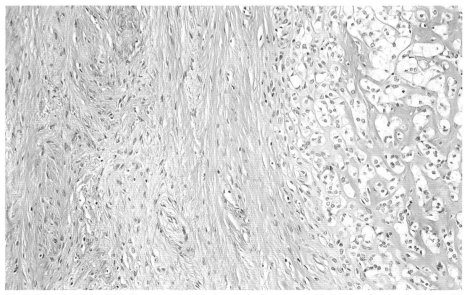

Fig. 3.106 Sclerosing epithelioid sarcoma showing abrupt transition to areas with features of low-grade fibromyxoid sarcoma (left). Shared molecular pathogenesis has been seen in a small subset of cases.

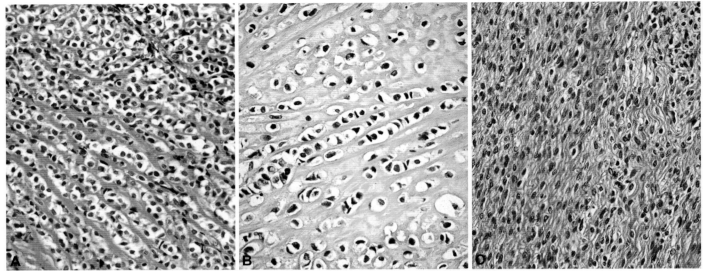

Fig. 3.107 Sclerosing epithelioid fibrosarcoma. **A, B** Typical nested, corded and pseudoalveolar growth patterns and prominent sclerotic collagen matrix. **C** Area of low-grade, conventional fibrosarcoma.

Genetics

Genetic information regarding SEF is limited. The three reported abnormal karyotypes all differ, but two share a rearrangement of band 10p11 {980,2100}. The t(7;16)(q33;p11), resulting in a *FUS-CREB3L2* fusion gene characteristic of low-grade fibromyxoid sarcoma, has been detected in low-grade fibromyxoid sarcoma with SEF-like foci, including four cases with exon 5, 6 or 7 of *FUS* joined with exon 5 or 6 of *CREB3L2* {696,740, 1059,2324}, leading some authors to postulate a potential relationship between SEF and low-grade fibromyxoid sarcoma. However, *FUS* rearrangement has been detected in only 2 of 22 cases of "pure" SEF by others {2902}.

Prognostic factors

SEF are prone to recur (> 50% of cases), sometimes on multiple occasions. Metastasis, reported in 40–80% of cases, has been reported in lung, pleura, bone and brain {82,1819}. Poor prognostic factors are large tumour size, proximal location, possibly male sex, and metastasis {1819}.

CHAPTER 4

So-called fibrohistiocytic tumours

Tenosynovial giant cell tumour, localized type

Tenosynovial giant cell tumour, diffuse type

Deep benign fibrous histiocytoma

Plexiform fibrohistiocytic tumour

Giant cell tumour of soft tissue

Tenosynovial giant cell tumour, localized type

N. de Saint Aubain Somerhausen
M. van de Rijn

Definition

The term "giant cell tumour of tendon sheath" encompasses a family of lesions most often arising from the synovium of joints, bursae and tendon sheaths {1314}. These tumours are usually divided according to their site (intra- or extra-articular) and growth pattern (localized or diffuse) into two main subtypes, which differ in their clinical features and biological behaviour, but appear to share a common pathogenesis. This family of lesions includes the localized giant cell tumour of tendon sheath/tenosynovial giant cell tumour, and the more diffuse and destructive variant called diffuse-type giant cell tumour/pigmented villonodular synovitis. The localized type of giant cell tumour of tendon sheath is a benign neoplasm composed of synovial-like mononuclear cells, accompanied by a variable number of multinucleate osteoclast-like cells, foam cells, siderophages and inflammatory cells, most commonly occurring in the digits.

ICD-O code 9252/0

Synonyms

Giant cell tumour of tendon sheath; nodular tenosynovitis

Epidemiology

The localized form is frequent and the most common subset of giant cell tumours. Tumours may occur at any age, but usually between 30 and 50 years, with a 2 : 1 female predominance {2824}.

Etiology

Tenosynovial giant cell tumours initially were regarded as an inflammatory process on the basis of animal models, the common history of trauma, the tendency to occur on the first three fingers of the right hand {1929} and one X-chromosome inactivation study suggesting polyclonality {2884}. However, the finding of aneuploidy in some cases {4}, the demonstration of clonal chromosomal abnormalities {533, 2052,2495,2942}, and the fact that these lesions are capable of autonomous growth are evidence of neoplastic origin.

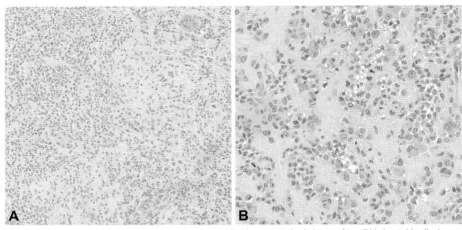

Fig. 4.01 Tenosynovial giant cell tumour, localized type, showing a typical admixture of small histiocytoid cells, larger epithelioid cells and osteoclastic giant cells. A In some cases, giant cells are scanty. B Mitotic figures are commonly seen.

Sites of involvement

Localized giant cell tumours occur predominantly in the hand. Approximately 85% of the tumours occur in the fingers, in close proximity to the synovium of the tendon sheath or interphalangeal joint. The lesions may rarely erode the nearby bone {2823}, or rarely involve the skin. Other sites include the wrist, ankle/foot, knee, and very rarely the elbow and the hip {1929,2824}. Intra-articular lesions, mostly in the knee, are recognized and should be distinguished from the diffuse type.

Clinical features

The most common presenting symptom is that of a painless swelling. The tumours develop gradually over a long period and a preoperative duration of several years is often mentioned. Antecedent trauma is reported in a variable number of cases (1–50%) {1929,2824}. Radiological studies usually demonstrate a well-circumscribed soft tissue mass, with occasional degenerative changes of the adjacent joint or pressure erosion of the adjacent bone {1342}.

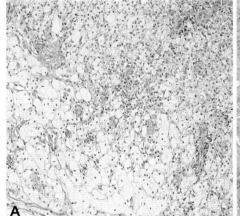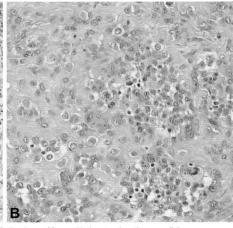

Fig. 4.02 Tenosynovial giant cell tumour, localized type. A Collections of foamy histiocytes (xanthoma cells) are common. B Occasional cases are composed of a predominance of large mononuclear cells with vesicular nuclei.

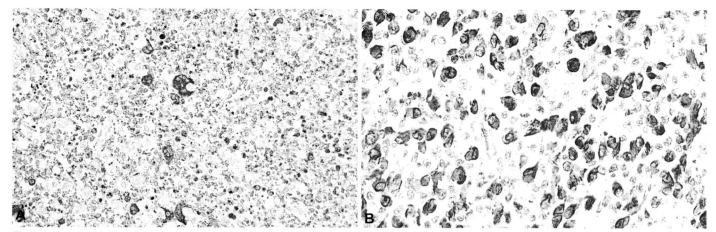

Fig. 4.03 Tenosynovial giant cell tumour, localized type. **A** Localized tumours are usually CD68-positive. **B** Some cases of both localized and diffuse type contain numerous desmin-positive mononuclear cells, sometimes with dendritic cytoplasmic processes.

Macroscopy

Grossly, most tenovial giant cell tumours of localized type are small (0.5–4 cm), although lesions of greater size may be found in large joints. Tumours are well circumscribed and typically lobulated, white to grey with yellowish and brown areas.

Histopathology

Tumours are lobulated, well circumscribed and at least partially covered by a fibrous capsule. Their microscopic appearance is variable, depending on the proportion of mononuclear cells, multinucleate giant cells, foamy macrophages, siderophages and the amount of stroma. Osteoclast-like giant cells, which contain a variable number of nuclei (from 3–4 to > 50), are usually readily apparent, but may be inconspicuous in highly cellular tumours. Most mononuclear cells are small, round to spindle-shaped. They are characterized by pale cytoplasm and round or reniform, often grooved nuclei. They are accompanied by larger epithelioid cells with glassy cytoplasm and rounded vesicular nuclei. Xanthoma cells are frequent, tend to aggregate locally near the periphery of nodules and may be associated with cholesterol clefts. Haemosiderin deposits are virtually always identified. The stroma shows variable degrees of hyalinization and may occasionally have an osteoid-like appearance. Cleft-like spaces are less frequent than in the diffuse form. Mitotic activity usually averages 3–5 mitoses per 10 HPF but may reach up to 20 per 10 HPF. Focal necrosis is rarely seen {2824}.

Immunophenotype

The larger mononuclear cells express clusterin, and in 45–80% of cases a small subset of these cells stains for desmin, which highlights their dendritic processes. Rarely, there are numerous desmin-positive cells, thereby mimicking rhabdomyosarcoma {894}. The smaller histiocyte-like cells are positive for CD68, CD163 and CD45. Multinucleate giant cells display an osteoclastic phenotype; they express CD68, CD45 and markers such as tartrate-resistant acid phosphatase {263,2736}.

Ultrastructure

Ultrastructural studies have revealed a heterogeneous cell population composed of a majority of histiocyte-like cells, accompanied by fibroblast-like cells, intermediate cells, foam cells and multinucleate giant cells {43,894,2824}.

Genetics

Cytogenetic studies have demonstrated relatively simple structural changes, most frequently translocations involving chromosome 1. The translocations of chromosome 1 involve the *CSF1* gene, encoding colony stimulating factor 1; the aberration is present in only a small subset of the tumoral cells. The translocation, most frequently with *COL6A3* on chromosome 2, results in high levels of CSF1 expression in the neoplastic cells, which attracts large numbers of macrophages to the tumour site {2942}. The presence of these numerous macrophages explains the failure of studies of X-chromosome inactivation to demonstrate clonality. A significant number of cases contain a fusion between *CSF1* and an as-yet-unidentified gene, distinct from *COL6A3* {533}.

Prognostic factors

Tenovial giant cell tumour of localized type is a benign lesion with a capacity for local recurrence. While 4–30% of cases recur {1942,2301,2318,2969}, these recurrences are usually non-destructive and are controlled by surgical re-excision.

Tenosynovial giant cell tumour, diffuse type

N. de Saint Aubain Somerhausen
M. van de Rijn

Definition

Tenosynovial giant cell tumour of diffuse type is a locally aggressive neoplasm composed of synovial-like mononuclear cells, admixed with multinucleate giant cells, foam cells, siderophages and inflammatory cells, which may be intra-articular or extra-articular. The very uncommon malignant tenovial giant cell tumour is defined by the coexistence of a benign giant cell tumour with overtly malignant areas or by recurrence of a typical giant cell tumour as a sarcoma.

ICD-O code

Tenosynovial giant cell tumour,
  diffuse type   9252/1
Tenosynovial giant cell tumour,
  diffuse type, malignant   9252/3

Synonyms

Diffuse-type giant cell tumour; pigmented villonodular synovitis; pigmented villonodular tenosynovitis

Epidemiology

Tenosynovial giant cell tumours of diffuse type tend to affect younger patients than their localized counterpart. The age of patients varies widely, but most lesions affect young adults, aged < 40 years. There is a slight female predominance {1988,2141, 2597}.

Etiology

See *Tenosynovial giant cell tumour, localized type*

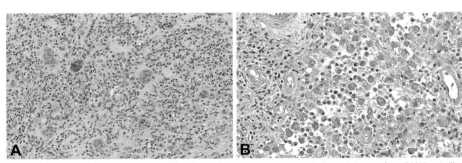

Fig. 4.04 Tenosynovial giant cell tumour, diffuse type. **A** Tumours are composed of an admixture of small histiocyte-like cells with cleaved nuclei, larger epithelioid cells with vesicular nuclei and osteoclast-like giant cells. **B** The cytoplasm of the large epithelioid cells often contains a peripheral rim of haemosiderin granules.

Sites of involvement

Intra-articular lesions affect predominantly the knee (75% of cases), followed by the hip (15%), ankle, elbow and shoulder. Rare cases are reported in the temporomandibular and spinal facet joints {973, 2141,2482}. Extra-articular tumours most commonly involve the knee region, thigh and foot. Uncommon locations include the finger, wrist, groin, elbow and toe {112,1983,2597}. Most extra-articular tumours are located in periarticular soft tissues, but these lesions can be purely intramuscular or predominantly subcutaneous {2597}.

Clinical features

Patients complain of pain, tenderness, swelling or limitation of motion. Haemorrhagic joint effusions are common. The symptoms are usually of relatively long duration (often several years) {1983}.

Radiographically, most tumours present as ill-defined peri-articular masses, frequently associated with degenerative joint disease and cystic lesions in the adjacent bone (often on both sides of the joint) {687,1983}. On MRI, giant cell tumours show decreased signal intensity in both T1- and T2-weighted images, with artefacts from haemosiderin deposition {1325,1983}.

Macroscopy

Diffuse-type tenosynovial giant cell tumours are usually large (often > 5 cm), firm or sponge-like. The typical villous pattern of so-called pigmented villonodular synovitis is usually lacking in extra-articular tumours. The latter have a multi-nodular appearance and a variegated colour, with alternation of white, yellowish and brownish areas {1983}.

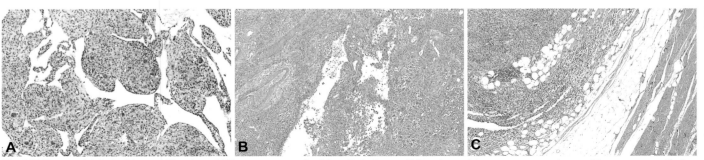

Fig. 4.05 Tenosynovial giant cell tumour, diffuse type. **A** Villous appearance of an intra-articular tumour. **B** Pseudosynovial spaces are commonly seen. **C** Low-power magnification of a completely extra-articular tumour showing infiltration of the muscular and adipose tissue.

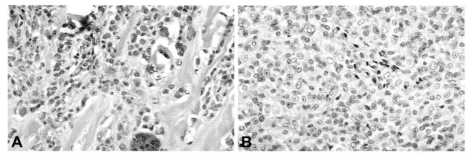

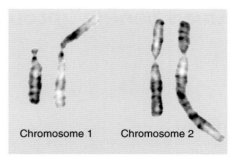

Chromosome 1   Chromosome 2

Fig. 4.06 Malignant tenosynovial giant cell tumour, diffuse type. **A** There is usually at least focal morphological overlap with usual giant cell tumour. **B** However, closer examination reveals increased cellularity and predominance of atypical large cells with prominent nucleoli.

Fig. 4.07 Tenosynovial giant cell tumour. Partial karyotype showing the characteristic t(1;2)(p13;q37) translocation. Arrows indicate breakpoints.

Histopathology

Most tumours are infiltrative and grow as diffuse, expansile sheets. Their cellularity is variable: compact areas alternate with pale, loose, discohesive zones. Cleft-like spaces are common and appear either as artefactual tears or as synovial-lined spaces. Blood-filled pseudoalveolar spaces are seen in approximately 10% of cases. Compared with the localized form, osteoclastic giant cells are less common and may be absent or extremely rare in up to 20% of cases. They are irregularly distributed throughout the lesions and are more easily found around haemorrhagic foci. The mononuclear component comprises two types of cells: small histiocyte-like cells, which represent the main cellular component, and larger cells. Histiocyte-like cells are ovoid or spindle-shaped, with palely eosinophilic cyto- plasm. Their nuclei are small, ovoid or angulated, contain fine chromatin, small nucleoli and frequently display longitudinal grooves. Larger cells are rounded or sometimes show dendritic cytoplasmic processes. Their cytoplasm is abundant, pale to deeply amphophilic, often contains a peripheral rim of haemosiderin granules and occasionally shows a paranuclear eosinophilic filamentous inclusion. Nuclei are characterized by reniform or lobulated shape, thick nuclear membranes, vesicular

chromatin and eosinophilic nuclei. The occasional predominance of these larger cells may obscure the typical features of giant cell tumour and lead to a diagnosis of sarcoma. Sheets of foam cells are frequently observed, usually in the periphery of lesions and variable amounts of haemosiderin are identified in most cases. Giant cell tumours may also contain a significant lymphocytic infiltrate. The stroma shows variable degrees of fibrosis and may appear hyalinized, although this is usually less marked than in the localized form. Mitoses are usually identifiable and mitotic activity of > 5 per 10 HPF is not uncommon {1983, 2597,2824}.

There have been several reports of typical giant cell tumours recurring as histologically malignant neoplasms and a few series included primary histologically malignant tenosynovial tumours of the tendon sheath resembling giant cell tumours {216,1604,2033,2597}. These neoplasms tended to show significantly increased mitotic rate (> 20 mitoses per 10 HPF), necrosis, enlarged nuclei with nucleoli, spindling of mononucleated cells, the presence of abundant eosinophilic cytoplasm in histiocyte-like cells, and stromal myxoid change, although none of these features could be used in isolation as a criterion for malignancy {216,1604,2597}. In addition, rare cases with banal histology

that developed metastatic disease (in the lungs or lymph nodes) have been reported {2597,2928}.

Immunophenotype
See *Tenosynovial giant cell tumour, localized type*

Genetics
See *Tenosynovial giant cell tumour, localized type*

Prognostic factors
Recurrences are common, often multiple and may severely compromise joint function. The recurrence rate has been estimated at 18–46% for intra-articular lesions and 33–50% for extra-articular tumours {216,2141,2482,2824}.

The risk of recurrence does not seem to be correlated with any histological parameter other than positive excision margins. Therefore, tenosynovial giant cell tumours of diffuse type should be regarded as locally aggressive but non-metastasizing neoplasms and wide excision is the treatment of choice. Although the number of cases is limited, malignant tenosynovial giant cell tumour showing obvious sarcomatous areas is potentially aggressive and may give rise to pulmonary metastasis {216,2033,2597}.

Deep benign fibrous histiocytoma

C.D.M. Fletcher
B.C. Gleason

Definition
A morphologically benign fibrous histiocytoma that arises entirely within subcutaneous or deep soft tissue and that may rarely metastasize.

ICD-O code   8831/0

Epidemiology
Deep-seated fibrous histiocytomas are rare, comprising < 1% of fibrohistiocytic tumours {857}. Their exact frequency is difficult to determine because some cases published as deep fibrous histiocytomas may represent solitary fibrous tumours {857,990}. They may develop at any age and show a slight predominance in males.

Sites of involvement
The most common site is the extremities, representing more than half of cases, followed by the head and neck region. Most deep fibrous histiocytomas are subcutaneous, but nearly 10% arise in visceral soft tissue (e.g. retroperitoneum, mediastinum, pelvis) {857,990}. Intramuscular tumours are uncommon, and tumours arising in visceral organs are exceedingly rare {2413}.

Clinical features
Most lesions present as a painless, slowly enlarging mass. The clinical impression is often that of a cyst {990}.

Macroscopy
These tumours form well-circumscribed nodules, with a median size of 2.5 cm for subcutaneous lesions. Deep-seated lesions may be larger {990}.

Histopathology
In contrast to their cutaneous counterparts, deep fibrous histiocytomas are well-circumscribed and often have a fibrous pseudocapsule. The lesions are more cellular than typical cutaneous fibrous histiocytomas, but share a storiform architecture. A minority of tumours have a predominantly short fascicular pattern – similar to that seen in cellular fibrous histiocytoma in skin – with only focal storiform areas. Many

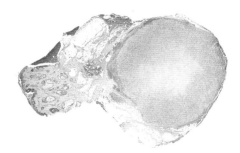

Fig. 4.08 Deep benign fibrous histiocytoma. These lesions arise most often in subcutis and are better circumscribed than their cutaneous counterparts.

lesions have a branching, haemangiopericytoma-like vascular pattern, which may cause confusion with solitary fibrous tumour, particularly when CD34 is expressed (see *Immunophenotype*). Generally, the uniform cellularity and storiform architecture of deep fibrous histiocytoma distinguish the two. The tumour cells are spindled with plump, ovoid to elongated vesicular nuclei and indistinct, palely eosinophilic cytoplasm. Nearly half of deep fibrous histiocytomas are cytologically monomorphic, lacking foamy histiocytes and giant cells. Stromal hyalinization is relatively common; less frequent findings include haemorrhage, myxoid change, cystic degeneration, central infarction and a peripheral lymphoid infiltrate. There is generally no nuclear pleomorphism or hyperchromasia, although rare examples of atypical deep fibrous histiocytoma (akin to atypical cutaneous fibrous histiocytoma) have been reported

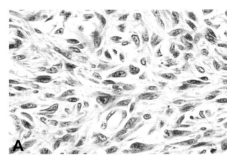

Fig. 4.09 Deep benign fibrous histiocytoma. These lesions show less cytological polymorphism than their dermal counterparts.

{990}. Mitoses typically number < 5 per 10 HPF but may be numerous (> 10 per 10 HPF). Tumour necrosis is rare.

Immunophenotype
Expression of CD34 is far more common in deep fibrous histiocytomas than those in the skin, with 40% of the former expressing this marker, sometimes diffusely {990}. Distinction from solitary fibrous tumour may be difficult. A similar number of cases express SMA, usually focally.

Genetics
A clonal t(16;17)(p13.3;q21.3) was reported in a single case {910}.

Prognostic factors
Deep fibrous histiocytomas recur locally in approximately 20% of cases, usually if incompletely or marginally excised {857, 990}. Rare examples of distant metastasis have been reported {990}.

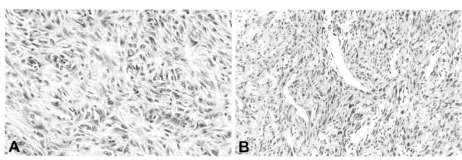

Fig.4.10 Deep benign fibrous histiocytoma. **A** A monomorphic storiform pattern is usually seen. **B** Branching haemangiopericytoma-like vessels are common.

Plexiform fibrohistiocytic tumour

J.C. Fanburg-Smith

Definition
Plexiform fibrohistiocytic tumour (PFHT) is a rarely metastasizing dermal-subcutaneous neoplasm composed of fibroblasts and histiocyte-like cells.

ICD-O code   8835/1

Epidemiology
PFHT preferentially affects children and young adults, with age ranging from birth (congenital presentation) to age 77 years, (median, 14.5–20 years) {759,1944}. Previously thought to be more common in females, {759,2328}, there are more recent data to suggest equal distribution between the sexes {1202,1944}.

Sites of involvement
PFHT most commonly involves the upper extremities {759}, especially forearm {1944}, followed by the lower extremity, trunk, and head and neck.

Clinical features
PFHT usually presents as a small, poorly delineated, painless dermal and subcutaneous mass or plaque that slowly enlarges over months to years. The overlying skin may be raised with a central depression {759}.

Macroscopy
PFHT is a multinodular, firm, poorly circumscribed dermal/subcutaneous interface tumour that can extend into skeletal muscle.

Grossly, it is a grey-white, fibrous or partially mucoid mass that ranges in size from 0.3 to 8.5 cm, but most examples are < 3.0 cm {759,2328}.

Histopathology
PFHT is characterized usually by a mass involving deep dermis/superficial subcutis that often demonstrates a plexiform architecture, with small to medium-sized whorling nodules or short fibroblastic fascicles extending further into subcutis. Three distinct cell types are present in variable proportions: mononuclear epithelioid histiocyte-like cells, spindled (myo)fibroblasts, and often osteoclast-type multinucleate giant cells. This results in several patterns: (i) fibroblast type, spindled and infiltrating, often with lymphocytic inflammation; (ii) histiocytoid type, epithelioid with cannonball nodularity and osteoclast-type giant cells, particularly in areas of haemorrhage; and (iii) mixed pattern. Adnexa are often spared {1944}. Stromal myxoid change, hyalinized collagen or metaplastic bone may be present {759,1944}, and perineural growth may be observed {1944}. Cytological atypia, atypical mitoses, and lymphovascular invasion are rare {759,1944}. Mitotic count is usually low and necrosis is absent. In rare pulmonary metastases, PFHT presents as small fibrohistiocytic nodules in subpleural and peribronchiolar locations {2328}.

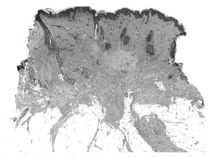

Fig. 4.11 Plexiform fibrohistiocytic tumour is a deep dermal to subcutaneous interface tumour with a plexiform growth pattern of dermal nodules and subcutaneous short fascicles, with predominant histiocytoid cells and/or fibroblastic cells.

Immunophenotype
PFHT displays immunoreactivity for CD68 (KP1) in multinucleated giant cells, and SMA in (myo)fibroblastic cells {1202}. Staining for S100 protein, desmin, and keratins is negative {759,1202,1944}.

Genetics
Only three plexiform fibrohistiocytic tumours with clonal chromosome aberrations have been reported, with no shared chromosome abnormalities found {1582, 2310, 2589}.

Prognostic factors
PFHT has been associated with a 13–38% rate of local recurrence and regional lymph-node metastasis in 6% of two series {759,1202}. Pulmonary metastasis is rare {1944,2328}.

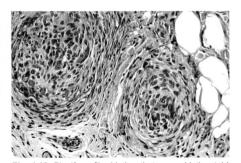

Fig. 4.12 Plexiform fibrohistiocytic tumour, histiocytoid type, with cannonball-like histiocytoid cells mixed with osteoclast-type giant cells, especially in areas of haemorrhage.

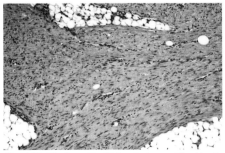

Fig. 4.13 Plexiform fibrohistiocytic tumour, fibroblastic type, with contiguous extension into subcutaneous tissue of spindled fibroblasts.

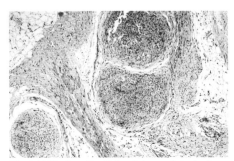

Fig. 4.14 Plexiform fibrohistiocytic tumour, mixed pattern, with ball-like histiocytoid cells and spindled fibroblasts, extending into subcutaneous tissue from dermis.

Giant cell tumour of soft tissue

A.M. Oliveira

Definition
Giant cell tumour of soft tissue (GCT-ST) is a primary soft tissue neoplasm that is clinically and histologically similar to giant cell tumour of bone; it very rarely metastasizes.

ICD-O code   9251/1

Synonyms
Osteoclastoma of soft tissue; giant cell tumour of low malignant potential

Epidemiology
GCT-ST occurs predominantly in the fifth decade of life, but can affect patients ranging in age from 5 to 89 years. GCT-ST shows no difference in incidence with regard to sex or ethnicity {891,2086, 2116}.

Sites of involvement
GCT-ST usually occurs in superficial soft tissues of the upper and lower extremities (70% of tumours). Affected less frequently are the trunk (20%) and head and neck (7%) regions {891,2086,2116,2217,2352}. A mediastinal case has been reported {999}.

Clinical features
The tumours present as painless growing masses {2086,2116} with an average duration of 6 months {2116}. Like giant cell

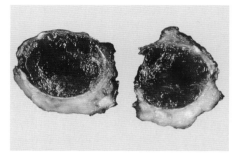

Fig. 4.15 Giant cell tumour of soft tissue presenting as a well-circumscribed, mostly solid, nodule with a fleshy, red-brown or grey cut surface.

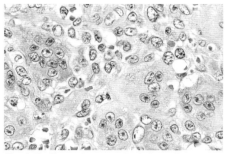

Fig. 4.16 Giant cell tumour of soft tissue. The cellular nodules contain a mixture of round/oval mononuclear and multinucleate osteoclast-like giant cells.

tumour of bone with soft tissue implants {509}, peripheral mineralization is common in GCT-ST, yielding a characteristic radiographic appearance.

Macroscopy
In the three major series of patients with GCT-ST reported to date {891,2086, 2116}, tumours ranged in size from 0.7 to 10 cm (mean, 3 cm). Subcutaneous adipose tissue or dermis was involved in 70% of tumours; 30% were situated deep to superficial fascia. GCT-ST is a well-circumscribed, mostly solid, nodular mass with a fleshy, red-brown or grey cut surface. Gritty regions of mineralized bone are frequently present at the periphery {2086}.

Histopathology
GCT-ST displays a strikingly multinodular architecture (85%), with nodules ranging in size up to 15 mm {2116}. Cellular nodules are separated by fibrous septa of varying thickness containing haemosiderin-laden macrophages {2086}. The nodules are composed of a mixture of round to oval mononuclear cells and osteoclast-like giant cells, with both cell types immersed in a richly vascularized stroma. Mitotic activity generally is present in every GCT-ST; typical mitoses range from 1 to 30 figures per 10 HPF {891,2086, 2116}. Atypia, nuclear pleomorphism and bizarre giant cells are absent, and necrosis is rarely found {891,2086,2116}. Metaplastic bone formation is present in

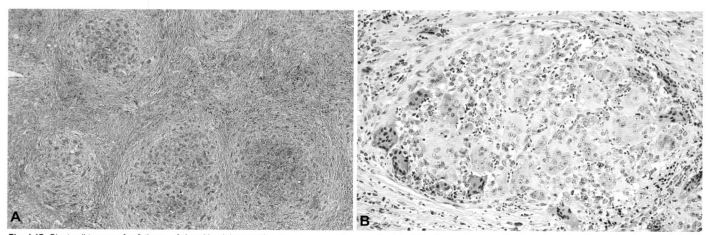

Fig. 4.17 Giant cell tumour of soft tissue. **A** A multinodular growth pattern is present in approximately 85% of these tumours. **B** A typical nodule with peripheral accumulation of osteoclast-like giant cells.

approximately 50% of tumours, frequently in the form of a peripheral shell of woven bone. Secondary cystic change and the formation of blood-filled lakes similar to aneurysmal bone cyst are present in approximately 30% of tumours. Vascular invasion is identified in about 30% of tumours {891,2116}. Additional histological features include stromal haemorrhage (50%) and regressive changes in the form of marked stromal fibrosis and clusters of foamy macrophages (70%).

Immunophenotype
GCT-ST displays immunoreactivity for CD68 and SMA {891,2086,2116}. CD68 is expressed by multinucleated giant cells; the mononuclear cells show focal expression only. SMA is expressed by a few mononuclear cells, but not the multinucleated giant cells. The mononuclear component expresses RANKL (ligand for receptor activator for nuclear factor kappa B), an important factor for osteoclastic recruitment and differentiation {1564}.

Genetics
Like giant cell tumour of bone, cytogenetic analysis of a single example showed multiple telomeric associations {1064}.

Prognostic factors
With follow-up of 3–4 years, GCT-ST is associated with a local recurrence rate of 12% and very rare cases of metastasis or death {891,2086,2116}. Incomplete surgical excision is associated with an increased risk for local recurrence. No clinicopathological factors are currently predictive of metastatic behaviour {891, 2086, 2116}.

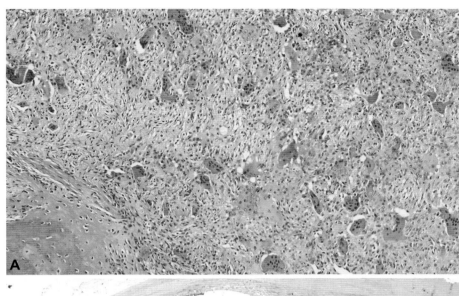

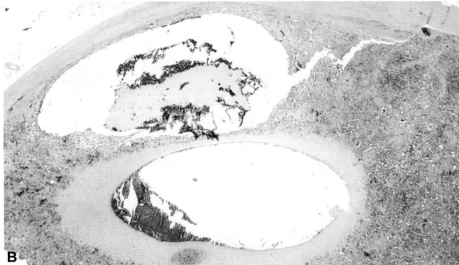

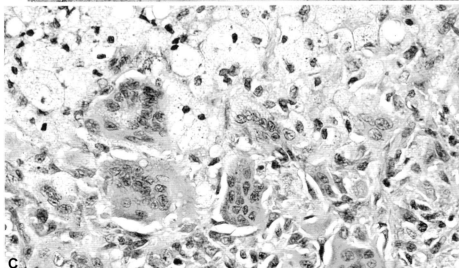

Fig. 4.18 Giant cell tumour of soft tissue. **A** Secondary cystic changes, similar to aneurysmal bone cystic changes, occur in approximately 30% of these tumours. **B** Metaplastic bone, frequently in the form of a peripheral shell of woven bone, is present in approximately 50% of tumours. **C** Clusters of foam macrophages reflecting regressive change.

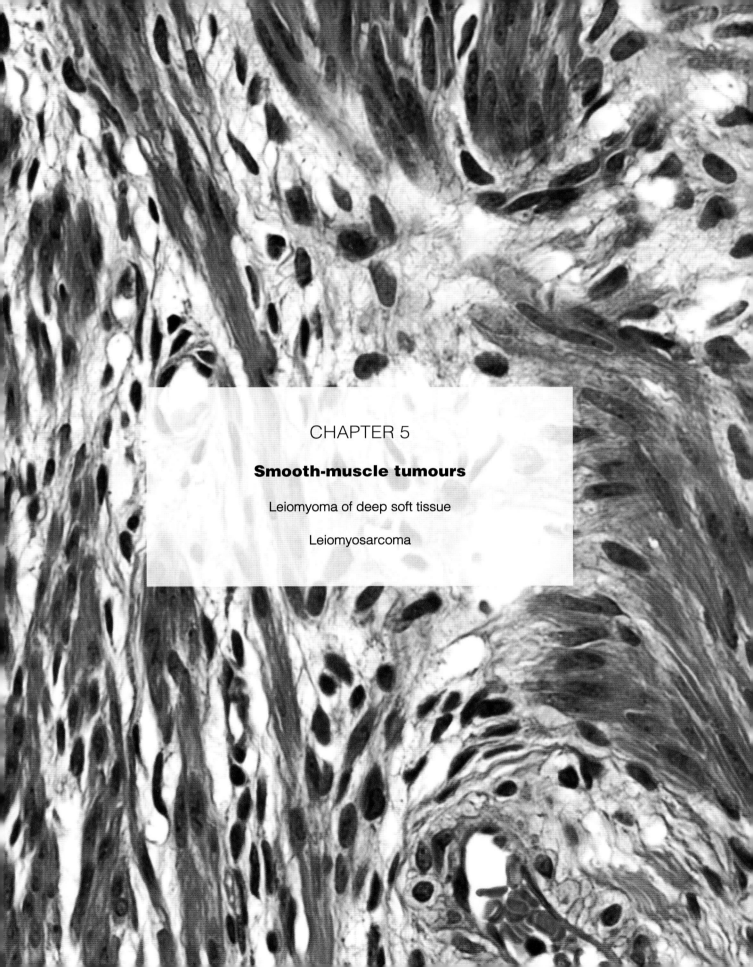

CHAPTER 5

Smooth-muscle tumours

Leiomyoma of deep soft tissue

Leiomyosarcoma

Leiomyoma of deep soft tissue

M.M. Miettinen
B. Quade

Definition

A rare type of leiomyoma that occurs in deep soft tissue in the retroperitoneum or abdominal cavity, mostly in women.

ICD-O code   8890/0

Epidemiology

Leiomyomas of the retroperitoneum or abdominal cavity occur almost exclusively in women, mostly in young adulthood or middle age {235,2147}. The very rare leiomyomas in deep peripheral soft tissue occur with equal frequency in men and women {1411}.

Sites of involvement

The vast majority of deep leiomyomas occur in the retroperitoneum and different parts of the abdominal cavity, such as the mesentery, omentum and in the abdominal wall. Similar tumours also occur in the inguinal region where they may originate from the round ligament. Occurrence in peripheral soft tissues is very rare.

Clinical features

These tumours may become very large and, in some patients, may be multiple. Calcifications may be detected radiographically.

Macroscopy

Leiomyomas of the abdomen and retroperitoneum form circumscribed, grey-white firm masses that may have mucoid or focal cystic change and that vary from a small nodule to >30 cm in size {235,2147}. Peripheral leiomyomas are

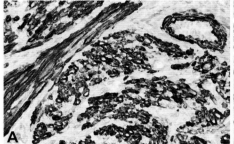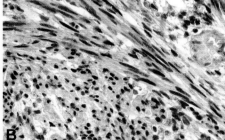

Fig. 5.01 Leiomyoma of deep soft tissue. There is strong immunoreactivity for h-caldesmon (similar to desmin and SMA) (**A**) and estrogen receptor (similar to WT1) (**B**).

grossly grey-white or yellowish in colour, with the greatest diameter of 11 leiomyomas reported from the deep somatic soft tissue ranging from 2.5 to 15 cm (mean, 7.7 cm) {1411}.

Histopathology

Leiomyomas of deep soft tissue and abdomen are composed of intersecting fascicles of spindled to slightly epithelioid cells that closely resemble normal smooth muscle cells with eosinophilic cytoplasm and uniform blunt-ended, cigar-shaped nuclei. There is no significant nuclear atypia and, at most, very low mitotic activity. In limb lesions and intra-abdominal lesions in males, mitoses number < 1 per 50 HPF. In peritoneal/retroperitoneal lesions in females (showing positivity for hormonal receptors) mitoses may number up to 5 per 50 HPF. Most lesions are paucicellular, and degenerative or regressive changes, such as fibrosis, calcification and myxoid change, are common in large lesions. Abdominal, retroperitoneal

and inguinal leiomyomas in women show a spectrum of patterns similar to uterine leiomyomas, with macro- and microtrabecular organization, hyalinization and focal myxoid or cystic change. Focal epithelioid or clear cell change, metaplastic bone, and fatty differentiation may also occur {1812}. The presence of focal nuclear atypia should prompt a careful search for mitoses and additional sampling, because some leiomyosarcomas can show only focal atypia and have very low mitotic activity. Peripheral deep soft-tissue smooth-muscle tumours should be approached with great caution and the possibility of metastasis from a uterine or soft tissue leiomyosarcoma should be considered in the differential diagnosis.

Immunophenotype

Tumour cells are positive for SMA, desmin (80% of cases) and h-caldesmon, but negative for S100 protein. Abdominal, retroperitoneal, and inguinal leiomyomas in women are almost uniformly positive

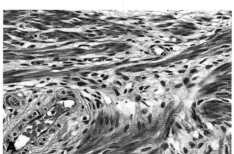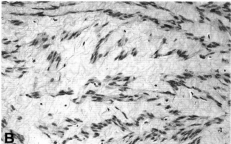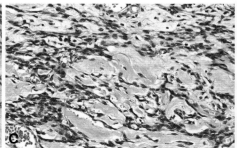

Fig. 5.02 Leiomyoma of deep soft tissue showing trabecular, myxoid, and hyalinizing features (**A**, **B**, **C**).

for estrogen and progesterone receptors and WT1 {235,2147,2197}. Deep leiomyomas occuring in the abdomen or retroperitoneum of women represent an estrogen receptor-positive subset of smooth muscle tumours analogous to uterine and pelvic leiomyomas. Peripheral leiomyomas {1411} or retroperitoneal leiomyosarcomas {2147} do not usually express these hormone-receptor proteins or WT1.

Prognostic factors
Tumours categorized as leiomyomas of deep soft tissue are usually cured by complete excision. Long-term follow-up has revealed non-destructive local recurrences in up to 10% of patients with retroperitoneal leiomyomas, but no progressive disease or metastases {235,2147}.

Leiomyosarcoma

A. Lazar
H.L. Evans
J. Shipley

Definition
Leiomyosarcoma is a malignant neoplasm showing pure smooth-muscle differentiation.

ICD-O code   8890/3

Epidemiology
Soft tissue leiomyosarcoma usually occurs in middle-aged or older persons, although it may develop in young adults and even in children {605}. Leiomyosarcoma forms a significant percentage of retroperitoneal (including pelvic) sarcomas {1129,2289,2547,2964} and is the predominant sarcoma arising from larger blood vessels {194,1404,1549,1596,2856}. Aside from these locations, it is less common, accounting for 10–15% of limb sarcomas {1752}.
Women constitute the clear majority of patients with retroperitoneal and inferior vena cava leiomyosarcomas, but not among patients with tumours at other sites.

Sites of involvement
The most common location of soft tissue leiomyosarcoma is the retroperitoneum, including the pelvis. Another distinctive subgroup arises in large blood vessels, most commonly the inferior vena cava, its major tributaries, and the large veins of the lower extremity. Leiomyosarcomas involving nonretroperitoneal soft tissue sites constitute a third group {541,761,817, 1127,2663}. These are found most frequently in the lower extremity, but may develop elsewhere. Tumours occur at intramuscular and subcutaneous localizations in approximately equal proportions, and some originate from a small to medium-sized vein.

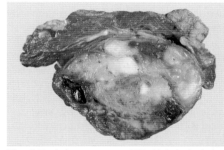

Fig. 5.03 Leiomyosarcoma. This high-grade lesion (19 cm) from the quadriceps muscle shows extensive necrosis and haemorrhage.

Clinical features
Leiomyosarcoma of the soft tissue generally presents as a mass lesion. Retroperitoneal tumours may be painful. The symptoms produced by leiomyosarcoma of the inferior vena cava depend on the portion involved. In the upper portion, it obstructs the hepatic veins and can evince Budd-Chiari syndrome, with hepatomegaly, jaundice, and ascites. Location in the middle portion may result in blockage of the renal veins and consequent renal dysfunction, while involvement of the lower portion may cause leg oedema. Imaging studies of leiomyosarcoma are nonspecific, but helpful in delineating the relationship to adjacent structures, particularly in the retroperitoneum.

Macroscopy
Leiomyosarcoma of soft tissue typically

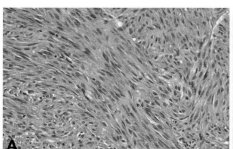 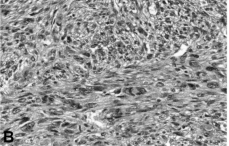

Fig. 5.04 Leiomyosarcoma. **A** This lesion shows distinctively well-differentiated histology. **B** Moderately differentiated features can be seen in this example.

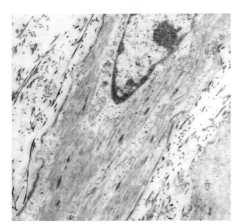

Fig. 5.05 Leiomyosarcoma. Tumour cells contain prominent longitudinal filament bundles with focal densities. Note also the external lamina.

forms a fleshy, grey to white to tan mass. A whorled appearance may be evident. Larger examples often display haemorrhage, necrosis, or cystic change. The tumour border frequently appears well-circumscribed, although obvious infiltration may also be found.

Histopathology

The typical histological pattern of leiomyosarcoma is that of intersecting, sharply marginated fascicles of spindle cells. This pattern may be less well-defined in some tumours, and occasionally there is a focal storiform, palisaded, or haemangiopericytoma-like arrangement. The tumours are usually compactly cellular, but fibrosis or myxoid change may be present. Hyalinized, hypocellular zones and coagulative tumour necrosis are frequent in larger leiomyosarcomas. The tumour-cell nuclei are characteristically elongated and blunt-ended and may be indented or lobated. Nuclear hyperchromasia and pleomorphism are generally notable, although they may be focal, mild, or occasionally absent. Mitotic figures can usually be found readily, although they may be few; atypical mitoses are often seen. The cytoplasm varies from typically brightly eosinophilic to pale, and in the former instance is often distinctly fibrillar. Epithelioid cytomorphology, multinucleated osteoclast-like giant cells {1832}, very prominent acute or chronic inflammatory cells {1848}, and granular cytoplasmic change {2066} are unusual findings that are normally present in only part of a tumour when identified. Occasional soft tissue leiomyosarcomas contain areas with a nonspecific, poorly differentiated,

pleomorphic appearance in addition to typical areas {2090}. These could be regarded as "dedifferentiated leiomyosarcoma" {435, 2032}. Rarely, an osteosarcomatous or rhabdomyosarcomatous component can be seen.

Immunophenotype

SMA, desmin and h-caldesmon are positive in a great majority (> 70%) of leiomyosarcomas. However, none of these is absolutely specific for smooth muscle, and positivity for two of these markers is more supportive than positivity for one alone. "Dedifferentiated" areas are negative for SMA and desmin {435}. Stains that may be positive, at least focally, include keratin, EMA, CD34, and S100 protein. CD117 (KIT) is typically negative. In general, the diagnosis of leiomyosarcoma should not be made on the basis of immunostains in the absence of appropriate morphological features.

Ultrastructure

Soft tissue leiomyosarcomas usually demonstrate at least some of the ultrastructural features of normal smooth muscle cells, namely bundles of cytoplasmic microfilaments with focal densities, cell junctions, pinocytotic vesicles, variable numbers of mitochondria, and discontinuous basement membrane.

Genetics

Karyotypes of soft tissue leiomyosarcomas are usually highly complex with genomic instability (http://www.ncbi.nlm.nih.gov/cancerchromosomes) {1449,2901} and often associated with defects in *TP53* or sometimes *FANCA* {173} and *ATM* {2814}. Frequent regions of chromosomal loss and, less frequently, gain have been reported {1718,2901,3020}.

Predisposition to tumours including leiomyosarcoma is found in the Li-Fraumeni syndrome, which is associated with

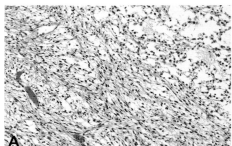
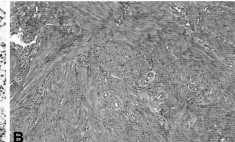

Fig. 5.06 Leiomyosarcoma. A This view shows the myxoid and reticular appearance. B The lesion is composed of nodules and bundles of eosinophilic spindle cells.

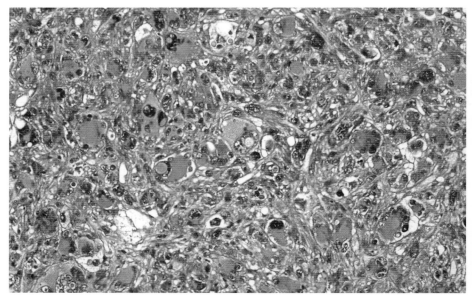

Fig. 5.07 Leiomyosarcoma with poorly differentiated features. To determine the diagnosis, the presence of areas more typical of leiomyosarcoma or very characteristic immunohistochemical results would be needed.

germline defects in *TP53* {2098}. *TP53* is mutated in about 25% of sporadic leiomyosarcomas and 50% of samples present with biallelic *TP53* inactivation {2221,2254}. There is frequent involvement of the retinoblastoma-cyclin D pathway with genomic loss at 13q14 centred on the *RB1* gene {626,2667}. Loss at 9p21 or promoter hypermethylation results in low expression of variously spliced *CDK2NA* transcripts that encode ARF and inhibitors of CDK4 {1380}. Loss of the 10q region that affects the *PTEN* tumour suppressor gene is a frequent alteration in leiomyosarcomas.

Myocardin (*MYOCD*) on 17p is amplified in about 70% of cases and encodes a smooth muscle-specific transcriptional co-activator {949,1418,2222}. Similarly, micro-RNAs show patterns of expression resembling those in smooth muscle and in mesenchymal stem cells {566}. Analysis of several gene-expression profiling datasets suggest that there are multiple molecular subgroups of leiomyosarcoma, including a "muscle-enriched" subtype, and less differentiated groupings with indications of differing frequencies of specific genomic changes and varying prognoses {173,443,975,2045}. Interestingly, some tumours classified as undifferentiated pleomorphic sarcoma cluster closely with a subset of leiomyosarcomas, suggesting similarity and perhaps supporting the existence of "dedifferentiated" leiomyosarcoma {173,640,975,1544,1590, 1904,2045,2504}.

Expression of ROR2 (receptor tyrosine kinase-like orphan receptor 2) has been shown to play a role in the invasiveness of leiomyosarcoma (gynaecological and non-gynaecological) in vitro and is predictive of a poor clinical outcome {723}.

Prognostic factors

Leiomyosarcomas of soft tissue are capable of both local recurrence and distant metastasis. The most important prognostic factors are tumour location and size, which are strongly interrelated. Retroperitoneal leiomyosarcomas are fatal in the great majority of cases; they are typically

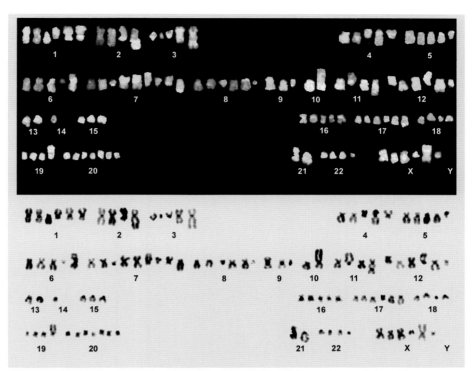

Fig. 5.08 A 24-colour karyotype and corresponding reverse DAPI-banded image from a soft tissue leiomyosarcoma; there are multiple copies of chromosomes and many rearrangements.

large (> 10 cm), often difficult or impossible to excise with clear margins, and prone to both local recurrence and metastasis. Leiomyosarcomas of large vessels also tend to have a poor prognosis, although local control rates are higher, except for those in the upper inferior vena cava, and very small examples (1–2 cm) may be less prone to metastasize. Non-retroperitoneal leiomyosarcomas are generally smaller than those in the retroperitoneum, more amenable to local control, and have a better prognosis. In some studies, intramuscular rather than subcutaneous location {1127} and larger tumour size {817,1917} were related to increased metastasis and poorer survival. Histological grading as well as osseous and vascular involvement are other reliable prognostic indicators. Leiomyosarcoma is the commonest sarcoma giving rise to metastases to skin; soft tissue and bone metastases are also seen {2903}.

Smooth muscle tumours in immunocompromised patients

Smooth muscle tumours in immunocompromised individuals form a distinctive subgroup. These usually involve parenchymal organs rather than soft tissue, occur predominantly in children and young adults who are HIV-positive or post-transplant, and are associated with EBV infection {413,1779,2278,2846}. Most cases are truly multicentric, based on independent EBV infection rather than metastasis {654,2599}. Histologically, they are relatively bland but can have a primitive-appearing round cell component. They show variable mitotic activity, a variable lymphocytic infiltrate and sometimes show a perivascular growth pattern, overlapping with similar myopericytic lesions. SMA reactivity is uniform, but desmin is less often expressed {654}. These tumours appear to behave better than conventional leiomyosarcoma in most cases.

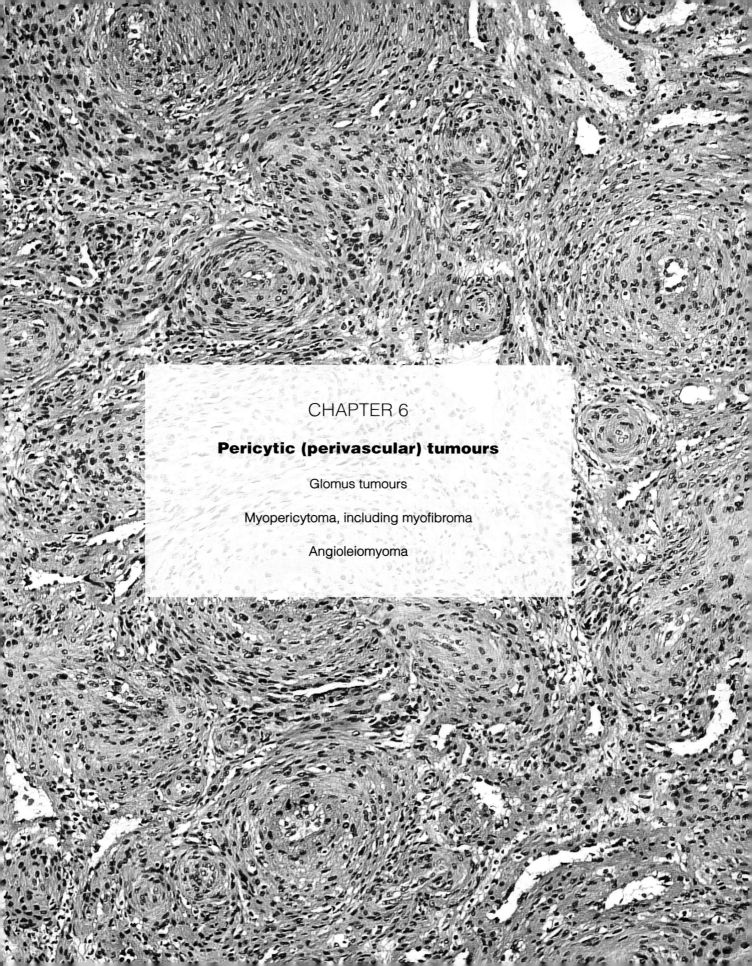

CHAPTER 6

Pericytic (perivascular) tumours

Glomus tumours

Myopericytoma, including myofibroma

Angioleiomyoma

Glomus tumours

A.L. Folpe
H. Brems
E. Legius

Definition
Glomus tumours are mesenchymal neo-plasms composed of cells resembling the modified smooth muscle cells of the normal glomus body.

ICD-O code
Glomus tumour	8711/0
Glomangiomatosis	8711/1
Malignant glomus tumour	8711/3

Synonyms
Glomangioma; glomangiomyoma; glomu-venous malformation

Epidemiology
Glomus tumours are rare, accounting for < 2% of soft tissue tumours {2548}. Multiple lesions may be seen in 10% of patients. Most are diagnosed in young adults, but may occur at any age.
Glomus tumours occur with equal frequency in men and women, except for subungual lesions, which are far more common in women {2704,2844}. Histologically, malignant glomus tumours are exceedingly rare and clinically malignant ones rarer still. Fewer than 40 histologically and/or clinically malignant tumours have

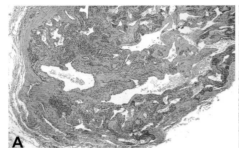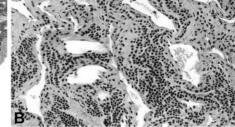

Fig. 6.01 Glomovenous malformation. **A** The lesion is composed of dilated, cavernous haemangioma-like vessels, surrounded by clusters of glomus cells. **B** Higher-power view of glomus cells in the glomovenous malformation.

been reported {407,473,885,1140,1533, 1753,1890,2103,2535,2601,2743,3061}.

Etiology
Multiple familial glomus tumours show autosomal dominant inheritance {1105,1771}. These tumours are caused by inactivating mutations in the glomulin gene (*GLMN*) in chromosome arm 1p, which is predominantly expressed in vascular smooth muscle cells {271,327,1792}. An association between digital glomus tumours and neurofibromatosis type I (NF1) has been reported, with frequent involvement of multiple digits {311,609,2111,2184,2447,2653,2654}.

Sites of involvement
The vast majority occur in the distal extremities, particularly the subungual region, the hand, the wrist and the foot {885, 2080,2548,2654}. Rare tumours have been reported in almost every location, including gastrointestinal tract {1890}, penis {1753, 2408}, bladder {2535}, mediastinum {1180}, nerve {359}, bone {2384} and lung {936}. Glomus tumours almost always occur in skin or superficial soft tissues, although rare cases occur in deep soft tissue or viscera. Malignant glomus tumours are usually deeply situated, but may be cutaneous {473,885}.

Clinical features
Cutaneous glomus tumours are typically small (< 1 cm), red-blue nodules often associated with a long history of pain, particularly with exposure to cold or minor tactile stimulation. Deeply seated or visceral glomus tumours present as a nonspecific mass. The vascular tumours in blue rubber bleb naevus syndrome are commonly glomovenous malformations.

Histopathology
Glomus cells are small, uniform, and rounded with a centrally placed, round nucleus and amphophilic to lightly eosinophilic cytoplasm. Each cell is surrounded by a sharply-defined basal lamina. Occasionally cases show oncocytic or epithelioid change {2275,2580}. Solid glomus tumours comprise approximately 75% of cases {2930}. They are composed of nests of glomus cells surrounding capillary

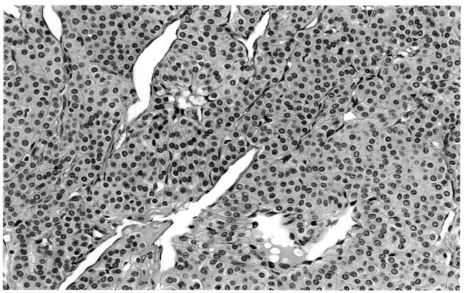

Fig. 6.02 A typical glomus tumour, consisting of uniform, round cells with well-defined cell membranes.

sized vessels. The stroma may show hyalinization or myxoid change. Glomovenous malformations, also known as glomangiomas and commonest in patients with multiple or familial lesions, comprise approximately 20% of cases and are characterized by cavernous haemangioma-like vascular structures surrounded by small clusters of glomus cells. Glomangiomyomas show transition from typical glomus cells to elongated cells resembling mature smooth muscle. In some glomus tumours, a branching, haemangiopericytoma-like vasculature is present ("glomangiopericytoma") {1026}. Glomangiomatosis is an extremely rare variant of glomus tumour with an overall architectural resemblance to diffuse angiomatosis, but containing nests of glomus cells investing vessel walls {885,1317,2181, 3068}. Symplastic glomus tumours show striking nuclear atypia in the absence of any other features indicative of negative outcome (e.g. large size, deep location, mitotic activity, necrosis) {111,454,885, 1358}.

The diagnosis of "malignant glomus tumour" should be reserved for tumours showing: (i) marked nuclear atypia and any level of mitotic activity; or (ii) atypical mitotic figures {885}. A component of pre-existing benign-appearing glomus tumour is often present. There are two types of malignant glomus tumour. In the first, the malignant component resembles a leiomyosarcoma or fibrosarcoma. In the second, the malignant component consists of sheets of highly malignant-appearing round cells. Immunohistochemical demonstration of SMA and pericellular type IV collagen is required for this diagnosis, in the absence of a clear-cut benign precursor. Glomus tumours not fulfilling the criteria for malignancy, but having at least one atypical feature other than nuclear pleomorphism should be labelled "glomus tumours of uncertain malignant potential". Although glomus tumours of > 2 cm in size and deep location were previously considered "malignant", subsequent experience suggests that these have "uncertain malignant potential".

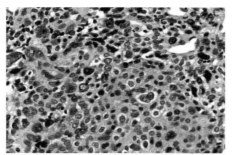

Fig. 6.03 Symplastic glomus tumour, showing scattered cells with marked nuclear atypia, but without mitotic activity.

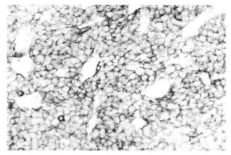

Fig. 6.04 Glomus tumour. Tumour cells show consistently strong immunoreactivity for SMA.

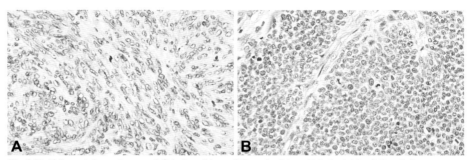

Fig. 6.05 Malignant glomus tumour. **A** Spindle-cell type. **B** Round-cell type. Note the brisk mitotic activity.

Immunophenotype

Glomus tumours of all types typically express SMA and have abundant pericellular production of type IV collagen. Staining for h-caldesmon is also positive {885}.

Ultrastructure

Ultrastructurally, glomus cells have short interdigitating cytoplasmic processes, bundles of thin actin-like filaments with dense bodies and occasional attachments plaques to the cytoplasmic membrane and prominent external lamina {1458}.

Genetics

In addition to a germline *GLMN* mutation, a second somatic mutation of the *GLMN* gene has been identified in the glomangioma tissue of a patient with multiple inherited glomus tumours {327}. Biallelic *NF1* inactivation underlies the pathogenesis of NF1-associated glomus tumours {311}. Mitotic recombination of chromosome arm 17q has been identified as another

somatic inactivation mechanism in NF1-associated glomus tumours and different NF1-associated glomus tumours have shown copy-number changes at other loci and even polyploidy {2653}. In contrast, there is no evidence for *NF1* inactivation or overactivation of the RAS-MAPK pathway in glomus cells from sporadic glomus tumours {311}.

Prognostic factors

Typical glomus tumours, glomovenous malformations, and symplastic glomus tumours are benign. Malignant glomus tumours are aggressive, with metastases and death from disease in up to 40% of patients. Some large, visceral glomus tumours without other atypical features (uncertain malignant potential) have behaved aggressively.

Myopericytoma, including myofibroma

T. Mentzel
J.A. Bridge

Definition
Myopericytoma represents a benign perivascular myoid neoplasm and forms a morphological spectrum with myofibroma, as well as with so-called infantile haemangiopericytoma, angioleiomyoma, and glomus tumour.

ICD-O code
Myopericytoma	8824/0
Myofibroma	8824/0
Myofibromatosis	8824/1

Synonyms
In the past, cases of myopericytoma may have been diagnosed as "haemangiopericytoma" or "solitary myofibroma". Myofibromas and myofibromatosis neoplasms were also called "infantile haemangiopericytoma" in the past {1833}.

Epidemiology
Myopericytoma may occur at any age; however, most are seen in adults {1835}. Myofibroma may be present at birth, appear in the first 2 years of life or arise in adults with a male predominance.

Etiology
An association between myopericytoma and EBV has been reported in patients with AIDS {1562}.
A subset of solitary and multiple (nonvisceral)

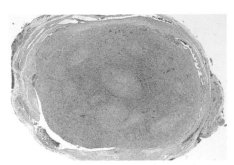

Fig. 6.06 An example of an intravascular myopericytoma.

forms of infantile myofibromatosis are familial. Familial infantile myofibromatosis appears to follow an autosomal-dominant mode of inheritance with variable penetrance and expressivity, although genetic heterogeneity has not been fully excluded as the presence of consanguinity in a few published pedigrees has led some authors to interpret the inheritance pattern as autosomal recessive {142,1280,2000, 2422,2582,3054}.

Sites of involvement
Myopericytoma generally arises in dermal or subcutaneous tissue, while involvement of deep soft tissues is seen more rarely. Lesions more commonly involve the distal extremities, followed by the proximal extremities, the neck, the trunk, and the oral cavity {576,1275}. Very

rarely, these neoplasms arise in visceral or intracranial sites {1563,2379}.
The majority of myofibromas arise in dermal and subcutaneous tissues, and the extremities, head and neck region and trunk are the usual sites.

Clinical features
Myopericytoma usually presents as a painless, slowly growing, superficially located nodule, than can be present for years. The majority of cases arise as a solitary lesion, but multiple lesions involving a particular anatomical region or different regions are sometimes seen {1026, 1835,3003}.
Myofibromas may present as solitary or multicentric lesions (myofibromatosis) and are seen mainly as congenital neoplasms or in the first years of life, often involving viscera or bone {1833}.

Macroscopy
In superficial locations, myopericytoma tends to form a well-circumscribed, nodule measuring < 2 cm in diameter, while larger neoplasms may be seen in deep soft tissues {1835}.

Histopathology
Myopericytoma
Myopericytomas are unencapsulated, usually well-circumscribed, nodular or

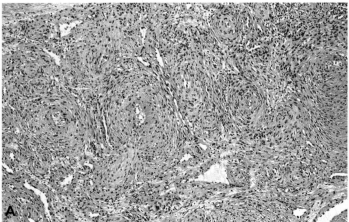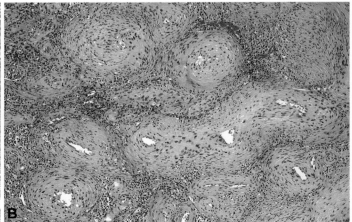

Fig. 6.07 Myopericytoma. **A** A concentric, perivascular growth of spindled, myoid tumour cells is characteristic. **B** Blood vessels are surrounded concentrically by plump spindled myoid tumour cells in the so-called classical, solid type of myopericytoma.

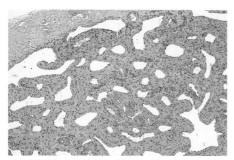

Fig. 6.08 Myopericytoma with branching vessels and a perivascular growth of eosinophilic myoid tumour cells.

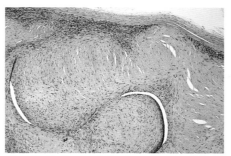

Fig. 6.09 Myofibroma. As in other myopericytic lesions, the spindle cells often bulge into vascular lumina beneath an intact layer of endothelium.

lobular lesions composed of cytologically uniform oval- to spindle-shaped myoid tumour cells that show a characteristic multi-layered, perivascular, concentric growth. Neoplastic cells contain eosinophilic cytoplasm and plump spindled nuclei. Cases of myopericytoma show variable cellularity ranging from cellular and solid-appearing examples to hypocellular neoplasms with prominent collagenous or myxoid stroma. Lesional blood vessels tend to be numerous and variable in size and, in addition to narrow vessels, thin-walled, branching vascular structures with a solitary fibrous tumour-like appearance are often seen. Blood vessels in the vicinity of the lesion may also show concentric perivascular proliferation of myoid, spindled cells {1835}. In some cases a more prominent fascicular or whorled arrangement of neoplastic cells resembling myofibroma or angioleiomyoma is present {698,1764}. Subendothelial proliferation of lesional cells in vessel walls is frequently seen, and cases of intramural and intravascular myopericytoma have been reported {1799,1835}. Some cases of myopericytoma have a cellular component with glomus-cell-like features composed of cuboidal cells with distinct cell borders and central, round, and sharply demarcated nuclei. For these hybrid cases, the term "glomangiopericytoma" has sometimes been used {1026}. Rarely, myopericytomas may show marked hyalinization, cystic change, metaplastic ossification, and coagulative, ischaemic necrosis, and degenerative cellular atypia may be seen in such cases {1835}.

Myofibroma

Myofibromas are nodular, well-circumscribed neoplasms, characterized by a biphasic growth of immature-appearing, plump spindled tumour cells associated with numerous thin-walled, branching solitary fibrous tumour-like vessels associated with more mature, spindled tumour cells with abundant eosinophilic cytoplasm, arranged in bundles or whorls. Tumour cells are set in a collagenous stroma with often characteristic myxohyaline changes. Mitoses are variable in number and, especially in the immature-appearing tumour areas, numerous mitoses as well as areas of necrosis may be present.

Although myofibroma, angioleiomyoma, glomus tumour and myopericytoma are distinct clinicopathological entities, the presence of hybrid cases and shared morphological and immunohistochemical features emphasizes the existence of a continuous spectrum of perivascular myoid neoplasms.

Immunophenotype

Myopericytomas stain positively for SMA and h-caldesmon, with staining being either generally diffuse or more prominent in perivascular cells. In contrast, neoplastic cells are negative or only focally positive for desmin, and focal positive staining for CD34 has also been reported. Lesional cells are negative for S100 protein and, in most cases, for keratin.

Immunohistochemically, neoplastic cells in both components of myofibroma stain positively for α-SMA, while h-caldesmon is negative or only focally positive.

Genetics

A discrete subgroup of tumours of soft tissue considered to fall within the myopericytic category exhibit a 7;12 translocation [t(7;12)(p22;q13)] that results in fusion of the *ACTB* (7p22) and *GLI1* (12q13) genes {544,545}.

Genetic reports of infantile myofibromatosis are rare. An interstitial deletion of 6q, del(6)(q12q15), was reported as the sole anomaly in a solitary infantile myofibromatosis and an unbalanced whole-arm translocation resulting in monosomy 9q and trisomy 16q in another {2570,2650}.

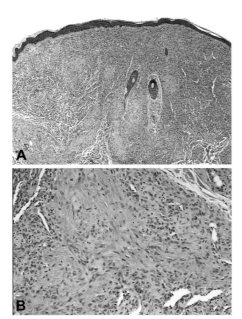

Fig. 6.10 Myofibroma. **A** Cutaneous myofibroma is characterized by multinodular growth and a biphasic growth pattern. **B** In addition to small, undifferentiated mesenchymal cells associated with branching, thin-walled vessels, more mature, spindled, eosinophilic tumour cells are seen in myofibroma.

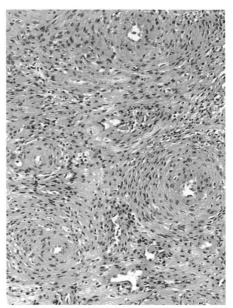

Fig. 6.11 Intravascular myopericytoma. A perivascular growth of myoid tumour cells is seen in this example.

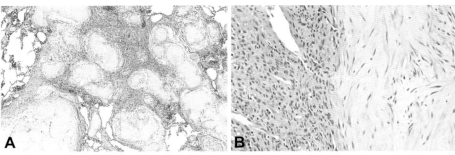

Fig. 6.12 Infantile myofibromatosis. **A** Lung is one of the more common visceral locations to be affected. Note the typically multinodular growth pattern. **B** High-power view showing typical cytological features, with rounded, less well-differentiated cells arranged around solitary fibrous tumour-like blood vessels on the left, and spindle-shaped myoid cells on the right.

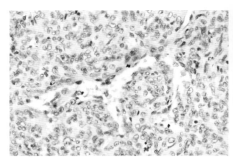

Fig. 6.13 Myofibroma/myofibromatosis. Primitive spindle cells with solitary fibrous tumour-like blood vessels.

Infantile myofibromatosis is negative for the *ETV6-NTRK3* gene fusion associated with infantile fibrosarcoma {29}.

Prognostic factors

Most cases of myopericytoma do not recur even if marginally or incompletely excised, and local recurrence may be related to poor circumscription and most likely represents continued local growth instead of a true recurrence. Very rarely, and mostly seen in deep soft tissues, examples of malignant myopericytoma have been reported {1802}. These malignant myopericytomas are characterized by a poor clinical outcome, and such infiltrative growing neoplasms are composed of atypical, perivascular myoid tumour cells with increased proliferative activity.

The overall prognosis in myofibroma is excellent; however, in cases with visceral involvement, poor outcome has been reported.

Angioleiomyoma

M. Hisaoka
B. Quade

Definition

A benign dermal or subcutaneous tumour composed of well-differentiated smooth muscle cells arranged around many vascular channels. A morphological continuum exists between angioleiomyoma and myopericytoma.

ICD-O code   8894/0

Synonyms

Angiomyoma; vascular leiomyoma

Epidemiology

Angioleiomyoma is a relatively common neoplasm, accounting for approximately 4–5% of benign soft tissue tumours {1072}. Lesions in the lower extremities occur in females twice as frequently as in males, whereas those in the upper extremities or head are more often seen in males than females. Lesions occur at all ages, but

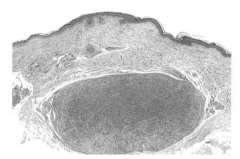

Fig. 6.14 Angioleiomyoma, solid type, showing sharp circumscription.

are commonest between the fourth and sixth decades of life.

Etiology

The etiology of these tumours remains largely unknown. Minor trauma and venous stasis have been proposed as potential causal factors {2293}. EBV infection has been reported in immunocompromised patients with angioleiomyoma or angioleiomyoma-like smooth muscle tumours {423,2228}.

Sites of involvement

Angioleiomyoma can occur anywhere in the body, but is most often seen in the extremities, particularly the lower leg, followed by the head and trunk {1072}. The lesions are usually located in the subcutis and less often in the deep dermis. Rare subfascial or intraosseous lesions have been described {2102,2827}.

Clinical features

Angioleiomyomas typically present as a small, slowly growing firm nodule. Pain is the major complaint in more than half of patients, is often paroxysmal and is provoked by exposure to wind or cold or by pressure, pregnancy or menses. MRI

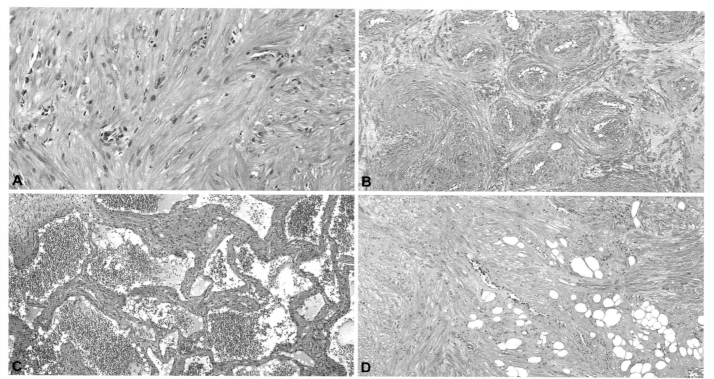

Fig. 6.15 Angioleiomyoma. **A** Solid type, showing compact fascicular proliferation of smooth muscle cells around slit-like vascular channels. **B** Venous type, composed of thick muscle-coated vascular elements and intervening smooth muscle. **C** Cavernous type, showing variably dilated vascular channels with attenuated walls of smooth muscle. **D** Angioleiomyoma with a mature fatty element.

demonstrates mixed hyperintense and isointense areas to skeletal muscle on T2-weighted images, and the hyperintense areas are strongly enhanced after intravenous contrast injection {3035}.

Macroscopy
Most angioleiomyomas are sharply circumscribed, grey-white or brown, rubbery, spherical nodules, measuring < 2 cm in diameter.

Histopathology
Angioleiomyoma is composed of well-differentiated smooth muscle cells with intervening vascular channels. Mitotic figures are usually absent or very scarce. Major histological variations of angioleiomyoma include solid, venous, and cavernous types {1072}. The solid type shows closely packed smooth muscle cells arranged in variably intersecting bundles between slit-like vascular channels. The venous type has variably gaping venous lumina surrounded by thick muscular coats blending with relatively loose intervascular smooth muscle bundles. The cavernous type has dilated vascular channels with thin or thick walls between

septa composed of smooth muscle, somewhat simulating cavernous haemangioma. In the largest reported series of 562 cases, it was found that the solid type was the most common (67%), followed by the venous (23%) and cavernous (11%) types. Other minor histological variations include angioleiomyomas with adipocytic metaplasia, some being erroneously described as (sub)cutaneous angiomyolipoma, and those with prominent hyalinization and/or calcification {1072}. Angioleiomyoma with focal degenerative atypia is rarely seen {1747}. There may be a perivascular concentric arrangement of smooth muscle cells, as typically found in myopericytoma {1764}.

Immunophenotype
The tumour cells are consistently and diffusely positive for SMA, MSA, calponin and variably for h-caldesmon {1764}. Although desmin is also expressed in a majority of the cases, the cells in the myopericytoma-like perivascular concentric structures or in thick muscular coats in the venous type are usually negative for desmin {1764}. HMB45 is negative {176}.

Ultrastructure
The lesional spindle cells show typical ultrastructural features of smooth muscle cells {2505}. The vessels, lined by endothelial cells with Weibel-Palade bodies, are enveloped by a basement membrane complex composed of multiple laminae. Unmyelinated nerve fibres are seen only sporadically in the vicinity of the vessels {2505}.

Genetics
Relatively simple karyotypes with varied structural rearrangements have been identified {2936}. Genomic array analysis of 23 angioleiomyomas showed that most cases were diploid; the most common loss involved 22q11.2, while the most common gain was low-level amplification of Xq {2063}.

Prognostic factors
Angioleiomyoma is benign. Simple excision is curative. Incomplete excision or a deeply situated lesion may exceptionally result in local recurrence {1703}.

CHAPTER 7

Skeletal-muscle tumours

Rhabdomyoma

Embryonal rhabdomyosarcoma

Alveolar rhabdomyosarcoma

Pleomorphic rhabdomyosarcoma

Spindle cell/sclerosing rhabdomyosarcoma

Rhabdomyoma

D.M. Parham
F.G. Barr

Adult rhabdomyoma

Definition
Adult rhabdomyoma is a benign soft-tissue neoplasm showing mature skeletal-muscle differentiation.

ICD-O code   8904/0

Synonyms
Adult extracardiac rhabdomyoma; rhabdomyomatous hamartoma; rhabdomyoma purum

Epidemiology
Adult rhabdomyomas are distinctly rare lesions; relatively few series exist {659,2173}. They represent < 2% of all muscular tumours {399}.

Etiology
Multicentric forms of adult rhabdomyoma {1470,1618} suggest a genetic origin, but no specific inherited gene alteration is known.

Sites of involvement
Most arise in the head and neck, e.g. the parapharyngeal space, salivary glands, larynx, mouth, and soft tissue of the neck. Rarely, they arise from other locations such as the mediastinum.

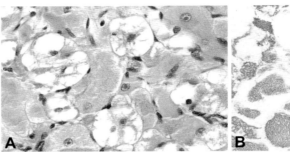
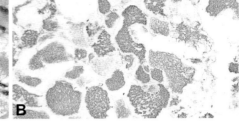

Fig. 7.01 Adult rhabdomyoma. **A** Vesicular nuclei and prominent round nucleoli are the hallmark of "spider" cells. **B** Cytoplasmic immunopositivity for myoglobin.

Clinical features
The median age is 60 years (range, 33–80 years), with a male to female ratio of 3 :1 {1470}. They usually present as slowly growing, painless masses {399}, but some grow rapidly {1104}. Other symptoms include hoarseness, obstructive sleep apnoea, and dysphagia. They arise as unifocal or multifocal lesions {1470}.

Macroscopy
They form well-circumscribed, soft, nodular or lobular, deep tan to red-brown masses. Tumour size ranges from 1.5 to 7.5 cm (median, 3 cm) {1370}.

Histopathology
These unencapsulated, lobular masses consist of large polygonal cells with abundant granular eosinophilic cytoplasm, small round vesicular nuclei, and well-defined cellular borders {1334}. The cytoplasm may be vacuolated ("spider cells") or contain rod-like inclusions or cross striations.

Immunophenotype
Positive markers include MSA, desmin, and myogenin {1334}. Occasional cells may express SMA or S100, but GFAP, keratin, EMA, and CD68 are negative.

Ultrastructure
Myofilaments, Z-bands, and glycogen are seen {3062}.

Genetics
Although adult rhabdomyomas are not

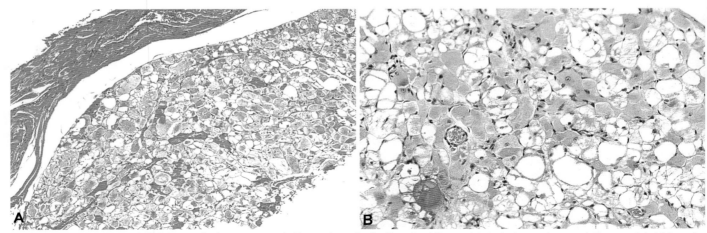

Fig. 7.02 Adult rhabdomyoma. **A** Well-circumscribed mass composed of large polygonal cells with eosinophilic vacuolated cytoplasm and surrounded by normal skeletal muscle. **B** Higher magnification shows large, polygonal cells with abundant granular and vacuolated cytoplasm.

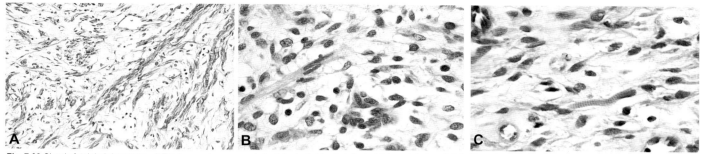

Fig. 7.03 Classic fetal rhabdomyoma. **A** The tumour is composed of cytologically bland, delicate fetal myotubules. **B** Primitive spindle cells in a myxoid stroma. **C** Occasional delicate rhabdomyoblasts display cross-striations.

associated with basal cell naevus syndrome {1015}, a few tumours show evidence of activation of the sonic hedgehog pathway {2773}. Cytogenetic analysis of one case revealed a t(15;17)(q24;p13) {974}.

Prognostic factors
Adult rhabdomyomas often recur, but do not deeply invade contiguous structures or metastasize {2173}.

Fetal rhabdomyoma

Definition
Fetal rhabdomyoma is a benign rhabdomyoblastic tumour with myotube-like differentiation.

ICD-O code 8903/0

Epidemiology
Fetal rhabdomyoma occurs rarely {621, 1370,1540}. All ages are affected. The mean age of affected children is 2.1 years {1540}; the male to female ratio is about 5:3. About 25% of cases are congenital {1370}.

Etiology
See Genetics

Sites of involvement
The great majority of cases (70–90%) {388} arise in the head and neck, particularly the posterior auricular region. A variety of subcutaneous, intranasal, and intra-oral sites are affected {2892}. Other sites include the chest, abdomen {2951}, pelvis, and extremities {1540}.

Clinical features
A growing mass may cause proptosis, decreased vision, airway obstruction, and hoarseness {1370}.

Macroscopy
Fetal rhabdomyoma forms a circumscribed, soft mass with glistening cut surfaces. Sessile or pedunculated polyps occur on mucosal surfaces. Tumour size ranges from 1.0 to 12.5 cm (median, 3.0 cm) {1370}.

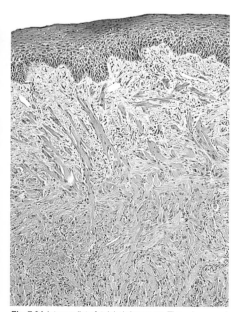

Fig. 7.04 Intermediate fetal rhabdomyoma. The submucosal mass shows broad strap-like rhabdomyoblasts with abundant eosinophilic cytoplasm.

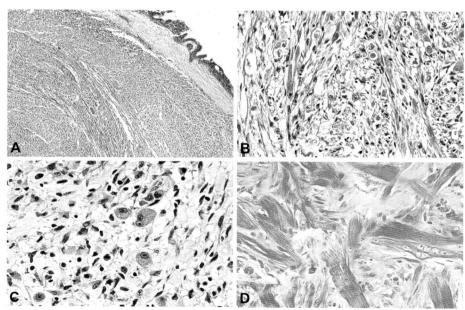

Fig. 7.05 Intermediate fetal rhabdomyoma. **A** Mucosal lesion showing more advanced rhabdomyoblastic maturation than the "classic" type. **B** Fascicles of spindled rhabdomyoblasts simulating smooth muscle cells. **C** Note the round ganglion cell-like rhabdomyoblasts. **D** Cytoplasmic cross-striations are highlighted by Masson trichrome stain.

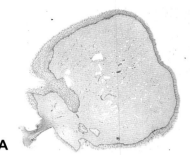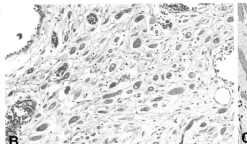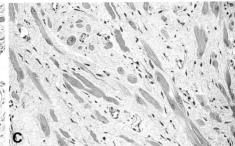

Fig. 7.06 Vaginal rhabdomyoma. **A** Whole mount shows a polypoid configuration and fibrous stroma. **B** Medium magnification displays fibrous stroma with dilated vessels and round or strap-like rhabdomyoblasts with abundant eosinophilic cytoplasm. **C** Cellular details of rhabdomyoblasts.

Histopathology

The classic form contains irregular bundles of immature skeletal muscle fibres within a myxoid background. Cells have features of fetal myotubes, i.e. spindly contours, central oblong nuclei, and eosinophilic cytoplasm. An intermediate (juvenile) subset shows greater cellularity, less myxoid stroma, cells with a smooth muscle phenotype, and differentiated rhabdomyoblasts {527}. The fetal cellular subtype contains a more uniform population of differentiating myoblasts. The myxoid variant shows a predominance of stroma {2218}. Mitoses can be relatively frequent (up to 14 per 50 HPF) {1370}, but tumours lack significant nuclear atypia, infiltrative margins, atypical mitoses or necrosis {2262}.

Immunophenotype

These tumours are positive for desmin, myogenin, and MSA, and often also for SMA and S100 {2892}.

Ultrastructure

Ultrastructural examination reveals differentiated rhabdomyoblasts with well-defined cytoplasmic myofilaments and prominent Z lines {621}.

Genetics

Fetal rhabdomyoma often occurs in association with basal cell naevus syndrome {1015}, caused by loss-of-function mutations in the tumour suppressor gene *PTCH1* {937,1075,1337}. *PTCH1* encodes an inhibitory receptor in the sonic hedgehog signalling pathway {2954}. Inactivation of the second *PTCH1* allele in syndromic fetal rhabdomyoma may fully inactivate PTCH1 function and thereby activate hedgehog signalling {2773}. Non-syndromic

fetal rhabdomyomas reveal evidence of hedgehog pathway activation by an unknown mechanism {2773}.

Prognostic factors

Complete excision of fetal rhabdomyoma is generally curative {2262,2829}.

Genital rhabdomyoma

Definition

Genital rhabdomyomas are benign rhabdomyoblastic neoplasms arising in the female or male genital tract.

ICD-O code   8905/0

Synonyms

Vaginal rhabdomyoma

Epidemiology

Genital rhabdomyomas are the rarest of the rhabdomyomas; only isolated case reports exist {1300,1625}. Most cases occur in women, typically adults, but males are also affected, including infants, adolescents, and adults {579}. It is likely that infantile lesions represent fetal rhabdomyomas {1505,2510}.

Sites of involvement

Most cases arise from the vagina {2672}; some affect the vulva and cervix {1462,1625}. Genital rhabdomyomas in males arise from the spermatic cord {1541}, tunica vaginalis {2717} or paratesticular soft tissues {1505}.

Clinical features

Genital lesions in females form symptomless masses discovered on clinical examination {1595} or cause postmenopausal

uterine bleeding {1625} or menorrhagia {935}. In males, tumours cause scrotal swelling {1541} or pain {579}.

Macroscopy

Genital rhabdomyomas in females form firm, lobulated, polypoid, non-ulcerated, epithelial-covered masses measuring 2–3 cm {1625}. Paratesticular rhabdomyomas may partially encase the testis and spermatic cord and have a pale, glistening surface {579}.

Histopathology

Genital rhabdomyomas in females contain loose fibrous connective tissue with differentiated spindled, polygonal, or elongate rhabdomyoblasts. Many contain eosinophilic cytoplasm with cross striations. The cells appear bland and lack mitoses {935}. Vaginal lesions have a polypoid configuration, but no cambium layer {935}. Genital tumours in males have features of adult {1541} or fetal {2510} rhabdomyomas, but may show prominent stromal fibrosis {508}.

Immunophenotype

These tumours show immunopositivity for desmin, myogenin, actin, and myosin.

Ultrastructure

Vaginal rhabdomyomas contain thick and thin myofilaments, A, I, and H bands, and prominent Z lines {1462,1595,1625}.

Prognostic factors

Genital rhabdomyomas in females typically do not recur after excision, with a single exception {1661}. Metastases have not been reported {1625}.

Embryonal rhabdomyosarcoma

D.M. Parham
F.G. Barr

Definition
A primitive, malignant soft-tissue tumour with phenotypical and biological features of embryonic skeletal-muscle cells.

ICD-O code   8910/3

Synonyms
Myosarcoma; malignant rhabdomyoma; rhabdopoietic sarcoma; rhabdosarcoma; embryonal sarcoma; botryoid rhabdomyosarcoma; sarcoma botryoides

Epidemiology
Rhabdomyosarcomas comprise the single largest category of soft-tissue sarcomas in children and adolescents, with 4.5 cases per million persons aged 0–20 years in the USA {2097}. Embryonal rhabdomyosarcoma (ERMS) is the most common subtype, occurring in 2.6 per million children aged < 15 years in the USA {2097}. Children aged < 10 years are typically affected, with most cases (36%) occurring in children aged < 5 years; only 18% cases of ERMS arise in adolescents {1068,2097}. About 4% of ERMS affect infants {1711}, and a few cases are congenital {1287}. ERMS also comprise about 20% of all adult rhabdomyosarcomas {2675}. In the USA, ERMS is more common in males than females (male to female ratio, 1.4 : 1) {2097}. Incidence figures in Europe resemble those in the USA, with a similar excess in males {2189}.
About 80% of rhabdomyosarcomas in North America occur in Caucasians, compared

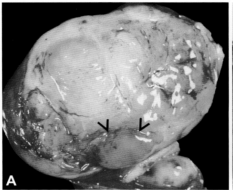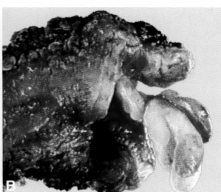

Fig. 7.07 **A** Large embryonal rhabdomyosarcoma involving the paratesticular soft tissues. The tumour forms a fleshy, pale tan mass with compression of the adjacent testis (arrows). **B** Botryoid rhabdomyosarcoma of distal vagina. A polypoid mass protrudes from the distal os of the resected specimen.

with 15% in African-Americans, 10% in Hispanics, and 6% in native Americans and Asians {2097}.

Etiology
A small subset of ERMS occurs with syndromes caused by germline mutations. ERMS is associated with several syndromes caused by mutations in the *RAS* signalling pathway, e.g. Costello syndrome (*HRAS* gene mutations) {90,1480}, neurofibromatosis 1 (*NF1* gene mutations) {1793, 3004} and Noonan syndrome (mutations in several genes) {1480}. A few are reported in association with Beckwith-Wiedemann syndrome, which is caused by dysregulation of imprinted genes in the 11p15.5 region {21,457}. ERMS of the uterine cervix occur with pleuropulmonary blastoma syndrome caused by *DICER1* mutations {904}. Rhabdomyosarcoma of unclassified histology occurs frequently in Li-Fraumeni syndrome, caused by *TP53* mutations {945}, and infrequently in Gorlin syndrome {1015}, in which *PTCH1* mutations activate the hedgehog signalling pathway {1337}.

Sites of involvement
Fewer than 9% of cases of ERMS arise within the skeletal musculature of the extremities. Approximately one half occur within head and neck, and one half within the genitourinary system {2298}. Common locations include the urinary bladder,

prostate, paratesticular soft tissues, periorbital soft tissues, oropharynx, parotid, auditory canal and middle ear, pterygoid fossa, nasopharynx, nasal passages and paranasal sinuses, tongue, and cheek. ERMS also occurs in the biliary tract {2624}, retroperitoneum, pelvis, perineum, and abdomen {108}, and in various viscera, such as the kidney and heart. ERMS infrequently involves the soft tissues of the trunk and extremities, compared with alveolar rhabdomyosarcomas. By definition, botryoid rhabdomyosarcomas are limited to epithelial-lined viscera such as the urinary bladder, biliary tract, pharynx, conjunctiva, or auditory canal {2024}.

Clinical features
ERMS produces a variety of clinical symptoms, generally related to mass effects and obstruction, but their presentation may be indolent {1788}. Head and neck lesions can cause proptosis, diplopia, sinusitis, or unilateral deafness; genitourinary lesions may produce a scrotal mass or urinary retention, and biliary tumours may cause jaundice.

Macroscopy
ERMS forms poorly circumscribed, fleshy, pale tan masses that impinge upon neighbouring structures. Botryoid tumours have a characteristic polypoid appearance with clusters of small, sessile

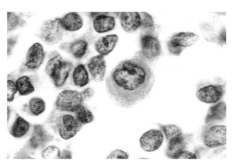

Fig. 7.08 Embryonal rhabdomyosarcoma. In the centre is a typical rhabdomyoblast, with an eccentric oval nucleus, central nucleolus, and eosinophilic cytoplasm.

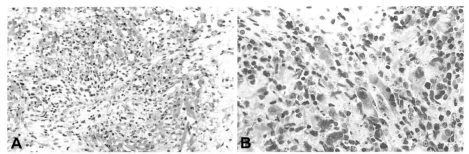
Fig. 7.09 Embryonal rhabdomyosarcoma. **A** Numerous rhabdomyoblasts with brightly eosinophilic cytoplasm and occasional multinucleated strap cells. **B** A compact area with rhabdomyoblastic differentiation adjacent to an area with loose, mucoid stroma.

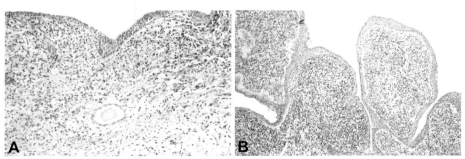
Fig. 7.10 Embryonal rhabdomyosacoma, botryoid variant. **A** A dense layer of tumour cells abuts an epithelial surface and forms a cambium layer. **B** Squamous epithelium outlines polypoid masses of tumour cells.

or pendunculated nodules that abut an epithelial surface.

Histopathology
Analogous to embryonic skeletal muscle, ERMS contains primitive mesenchymal cells in various stages of myogenesis, with a variable content of rhabdomyoblasts. Stellate cells with sparse, amphophilic cytoplasm and central nuclei represent the most primitive end of this spectrum. Coincident with cytodifferentation, rhabdomyoblasts progressively acquire more cytoplasmic eosinophilia and elongation, manifested by "tadpole", "strap", and "spider" cells. Bright eosinophilia, peripheral nuclei, cytoplasmic cross-striations, and multinucleation indicate terminal differentiation, and myotube forms may be evident. Differentiation often becomes more evident after chemotherapy {107}. ERMS forms embryoid aggregates of myoblasts amid loose, myxoid mesenchyme, creating alternating dense and loose cellularity {2175}. Some contain an abundant, myxoid stroma resembling myxomas, while others comprise compact, patternless sheets of spindle and round cells. Particularly on a limited biopsy, ERMS may only contain densely cellular sheets of round cells, inviting confusion with alveolar rhabdomyosarcoma.

The botryoid variant of ERMS contains linear aggregates of tumour cells (the "cambium layer") that tightly abut an epithelial surface {2024}, along with variable numbers of polypoid nodules that can appear deceptively benign.

Traditionally, spindle cell rhabdomyosarcoma was included as a variant of ERMS, but it is now provisionally listed as a separate subtype (see *Spindle cell/sclerosing rhabdomyosarcoma*). Occasional tumours have mixed spindle cell and ERMS histology {1597}.

The presence of markedly enlarged, atypical cells with hyperchromatic nuclei defines the anaplastic variant of rhabdomyosarcoma {2281}. Bizarre, multipolar mitoses are also often present. Heterologous cartilaginous differentiation may be seen, most often in female genital lesions.

Immunophenotype
Markers of skeletal-muscle differentiation typify ERMS {410,879,1952,2175}. These markers correlate with the degree of tumour cell differentiation. Only vimentin is present in the cytoplasm of the most primitive cells, and desmin and actin are acquired by developing rhabdomyoblasts. Differentiated cells exhibit markers of terminal differentiation, such as creatine kinase M. Antibodies against MyoD and myogenin are highly specific and sensitive for rhabdomyosarcoma and are currently used for diagnosis {410,1952}. However, only nuclear staining is specific, as nonspecific cytoplasmic MyoD positivity is common in paraffin-embedded tissues {2900}. ERMS typically shows negative, weak focal, or moderate staining for myogenin that differs from the diffusely strong positivity of most alveolar rhabdomyosarcomas {2175}. ERMS may show aberrant staining with a variety of immunohistochemical markers, including keratin, S100 protein, and neurofilament {495,1891}. SMA positivity is not uncommon {2177, 2178}.

Ultrastructure
Rhabdomyosarcomas with differentiating cells contain bundles of 5 and 15 nm thickness and thin filaments punctuated by abortive Z-bands. Parallel arrays of 15 nm filaments and ribosomes (myosin-ribosome complexes) comprise the earliest diagnostic stage {768}. Non-specific features include discontinuous basal lamina, phagocytosed collagen, and ergastoplasm {666}.

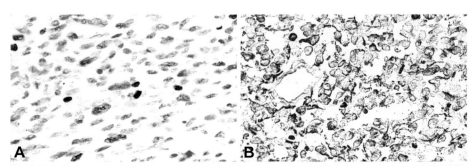
Fig. 7.11 Embryonal rhabdomyosarcoma. **A** Some tumour cells show nuclear immunopositivity for myogenin (MYOG). **B** Desmin staining. Scattered tumour cells contain strongly positive cytoplasmic tails.

Genetics

Sporadic cases of ERMS are aneuploid with multiple numerical chromosome changes {318,1014,2200,2911}. Whole-chromosome gains are common, with polysomy 8 occurring in most cases, and frequent extra copies of chromosomes 2, 11, 12, 13, and 20. Common whole-chromosome losses include monosomies involving chromosomes 10 and 15. Genomic amplification is relatively infrequent, particularly when compared with alveolar rhabdomyosarcoma {2911}. However, multiple amplified regions were found in ERMS with anaplastic features in one small study {318}.

In most cases of ERMS, a genomic event such as chromosome loss, deletion, or uniparental disomy results in loss of one of the two alleles of many chromosome 11 loci {1467,2499}. This loss of heterozygosity localizes to chromosomal region 11p15.5, which contains imprinted genes that encode the growth factor IGF2 and the growth suppressors H19, CDKN1C and HOTS {457,2127}. These findings suggest that an imprinted tumour suppressor gene is inactivated during ERMS tumorigenesis by allelic loss of the active allele and retention of the inactive allele. Analyses of individual genes in sporadic ERMS have implicated several important oncogenic pathways in subsets of ERMS. Deregulation of the RB1 and TP53 pathways is suggested by the finding of inactivating mutations of *TP53* and *CDKN2A/CDKN2B* {1284,2200,2703}. The RAS pathway is activated by either mutations of RAS family genes or *NF1* deletions {2200}. Activation of the hedgehog signalling pathway may be explained by low-level gains of the 12q13 region containing the *GLI1* gene {2200,2773,3069}. Activating oncogenic mutations of the *FGFR4* gene occur with or without accompanying gene amplification {2200}. In addition to *RAS* and *FGFR4* mutations, *PIK3CA* and *CTNNB1* (β-catenin) mutations have been identified in a subset of ERMS {2549}. In primary ERMS, copy-number gain at the *ALK* gene locus is a genetic feature that may correlate with metastatic disease and poor disease-specific survival {2843}. Finally, several known or putative tumour suppressor genes and differentiation-related genes are hypermethylated and thereby epigenetically inactivated {1107,1108, 1704,2306}. Cluster analysis from one genome-wide methylation study revealed that embryonal and alveolar subtypes had distinct DNA methylation patterns, suggesting that DNA methylation signatures may be useful in the diagnostic classification and risk stratification of paediatric rhabdomyosarcoma {1704}.

Prognostic factors

Prognosis can be determined by stage, histological classification, age, and site of origin. Staging is accomplished by clinical evaluation (stage) or surgicopathological evaluation (group) {1861}. Using these features, the Intergroup Rhabdomyosarcoma Study Group (IRSG) subdivided rhabdomyosarcomas into low-, intermediate-, and high-risk groups for purposes of protocol-based therapy {1861}. Age tends to be an independent risk factor, with patients aged 1–9 years having better outcomes than infants or adolescents {1346}. Similarly, children have a better outcome than adults {2675}. Histological classification in paediatric patients has traditionally been an independent predictor of outcome {1861}, with embryonal tumours having a better prognosis than alveolar tumours {108,2295}. However, this effect is likely to be related to the cytogenetic aberrations associated with alveolar rhabdomyosarcoma {577, 2946}. Botryoid variants have a superior outcome to other paediatric rhabdomyosarcomas {2946}. Univariate analysis shows that ERMS with anaplasia have a worse outcome than non-anaplastic ones {2281}. The outcome for parameningeal and extremity tumours is poor, whereas that for orbital and paratesticular tumours is favourable {1861}.

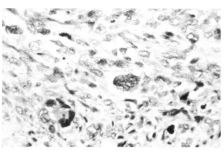

Fig. 7.12 Anaplastic embryonal rhabdomyosarcoma. Some cells contain enlarged, hyperchromatic nuclei.

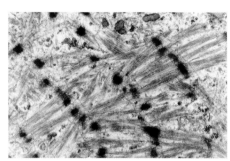

Fig. 7.13 Electron microscopic appearance of embryonal rhabdomyosarcoma showing well-formed Z-bands.

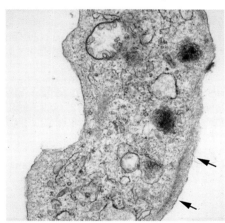

Fig. 7.14 Electron micrograph of an uncommitted mesenchymal cell in embryonal rhabdomyosarcoma. There are no features of myoblastic differentiation. Note the subplasmalemmal microfilaments (arrows).

Alveolar rhabdomyosarcoma

D.M. Parham
F.G. Barr

Definition
Alveolar rhabdomyosarcoma (ARMS) is a highly cellular, malignant neoplasm containing a monomorphous population of primitive cells with round nuclei and features of arrested myogenesis. Most cases exhibit either *PAX3-FOXO1* or *PAX7-FOXO1* fusion genes.

ICD-O code
8920/3

Synonyms
Monomorphous round cell rhabdomyosarcoma

Epidemiology
ARMS occurs at all ages. It occurs more often in adolescents and young adults than embryonal rhabdomyosarcoma (ERMS) and is less common in younger children; very rare cases may be congenital. The median age of affected patients is between 6.8 and 9.0 years {355,2026}. ARMS occurs less frequently than ERMS and comprises about 20% of all paediatric rhabdomyosarcomas. The male to female ratio is approximately even, and no geographical or racial bias has been reported.

Etiology
Rarely, ARMS occurs as part of recognizable genetic syndromes associated with germline mutations. ARMS infrequently arises as a secondary tumour in hereditary retinoblastoma syndrome, caused by *RB1* mutations {1120}. A few cases have occurred in Beckwith-Wiedemann syndrome, caused by dysregulation of imprinted genes in the 11p15.5 region {457,2583}. In both syndromes, ARMS gives negative results in assays for gene fusions.

Sites of involvement
ARMS most commonly arises in the extremities {1113}. Additional sites include the paraspinal and the perineal regions {1143}, paranasal sinuses {2297}, and female breast {1142}.

Clinical features
ARMS typically causes rapidly growing masses in the extremities {1861}. Lesions with meningeal extension often cause cranial nerve deficits {2297}. Perirectal tumours can cause constipation. Rare examples occur as disseminated lesions with no obvious primary, resembling leukaemia {1508}. ARMS tends to be of high stage at presentation {1143,1465}, but many cases are localized {2296}.

Macroscopy
ARMS forms an expansile, rapidly growing soft tissue tumour with a fleshy quality, grey-tan in colour and containing variable amounts of fibrous tissue.

Histopathology
ARMS is highly cellular and composed of primitive cells with monomorphous round nuclei {2175}. Morphological features vary, depending on the presence or absence of fibrous stroma. Typical ARMS produces fibrovascular septa that separate tumour cells into discrete nests containing central clusters and a discohesive periphery. Cells align along the septa in a "picket fence" pattern. Wreath-like multinucleate cells with rhabdomyoblastic differentiation may be seen. The solid variant of ARMS lacks the fibrovascular stroma and forms sheets of round cells with variable rhabdomyoblastic differentiation (often little). Occasional small

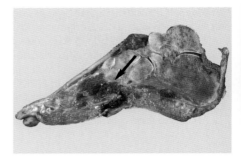

Fig. 7.15 Sagittal section of foot containing alveolar rhabdomyosarcoma. An infiltrative, haemorrhagic mass arises in the plantar and metatarsal soft tissues (arrow).

nests may be seen, particularly with larger samples. The cytological features of solid-variant tumours do not differ from those of typical lesions {2792}. Rare cases may show clear-cell morphology. Tumours with mixed embryonal and alveolar features were previously considered to be variants of ARMS {1113}, but most of these lack *PAX3-FOXO1* fusions {2060}, thus appearing to be clinically and biologically more akin to embryonal rhabdomyosarcoma (ERMS) {2972}. However, fusion genes have been detected in rare cases of mixed ERMS/ARMS {226}.

Immunophenotype
ARMS stains with antibodies against muscle proteins (see *Embryonal rhabdomyosarcoma*), although primitive tumours may have focal staining or lack positivity for markers of differentiation such as myoglobin or actin. Staining for myogenin usually shows a diffuse, strong nuclear pattern {2501}, which correlates with decreased survival {1154}. Positivity for keratin and neuroendocrine markers is not uncommon and may cause diagnostic confusion.

Ultrastructure
See *Embryonal rhabdomyosarcoma*

Genetics
Cytogenetics
Cytogenetic analyses demonstrate recurrent translocations that are consistently and specifically associated with ARMS. A t(2;13)(q35;q14) occurs in most cases of

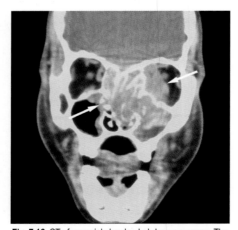

Fig. 7.16 CT of a cranial alveolar rhabdomyosarcoma. The expansile lesion destroys the nasal and paranasal bone and extends into the orbit and parameningeal tissues (arrows).

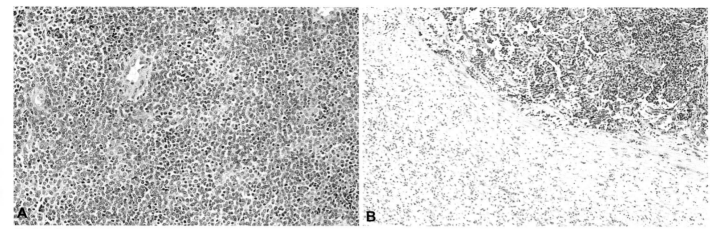

Fig. 7.17 Alveolar rhabdomyosarcoma. **A** The solid variant displays sheets of undifferentiated rhabdomyosarcoma cells without fibrovascular septa. Cytogenetic analysis revealed a t(2;13) translocation, characteristic of alveolar rhabdomyosarcoma. **B** Mixed alveolar-embryonal rhabdomyosarcoma. A discrete, highly cellular focus of alveolar rhabdomyosarcoma contrasts with the adjacent loose embryonal histology.

ARMS, while a t(1;13)(p36;q14) occurs in a smaller subset {153}. These translocations juxtapose *PAX3* or *PAX7* on chromosomes 2 and 1, respectively, with *FOXO1* on chromosome 13, to generate chimeric genes that encode PAX3- and PAX7-FOXO1 fusion proteins {585,939}. These fusion proteins function as potent transcriptional activators with oncogenic effects {190,1395,1532}. Moreover, the fusion products are expressed at high levels in a gene-specific manner; *PAX3-FOXO1* is usually upregulated by a transcriptional mechanism, whereas *PAX7-FOXO1* is generally upregulated by fusion-gene amplification {584}.

Fusion-positive ARMS is notable for the frequent occurrence of genomic amplification {2911}. In addition to *PAX7-FOXO1* amplification, there are several other common amplification events. Amplification of the *MYCN* oncogene on 2p24 occurs in both *PAX3-* and *PAX7-FOXO1*-positive subsets (about 20%) {154}. Amplification of a 12q13–14 region containing 27 genes, including *CDK4*, occurs almost exclusively in *PAX3-FOXO1*-positive cases (about 25%) {154}. Finally, amplification of the miR-17-92 microRNA cluster-encoding *MIR17HG* gene within the 13q31 region has a marked preference for *PAX7-FOXO1*-positive cases (about 70%) {2315}.

Molecular genetics
Analyses of individual genes in sporadic ARMS tumours have implicated several important oncogenic pathways. Inactivating mutations of *TP53* and *CDKN2A/CDKN2B* {1284,2703} and activating mutations of *FGFR4* are present in a small subset {2734}. *ALK* gene copy-number gain and strong cytoplasmic expression of ALK protein reportedly occur in the vast majority of ARMS {2843}. Several known or putative tumour suppressor genes (*RASSF1*, *HIC1*, and *CASP8*) are hypermethylated and thereby epigenetically inactivated {1107,1108,2306}. Studies of genome-wide DNA methylation have suggested that ARMS and ERMS show distinct patterns, with the alveolar subtype being enriched in DNA hypermethylation of polycomb target genes {1704}.

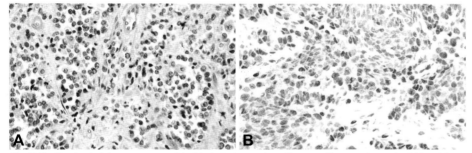

Fig. 7.18 Alveolar rhabdomyosarcoma. **A** In this typical example, collagenous fibrovascular septa divide mixtures of undifferentiated tumour cells and rhabdomyoblasts into discrete nests. **B** Many tumour-cell nuclei show strong immuno-positivity for myogenin.

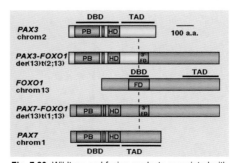

Fig. 7.19 Alveolar rhabdomyosarcoma. Interphase FISH analysis showing amplification of the *PAX7-FOXO1* fusion gene (juxtaposed red and green signals) by 1;13 translocation breakpoint-flanking probes.

Fig. 7.20 Wildtype and fusion products associated with 2;13 and 1;13 translocations. The paired box, octapeptide, homeobox and forkhead domain (PB, HD, FD) are shown as grey boxes. Transcriptional domains (DNA binding domain, DBD; transcriptional activation domain, TAD) are indicated as solid horizontal bars. The translocation fusion point is shown as a vertical dashed line.

There is a subset of ARMS cases without *PAX3*- or *PAX7-FOXO1* fusions {2605}. In a few of these cases, variant rearrangements generate novel fusions such as *PAX3* fused to *FOXO4, NCOA1* or *NCOA2* {155,2677} or *FOXO1* fused to *FGFR1* {1637A}. Some of these variant fusions (*PAX3-NCOA1, FOXO1-FGFR1*) are also amplified. However, most cases appear to represent true fusion-negative cases {155}. Similarly, the gene-expression profiles of these fusion-negative ARMS cases differ from those of fusion-positive ARMS, but are similar to those of ERMS {2889,2972}. Like ERMS, fusion-negative ARMS demonstrates few amplification events and a pattern of whole chromosome gains and losses with 11p15 allelic loss {577,2972}.

Prognostic factors
ARMS is a high-grade neoplasm that is inherently more aggressive than ERMS {2295}, probably because of *PAX-FOXO1* fusions {2972}. As with ERMS, surgicopathological staging (Intergroup Rhabdomyosarcoma Study [IRS] grouping) is predictive of outcome {1861}. Some data indicate that metastatic *PAX7-FOXO1*-positive tumours behave in a more benign fashion than do *PAX3-FOXO1*-positive tumours {2605}. Fusion-negative ARMS has an outcome similar to that of ERMS {2972}.

Pleomorphic rhabdomyosarcoma

E.A. Montgomery
F.G. Barr

Definition
A high-grade sarcoma composed of bizarre polygonal, round and spindle cells that display skeletal-muscle differentiation without embryonal or alveolar components.

ICD-O code   8901/3

Epidemiology
These are tumours of adults and are most common in the sixth to seventh decades of life, occurring more frequently in men than in women {932,2657}. Exceptional (and controversial) paediatric cases have been reported {929}.

Sites of involvement
These tumours arise in the deep soft tissue, most often in the lower extremity, but also the chest/abdominal wall, upper extremity, abdomen/retroperitoneum, and head and neck {932,2657}. They can arise in a host of other locations, including the uterus {796}.

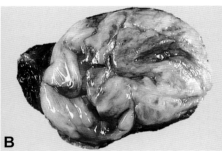

Fig. 7.21 Pleomorphic rhabdomyosarcoma. **A** CT without contrast enhancement of a recurrent tumour, which is similar in consistency to the adjacent skeletal muscles. **B** This mass, which displays zones of necrosis, was excised from the thigh of a man aged 56 years. The lesion extended into the pelvis and recurred quickly following the initial resection.

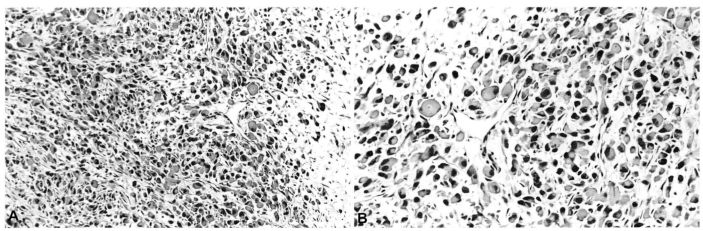

Fig. 7.22 Pleomorphic rhabdomyosarcoma. **A** This tumour is composed of intensely eosinophilic polygonal cells. **B** Note the wide range of cell shapes, from round to tadpole-like.

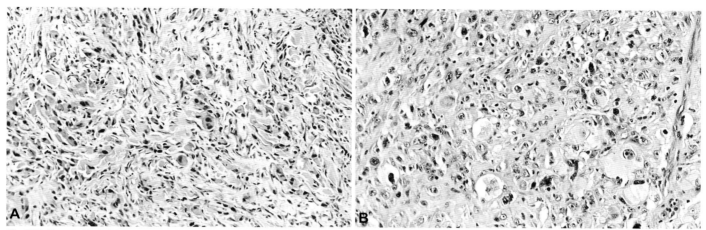

Fig. 7.23 Pleomorphic rhabdomyosarcoma. **A** The tumour comprises spindled and polygonal cells. **B** Bizarre nuclei and abundant cytoplasm are seen in this example.

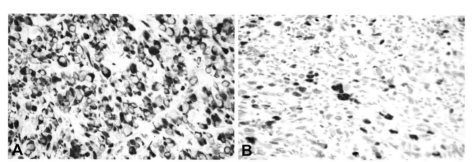

Fig. 7.24 Pleomorphic rhabdomyosarcoma. **A** Note the strong diffuse labelling of desmin. **B** There is strong nuclear expression of myogenin in this example.

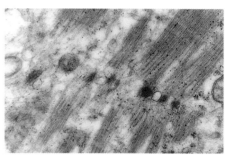

Fig. 7.25 Pleomorphic rhabdomyosarcoma. On electron microscopy, rudimentary sarcomere formation is the key criterion. Such sarcomeres consist of Z-bands or irregular masses of Z-band material with converging thick (16 nm) and thin (8 nm) filaments.

Clinical features

Patients present with rapid growth of an often painful mass {932}.

Macroscopy

These tumours are well-marginated, large (5–15 cm), with a pseudocapsule and a whitish or fleshy cut surface, often with necrosis.

Histopathology

Tumours are composed of sheets of large, atypical, and frequently multinucleated polygonal eosinophilic cells or of undifferentiated round to spindle cells. Cross-striations are seldom detected. Similar morphology is more commonly seen as a heterologous component in tumours such as malignant mixed mullerian tumour and dedifferentiated liposarcoma, among others.

Immunophenotype

These tumours may express desmin, MyoD1, skeletal-muscle (fast) myosin, and myogenin {932,2657}, with variable SMA and focal keratin AE1/3 and EMA positivity. MDM2 nuclear labelling without *MDM2* amplification has been reported {2657}.

Ultrastructure

There is rudimentary sarcomere formation with Z-bands or irregular masses of Z-band material in a minority of cells {2309}.

Genetics

Pleomorphic rhabdomyosarcomas have complex karyotypes with numerical and unbalanced structural changes, but no recurrent structural alterations {1608}. Genome-wide surveys have identified recurrent losses of DNA (e.g. 10q23), gains (e.g. 1p22–23), and amplifications {1013}. This copy-number pattern differs from that found in either alveolar or embryonal rhabdomyosarcoma.

Prognostic factors

These are aggressive lesions, the majority of which metastasize within 5 years {932,2657}. Increasing age is an adverse factor {2096,2675}.

Spindle cell/sclerosing rhabdomyosarcoma

A.F. Nascimento
F.G. Barr

Definition

Spindle cell/sclerosing rhabdomyosarcoma (RMS) is an uncommon variant of rhabdomyosarcoma that has spindle cell morphology. Affecting both children and adults, spindle cell/sclerosing RMS is distinctly more frequent in males. The nosological status of this subgroup remains somewhat uncertain.

ICD-O code   8912/3

Synonyms

Spindle cell rhabdomyosarcoma; sclerosing rhabdomyosarcoma

Epidemiology

Spindle cell/sclerosing RMS is an uncommon subtype of RMS, accounting for 5–10% of all cases of RMS. It affects both children and adults, with a male to female ratio of up to 6 : 1) {401,448,889,1597, 1837,1838,2003,2388,2657}.

Sites of involvement

In the paediatric population, tumours with spindle cell morphology arise predominantly in the paratesticular region, while in adults > 50% of cases affect the deep soft tissues in the head and neck. Lesions with sclerosing morphology in both age groups are most common in the limbs. Other rarely affected anatomical locations include the

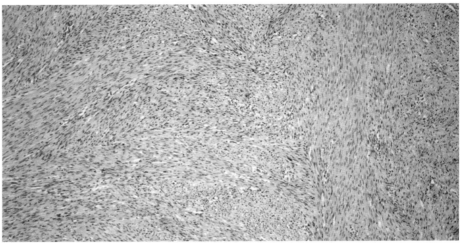

Fig. 7.26 Spindle cell rhabdomyosarcoma. Tumours are frequently composed of long fascicles of spindled cells.

viscera and retroperitoneum {401,448, 1597,1837,1838,2003,2388,2657}.

Clinical features

Spindle cell/sclerosing RMS most commonly presents as a painless mass. Occasionally, tumours may also lead to local compressive symptoms.

Macroscopy

Grossly, tumours appear well-circumscribed but unencapsulated, with an average size of 4–6 cm (range, 2–35 cm)

{401,2003}. The cut surface is grey and white, and whorled. Necrosis and haemorrhage may be seen, but are not consistent features.

Histopathology

Microscopically, tumours are characterized by infiltrative edges and show a fascicular or storiform growth pattern.
Spindle cell RMS is composed of a predominant population of spindled neoplastic cells with ovoid or elongated nuclei, vesicular chromatin, inconspicuous

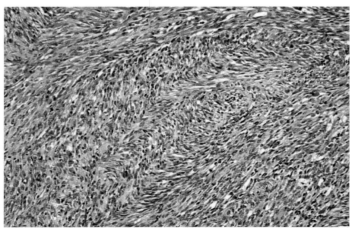

Fig. 7.27 Spindle cell rhabdomyosarcoma. Polygonal rhabdomyoblasts are usually noted throughout the tumour.

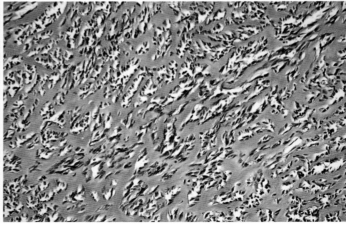

Fig. 7.28 Sclerosing rhabdomyosarcoma. Dense stromal sclerosis imparts a pseudovascular appearance.

nucleoli and scant, palely eosinophilic cytoplasm. Rare to scattered eosinophilic rhabdomyoblasts with eccentrically placed, hyperchromatic nuclei are usually present throughout the tumour. Cross-striations may sometimes be apparent. Nuclear atypia, hyperchromasia and mitotic figures are common. Occasionally, RMS with spindle cell morphology may show focal, subtotal or total stromal hyalinization with tumour cells arranged in nests, microalveoli, or trabeculae, imparting a pseudovascular appearance, and characterizing the sclerosing variant of RMS (when sclerosis is extensive) {889,1837}.

Immunophenotype

Spindle cell RMS is characterized by diffuse expression of desmin, with most cases also expressing SMA and MSA. Nuclear expression of myogenin (MYF4) is seen in almost all cases. This marker is positive in the large polygonal rhabdomyoblasts and in a variable subset of the spindled cells. Rarely, spindle cell/sclerosing RMS may be focally positive for S100 and keratins. Sclerosing RMS may show only very limited expression of desmin and myogenin, but is often strongly positive for myoD1.

Ultrastructure

By electron microscopy, the neoplastic cells contain thick and thin filaments in tangles and/or forming Z bands, and occasional

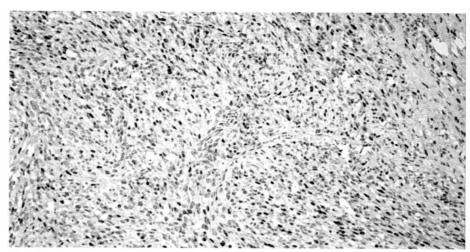

Fig. 7.29 Staining for myogenin (MYF4) is positive in spindle cell/sclerosing rhabdomyosarcoma.

myosin–ribosome complexes {1597}. Collagen is present surrounding tumour cells {1597}.

Genetics

Cytogenetic studies of a limited number of cases has revealed aneuploidy with mostly whole chromosome gains, as well as non-recurrent structural changes {448,526,3049}. Genome-wide surveys of two cases identified whole-chromosome losses in addition to gains, but no recurrent changes {279,1490}. *PAX3*- and *PAX7-FOXO1* fusions are virtually always absent {448,526,889,1750,1759,2826}.

Prognostic factors

In the paediatric population, spindle cell RMS is usually diagnosed at an early stage (IRS stage I and II) and, in contrast to other RMS types, lymph-node metastasis is only seen in a small subset of cases (approximately 16%) {1597}. Patients in this group have a limited disease burden and a favourable outcome, with 95% survival at 5 years {401,1597}.

In adults with spindle cell/sclerosing RMS, the outcome is significantly worse, with a rate of recurrence and metastasis of approximately 40–50%.

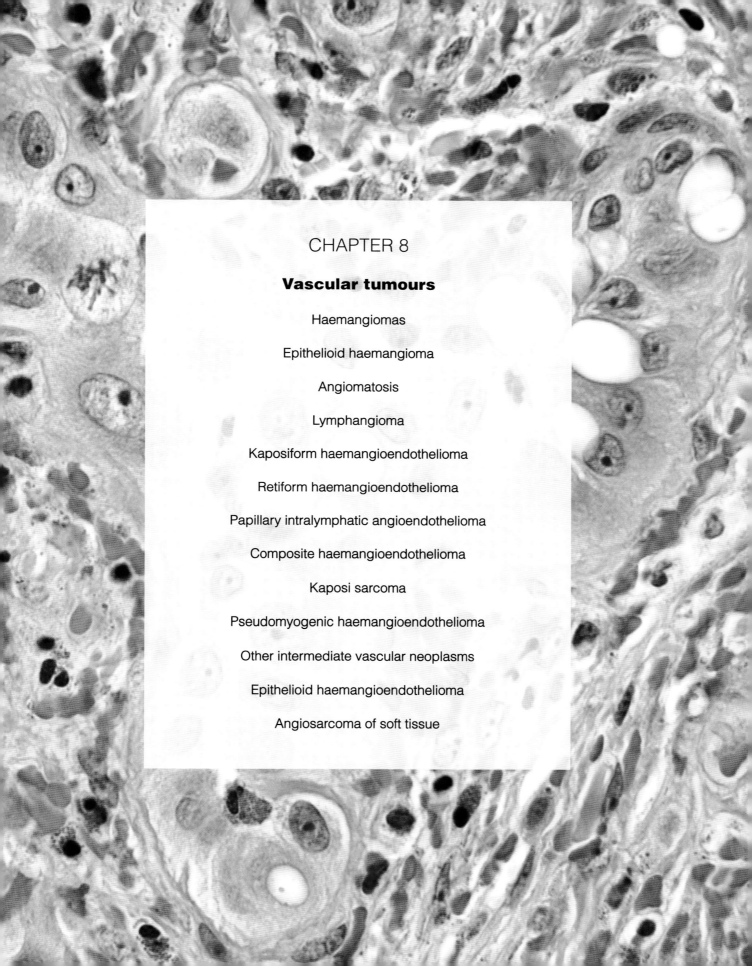

CHAPTER 8

Vascular tumours

Haemangiomas

Epithelioid haemangioma

Angiomatosis

Lymphangioma

Kaposiform haemangioendothelioma

Retiform haemangioendothelioma

Papillary intralymphatic angioendothelioma

Composite haemangioendothelioma

Kaposi sarcoma

Pseudomyogenic haemangioendothelioma

Other intermediate vascular neoplasms

Epithelioid haemangioendothelioma

Angiosarcoma of soft tissue

Haemangiomas

J.E. Calonje

Synovial haemangioma

Definition
Synovial haemangioma (SH) is a benign proliferation of blood vessels arising in a synovium-lined surface, including the intra-articular space or a bursa. Similar lesions occurring within the tendon sheath do not fall into this category.

Epidemiology
SH is very rare. Most patients are children or adolescents and males are affected more commonly than females {648}.

Etiology
The presentation of most lesions at a young age suggests that SH is a form of vascular malformation. Trauma is unlikely to be of relevance in pathogenesis.

Sites of involvement
The most common site by far is the knee, followed much less commonly by the elbow and hand.

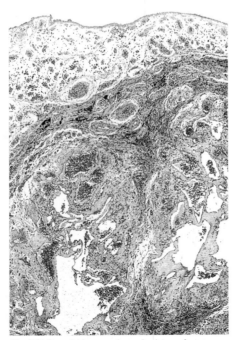

Fig. 8.01 Synovial haemangioma. A mixture of cavernous and capillary vascular channels underlie the synovium.

Clinical features
The tumour presents as a slowly growing lesion, often associated with swelling and joint effusion {648}. Recurrent haemarthrosis has been reported {387,1626} and recurrent pain is a frequent symptom. In about one third of cases, the lesion is painless. Rarely, destructive growth may be seen {2828}, exceptionally with extra-articular extension, bone involvement and pathological fracture of bone {5,1205}. MRI is the best radiological technique to identify the lesion, particularly with regard to the extent of involvement {1032}.

Macroscopy
Numerous congested, variably dilated vessels of different calibre can be seen and the tumour can be fairly circumscribed or diffuse.

Histopathology
The tumour often has the appearance of a cavernous haemangioma with multiple dilated thin-walled vascular channels. A smaller percentage of cases have the appearance of either a capillary or arteriovenous haemangioma. The vascular channels are located beneath the synovial membrane and are surrounded by myxoid or fibrotic stroma. Haemosiderin deposition can be prominent. Secondary villous hyperplasia of the synovium is present in some cases.

Prognostic factors
Small lesions are usually easy to remove completely with no risk of local recurrence. When more diffuse involvement of the joint is present, complete excision can be difficult to achieve and may predispose to recurrence.

Intramuscular angioma

Definition
Intramuscular angioma is defined as a proliferation of benign vascular channels within skeletal muscle and is associated in most instances with variable amounts of mature adipose tissue.

ICD-O code   9132/0

Synonyms
Intramuscular haemangioma; intramuscular-infiltrating angiolipoma

Epidemiology
Although relatively uncommon, intramuscular angioma is one of the most frequent deep-seated soft tissue tumours. The age range is wide, but adolescents and young adults are most commonly affected (up to 90% of cases) {48,180,825}. Lesions have often been present for many years and it is therefore likely that many examples are congenital. The incidence of intramuscular angioma is similar in males and females.

Etiology
It is likely that these lesions are malformations and there is no relationship to trauma.

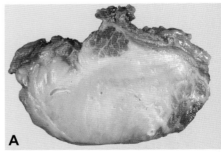

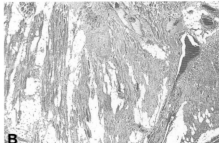

Fig. 8.02 Intramuscular angioma. **A** This lesion was excised from the rectus abdominis muscle of a young woman. Note the poorly circumscribed margins and prominent fatty stroma. **B** Extensive replacement of the muscle by dilated vascular channels with focal thrombosis. There is a prominent adipocytic component.

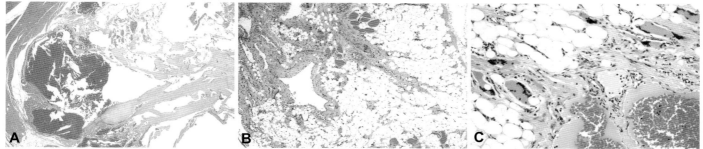

Fig. 8.03 Intramuscular angioma. **A** Predominance of cavernous-like vascular spaces. **B** Extensive adipocytic component with muscle atrophy. **C** Entrapped muscle fibres with hyperchromatic, reactive nuclei.

Sites of involvement

Intramuscular angioma most commonly affects the lower limbs, particularly the thigh, followed by the head and neck, upper limbs and trunk. Rare cases can present in the mediastinum and retroperitoneum and, exceptionally, within cardiac muscle {2608}.

Clinical features

Typical presentation is of a slowly growing mass that is often painful, particularly after exercise. Pain is mainly present in tumours located in the limbs. Giant lesions may exceptionally induce osteolysis {1763}. Radiological examination often reveals the presence of calcification secondary to phleboliths or metaplastic ossification. MRI is the most important radiological technique to establish the diagnosis {1979}.

Macroscopy

Tumours are often large and there is diffuse infiltration of the involved muscle. Variably sized vascular channels with thrombosis and haemorrhage are usually readily seen. The appearance of the tumour can be solid and yellowish as a result of the presence of adipose tissue. Lesions also appear solid when capillaries predominate.

Histopathology

Intramuscular angioma has been traditionally classified according to vessel size into small (capillary) and large (cavernous), although most are mixed {48}, also including lymphatics. Intramuscular angioma usually consists of large thick-walled veins, a mixture of cavernous-like vascular spaces and capillaries or a prominent arteriovenous component. Tumours purely composed of capillaries are more common in the head and neck area and those with a predominant cavernous lymphatic component are seen mainly on

the trunk, proximal upper limb and head. Variable amounts of mature adipose tissue are almost always present and may be very prominent. This explains why intramuscular angioma was sometimes known in the past as "deep" or "infiltrating" angiolipoma {1627}. Atrophy of muscle fibres secondary to tumour infiltration often results in degenerative/reactive sarcolemmal changes with hyperchromatic nuclei. Perineural involvement may be present.

Prognostic factors

The rate of local recurrence is high (30–50%) and therefore wide local excision is recommended. Local recurrence seems to be determined only by size of the tumour and excision margins {183}.

Venous haemangioma

Definition

Venous haemangioma (VH) is composed of veins of variable size, often having thick muscular walls. Intramuscular angiomas and angiomatosis, which are described separately, can be composed almost exclusively of veins but are usually intermixed with other vessel types.

ICD-O code   9122/0

Epidemiology

Venous haemangioma is rare and data are limited, but these lesions occur mainly in adults.

Etiology

The clinical evolution and clinicopathological features suggest that these lesions represent vascular malformations.

Sites of involvement

Tumours present in the subcutaneous or deeper soft tissues, and are commonly

located in the limbs. Rarely, lesions have been described elsewhere, including the mandibular division of the trigeminal nerve {1803}, the orbit {1489}, the superior sulcus of the lung {3040}, the mediastinum {1179}, the retroperitoneum {1450}, the breast {1416}, the brain {1063} and parapharyngeal space {451}.

Clinical features

VH often presents as a long-standing slowly growing tumour. Radiological examination often shows the presence of calcification due to phleboliths.

Macroscopy

VH is ill defined and consists of dilated congested vascular spaces with areas of haemorrhage.

Histopathology

VH typically consists of large thick-walled muscular vessels, which are variably dilated and commonly display thrombosis with occasional formation of phleboliths. Widely dilated vessels can show attenuation of their walls, mimicking a cavernous haemangioma. Elastic stains reveal the absence of an internal elastic lamina. This aids in the distinction from an arterio-venous haemangioma.

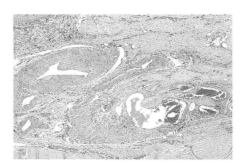

Fig. 8.04 Venous haemangioma with typically numerous prominent thick-walled veins.

Prognostic factors

Deep-seated tumours are difficult to excise and can recur locally but subcutaneous tumours do not usually recur.

Arteriovenous malformation/ haemangioma

Definition

Arteriovenous malformation/haemangioma (AVMH) is a benign vascular lesion characterized by the presence of arteriovenous shunts. There are two distinctive variants: deep-seated and cutaneous (cirsoid aneurysm, or acral arteriovenous tumour {67,1581,2392}). When these lesions involve multiple tissue planes, they are termed "angiomatosis". AVMH should not be confused with juvenile, cutaneous (cellular) haemangiomas since they do not usually regress spontaneously. Spontaneous regression of AVMH is exceptional {2480}.

ICD-O code   9123/0

Epidemiology

Deep-seated AVMH is uncommon and affects children and young adults. AVMH represent about 14.3% of all vascular anomalies in children {1031}. Although a large proportion of lesions (particularly those that are deep-seated) are congenital, acquired lesions are increasingly being recognized {1700}.

Sites of involvement

AVMH affects predominantly the head and neck (including the brain), followed by the limbs. Internal organs including the lungs and uterus may be involved {568}.

Clinical features

Angiography is an essential tool to confirm the diagnosis and establish the extent of disease. Lesions are often associated with a variable degree of arteriovenous shunting and this can be severe enough to induce limb hypertrophy, heart failure, and consumption coagulopathy (Kasabach-Merritt syndrome). Pain is also a frequent symptom and superficial cutaneous changes mimicking Kaposi sarcoma clinically and histologically can be seen (pseudo-Kaposi sarcoma or acroangiodermatitis) {2669}. The presence of shunting can be confirmed clinically by auscultation. AVMH is common in the lungs and brain of patients with hereditary haemorrhagic telangiectasia {28}.

Macroscopy

Tumours are ill-defined and contain variable numbers of small and large blood vessels, many of which are dilated.

Histopathology

This diagnosis always requires clinicopathological and radiological correlation. AVMH is characterized by large numbers of vessels of different sizes, including veins and arteries, with the former largely outnumbering the latter. Areas resembling a cavernous or capillary haemangioma are frequent, as are thrombosis and calcification. Lymphatic vessels may be present. Recognition of arteriovenous shunts is difficult and requires examination of numerous serial sections. Fibrointimal thickening in veins is a useful diagnostic clue. Elastic stains are helpful in distinguishing between arteries and veins. True arteriovenous shunts are sometimes impossible to demonstrate in superficial lesions. Some malformations may be purely venous (see *Venous haemangioma*).

Immunophenotype

Negative staining for GLUT1 may facilitate distinction from juvenile haemangioma {2074}. Wilms tumour 1 (WT1) protein, a marker that is usually positive in haemangiomas, tends to be negative or focally positive in other vascular malformations {25}. However, this marker has recently been reported to be positive in AVMH {2777}.

Prognostic factors

Treatment is sometimes difficult because of the extent of tumour involvement, which has to be determined by angiographic examination. Local recurrence is common because of difficulty in achieving complete excision.

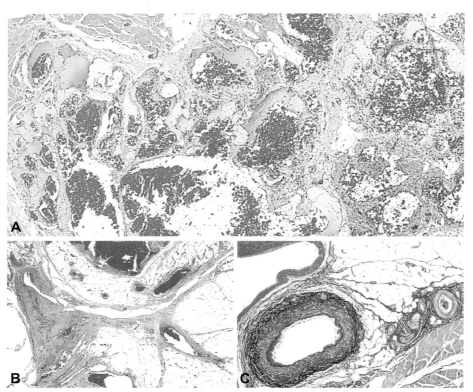

Fig. 8.05 Arteriovenous malformation/haemangioma. **A** In some cases, cavernous vascular spaces predominate. **B** There is extensive infiltration of the subcutaneous tissue by large vessels. **C** An elastic stain (elastic van Gieson) is useful to determine the type of vessels involved.

Epithelioid haemangioma

J.F. Fetsch

Definition

Epithelioid haemangioma is a benign vascular neoplasm with well-formed vessels lined by plump, epithelioid (histiocytoid) endothelial cells with copious amphophilic or eosinophilic cytoplasm. Subcutaneous examples are usually associated with a small artery. Many lesions are rich in lymphocytes and eosinophils.

ICD-O code   9125/0

Synonyms

Angiolymphoid hyperplasia with eosinophilia {398,845,1809,2125,2364,2937}; nodular angioblastic hyperplasia with eosinophilia and lymphofolliculosis {186}; subcutaneous angioblastic lymphoid hyperplasia with eosinophilia {2312}; atypical pyogenic granuloma {2227}; inflammatory angiomatous nodule {1341}; histiocytoid haemangioma {2365}

Epidemiology

Epithelioid haemangioma affects a wide age range, peaking in the third through fifth decades {845,2125}, with a slight predominance in females.

Etiology

It has been controversial as to whether epithelioid haemangioma is a reactive lesion or a true neoplasm, although most available data favour the latter {845,2125, 2364,2789}.

Sites of involvement

Most frequent sites are the head, especially the forehead, preauricular area and scalp, and distal extremities, especially the digits {845,2125}. The penis is an uncommon but noteworthy site of involvement, because lesions in this location are often confused with epithelioid haemangioendothelioma {842,2630}. Epithelioid haemangiomas of bone {875,2043,2084} and various deep soft-tissue sites {845,1955, 2364} have also been documented, but it is unclear if all these lesions have similar behaviour and share a common pathogenesis with superficial lesions {785,790,875,2369}.

Clinical features

Most patients present with a mass of up to 1 year in duration. However, rare examples have been present for up to 15 years {845,2125}. Multifocality in the same anatomical region is encountered with some frequency. Most lesions are subcutaneous, with dermal examples being less frequent, and deep-seated lesions being rare {845,2125}.

Macroscopy

Epithelioid haemangiomas of superficial soft tissue origin are usually 0.5–2.0 cm in size, only rarely exceeding 5 cm {2125}. Most have a nonspecific nodular appearance; some with retained blood may suggest a haemangioma. Occasional subcutaneous lesions may be confused with lymph nodes because of circumscription and a peripheral lymphoid reaction.

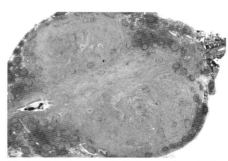

Fig. 8.06 Subcutaneous epithelioid haemangioma showing circumscription, a peripheral lymphoid reaction and symmetrical growth around a small artery.

Histopathology

Subcutaneous epithelioid haemangiomas are characterized by a proliferation of small, capillary-sized vessels lined by plump, epithelioid endothelial cells. The vessels may lack a well-defined lumen, but they are well formed with monolayered endothelium and an intact myopericytic/smooth-muscle layer {842}. The endothelial cells have abundant amphophilic or eosinophilic cytoplasm that is sometimes vacuolated, and they have a single large nucleus with a central nucleolus. The process is usually well demarcated and commonly is intimately associated with a small artery. Numerous eosinophils and lymphocytes are present in most cases, and many examples are bordered by a prominent lymphoid reaction with follicles. Identification of the involved arterial segment is dependent on adequate sampling and aided by a pentachrome stain

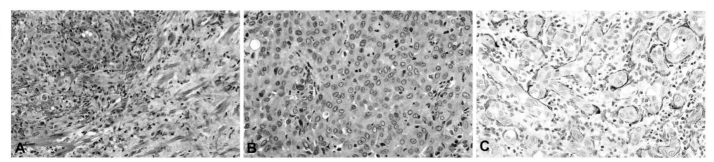

Fig. 8.07 Epithelioid haemangioma. **A** The lesion is growing within the lumen of a damaged artery. Residual smooth muscle of the arterial wall is evident peripherally. **B** Some "exuberant" examples of epithelioid haemangioma have high central cellularity. These lesions have conventional cytology, and typically show peripheral maturation. **C** An intact myopericytic layer, highlighted with staining for SMA, will be evident in the peripheral zones of the tumour.

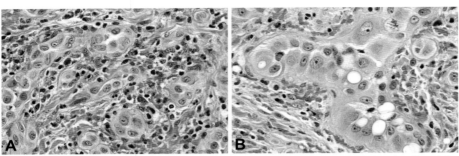

Fig. 8.08 Subcutaneous epithelioid haemangioma. Intermediate and high-power views (**A**, **B**) show that although the vessels are immature, they are well-formed. Note the characteristic cytomorphological features of the endothelial cells and the presence of occasional cytoplasmic vacuoles.

that highlights residual vessel wall. It is common to encounter epithelioid endothelial cells within the lumen of the affected artery, either replacing part of the normal endothelial lining or "coating" fibrin fronds. Cross-sections of the artery may reveal epithelioid endothelial-lined channels transgressing the vessel wall and communicating with the surrounding vascular proliferation. Some lesions are hypercellular centrally but cytological features of malignancy are absent {842}.

Dermal epithelioid haemangiomas feature an often lobular proliferation of small vessels, lined by epithelioid endothelial cells,

associated with lymphocytes and eosinophils. However, in this location, the vessels often have a more mature appearance with a well-canalized lumen, and the endothelial cells are somewhat less plump, frequently being more cobblestone-like in appearance. Dermal examples are less well-marginated and lack association with an artery.

Immunophenotype

The epithelioid endothelial cells are immunoreactive for ERG {1897} and CD31 {842, 2125,2630,2820}. Immunoreactivity for CD34 is also present, though to a lesser

degree. Focal expression of keratin may be seen {842}. Immunostaining for SMA highlights an intact myopericytic layer around the vessels {842}.

Genetics

A somatic Y897C mutation was identified in exon 17 of the *TEK* gene in an epithelioid haemangioma of cutaneous localization {3029}.

Prognostic factors

Local recurrence occurs in up to one third of patients {2125,2789}. Whether this is due to persistence of an underlying vascular anomaly (e.g. an arteriovenous shunt) that incites regrowth or an indication of true neoplastic potential is unresolved. The vast majority of recurrences are indolent and cured by re-excision, but very rarely recurrences can be locally aggressive. Recurrences may appear to be anatomically separate, perhaps reflecting multicentricity, but they characteristically occur along the distribution of the initially affected vessel. There is one report of regional lymph-node seeding that had no adverse effect on outcome with 5 years follow-up {2312}. There are no reports of distant metastases.

Angiomatosis

S.W. Weiss

Definition
Angiomatosis is a diffuse proliferation of benign, architecturally well-developed blood vessels that, by definition, affects a large segment of the body in a contiguous fashion, either by vertical extension to involve multiple tissue plans (e.g. skin, subcutis) or by crossing muscle compartments to involve similar tissue types (e.g. multiple muscles) {2304}.

Epidemiology
About two thirds of cases of angiomatosis present in the first two decades of life {649,1234,2304}. Females are affected slightly more often than males.

Etiology
Angiomatosis was once classified as a neoplasm, but currently is considered a vascular malformation because it: (i) presents early in life; (ii) grows proportionately with the host; (iii) is composed of mitotically quiescent vessels; and (iv) shows no tendency to regress {1977}.

Sites of involvement
More than one half of cases occur in the lower extremities, followed by the chest wall, abdomen, and upper extremity.

Clinical features
Most lesions are likely congenital but, because of their deep location, become apparent at adolescence or in early adult life. Patients with angiomatosis present with diffuse persistent swelling of the affected part, which may wax and wane in size, and is affected by strenuous activity. If significant arteriovenous shunting is present, the patient displays increased skin temperature, thrill, pulsation or hypertrophy of the affected part.

Macroscopy
The lesions are ill-defined masses that vary from a few to many centimetres in diameter.

Histopathology
Angiomatosis contains a mixture of large arteries, veins, and small capillaries. The

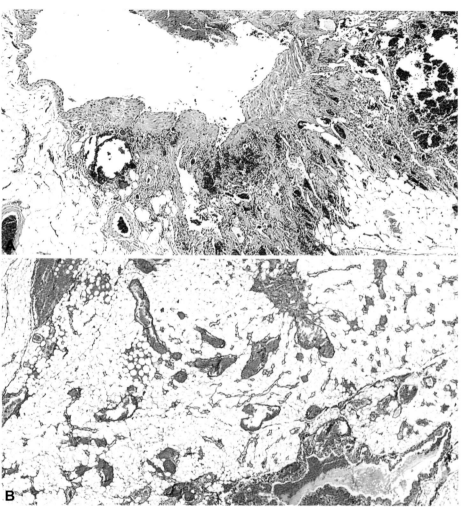

Fig. 8.09 Angiomatosis. **A** Clusters of small vessels radiate from a vein. **B** Note the diffuse growth pattern.

proportion is influenced by whether the angiomatosis is clinically/radiographically an arteriovenous or venous malformation. The most common pattern observed in the majority of surgically resected cases of angiomatosis is that of thick and thin-walled veins associated with capillary-sized vessels scattered haphazardly throughout the tissue {2304}. The veins have irregularly attenuated walls from which sprout clusters of small venules or capillaries. A less common pattern of angiomatosis consists of infiltrating nodules of capillary vessels. Whether these are two

distinct patterns or regional variations within a tumour is not clear.

Immunophenotype
These lesions are GLUT1-negative.

Prognostic factors
Although biologically benign, nearly 90% of lesions persist after surgical excision, and 50% recur multiple times {2304}. Recurrence is related to incomplete excision as well as recruitment of collateral arterial flow into a low-resistance vascular bed.

Lymphangioma

A. Beham

Definition
A benign, cavernous/cystic vascular lesion composed of dilated lymphatic channels.

ICD-O code   9170/0

Synonyms
Cystic hygroma; lymphatic malformation

Epidemiology
Lymphangiomas are common paediatric lesions, presenting most often at birth or during the first years of life {50}. Some cases are identified in the context of Turner syndrome (or other malformative syndromes) and may be found in abortuses {184,351,440}. Cavernous/cystic lymphangioma of head and neck represents the most frequent subtype.

Etiology
Early or even congenital appearance in life and lesional architecture favour a developmental malformation, with genetic abnormalities playing an additional role {2959}.

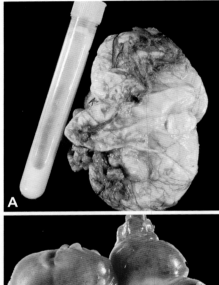

Fig. 8.10 Cystic lymphangioma. **A** The tube shows the milky lymph removed from the collapsed lesion. **B** Lesion located in the lower neck of a fetus with Turner syndrome. **C** Large, partly cystic lymphangioma from mesentery and partially covered by adipose tissue.

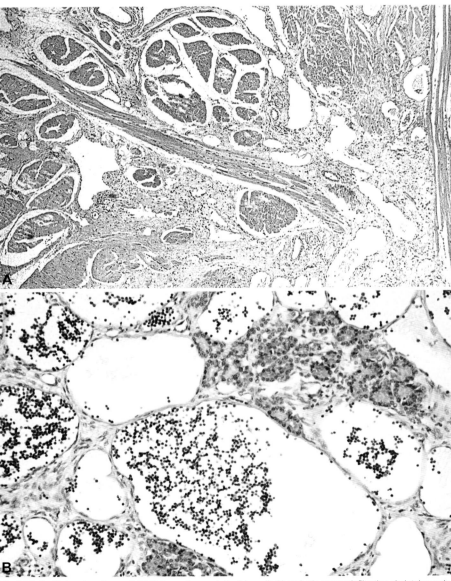

Fig. 8.11 Cystic lymphangioma. **A** Multiple, cystic or ectatic, thin-walled lymphatic spaces infiltrating skeletal muscle. **B** Thin-walled spaces of varying diameter, containing lymph and/or lymphocytes, and lined by flattened endothelium.

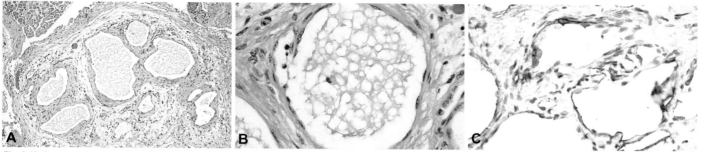

Fig. 8.12 Cavernous lymphangioma. **A** Note the prominent smooth muscle in the vessel walls. **B** There is no endothelial multilayering or atypia. **C** Immunoreactivity of the lymphatic endothelium to the antibody D2-40.

Sites of involvement
Cystic lymphangiomas are mostly located in the neck, axilla and groin, whereas the cavernous type occurs additionally in the oral cavity, upper trunk, limbs and abdominal sites, including mesentery and retroperitoneum {50,1219}.

Clinical features
The lesions present as rather circumscribed painless swellings, which are soft and fluctuant on palpation, and show displacement of surrounding organs at mediastinal (compression of trachea and oesophagus) or intra-abdominal sites (intestinal obstruction).

Macroscopy
Cavernous/cystic lymphangiomas correspond to a multicystic or spongy mass, with cavities containing watery/milky fluid.

Histopathology
Cavernous/cystic lymphangiomas are characterized by thin-walled, dilated lymphatic vessels of different sizes, lined by flattened endothelium, and frequently surrounded by lymphocytic aggregates. The lumina may be empty, or contain proteinaceous fluid, lymphocytes and sometimes erythrocytes. Larger vessels can be invested by a smooth-muscle layer, and longstanding lesions may show interstitial fibrosis and stromal inflammation {1219}. Stromal mast cells and haemosiderin deposition are common.

Immunophenotype
The endothelium expresses podoplanin (D2-40) and PROX1 {1895} selectively, CD31 consistently, and CD34 variably {922,1219}.

Prognostic factors
Rare recurrences are due to incomplete surgical removal. Malignant transformation does not occur.

Kaposiform haemangioendothelioma
S.W. Weiss

Definition
Kaposiform haemangioendothelioma is a locally aggressive vascular tumour often associated with Kasabach-Merritt phenomenon and displaying features reminiscent of both capillary haemangioma and Kaposi sarcoma {1682,3076}.

ICD-O code   9130/1

Synonyms
Kaposi-like haemangioendothelioma; haemangioma with Kaposi-like features

Epidemiology
This tumour occurs nearly exclusively in children. More than half present during the first year of life. Males are more often affected than females. Cases in adults are distinctly rare {1840}.

Etiology
The etiology is unknown; the tumour is not related to HHV8 infection or Kaposi sarcoma.

Sites of involvement
The tumour occurs most often in soft tissues of the extremity. A small subset occur in body cavities, e.g. retroperitoneum.

Clinical features
These tumours are typically ill-defined, violaceous lesions on the extremities. Large lesions at any site may present with thrombocytopenia (Kasabach-Merritt phenomenon) {2787}. A subset of patients have signs and symptoms of lymphangiomatosis.

Histopathology
The tumours consist of irregular vascular lobules that infiltrate soft tissue in a "cannon-ball" fashion and that may evoke striking desmoplasia. The tumour modulates between areas having features of a capillary haemangioma and Kaposi sarcoma.

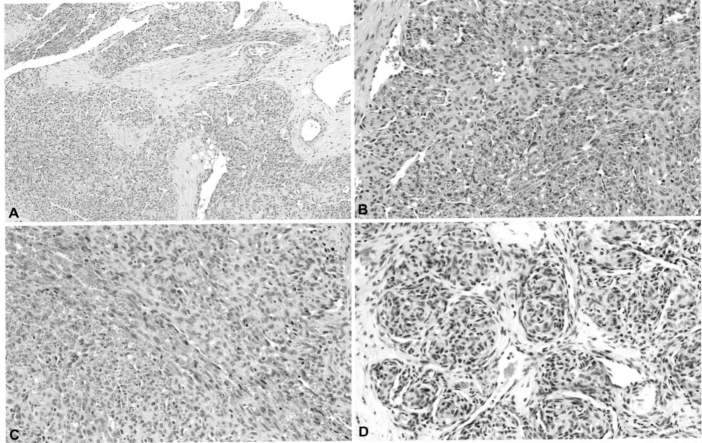

Fig. 8.13 Kaposiform haemangioendothelioma. **A** Low-power view illustrating large, irregularly shaped tumour nodules. **B** A capillary haemangioma-like area. **C** A spindled, Kaposi-like area. **D** Glomeruloid clusters of vessels.

A signature feature of the lesions is glomeruloid structures, which comprise tightly coiled, CD31-positive capillary vessels invested with actin-positive pericytes. They contain CD61-positive fibrin thrombi and probably represent the site of platelet sequestration {1682}. Adjacent to these bodies are compressed rims of slit-like vessels. Large lymphatic vessels are present adjacent to the tumour. In the extreme case, the number and size of the lymphatic vessels qualifies as a lymphangioma/lymphangiomatosis. This lesion is morphologically identical to tufted angioma.

Immunophenotype

Immunohistochemical studies have documented the participation of blood vascular and lymphatic components {1577}. Lymphatic markers (PROX1, LYVE1, podoplanin, and VEGFR3) are highly expressed in the slit-like Kaposi-like vessels, whereas the glomeruloid structures lack these antigens and express only CD31 and CD34 {1577}. The endothelium within Kaposiform haemangioendothelioma does not express GLUT1, the glucose transport protein expressed in infantile haemangioma.

Prognostic factors

Kaposiform haemangioendothelioma shows no tendency to regress. Patient outcome is highly dependent on site, clinical extent and whether there is supervening thrombocytopenia. Mortality from this disease is approximately 10% and is attributable to extensive local disease or thrombocytopenia. One case of regional lymph-node metastasis has been reported, but there have been no reports of disseminated disease {1682}.

Retiform haemangioendothelioma

J.E. Calonje

Definition

Retiform haemangioendothelioma (RH) is a locally aggressive, rarely metastasizing vascular lesion, characterized by distinctive arborizing blood vessels lined by endothelial cells with characteristic hobnail morphology.

ICD-O code   9137/1

Synonym

Hobnail haemangioendothelioma

Epidemiology

RH is uncommon. Since its original description in 1994, only about 35 cases have been reported {39,361,923,1845, 2712}. The age range is wide, but it usually affects young adults or children; males and females are affected equally frequently.

Sites of involvement

The tumour involves predominantly the skin and subcutaneous tissue and is most commonly found in the distal extremities, particularly the lower limb.

Clinical features

RH presents as a red/bluish slowly growing plaque or nodule usually < 3 cm in maximum dimension. A case with multiple lesions has been described {711}. Exceptional cases occur in the setting of previous radiotherapy {361}, pre-existing lymphoedema {361} and in association with a cystic lymphangioma {39}.

Macroscopy

Macroscopic examination reveals diffuse, sometimes discoloured, induration of the dermis with frequent involvement of the underlying subcutaneous tissue.

Histopathology

Scanning magnification reveals characteristic elongated and narrow arborizing vascular channels with a striking resemblance to normal rete testis. Although this pattern is usually readily apparent, if the vascular channels are small or collapsed, then the retiform architecture may be difficult to recognize. Monomorphic hyperchromatic endothelial cells with prominent protuberant nuclei having a characteristic "tombstone" or "hobnail" appearance line the blood vessels. These cells have scanty cytoplasm, which seems to blend with the underlying stroma. Pleomorphism is absent and mitotic figures are rare. A prominent stromal and often intravascular lymphocytic infiltrate is present in around half of the cases. The stroma surrounding the tumour tends to be sclerotic. Focal solid areas composed of sheets of endothelial cells are often identified. Vacuolated cells are uncommonly seen. Monomorphic endothelial spindle-shaped cells are also a rare feature and were described in a case of metastatic disease in a lymph node {361}. In some cases there are intravascular papillae with hyaline collagenous cores similar to those seen in papillary intralymphatic angioendothelioma {39}. Retiform haemangioendothelioma can be one of the components of a composite haemangioendothelioma.

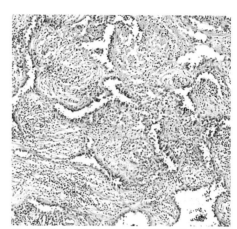

Fig. 8.14 Retiform haemangioendothelioma. Characteristic arborizing channels simulating the rete testis and with a prominent stromal lymphocytic infiltrate.

Immunophenotype

The neoplastic cells in RH stain for vascular markers including CD31, CD34, and ERG. Staining for CD34 is often stronger than that for other vascular markers. Claudin-5 (CLDN5), a tight-junction protein,

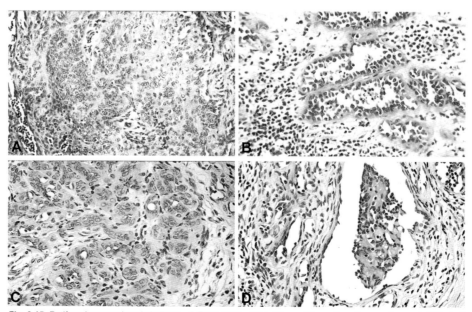

Fig. 8.15 Retiform haemangioendothelioma. **A** Focal areas with a more solid growth pattern are frequent. **B** Typical hobnail endothelial cells with prominent nuclei. Vacuolated cells (**C**) and intraluminal papillae (**D**) with collagenous cores similar to those seen in Dabska tumour are seen in some cases.

has recently been proposed as a reliable marker in vascular tumours including RH {1892}. A number of the histological features of the neoplasm suggest that the tumour is of lymphatic lineage. Although the lymphatic marker PROX1 is positive in RH, other lymphatic markers, including podoplanin (D2-40) and the less specific VEGFR3 are usually but not always negative {742,1895,2191}. In general experience, these lesions are negative for HHV8.

Prognostic factors
Multiple local recurrences (in up to 60% of cases), often over many years, are the rule, unless wide local excision is performed {361}. So far two patients have been reported as having developed a metastasis to a regional lymph node {221,361}. An additional patient developed a local soft tissue metastasis from a primary in the right big toe {1845}. To date, no patients have developed distant metastases or died from this disease.

Papillary intralymphatic angioendothelioma

J.C. Fanburg-Smith

Definition
Papillary intralymphatic angioendothelioma (PILA) {811} is a rarely metastasizing lymphatic vascular neoplasm {537,2485} that may be related to retiform haemangioendothelioma.

ICD-O code   9135/1

Synonyms
Dabska tumour {537,2486}; malignant endothelial papillary angioendothelioma; hobnail haemangioendothelioma

Epidemiology
Originally described in 1969 {537} and renamed 30 years later for its borderline behaviour and prominent lymphatic phenotype {811}.
PILA is very rare, occurring more commonly in infants and children, with about 25% of cases presenting in adults {811}.

These tumours occur equally frequently in males and females

Sites of involvement
Most PILA involve the extremities (especially thigh/buttocks) {811}, less commonly elsewhere on the trunk, head and neck, intra-abdominal, parenchymal (spleen) {1378} and intraosseous {1777} locations.

Clinical features
PILA presents as a slowly growing asymptomatic cutaneous induration, plaque, or rarely nodule, often with unremarkable overlying skin {811}.

Macroscopy
Tumours are ill defined and usually involve dermis and subcutaneous tissue. Grossly, grey-white to pink streaks or cystic change in otherwise normal dermis and subcutis may be visualized; haemorrhage

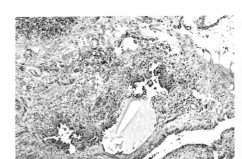

Fig. 8.16 Papillary intralymphatic angioendothelioma is an extensive dermal and subcutaneous lymphatic vascular proliferation, often with obvious lymphangioma with proteinaceous luminal fluid in addition to intraluminal columnar endothelial-cell proliferation.

or necrosis is not present. Tumour size ranges from 1 to > 40 cm (mean, 7 cm) {811}.

Histopathology
PILA is an extensive, poorly delineated

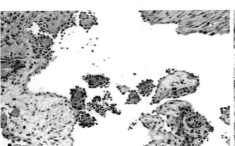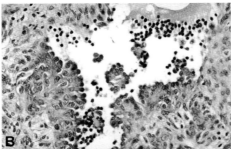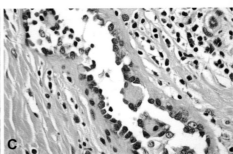

Fig. 8.17 Papillary intralymphatic angioendothelioma (PILA). **A, B** PILA is characterized by a matchstick-like, columnar or hobnail endothelial proliferation into lymphatic-channel lumina, at progressive higher magnifications. **C** The intraluminal endothelial tufting can have hyaline cores.

dermal and/or subcutaneous proliferation of lymphatic channels: a cavernous lymphangioma may be present adjacent to either cavernous or slit-like vascular channels with intraluminal proliferations of columnar/matchstick-like/hobnail endothelial cells with eosinophilic cytoplasm, indistinct nucleoli, lack of frank cytological atypia and relative absence of mitotic activity {811}. The intraluminal papillary tufts have hyaline cores and intermixed intraluminal lymphocytes. Accompanying rare epithelioid endothelial cells and glomeruloid-like pericytic proliferations may suggest a capillary component.

Immunophenotype
The lymphatic phenotype of PILA is confirmed by immunostaining of tumour cells by podoplanin (D2-40) {922} and VEGFR3 {811}, as well as endothelial markers, CD31 more strongly than CD34 {811}.

Prognostic factors
In the original series, two patients had lymph-node metastasis and one died of disease during long-term follow-up {537, 2485}. However, follow-up in more recent series demonstrates no local recurrence or metastasis {811}, and most cases have excellent prognosis with complete, wide excision {1777}.

Composite haemangioendothelioma

B.P. Rubin

Definition
Composite haemangioendothelioma is a locally aggressive, rarely metastasizing vascular neoplasm, containing an admixture of histologically distinct components.

ICD-O code   9130/1

Epidemiology
Composite haemangioendothelioma is an extremely rare neoplasm, with 28 cases reported in the English language literature to date {125,926,2017,2320,2329, 2785}. There is a female predominance (18 females : 10 males) and the majority of cases occur in adults with a median age of 42.5 years. However, three cases first developed in infancy and another two cases developed in childhood {926,2017, 2320,2329}. One case that developed in infancy arose in a patient with Maffucci syndrome {926}.

Sites of involvement
Most cases occur on the distal extremities, especially the hands and feet. Other sites

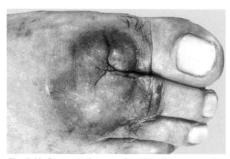

Fig. 8.18 Composite haemangioendothelioma presenting as a bluish-purple multinodular mass.

have included tongue, mandibular vestibule, cheek, hypopharynx, back and inguinal lymph node.

Clinical features
Several patients with composite haemangioendothelioma had a history of lymphoedema. Lesions are usually longstanding (up to several decades) and have a reddish-blue, variably nodular appearance.

Macroscopy
Composite haemangioendothelioma presents as an infiltrative, uninodular or multinodular mass (individual nodules measure 0.7–30 cm; median, 3.2 cm), or as an area of ill-defined "swelling". Some of the lesions are associated with reddish purple skin discoloration, suggestive of a vascular neoplasm.

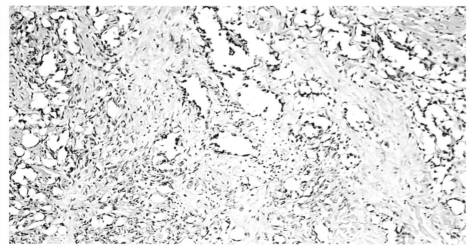

Fig. 8.19 Composite haemangioendothelioma. This complex lesion had areas consistent with retiform haemangioendothelioma, as well as more solid areas consistent with epithelioid haemangioendothelioma.

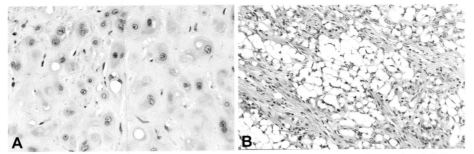

Fig. 8.20 Composite haemangioendothelioma. **A** Typical appearance of the epithelioid haemangioendothelioma component. **B** Sheets of vacuolated endothelial cells are not unusual.

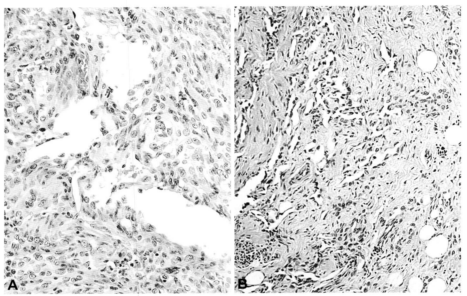

Fig. 8.21 Composite haemangioendothelioma. **A** Some lesions have areas consistent with spindle cell haemangioma. **B** These areas are consistent histologically with well-differentiated angiosarcoma.

Histopathology

Composite haemangioendothelioma is a poorly circumscribed, infiltrative lesion, which is centred in the dermis and subcutis. It comprises a complex admixture of histologically benign and malignant vascular components that vary greatly in their relative proportions. These lesions are unified by a similar admixture of the different components, which include epithelioid haemangioendothelioma, retiform haemangioendothelioma, spindle cell haemangioma, "angiosarcoma-like" areas, and benign vascular lesions (lymphangioma, angiomatatosis, arteriovenous malformation, cavernous haemangioma, and lymphangioma circumscriptum). Not all cases contain every component. Another interesting feature, seen in several cases, is the presence of large numbers of vacuolated endothelial cells that impart a pseudolipoblastic appearance. The "angiosarcoma-like" areas are usually characterized by a low-grade angiosarcomatous appearance composed of complex dissecting vascular channels with endothelial atypia and relatively few mitotic figures.

Prognostic factors

Several lesions recurred locally between 4 months and 10 years after excision of the primary mass, often with multiple recurrences. Two cases developed lymphnode metastases within months to 2 years and in the patient with the tongue lesion, metastasis occurred to a submandibular lymph node and to the soft tissue of the thigh at 9 and 11 years after excision of the primary, respectively {125,2017, 2329}. Thus, the behaviour of this lesion appears to be much less aggressive than that of conventional angiosarcoma.

Kaposi sarcoma

T. Mentzel
S. Knuutila
J. Lamovec

Definition

Kaposi sarcoma (KS) is a locally aggressive, endothelial tumour or a tumour-like lesion that usually presents with cutaneous lesions in the form of multiple patches, plaques or nodules, but may also involve different mucosal sites, lymph nodes and visceral organs. The disease is uniformly associated with human herpesvirus (HHV8) infection {425,1943}, and most likely represents an example of virus-induced vascular proliferation.

ICD-O code   9140/3

Synonyms

Idiopathic multiple pigmented sarcoma of the skin; angiosarcoma multiplex; granuloma multiplex haemorrhagicum

Epidemiology

Four different clinical and epidemiological forms of KS are recognized:
(i) *classic indolent KS*, which occurs predominantly in elderly men of Mediterranean/East European or Ashkenazi descent; (ii) *endemic African KS*, which occurs in middle-aged adults and children in equatorial Africa who are not infected with HIV; (iii) *iatrogenic KS*, which arises in solid-organ transplant recipients treated with immunosuppressive therapy and also in patients treated by immunosuppressive agents, notably corticosteroids, for various diseases {2776}; and (iv) *AIDS-associated KS* (AIDS KS), the most aggressive form of the disease, found in individuals infected with HIV-1, which is particularly frequent in homosexual and bisexual men. The relative risk of acquiring KS in the latter patients is > 10 000 {996}; the risk has been reduced with the advent of highly active antiretroviral therapy (HAART) {232}.

Etiology

The long-sought-after infectious agent causing KS was identified in 1994 by Chang et al. and was named as KS-associated herpesvirus (KSHV) or HHV8 (532). The virus is found in KS cells of all epidemiological-clinical forms of the disease

and is detected in the peripheral blood before the development of KS {943,2948}; the disease itself is the result of the complex interplay of HHV8 with immunological, genetic and environmental factors {747,1447}.

Sites of involvement

The most typical site of involvement by KS is the skin. During the course of the disease, or initially, mucosal membranes (e.g. oral mucosa), lymph nodes, and visceral organs may be affected, sometimes without skin involvement. The involvement of a variety of tissues and organs has been described and essentially no organ is invariably spared {1283}, although brain and bone involvement is rare, even in disseminated disease.

Clinical features

The classic type of KS is characterized by the appearance of purplish, reddish blue or dark brown macules, plaques and nodules that may ulcerate. They are particularly frequent in distal extremities and may be accompanied by lymphoedema. The disease is usually indolent; lymph-node and visceral involvement occurs only rarely.
In the endemic form of KS, the disease may be localized to skin and shows a protracted course. A variant of endemic disease, a lymphadenopatic form in children, is rapidly progressive and highly lethal.
Iatrogenic KS is relatively infrequent. It develops within a few months to several years after the transplantation of solid organs or immunosuppressive treatment for a variety of conditions. The disease may resolve upon withdrawal of immunosuppressive treatment, although its course is somewhat unpredictable. Patients who develop visceral lesions may succumb to their disease {2214}.
AIDS-associated KS is the most aggressive type. In the skin, lesions are most common on the face, genitals, and lower extremities; oral mucosa, lymph nodes, gastrointestinal tract and lungs are frequently involved. Lymph-node and visceral disease without mucocutaneous lesions may occur.

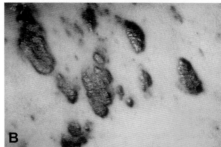
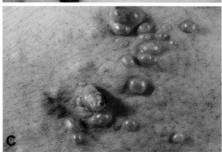

Fig. 8.22 Kaposi sarcoma. **A** Patch lesion. **B** Plaque-stage lesion. **C** Nodular-stage lesion.

While skin lesions and lymphadenopathy are obvious signs of the disease in various types of KS, the involvement of visceral organs may be silent or symptomatic, depending on the extent and particular location of the lesions.

Macroscopy

The lesions in the skin (patches, plaques, nodules) range in size from very small to several centimetres in diameter. Involvement of the mucosa, soft tissues, lymph nodes and visceral organs presents as haemorrhagic nodules of various sizes that may coalesce.

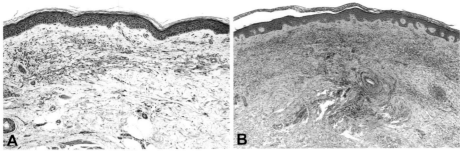

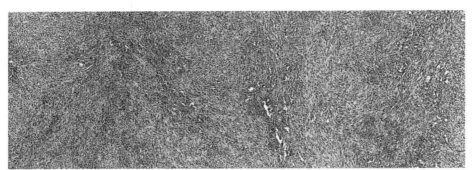

Fig. 8.23 Kaposi sarcoma. **A** The early form shows scattered spindled cells, dilated and narrow vascular spaces and inflammatory cells. Note that the upper part of the papillary dermis is not involved, which represents an important finding in the differential diagnosis. **B** An increase in the number of spindled cells, vascular spaces and inflammatory cells is seen in plaque-stage lesions.

Fig. 8.24 An example of nodular stage Kaposi sarcoma composed of cellular bundles and fascicles of spindled cells as well as slit- and sieve-like vascular spaces.

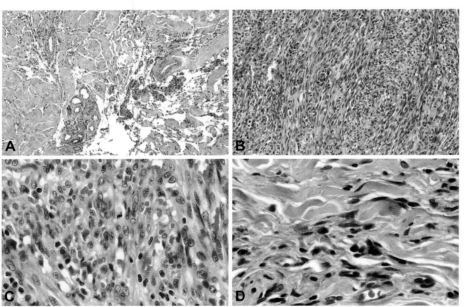

Fig. 8.25 Kaposi sarcoma. **A** Numerous dilated, lymphatic-like vascular spaces resembling lymphangioendothelioma are seen. **B** Cytologically bland spindled cells and scattered inflammatory cells are closely associated with narrow vascular spaces. Note the numerous erythrocytes. **C** Despite the bland cytology of spindled tumour cells at the nodular stage, mitoses are easily identified. **D** Note that inflammatory cells, especially plasma cells, are closely associated with spindled cells and small vascular spaces.

Histopathology

All four different epidemiological-clinical types of KS show identical morphological features. Early lesions of the skin are uncharacteristic and present with subtle vascular proliferation {2396}.

In the patch stage, vascular spaces are increased in number, and dissect collagen fibres in the upper reticular dermis. Lining endothelial cells are flattened or more oval, with no or little atypia. Pre-existing blood vessels may protrude into the lumen of new vessels. In addition a proliferation of oval to spindle-shaped endothelial cells surrounding pre-existing blood vessels is noted. An admixed infiltrate of lymphocytes and plasma cells and frequently extravasated erythrocytes and haemosiderin deposits is seen. Rarely lymphangioma or haemangioma-like lesions may be present causing considerable problems in the differential diagnosis. The papillary dermis is not involved in early stages.

In the plaque stage, all characteristics of the patch stage are exaggerated, angio-proliferation is extensive with vascular spaces showing jagged outlines. The inflammatory infiltrate is denser and extravascular erythrocytes and siderophages are numerous. Hyaline globules are frequently found. The nodular stage is characterized by well-circumscribed, cellular nodules of intersecting fascicles of spindle cells with no or little cytological atypia and numerous slit-like spaces containing erythrocytes. Peripherally, there are ectatic blood vessels. Hyaline droplets are present inside and outside the spindle cells.

Rare histological variants include anaplastic Kaposi sarcoma characterized by an aggressive clinical course and increased metastatic potential {1266,3044}, intravascular Kaposi sarcoma {1678} and lymphangioma-like Kaposi sarcoma.

In lymph nodes, the infiltrate may be uni- or multifocal and lymph nodes may be entirely effaced by the tumour. Early lesions may be subtle, showing only increased numbers of vascular channels accompanied by plasma-cell infiltration in the sinusoids {1668}. In visceral organs, the lesions tend to respect the architecture of the organs involved and spread along vascular structures, bronchi, portal areas in the liver etc., and from these sites they involve surrounding parenchyma {801}.

Immunophenotype

The lining cells of vascular structures and the spindled tumour cells are positive for pan-endothelial markers including CD31, CD34 and ERG, as well as lymphatic markers such as podoplanin (D2-40), and show almost invariable nuclear expression of HHV8 {882}. In rare negative cases, PCR confirmation may be helpful.

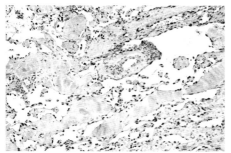

Fig. 8.26 A rare example of lymphangioendothelioma-like Kaposi sarcoma. Note the nuclear expression of HHV8 in endothelial cells.

Genetics

No clinically relevant genetic changes have been reported. Earlier CGH analyses indicated a recurrent involvement of 11q13 {1431} including the target genes *FGF4* and *FGF3*. A more recent CGH study showed loss of the Y chromosome to be recurrent in early phases of the disease, while additional changes of chromosomes 16, 17, 21, X, and Y appeared during tumour growth {2279}. *KRAS* and *TP53* alterations have been reported {2031,2489} in addition to aberrant expression of numerous genes related to neoangiogenesis and proliferation that

may have an impact on endothelial cell transformation by KSHV {1959,2288, 2679}. Both viral and cellular DNA encoded microRNAs have been shown to play an important role in KS pathogenesis {942, 1033,2429}.

Prognostic factors

The evolution of disease depends on the epidemiological–clinical type of KS and on its clinical extent (see above). It is also modified by treatment that includes surgery, radio- and chemotherapy. Cases with widespread visceral involvement are commonly poorly responsive to treatment.

Pseudomyogenic haemangioendothelioma

J.L. Hornick
C.D.M. Fletcher
F. Mertens

Definition

Pseudomyogenic haemangioendothelioma is a distinctive, rarely metastasizing endothelial neoplasm that occurs more frequently in young adult males, and that often presents as multiple discontiguous nodules in different tissue planes of a limb and histologically mimics a myoid tumour or epithelioid sarcoma.

ICD-O code   9138/1

Synonym

Epithelioid sarcoma-like haemangioendothelioma

Epidemiology

This lesion is rare, with just over 60 reported cases {236,1224,1911}. There is a

marked male predominance (male to female ratio, 4 : 1), with peak incidence in young adults (mean age, 30 years). Only 20% of patients are older than 40 years at presentation.

Sites of involvement

Pseudomyogenic (epithelioid sarcoma-like) haemangioendothelioma usually arises on the lower limbs (60% of patients); upper limbs and trunk are less commonly affected {236,1224,1911} and lesions rarely occur on the face or scalp.

Clinical features

The preoperative duration is typically short (< 18 months). About half of affected patients present with painless and half with painful nodules. In approximately two

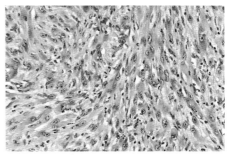

Fig. 8.27 Pseudomyogenic haemangioendothelioma. The tumour cells contain abundant brightly eosinophilic cytoplasm. Note the uniform nuclear morphology.

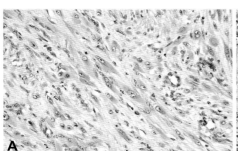
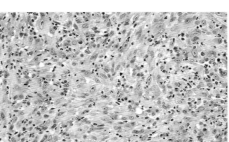
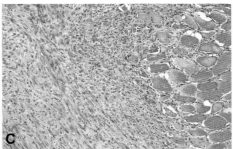

Fig. 8.28 Pseudomyogenic haemangioendothelioma. **A** Some tumour cells with brightly eosinophilic cytoplasm resemble rhabdomyoblasts. **B** Prominent stromal neutrophils can be seen in this example. Note the scattered tumour cells with a more epithelioid appearance. **C** The tumour shows infiltrative margins into adjacent skeletal muscle.

thirds of patients, this disease is multifocal, often involving multiple tissue planes {1224}. Most patients present with cutaneous and subcutaneous nodules. About 50% of affected patients have intramuscular lesions, and 20% of patients have lytic bony lesions {1224,1911}. By PET, the tumours in most patients are highly avid for 18F-fluorodeoxyglucose {1224}; this technique can be used to visualize clinically occult deep lesions in patients who present with cutaneous nodules.

Macroscopy
Grossly, margins are ill-defined and the cut surface is firm, grey or white. Most tumour nodules are between 1 and 2.5 cm in greatest dimension; only 10% of tumours are > 3 cm in size {1224}.

Histopathology
The tumour is composed of sheets and loose fascicles of plump spindle cells with abundant brightly eosinophilic cytoplasm, sometimes mimicking rhabdomyoblasts. The tumour cells contain vesicular nuclei with generally small nucleoli. A minor component of cells with epithelioid cytomorphology is often present. The degree of nuclear atypia is usually mild, and mitotic activity is scarce. About 10% of tumours show notable pleomorphism. Occasional tumours contain focally myxoid stroma. About 50% of cases contain prominent stromal neutrophils. The tumours show infiltrative margins.

Immunophenotype
These tumours show diffuse expression of keratin AE1/AE3 and the endothelial transcription factors FLI1 and ERG. About 50% of cases are positive for CD31. Focal expression of SMA is observed in one third of tumours. Staining for keratin MNF-116, EMA, S100 protein, CD34, and desmin is consistently negative. In contrast to epithelioid sarcoma, INI1 expression is retained in tumour cells {1224}.

Ultrastructure
The cytoplasm contains prominent rough endoplasmic reticulum and aggregates of intermediate filaments {1224,1911}. Subplasmalemmal pinocytotic vesicles are numerous in some cells, and scattered desmosome-like junctions are seen. An external lamina is prominent in some cases.

Genetics
Cytogenetic information is restricted to a single case showing a balanced t(7;19)(q22;q13) as the sole change. Interphase FISH analysis identified an unbalanced der(7)t(7;19) in one of nine additional cases {2781}.

Prognostic factors
Approximately 60% of patients with this tumour experience local recurrences (often multiple) or develop additional nodules in the same anatomical region {236,1224, 1911}. The interval between excision of the primary tumour and recurrence is usually

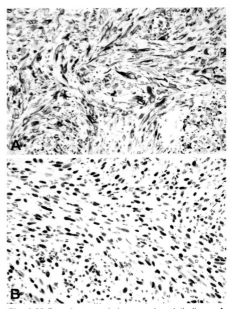

Fig. 8.29 Pseudomyogenic haemangioendothelioma. **A** Diffuse expression of keratin AE1/AE3. **B** Strong nuclear staining for the endothelial transcription factor ERG.

short, within 1–2 years. The relationship between margin status and recurrence has not been established. A regional lymph-node metastasis has been detected in only one patient, and only two patients thus far have developed distant metastases, 7 years and 16 years after excision of the primary, and died of disease {1224,1911}. Metastatic sites included lungs (both cases), bones, scalp, and soft tissues.

Other intermediate vascular neoplasms

C.D.M. Fletcher
B.P. Rubin
W.Y.W. Tsang

The Working Group also considered two other tumours – polymorphous haemangioendothelioma and giant cell angioblastoma – for possible inclusion in this edition of the WHO classification, but decided that the available data were insufficient to allow definitive classification of these lesions. Specifically, very few cases have been reported to date, there are as yet no clear diagnostic criteria and there are uncertainties regarding the biological potential of these lesions. Giant cell angioblastoma, of which fewer than 10 cases have been reported, arises in soft tissue of infants, is comprised of nodular aggregates of histiocytoid cells arranged around bland angiomatous vessels and may show persistent growth {1009,2857}.

As yet, it is not certain that this is primarily an endothelial tumour. Polymorphous haemangioendothelioma, of which fewer than 10 convincing cases have been reported, may primarily involve soft tissue or lymph nodes, affects adults, has morphological features that are complex and suggestive of poor outcome, and metastasizes in some cases {418,2008, 2199,2314}.

Epithelioid haemangioendothelioma

S.W. Weiss
C.R. Antonescu
J.A. Bridge
A.T. Deyrup

Definition
Epithelioid haemangioendothelioma is a malignant angiocentric vascular neoplasm composed of cords of epithelioid endothelial cells in a distinctively myxohyaline stroma and characterized by a *WWTR1-CAMTA1* fusion.

ICD-O code   9133/3

Synonym
Intravascular bronchioloalveolar tumour (IVBAT) is an archaic term for epithelioid haemangioendothelioma in the lungs.

Epidemiology
Epithelioid haemangioendothelioma affects patients of all ages, but is most common after the second decade of life. There is a slight predominance in females {657, 1828,2927,2931}.

Sites of involvement
The tumour arises as a solitary soft tissue mass usually on the extremities but, given its angiocentricity, can be found in virtually any body site.

Clinical features
The tumour develops as a slightly painful mass in soft tissue. Those arising from large vessels can give rise to symptoms of vascular occlusion. Longstanding tumours may ossify and therefore be identified on plain-film radiography.

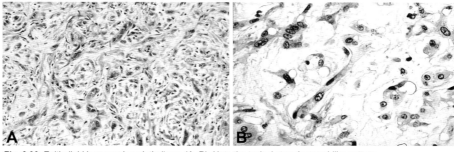

Fig. 8.30 Epithelioid haemangioendothelioma (**A**, **B**). Note the typical strand or cord-like pattern.

Macroscopy
Angiocentric tumours appear as a firm, tan-tinged mass circumscribed by the vessel wall.

Histopathology
Angiocentric tumours expand the vessel wall, obliterate the lumen, and spread centrifugally into surrounding tissue where they induce a sclerotic response. The tumour is characterized by chains and cords of epithelioid endothelial cells distributed in a myxohyaline stroma. The cells have eosinophilic cytoplasm containing vacuoles that deform the cytoplasm (blister cells). Some vacuoles contain fragmented erythrocytes. The sulfated acid-rich matrix varies from light blue (chondroid) to deep pink (hyaline). In most cases the cells are of low nuclear grade. However, a subset has higher-grade morphology and are labelled by some as "malignant epithelioid haemangioendothelioma."

Immunophenotype
Epithelioid haemangioendotheliomas express typical vascular markers including CD34, CD31, FLI1, and ERG transcription factor {882,1897,2375}. In 25–40% of cases, epithelial antigens are also expressed (keratins 7, 8, 18 and EMA) {1828,1880}.

Ultrastructure
Vascular differentiation has been documented by investiture of cells with basal lamina, surface-oriented pinocytotic vesicles, and Weibel-Palade bodies.

Genetics
Epithelioid haemangioendothelioma has a t(1;3)(p36;q23-25) that results in a fusion of *WWTR1* in 3q23-24 with *CAMTA1* in 1p36 in virtually all cases {773,1825, 2716}. This fusion event is unique to this tumour and is not found in its mimics. Three fusion-transcript variants have been described: exon 3 or 4 of *WWTR1* fused to

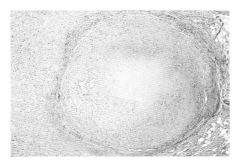

Fig. 8.31 Epithelioid haemangioendothelioma involving the lumen of a small vein and extending into adjacent tissue. Origin from a vessel is evident in about 30% of cases.

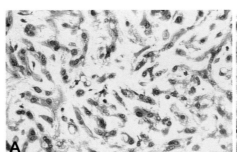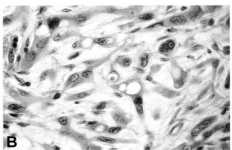

Fig. 8.32 Epithelioid haemangioendothelioma. Note the myxoid matrix (**A**) and intracytoplasmic lumina (**B**).

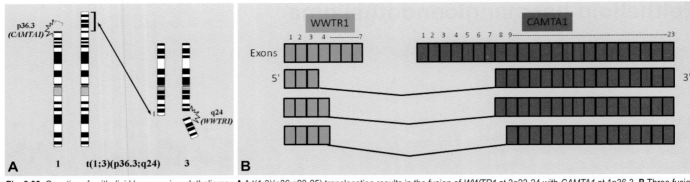

Fig. 8.33 Genetics of epithelioid haemangioendothelioma. **A** A t(1;3)(p36;q23-25) translocation results in the fusion of *WWTR1* at 3q23-24 with *CAMTA1* at 1p36.3. **B** Three fusion-transcript variants have been described in which exon 3 or 4 of *WWTR1* is fused to either exon 8 or 9 of *CAMTA1*.

either exon 8 or 9 of *CAMTA1*. The fusion gene encodes a putative transcription factor that places *CAMTA1* under control of the *WWTR1* promoter and results in over-expression of the C-terminus of CAMTA1, thereby activating a novel transcriptional programme. The monoclonal origin of "multifocal" epithelioid haemangioendotheliomas has also been established using *WWTR1-CAMTA1* breakpoint analysis. This indicates that multiple lesions arise from local or metastatic spread from a single primary as opposed to multiple independent primaries {771}.

Prognostic factors

Most soft tissue epithelioid haemangioendotheliomas are indolent; however, 20–30% of tumours metastasize and about 15% of patients die of their disease {1828,2927,2931}. This contrasts with the behaviour of most angiosarcomas. Overtly malignant lesions, as described above, pursue an aggressive course. Recently, a combination of mitotic activity and tumour size has been used to stratify tumours into low- and high-risk groups: patients with tumours of > 3 cm in diameter and having > 3 mitoses per 50 HPF have a 5-year disease-specific survival of 59% compared with 100% survival in patients whose tumours lacked these features {657}.

Angiosarcoma of soft tissue

S.W. Weiss
C.R. Antonescu
A.T. Deyrup

Definition

Angiosarcoma is a malignant tumour that recapitulates the morphological and functional features of endothelium to a variable degree.

ICD-O code 9120/3

Synonyms

Angiosarcoma: haemangiosarcoma; malignant haemangioendothelioma; malignant angioendothelioma
Lymphoedema-associated angiosarcoma: lymphangiosarcoma

Epidemiology

Angiosarcomas of soft tissue affect patients

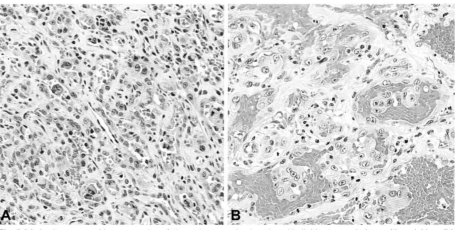

Fig. 8.34 Angiosarcoma. Many cases in soft tissue have predominantly epithelioid cytomorphology with variably solid or vasoformative architecture (**A**, **B**).

of all ages and have a peak incidence in the seventh decade of life. More cases occur in males than in females {863, 1818}. Angiosarcomas of deep soft tissue in children are extremely rare {655}.

Etiology
The etiology is unknown in most cases. A subset of cases is associated with exposure to radiation. A smaller subset occur adjacent to synthetic (graft) or foreign material, in the vicinity of arteriovenous fistulas in patients who have undergone renal transplant, in certain syndromes (neurofibromatosis, Maffucci syndrome) and, rarely, within other tumours. These associations suggest more than a fortuitous occurrence.

Sites of involvement
Angiosarcomas of soft tissue arise most commonly in the deep muscles of the lower extremities (approximately 40% of cases), followed by the retroperitoneum, mediastinum and mesentery {863,1818}.

Clinical features
The tumour presents as a painful enlarging mass of several months duration, associated in one third of cases with other symptoms, such as coagulopathy, anaemia, or persistent haematoma.

Macroscopy
Angiosarcomas of soft tissue are multinodular haemorrhagic masses often with secondary cystic degeneration and necrosis.

Histopathology
Angiosarcomas of soft tissue display a wide range of morphological appearances ranging from areas of well-formed, anastomosing vessels to solid sheets of high-grade epithelioid or spindled cells without clear vasoformation. Multiple patterns may be present in the same tumour. Vasoformative areas consist of ramifying channels lined by atypical endothelial cells forming intraluminal buds and papillations. Solid areas lacking vasoformation are composed of high-grade spindled and epithelioid cells with abundant amphophilic to lightly eosinophilic cytoplasm, large vesicular nucleoli and prominent nucleoli. Tumours in which these epithelioid cells predominate are classified as "epithelioid angiosarcomas." They are commonly confused with carcinomas because of morphological and immunophenotypical

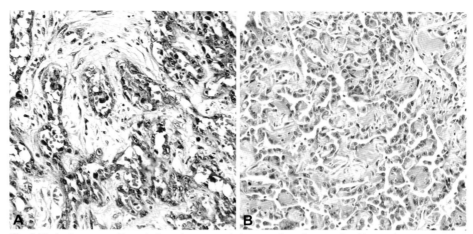

Fig. 8.35 Angiosarcoma. These lesions show more obvious vasoformative growth, with complex anastomosing channels (**A**, **B**).

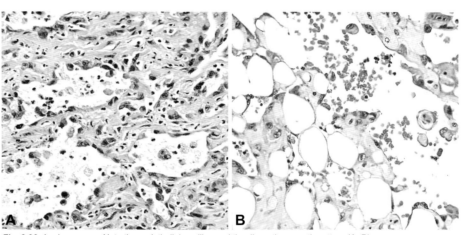

Fig. 8.36 Angiosarcoma. Note the endothelial papillae and the dissecting growth pattern (**A**, **B**).

similarities {26,863, 1880}. The vast majority of angiosarcomas of soft tissue are high-grade neoplasms with brisk mitotic activity, coagulative necrosis and significant nuclear atypia. Extensive haemorrhage is commonly present and may suggest a haematoma. Careful sampling may be necessary to document malignant cells.

Immunophenotype
Angiosarcomas express the typical vascular markers: CD34, CD31, ERG, FLI1 and occasionally podoplanin (D2-40), a lymphatic marker {653,882,1888,1897}. Given differences in sensitivity and specificity, a panel of antibodies should be used {653,882,1888}. Some angiosarcomas co-express epithelial antigens (keratins and, less often, EMA), a fact that should be considered in distinguishing

them from carcinoma. Immunostaining for HHV8 is negative.

Ultrastructure
Because of the superior performance of immunohistochemistry in the diagnosis of angiosarcoma, ultrastructural analysis is now rarely used. In well-differentiated tumours, plump endothelial cells are invested with basal lamina and an incomplete rim of pericytes. The cells possess tight junctions, surface-oriented pinocytotic vesicles, and occasional intracytoplasmic erythrocytes. Weibel-Palade bodies, a specific organelle of endothelium, are rarely identified within angiosarcomas.

Genetics
Angiosarcomas in general show distinct upregulation of vascular-specific receptor

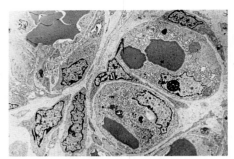

Fig. 8.37 High-grade angiosarcoma with epithelioid features, showing an ill-formed vessel lined by plump endothelial cells and containing erythrocytes.

tyrosine kinases, including TIE1, KDR, TEK and FLT1, compared with other types of sarcoma. In a subset (10%) of tumours, mutations in *KDR* (also known as *VEGFR*) are identified {85} and correlate with strong expression of KDR protein and location in the breast, irrespective of exposure to radiation. Furthermore, high-level amplification of *MYC* in 8q24 is a consistent hallmark of radiation-induced and lymphoedema-associated angiosarcoma {1065,1728}. *FLT4* (also known as *VEGFR3*) coamplification in 5q35 is detected in 25% of secondary angiosarcomas. Neither *MYC* nor *FLT4* gene abnormalities have been reported in primary deep-seated soft tissue angiosarcoma or radiation-associated atypical vascular lesions thus far {1065,1844}.

Prognostic factors

Angiosarcomas of soft tissue are aggressive malignancies with a high rate of tumour-related death. More than half of patients die within the first year {1818}. Features that are associated with poor outcome include older age, retroperitoneal location, large size and high Ki67 values {818,1818}. Other factors, which have been shown to have prognostic import for angiosarcomas in general, such as necrosis, margin status, and epithelioid change, have not been specifically validated for angiosarcomas in soft tissue {818,1528}.

CHAPTER 9

Chondro-osseous tumours

Soft-tissue chondroma

Extraskeletal osteosarcoma

Soft-tissue chondroma

A.E. Rosenberg
N. Mandahl

Definition
Soft-tissue chondroma is a benign mesenchymal neoplasm composed of cells that have a chondrocyte phenotype, secrete cartilage matrix and arise in extraosseous and extrasynovial tissues.

ICD-O code   9220/0

Synonyms
Extraskeletal chondroma; chondroma of soft parts

Epidemiology
These tumours arise over a broad age range, but most patients are middle-aged (mean, 34.5 years) {468,2252}. Males are affected more frequently than females (3 : 2) {468}.

Sites of involvement
Two thirds of tumours occur on the fingers {1249,1406,2252}. The remainder arise on the hands, followed by toes and feet, with origin in the trunk, head and neck region {802} being uncommon. Rare examples have been described in the skin {1413}, intracranial structures {3057} and, exceptionally, the fallopian tube {2861}.

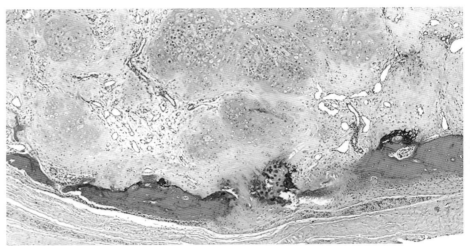
Fig. 9.01 Soft tissue chondroma surrounded by a rim of bone formed by enchondral ossification.

Clinical features
Most tumours are solitary and present as a painless mass in soft tissue in the vicinity of tendons and joints. Radiologically, they are well-demarcated, lobulated, and have central and peripheral calcifications that range from arch-like to punctate and spiculated to coarsely geometrical {1206}.

Macroscopy
Soft-tissue chondromas are well-circumscribed, nodular masses that are grey-white and sometimes focally myxoid. Most tumours are solid and are 1–2 cm in size.

Histopathology
Soft-tissue chondromas are typically composed of lobules of mature, hyaline cartilage {468,1249,1406,2252}. The lobules may be demarcated by fibrous connective tissue and are often hypercellular and contain chondrocytes that reside within lacunar spaces. The chondrocyte nuclei may be small, round, and dark or large with fine or coarse chromatin, small nucleoli and exhibit mild to moderate pleomorphism. Cartilage may undergo coarse calcification or endochondral ossification and become surrounded by bone. The chondrocytes in the mineralized areas may undergo necrosis, and tumours that are heavily calcified may have an infiltrate of histiocytes that can obscure the nature of the lesion. In a minority of cases the cartilage is myxoid with stellate chondrocytes "floating" in the mucinous stroma.

The chondroblastoma-like variant is composed of chondrocytes with moderate amounts of eosinophilic cytoplasm and nuclei that are often grooved or cleaved; the matrix contains scattered osteoclast-like giant cells and undergoes fine calcification that surrounds individual chondrocytes, thereby mimicking chondroblastoma {400}. Regardless of the morphology, mitotic activity is limited and abnormal mitotic figures are not observed.

Genetics
Cytogenetic analyses of 11 Soft-tissue chondromas revealed rearrangements of 12q13–15 in 6 cases, trisomy of chromosome 5 in 3 cases, and involvement of chromosome 11 in incompletely described, unbalanced karyotypes in 2 cases, possibly with loss of 11q21-qter in common {312,546,2517, 2708}. These aberrations seem to be mutually exclusive. One oral tumour displaying 2–5 supernumerary ring chromosomes

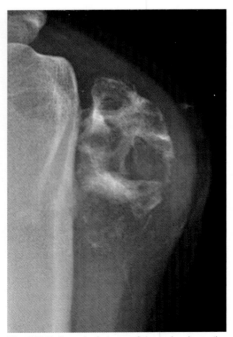
Fig. 9.02 Radiograph of a large soft tissue chondroma; the mineralized portion has undergone enchondral ossification.

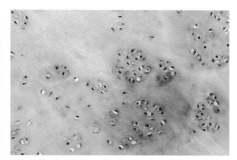

Fig. 9.03 Soft tissue chondroma: the hyaline cartilage shows abundant matrix and groups of chondrocytes.

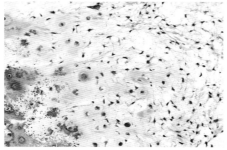

Fig. 9.04 Cellular soft tissue chondroma composed of hyaline and myxoid cartilage.

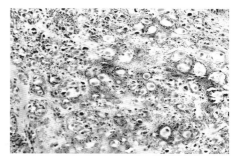

Fig. 9.05 Soft tissue chondroblastoma-like chondroma with abundant calcification with some surrounding individual cells.

had amplification of 12q sequences, including 12q13–15 {2517}. In a set of tumours with rearrangements of 12q13–15, a truncated or full-length *HMGA2* transcript was found {546}. One of these cases had a t(3;12)(q27;q15) resulting in a *HMGA2-LPP* fusion transcript composed of *HMGA2* exons 1–3 and *LPP* exons 9–11; this is identical to fusion transcripts found in lipoma and pulmonary chondroid hamartoma.

Prognostic factors
Soft-tissue chondromas are appropriately treated by simple excision. The prognosis is excellent, with the recurrence rate being 15–20% {468}.

Extraskeletal osteosarcoma

A.E. Rosenberg

Definition
Extraskeletal osteosarcoma is a malignant neoplasm composed of neoplastic cells that secrete organic bone matrix, which may mineralize. The tumour cells may also demonstrate chondroblastic and fibroblastic differentiation.

ICD-O code   9180/3

Synonym
Soft tissue osteosarcoma

Epidemiology
Extraskeletal osteosarcoma is rare, accounting for 1–2% of all soft tissue sarcomas and approximately 2–5% of all osteosarcomas {471,1586,1610,2769}. It typically arises during mid and late adulthood, with most patients being in the fifth to seventh decades of life at diagnosis; occurrence in children is uncommon

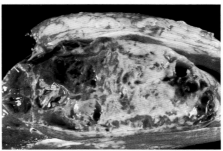

Fig. 9.06 Extraskeletal osteosarcoma is usually large, tan-white, haemorrhagic and often cystic.

{171,471,1586,1610}. Males are affected more frequently than females (1.9 : 1) {1586}.

Etiology
Most cases develop de novo, but 5–10% are associated with previous exposure to radiation; many patients have a history of previous trauma, but this probably has no etiological role {171,471,1586,1610, 2133}. Radiation-induced extraskeletal osteosarcoma usually develops at least 2 years after radiotherapy for another malignancy {2133}.

Sites of involvement
The majority of these tumours arise in the deep soft tissues and < 10% of cases are superficial, originating in the dermis or subcutis. The most common location is the thigh (50%); other frequent sites include the buttock, shoulder girdle, trunk, and retroperitoneum.

Clinical features
Most patients present with a progressively enlarging mass that may be associated with pain. Plain radiographs, CT and MRI usually reveal a large deep-seated soft-tissue mass with variable mineralization

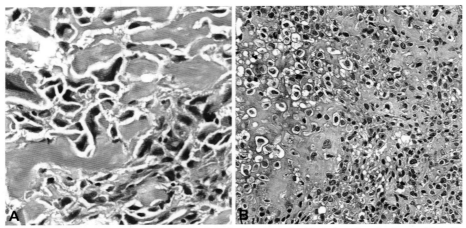

Fig. 9.07 Extraskeletal osteosarcoma. **A** Osteoblastic variant consisting of cytologically malignant cells associated with lace-like tumour bone. **B** Chondroblastic variant. The cellular malignant hyaline cartilage merges peripherally with tumour bone.

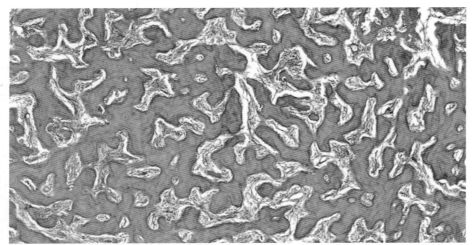

Fig. 9.08 Extraskeletal well-differentiated osteosarcoma; there are numerous interconnecting trabeculae.

{1773}. By definition these tumours do not arise from bone, but may secondarily involve osseous structures.

Macroscopy

These tumours range in size from 1 cm to 50 cm (mean, 8–10 cm) and are circumscribed, tan-white, haemorrhagic and focally necrotic gritty masses. The tumour bone is frequently most prominent in the centre of the lesion. Extensive haemorrhagic cystic change is present in a minority (10%) of cases.

Histopathology

All the major subtypes of osteosarcoma that arise in bone are seen in extraskeletal osteosarcoma. The most common is the osteoblastic variant, followed by the fibroblastic, chondroblastic, telangiectatic, small cell, and well-differentiated types {171,471,1586,1610,3023}. The tumour cells are variably pleomorphic spindle or polyhedral cells that are cytologically atypical, mitotically active and frequently demonstrate atypical mitotic figures.

Common to all variants is the presence of neoplastic bone, intimately associated with tumour cells, which may be deposited in lacy, trabecular or sheet-like patterns. The bone is usually most prominent in the centre of the tumour, with the more densely cellular areas located in the periphery, a pattern that is the reverse of myositis ossificans.

In the osteoblastic variant, the tumour cells resemble malignant osteoblasts and bone matrix is abundant. Spindle cells arranged in a herringbone or storiform pattern characterize the fibroblastic subtype and malignant cartilage predominates in the chondroblastic variant. Telangiectatic extraskeletal osteosarcomas contain numerous large blood-filled spaces lined by malignant cells. Sheets of small round cells that mimic Ewing sarcoma or lymphoma are typical of the small cell variant. The extremely rare well-differentiated subtype contains abundant bone deposited in well-formed trabeculae, surrounded by a minimally atypical spindle-cell component similar to parosteal osteosarcoma {3032}.

Immunophenotype

The immunophenotype of extraskeletal osteosarcoma is nonspecific {807,1118, 1610}.

Genetics

Only three cases with clonal chromosomal aberrations have been reported. In two tumours {1722,1852}, highly complex aberrations were seen, whereas the third {1923} had a moderately hyperdiploid karyotype with relatively few chromosomal abnormalities. Genomic changes assessed in a case of primary pulmonary osteosarcoma by CGH analysis revealed multiple regions of loss and gain, such as gain of 1q and 8q and loss of 13q and 15q {426}. Nothing indicates that systematic genetic differences exist between osteosarcomas of bone and soft tissues.

Prognostic factors

Extraskeletal osteosarcoma has a very poor prognosis and approximately 75% of patients die of their disease within 5 years of diagnosis {171,1586,1610,2769}. Tumours of small size (< 5 cm) or those that are of low grade have a better prognosis.

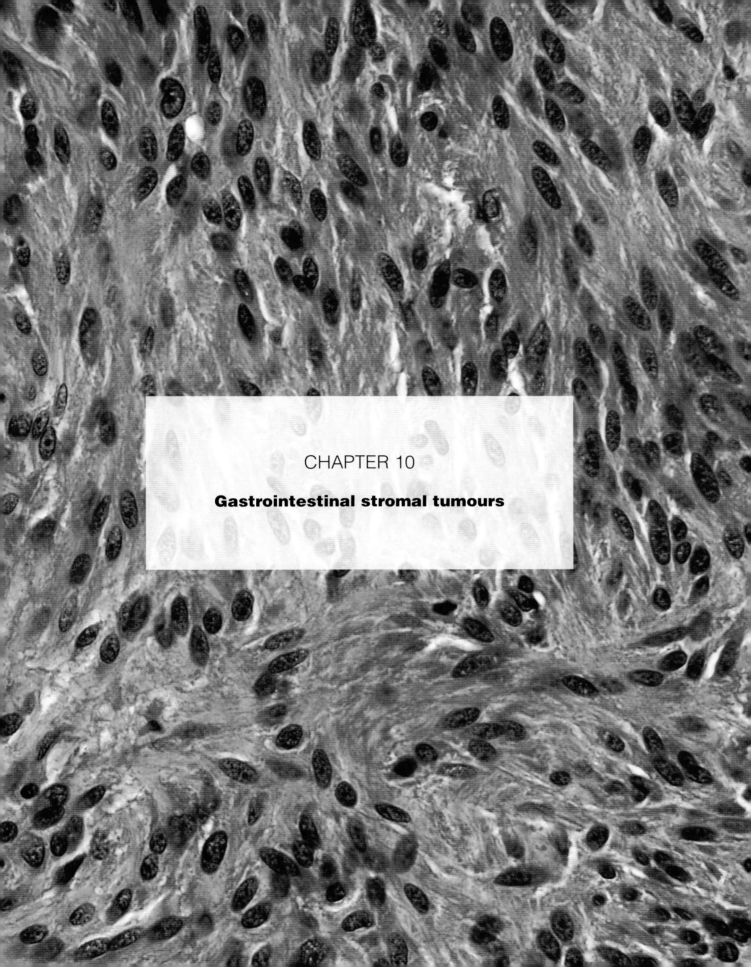

CHAPTER 10

Gastrointestinal stromal tumours

Gastrointestinal stromal tumours

M.M. Miettinen
C.L. Corless
M. Debiec-Rychter
J.A. Fletcher

J. Lasota
B.P. Rubin
R. Sciot

Definition

Gastrointestinal stromal tumour (GIST) is the most common primary mesenchymal tumour in the gastrointestinal tract and spans a clinical spectrum from benign to malignant. It is generally immunopositive for CD117 (KIT), phenotypically paralleling Cajal-cell differentiation, and most examples contain *KIT*- or *PDGFRA*-activating mutations. Most gastric smooth muscle and nerve sheath tumours defined before the current concept of GIST are actually GISTs, as are tumours formerly designated as leiomyoblastomas and gastrointestinal autonomic nerve tumours (GANTs).

ICD-O code

Gastrointestinal stromal tumour	8936/1
Benign	
(prognostic groups 1, 2, 3a)	8936/0
Uncertain malignant potential	
(group 4)	8936/1
Malignant	8936/3
(groups 3b, 5, 6a, 6b)	

Epidemiology

Population-based studies in Scandinavia have suggested an annual incidence of GIST of 11–15 per 100 000; approximately 55% of these tumours arise in the stomach {2050}. However, incidental microscopic GISTs are more common: a frequency of 10% was reported in gastro-oesophageal carcinoma specimens {6}. Autopsy studies report an even higher frequency of small gastric GIST. We estimate that approximately 25% of gastric GISTs (excluding minimal incidental tumours) are clinically malignant {17}. SEER data indicate that GISTs (interpolated from data on leiomyosarcomas) account for 2.2% of all malignant gastric tumours {2751}. GISTs typically occur in older adults (median age, 60–65 years) without distinction between men and women. Rarely, GISTs occur in children, nearly always in the stomach.

Etiology

Most GISTs are sporadic, but 10% are associated with a variety of syndromes. Most common among these are deficiencies in succinate dehydrogenase complex that occur only in gastric GISTs, especially in young age groups with female predominance (estimated frequency of all gastric GISTs, 8%), sometimes in connection with the non-hereditary Carney triad (GIST, pulmonary chondroma, paraganglioma) or the autosomal dominant Carney-Stratakis syndrome (GIST plus paraganglioma and germline mutation in one of the SDH-subunit genes). Neurofibromatosis type 1 (NF1) is associated with intestinal GISTs that are often multiple and usually indolent. A minute subset of GISTs occur

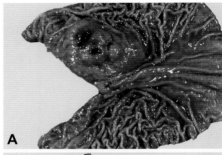
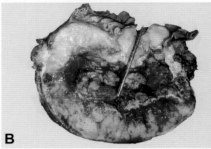

Fig. 10.01 Gross appearance of gastrointestinal stromal tumour (GIST). **A** Multinodular gastric GIST. **B** Jejunal GIST with large central necrosis and cystic change, with the cyst communicating with the intestinal lumen.

in familial GIST syndrome caused by *KIT*- or rarely *PDGFRA*-activating germline mutations. These patients can develop multiple or diffuse GISTs that often evolve into a malignancy {296,1000,1889,2806}.

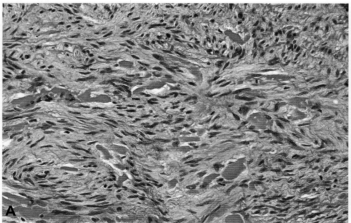
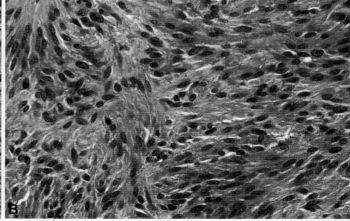

Fig. 10.02 Gastrointestinal stromal tumour (GIST) of the small intestine. **A** An example with extracellular collagen globules (skeinoid fibres). **B** This example has anuclear zones resembling Veracay bodies or neuropil.

Sites of involvement

Approximately 54% of all GISTs occur in the stomach, 32% in the small intestine, including duodenum, 5% in the colon and rectum, around 1% in the oesophagus, and 9% are primarily disseminated with unspecified site or origin. Isolated cases have been reported in the appendix. Rarely, GISTs form solitary masses in the omentum or the mesentery ("extragastrointestinal GIST"). However, most such extragastrointestinal GISTs are metastatic or may be detached from a gastrointestinal primary source.

Clinical features

Common presentations include vague abdominal complaints or ulcer symptoms, acute or chronic bleeding, abdominal mass, obstruction, or tumour perforation. Many smaller GISTs are detected incidentally during endoscopy, surgery, or CT scan. Malignant GISTs spread into peritoneal cavity and retroperitoneal space, and often metastasize to the liver. Bone and peripheral skin or soft tissue metastases occur infrequently, but pulmonary metastases are distinctly rare, in contrast with leiomyosarcomas. GISTs may metastasize after a long delay and, in some cases, patients survive long periods even with liver metastases. For anatomical reasons, gastric GISTs can recur locally, whereas intestinal GISTs removed by segmental resections do not recur locally.

Macroscopy

GISTs vary from minimal mural nodules to large complex masses of > 20–30 cm with variable intra- and extraluminal components. Gastric GISTs often have substantial intraluminal components, whereas serosal masses are more commonly seen with intestinal GISTs. Extragastrointestinal GISTs are connected only by a narrow pedicle or are disconnected from any gastrointestinal site of origin. Malignant GISTs frequently extend into surrounding structures, such as spleen and pancreas. Spread in the omentum, mesentery and retroperitoneal space can involve the abdominal cavity from the diaphragm to the pelvis. On sectioning, GISTs vary in colour from pale to pink tan and often show microcystic change. Haemorrhage and cystic change are typical of larger tumours {1889,1894,2986}.

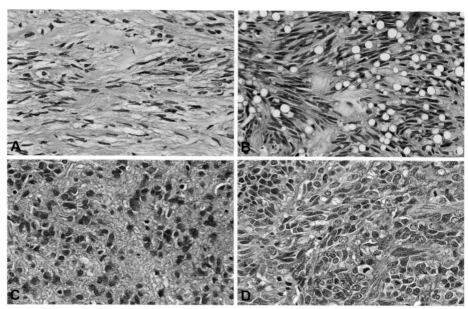

Fig. 10.03 Histological features of the most common subtypes of gastrointestinal stromal tumour (GIST) in the stomach (gastric GIST). **A** Spindle cell sclerosing subtype. **B** Palisaded-vacuolated subtype. **C** Epithelioid subtype with sclerosing morphology. **D** Sarcomatous subtype, composed of spindled to ovoid cells with significant mitotic activity.

Histopathology

Gastric GISTs have a broad morphological spectrum. Most are spindle cell tumours, while epithelioid histology is seen in 20–25% of cases, with some cases showing mixed histology. Nuclear pleomorphism is relatively uncommon, and occurs more often in epithelioid tumours. Distinctive histological patterns among spindle cell GISTs include sclerosing type, seen especially in small tumours that often contain calcifications. The palisaded-vacuolated subtype is one of the most common, while some examples show diffuse hypercellularity, and others show sarcomatoid features with significant nuclear atypia and mitotic activity. Epithelioid GISTs may show sclerosing, discohesive, hypercellular, sometimes with pseudopapillary pattern, or sarcomatous morphology with significant atypia and mitotic activity {1894}. SDH-deficient GISTs characteristically show epithelioid morphology and are typically multinodular with "plexiform" mural involvement. They often feature lymphovascular invasion and occasionally lymph-node metastases, not seen with usual GISTs {1898}.

Small-intestinal and colonic GISTs are usually composed of spindled or ovoid cells, and many show distinct extracellular collagen fibres (so-called "skeinoid fibres"). Epithelioid morphology may be associated with higher mitotic activity, reflecting malignancy. Intestinal GISTs also often contain anuclear zones similar to Verocay bodies or neuropil, reflecting entangled complex cell processes. Vascular hyalinization and thrombosis similar to that of schwannoma are common in intestinal GISTs. While nuclear palisading is fairly common, cytoplasmic vacuolization is less prominent than in gastric GISTs. Rectal GISTs usually show spindle cell morphology {1883,1889,1894}. Divergent skeletal muscle differentiation may be seen after imatinib therapy {1615}.

Immunophenotype

Immunohistochemically most GISTs show strong positivity for CD117 (KIT), which can be cytoplasmic, membrane-associated, or sometimes seen as perinuclear dots. However, 5% of GISTs, especially those gastric GISTs with mutant *PDGFRA*, may have very limited, if any, CD117 positivity {1805}. Anoctamin-1 (Ano-1), a chloride-channel protein detected by DOG1-antibody, is an equally sensitive and specific marker that often reacts with CD117-negative GISTs {775,1896}. Most spindle cell GISTs (especially the gastric ones) are positive for CD34, whereas epithelioid examples are less consistently positive. Some GISTs express h-caldesmon, a minority expresses SMA, and rare examples show positivity for desmin, keratins (usually keratin 18 only), or S100 protein {1885}.

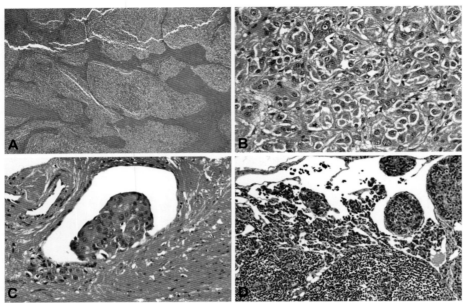

Fig. 10.04 Paediatric gastrointestinal stromal tumour (GIST), succinate dehydrogenase (SDH)-deficient. Most paediatric and SDH-deficient gastric GISTs are multinodular, feature epithelioid cytology, and often demonstrate lymphovascular invasion and sometimes regional lymph-node metastases (**A, B, C, D**).

Immunohistochemical loss of succinate dehydrogenase subunit B (SDHB) is a practical marker to identify SDH-deficient GISTs, some of which have loss-of-function germline mutations in one of the SDH subunits (A, B, C or D) in the mitochondrial membranes. The best criterion for interpreting SDH loss is observing a contrast between positive fibrovascular septa and tumour cells. The latter can be nega-tive or weakly positive in a diffuse, non-granular pattern {934,976,1898}.

Genetics

KIT oncogenic mutations, leading to con-stitutive activation of KIT-dependent sig-nalling pathways, are detected in approx-imately 80% of sporadic GISTs. Mutations most frequently occur in exon 11 (67%) and are variable in type and location, ranging from in-frame deletions (often in-volving codons 557 and 558) to missense mutations (W557, V559, V560) to tandem duplications. The latter typically involve the 3' portion of exon 11 and are associ-ated with gastric location and a favourable prognosis. Complex mutations combining the above types may also occur. Gastric GISTs with exon 11 deletions have a worse prognosis than those with missense mutations. *KIT* exon 9 mutations are also common (10% of cases) and are almost invariably found in intestinal tumours. These mutations generally result in tandem duplication of amino acids AY502–503. *KIT* exons 13 and 17 are rarely involved. Such mutations include K642E and N822K, among others. Most exon 11 and some other *KIT* mutants are extremely sensitive to imatinib mesylate, a KIT/PDGFRA/ABL tyrosine kinase inhibitor widely used in treatment of metastatic and unresectable GISTs, and for adjuvant therapy. *KIT* exon 9 mutant GISTs respond less well to ima-tinib, prompting dose escalation or use of alternative inhibitors, such as sunitinib or nilotinib.

A subset of gastric GISTs, especially tu-mours with epithelioid morphology, have mutations in *PDGFRA*, which is closely homologous to *KIT*. Most common of these is exon 18 substitution D842V, and these mutant tumours are notably resistant to imatinib. *PDGFRA* exon 12 deletions and exon 14 substitutions are rare muta-tions. Most *KIT* mutations are heterozyg-ous, but homozygous mutations can occur (via hemizygosity), and these tumours are often more aggressive than correspon-ding heterozygous mutants {511,873, 1557}.

Recurrent cytogenetic changes in sporadic GISTs include deletions/monosomy of chro-mosomes 14 (70%) and 22 (50%). Dele-tions in 1p, 9p (*CDNK2A/B*), 9q, 10, 11p and 13q, and gains or amplifications on 5p, 3q, 8q, and 17q are associated with malignant behaviour {735,1158}. High ex-pression of ROR2 (receptor tyrosine ki-nase-like orphan receptor 2) has been identified in a subset of GISTs; this is as-sociated with increased invasiveness in vitro and a poor clinical outcome {723}.

The secondary mutations conferring ima-tinib-resistance mutations are concen-trated in two regions of the KIT kinase do-main. One is the ATP-binding pocket, en-coded by exons 13 and 14, mutations of which directly interfere with drug binding. The second is the activation loop, where

Table 10.01 Prognosis for patients with gastrointestinal stromal tumours (GIST), based on long-term follow-up

Prognostic group	Size	Mitotic rate per 50 HPFs	Progressive disease during follow-up (% of patients)[a]	
			Gastric GISTs	Small-intestinal GISTs
1	≤ 2	≤ 5	0	0
2	> 2 ≤ 5	≤ 5	1.9	4.3
3a	> 5 ≤ 10	≤ 5	3.6	24
3b	> 10	≤ 5	12	52
4	≤ 2	> 5	0[b]	50[b]
5	> 2 ≤ 5	> 5	16	73
6a	> 5 ≤ 10	> 5	55	85
6b	> 10	> 5	86	90

HPF, high-power field

[a] Based on observation of 1784 patients in studies carried out by the Armed Force Institute of Pathology (AFIP). Intestinal GISTs generally follow the behaviour of small-intestinal GISTs.
[b] Denotes tumour categories with very small numbers of cases. Data based on reference {1885}.

mutations can stabilize KIT in the active conformation and thereby hinder drug interaction {511,1617}.

GISTs that are deficient in SDH or associated with NF1 do not contain *KIT* or *PDGFRA* mutations {1886,2260}. SDH-deficient GISTs in Carney-Stratakis syndrome are associated with germline mutations of SDH subunits A, B, C, and D {1318,2193}. The genetic basis for the Carney triad as well as pathogenesis of the SDH loss in most SDH-deficient GISTs remains unknown to date {381,2664}.

Prognostic factors

The best documented prognostic factors are tumour size, mitotic activity, and anatomical site {1885}. It should be noted that mitotic counts have been defined with small-field microscope with a total area of 5 mm^2 per 50 HPFs. Therefore, one should generally count a smaller number of wide fields to reach a comparable total area (usually about 25 fields). In the TNM classification, grading is based on mitotic rate (5 mitoses per 50 HPFs is considered to be a low mitotic rate, while > 5 mitoses per 50 HPFs is considered a high mitotic rate). The stage combines tumour size and mitotic activity. Estimates of metastatic rate for prognostic groups defined by tumour size and mitotic rate are shown in Table 10.01. It should be noted that staging criteria are different for gastric and small-intestinal GISTs to reflect the more aggressive course of small-intestinal GISTs with

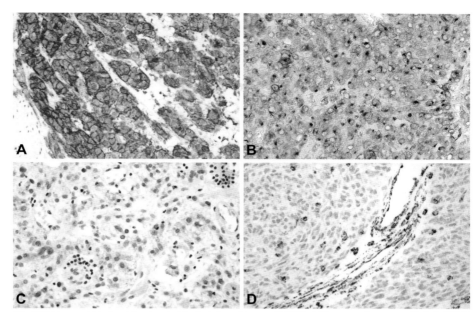

Fig. 10.05 Immunohistochemistry of gastrointestinal stromal tumours (GISTs). **A** Strong membranous positivity for KIT. **B** Some GISTs show perinuclear dot-like positivity for KIT. **C** Some gastric GISTs, especially those that are *PDGFRA*-mutant, may show limited focal/weak or no positivity for KIT. **D** GIST with negative immunostaining for succinate dehydrogenase subunit B (SDHB). Note the strong contrast between positive fibrovascular septa and negative tumour cells.

similar parameters. SDH-deficient GISTs are more unpredictable. Even tumours with low mitotic counts in this group can develop liver metastases, while tumours with high mitotic counts may never metastasize. In this group, latency between primary tumour and metastasis can also be long, > 40 years, and patients with metastases can survive for long periods even without specific treatment. While many metastatic GISTs were formerly fatal within 1–2 years, these patients often now survive 5 years or more with tyrosine-kinase inhibitor treatment.

There is no formal grading system for GISTs; grading for soft tissue sarcoma is not applicable because relatively low levels of mitotic activity may confer high malignant potential. Rare tumours that rupture are at high risk for peritoneal metastasis.

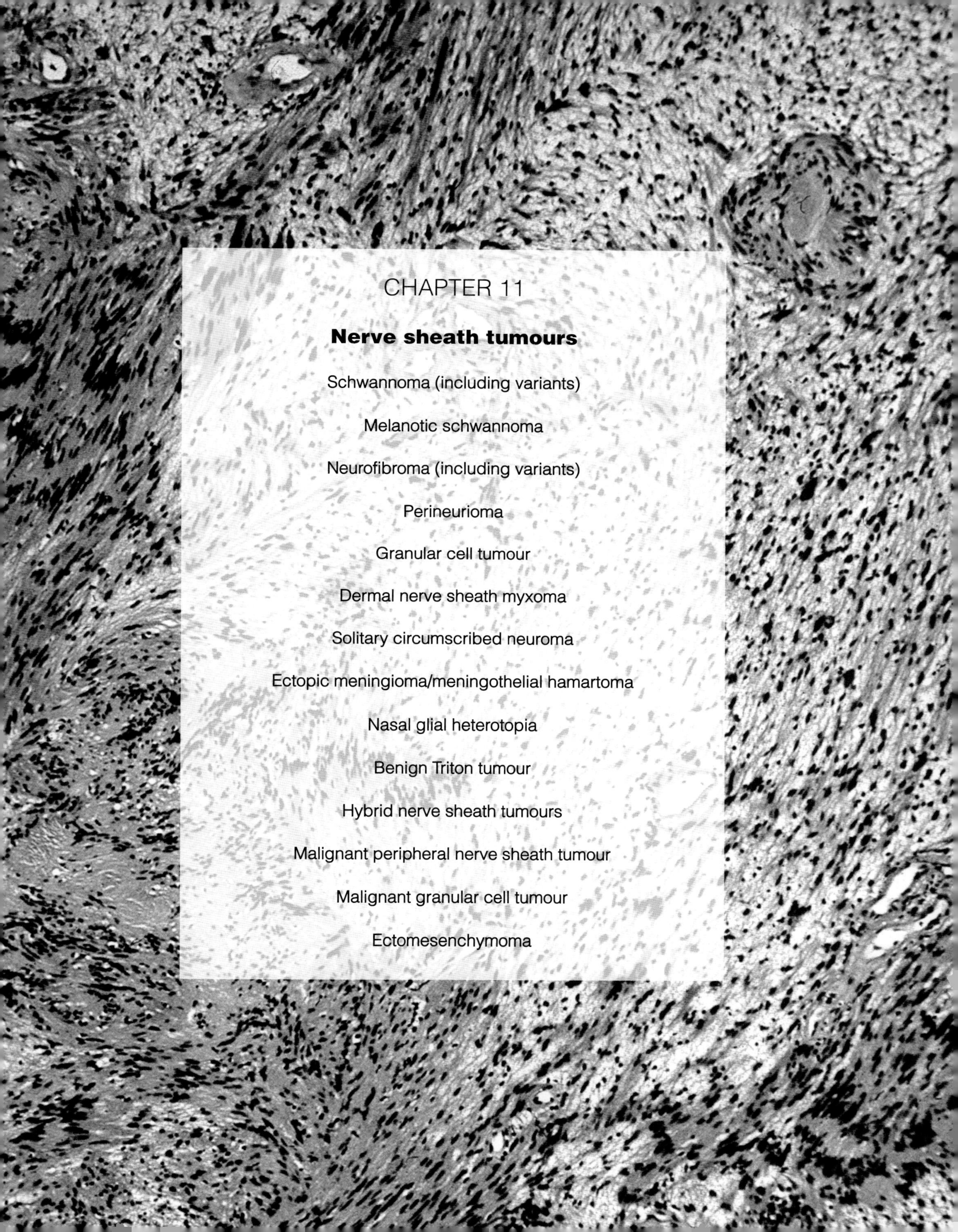

CHAPTER 11

Nerve sheath tumours

Schwannoma (including variants)

Melanotic schwannoma

Neurofibroma (including variants)

Perineurioma

Granular cell tumour

Dermal nerve sheath myxoma

Solitary circumscribed neuroma

Ectopic meningioma/meningothelial hamartoma

Nasal glial heterotopia

Benign Triton tumour

Hybrid nerve sheath tumours

Malignant peripheral nerve sheath tumour

Malignant granular cell tumour

Ectomesenchymoma

Schwannoma (including variants)

C.R. Antonescu
A. Perry
J.M. Woodruff

Definition

This group of nerve sheath tumours, composed entirely of differentiated neoplastic Schwann cells, is divided into two clinically, morphologically, and genetically different entities. One, common and benign, rarely develops malignant changes (conventional schwannoma); the other, rare, has a low malignant potential (melanotic schwannoma).

ICD-O code   9560/0

Synonyms

Schwannoma; neurilemoma; neurinoma

Epidemiology

More than 90% of these lesions are solitary and sporadic, affect all ages, and have a peak incidence in the fourth to sixth decades of life. There is no known predisposition with regard to race or sex.

Etiology

The etiology of sporadic schwannoma is not known. Multiple schwannomas are a feature of neurofibromatosis type 2 (NF2), schwannomatosis, and Gorlin-Koutlas syndrome. NF2-associated schwannomas commonly present before the age of 30 years, whereas in schwannomatosis the tumours usually do not manifest until adulthood. Bilateral vestibular schwannoma {737,1368} is the hallmark of NF2, often showing multifocal nerve involvement and nodular microscopic growth pattern. In addition, patients with the more severe Wishart form of NF2 typically have

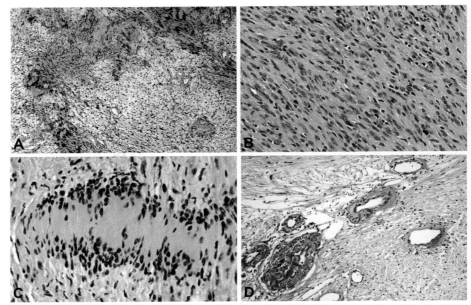

Fig. 11.01 Conventional schwannoma. **A** Compact Antoni A and loose Antoni B areas, creating a biphasic pattern. **B** Detail of Antoni A tissue. **C** Verocay body, formed by palisaded Schwann cells. **D** Hyalinized thick-walled vessels in Antoni A area.

meningiomas, which are often multiple and are associated with increased morbidity and mortality {1020}. Gliomas, most frequently ependymoma of the cervical spinal cord, develop less commonly {2354}. NF2 is inherited in an autosomal dominant manner and 50% of cases represent new or sporadic mutations.

Schwannomatosis is characterized by the presence of multiple schwannomas, mostly in the absence of vestibular nerve involvement and meningiomas {164,1686}. Cranial and cutaneous nerves are infrequently affected. In contrast to NF2 patients, only about 15% of schwannomatosis cases are familial. Schwannomas in schwannomatosis also have biallelic inactivation of the *NF2* gene. The mutation, however, is not germline but somatic, and differs among schwannomas in any one patient as well between family members {1308}. Linkage studies of schwannomatosis kindreds has led to the identification of the *SMARCB1* (*INI1*) gene, located centromeric to *NF2* on chromosome 22, which when mutated predisposes individuals to schwannomatosis {1248}.

Sites of involvement

Leading sites of origin are peripheral nerves in the skin and subcutaneous tissue of the head and neck or along the flexor surfaces of the extremities. Spinal intradural extramedullary examples are also common and form "dumb-bell" tumours when growing through neural foramina. Intracranial nerve involvement, although less common, is significant, 85%

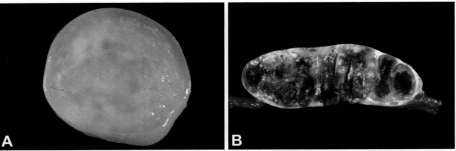

Fig. 11.02 Conventional schwannoma. **A** Sectioned surface of globoid schwannoma. **B** Splaying of uninvolved nerve fascicles over the capsule of a schwannoma involving a sizeable nerve.

of intracranial schwannomas being cerebellopontine angle tumours, emanating from the vestibular division of the eighth cranial nerve {2393}. Spinal intramedullary and CNS sites are rare {393,574}, as are those involving viscera (such as the gastrointestinal tract) and bone {1893,2267}.

Clinical features

Schwannomas are slowly growing tumours, often present as asymptomatic masses or incidental findings on imaging studies and, particularly in the setting of schwannomatosis, may be painful. Spinal schwannomas may elicit sensory symptoms such as radicular pain and motor signs if growing intraspinally. Hearing loss and vertigo most often precede discovery of a vestibular schwannoma.

Macroscopy

These tumours are mainly solitary and globoid, have a smooth surface and measure < 10 cm in greatest dimension. Fewer than half have an evident attached nerve, which is most often small. The uninvolved nerve fascicles are often found draped over the tumour capsule. Excepting those arising in intraparenchymal CNS sites, skin, viscera and bone, tumours are usually encapsulated. Sectioned tumours reveal firm, light tan glistening tissue, interrupted by white/yellow areas or patches of haemorrhage.

Histopathology

Conventional schwannoma is a common, benign, usually encapsulated, nerve sheath tumour that is composed of well-differentiated Schwann cells. Schwannomas have a broad morphological range. The large majority are encapsulated biphasic tumours with compact areas of spindle cells (Antoni A tissue) showing occasional palisading (Verocay bodies), alternating with loosely arranged foci (Antoni B tissue). Cells of Antoni A tissue possess modest amounts of eosinophilic cytoplasm, no discernible cell borders, and normochromatic elongated tapered nuclei. Cytoplasmic nuclear inclusions, nuclear pleomorphism and mitotic figures may be seen. Palisading (Verocay bodies) takes the form of parallel rows of Schwann cell nuclei separated by their aligned cell processes. Antoni B tissue commonly contains collections of lipid-laden histiocytes and thick-walled, hyalinized blood vessels.

A minority of schwannomas deviate from a readily recognized biphasic pattern. Tumours of the eighth cranial nerve show predominantly Antoni B tissue, while intestinal schwannomas typically lack Antoni B tissue. The most extreme deviation from biphasic histology is seen among conventional variants of schwannoma. Cases with degenerative nuclear atypia or extensive hyalinization are often referred to as "ancient" schwannoma. Rare cases with rosette-like structures may be referred to as "neuroblastoma-like".

Cellular schwannoma

This variant is composed exclusively or predominantly of Antoni A tissue and is devoid of Verocay bodies. The tumours most commonly present at paravertebral sites, mediastinum, retroperitoneum and pelvis {865,2988}. Cranial nerves may be affected {641}, especially the fifth and eighth {394}. In addition to the cells being closely packed, they are not uncommonly hyperchromatic and mitotically active. Small areas of microscopic necrosis, identified in a few cases, were considered trauma-induced {2950}. Other histological findings are cellular whorls and perivascular and capsular lymphoid aggregates. Tumour erosion of nearby bone may occur.

Plexiform schwannoma

This is the designation for schwannomas, either biphasic or cellular, that, involving multiple nerve fascicles or a nerve plexus, grow as thinly encapsulated plexiform or multinodular tumours {2989}. The tumours come to clinical attention earlier in life, being described both in childhood and at birth {2990}. The majority of plexiform

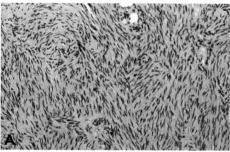
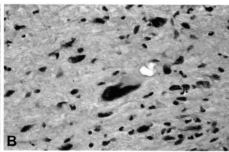
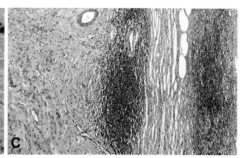

Fig. 11.03 Common features of "ancient" schwannoma. **A** Hypercellularity. **B** Cell pleomorphism. **C** Paracapsular and intracapsular lymphoid aggregates.

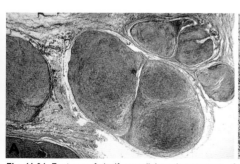
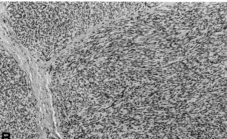
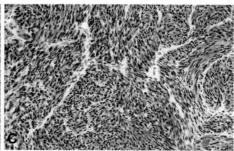

Fig. 11.04 Features of plexiform cellular schwannomas. **A** Nodules are uniformly cellular and lined by a thin fibrous capsule. **B** Lobules of tumour in circumscribed lesions are separated by thin fibrous bands. **C** Immunostaining for S100 protein is characteristically strong and diffuse.

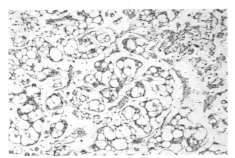

Fig. 11.05 Histological features of the microscopic/reticular variant of schwannoma. Note the reticular growth pattern with formation of microcysts and presence of myxoid stroma.

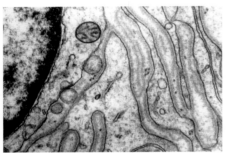

Fig. 11.06 Ultrastructure of schwannoma with long cell processes lined by reduplicated deposits of external lamina.

schwannomas arise in skin or subcutaneous tissue. There is a weak association with NF2 and occasionally reported in patients with schwannomatosis {2515}. Biphasic plexiform schwannomas are more readily identified pathologically than plexiform cellular examples. The latter are composed of solid nodules separated by thin fibrous bands, or more infiltrative nodules with entrapped axons. The tumours differ from the non-plexiform cellular schwannoma in the absence of a well-formed capsule and thick-walled vessels.

Microcystic/reticular schwannoma
The rarest variant of schwannoma, this form is represented by the recently described microcystic/reticular schwannoma {1613}. The 10 reported patients ranged widely in age, with tumours preferentially located in the gastrointestinal submucosa or subcutaneous tissue. All were circumscribed and encapsulated except for visceral examples. Microscopically, there was a microcyst-rich network of interconnected bland spindle cells with scant eosinophilic cytoplasm. Tumour cells showed a myxoid, fibrillary, and/or hyalinized collagenous stroma. Generally absent were hyalinized blood vessels, foamy histiocytes, and Verocay bodies. Supporting the tumour's classification as schwannoma was the presence of Antoni A tissue and strong and diffuse expression of S100 protein.

Immunophenotype
Diffuse staining for S100 protein in cell nuclei and cytoplasm, which is more prominent in Antoni A than in Antoni B areas, is found in all tumours {2932}. Expression of GFAP is less frequent and more variable, while collagen IV and laminin is often diffuse. Retroperitoneal and mediastinal lesions are commonly positive for keratin AE1/AE3 due to cross-reactivity with GFAP. CD34 is commonly positive in subcapsular areas. Staining for neurofilament protein is helpful in identifying entrapped intratumoral axons, found in one third of assorted forms of sporadic schwannomas {2004}.

Ultrastructure
Smooth contoured nuclei and long entangled thin cytoplasmic processes are joined by rudimentary cell junctions and lined by continuous basal lamina {769}. Long-spacing collagen (Luse body) is a common finding.

Genetics
Complete or partial loss of chromosome 22, the most common cytogenetic anomaly in schwannoma, has also been reported in cellular schwannoma {1647}. Trisomy 17 has been identified as recurrent in plexiform cellular schwannoma {1347, 2731}. A causal relationship exists between schwannoma tumorigenesis and loss of expression of merlin (schwannomin), the growth inhibitory protein product of the *NF2* tumour suppressor gene located at 22q12 {2647}. *NF2*-inactivating mutations have been detected in approximately 60% of sporadic cases {233,1309, 1310,2378,2779}. Underlying genetic events are predominantly small frameshift mutations {1664} and loss of the remaining wildtype allele on chromosome 22. Mutation of the wildtype *SMARCB1* allele has been detected and the corresponding schwannomas shown to have a mosaic immunohistochemical staining pattern for SMARCB1 {2198}. This has led to a recent "four-hit" or possibly "three-hit" hypothesis for tumorigenesis, with one mutation occurring in *NF2*, one in *SMARCB1* and a third hit that deletes the remaining wildtype alleles of both genes on chromosome 22 simultaneously {2515}.

Prognostic factors
Schwannomas are benign, and do not usually recur if treated by gross total resection. Cellular and plexiform examples are least amenable to total removal and sometimes can only be debulked. Due to occasional involvement of multiple nerves, erosion of bone, increased cellularity, hyperchromasia, presence of pleomorphic nuclei, and frequent mitotic figures, examples of both these variants are subject to misinterpretation as malignant tumours. Schwannoma does not represent a precursor of spindle cell malignant peripheral nerve sheath tumour (MPNST).

Malignant transformation of conventional schwannoma is exceptionally rare. In the small number of cases thus far reported, it has most often taken the form of epithelioid MPNST {1800,2991}, primitive neuroectodermal cells {2991}, in one case rhabdomyosarcoma {1502} and in others, epithelioid angiosarcoma {2389,2775}.

Melanotic schwannoma

C.R. Antonescu
C.A. Stratakis
J.M. Woodruff

Definition
A rarely metastasizing nerve sheath tumour with a uniform composition of variably melanin-producing Schwann cells.

ICD-O code   9560/1

Epidemiology
Melanotic schwannoma is a rare tumour occurring mainly in adults, with peak incidence in the fourth decade of life and a slight predominance in females.

Etiology
As many as half of patients have the Carney complex, an often familial, autosomal dominant, multiple neoplasia syndrome {380,383, 384,2666}. The Carney complex is a genetically heterogeneous disorder with two identified genetic loci: *CNC1* and *CNC2*, mapping to chromosome bands 17q22–24 and 2p16, respectively {2665, 2666}. *CNC1* harbours the tumour suppressor gene *PRKAR1A*, which is inactivated in half of the Carney-complex kindreds {1766,2666}.

Site of involvement
About half of tumours arise from spinal nerves {899} and paraspinal ganglia, particularly at the cervical and thoracic levels. The second most common site of origin is the gastrointestinal tract, where autonomic nerves are involved.

Clinical features
Symptoms include pain, sensory abnormality, and mass effects. Spinal-root tumours may cause bone erosion. Lung metastases may present with respiratory failure, while stomach, liver and adrenal metastases may affect organ function. Brain metastases are often fatal, with diffuse invasion of the cerebrospinal space.

Macroscopy
Most melanotic schwannomas are solitary lesions, but may occasionally be multiple and multicentric, notably in Carney complex. Sectioned tumours are usually pigmented, ranging from brown discoloration to uniformly black, and texture ranging from soft to hard. Heavily pigmented examples, especially in Carney complex, have the appearance and consistency of dried tar.

Histopathology
Typically, the tumours are cellular, unencapsulated, and lined externally by a thin fibrous capsule. They are composed of closely packed variably pigmented plump spindle and epithelioid cells, arranged in short fascicles or nests. Tumour cells have eosinophilic to amphophilic cytoplasm and mostly round nuclei with a distinct small nucleolus and striking nuclear grooves. Intranuclear cytoplasmic inclusions are often found. Multinucleated cells and cells with large vesicular nuclei and prominent eosinophilic macronucleoli may also be present occasionally. The pigment, in the form of brown to black granules in tumour cells and macrophages, is Fontana–Masson-positive. Half the cases contain psammoma bodies (psammomatous melanotic schwannomas) and half these individuals have Carney complex. There are no pathognomonic features of malignancy, but malignant forms often have large vesicular nuclei, prominent eosinophilic nucleoli, mitotic figures, and necrosis.

Immunophenotype
Tumours are diffusely and strongly immunoreactive for S100 protein, HMB45 and Melan-A. There is also consistent positivity for laminin and collagen IV.

Ultrastructure
Tumour cells have long interdigitating cytoplasmic processes, coated by a continuous often reduplicated basal lamina {767}. Melanosomes, primarily late-stage forms, are routinely found {899,1320,1328}.

Genetics
In a study of tumours from 46 patients with or without Carney complex, amplification or deletion of the 2p16 region was shown in about 80% of the specimens, both familial and sporadic {1766}.

Prognostic factors
Data are limited mainly to case reports. Melanotic schwannomas have a tendency for late metastasis, although they initially appear clinically benign. Most young patients with Carney complex presenting with this tumour develop metastases in later life. Mortality is about 15% for patients having either non-psammomatous or psammomatous tumours {380}.

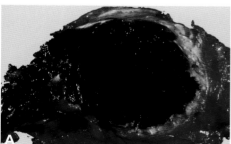
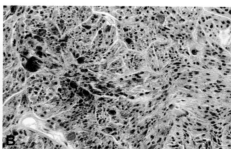
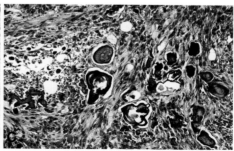

Fig. 11.07 Melanotic schwannoma. **A** Malignant tumour arising in a thoracic nerve root. The sectioned tumour had the appearance and texture of dried tar, and was circumscribed, except for a portion (left) that invaded nearby soft tissues and vertebral bone. **B** Commonly found clusters of plump, spindled, and heavily pigmented tumour cells. **C** The presence of calcospherites is required for a diagnosis of psammomatous melanotic schwannoma.

Neurofibroma (including variants)

C.R. Antonescu
H. Brems
E. Legius
J.M. Woodruff

Definition

A benign peripheral nerve sheath tumour (PNST) consisting of differentiated Schwann cells, perineurial-like cells, fibroblasts, mast cells and residual interspersed myelinated and unmyelinated axons embedded in extracellular matrix.

ICD-O code

Neurofibroma	9540/0
Plexiform neurofibroma	9550/0

Epidemiology

Neurofibromas are the most common PNST, the majority occurring sporadically as solitary lesions. Less often they occur as multiple or numerous tumours in individuals with neurofibromatosis type 1 (NF1). The diffuse cutaneous and plexiform tumours are presumably of congenital origin {1579} and, in NF1, the localized cutaneous and localized intraneural neurofibromas begin to appear in the second half of the first decade of life {2332}. All races, ages and both sexes are affected.

Etiology

Localized cutaneous or solitary intraneural neurofibromas, when multiple, and also massive soft tissue and most plexiform neurofibromas are caused by inactivation of the NF1 gene {1775}.

Sites of involvement

The commonest site of involvement is the skin, where the tumours are associated with small nerves. Less often involved are more deeply situated nerves of medium size, a nerve plexus, or major nerve trunk. Rarely, the tumours arise from spinal nerve roots and cranial nerves.

Clinical features

Cutaneous neurofibromas are usually asymptomatic (rarely painful) and most commonly present as a mass. They are mobile, soft, hemispheric to pedunculated lesions, without particular anatomical distribution. Deep tumours often present with motor or sensory symptoms in the distribution of the affected nerve. Least commonly, the tumour presents as a plaque-like cutaneous and subcutaneous mass, mainly in the head and neck region, or as massive soft tissue enlargement of a body region, such as shoulder or pelvic girdle. Neurofibromas can be multiple, an indication of the patient having NF1. In this case, there may be associated findings such as pigmented cutaneous macules (café-au-lait spots in fair-skinned individuals but brown spots in those of African descent), axillary or inguinal freckling, Lisch nodules, optic pathway gliomas, and bone dysplasia.

Macroscopy

Five macroscopic forms are distinguished: (i) localized cutaneous; (ii) diffuse cutaneous; (iii) localized intraneural; (iv) plexiform intraneural; and (v) massive diffuse soft tissue plexiform tumour. Localized cutaneous neurofibromas are nodular or polypoid lesions, up to 2 cm in size. Diffuse cutaneous neurofibromas are plaque-like and may extend into subcutaneous tissue and be associated with overlying

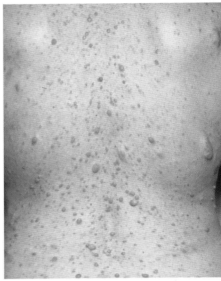

Fig. 11.08 Multiple solitary cutaneous neurofibromas and some background freckling in a patient with NF1.

hyperpigmentation. Intraneural neurofibromas present as solitary segmental fusiform enlargements of sizeable nerves, or as a series of lumpy masses or worm-like growths involving a plexus of nerves, or multiple fascicles of a single nerve. Massive soft tissue neurofibromas range in shape from a relatively uniform regional soft tissue enlargement to pendulous bag-like, or cape-like masses. The skin overlying massive tumours commonly shows widespread hyperpigmentation. Cut surfaces of neurofibromas are most often uniformly tan or grey-tan, glistening, mucoid, semi-translucent, and firm.

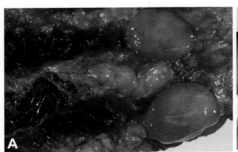
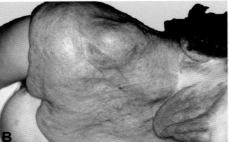
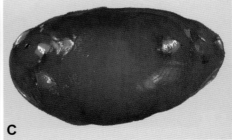

Fig. 11.09 Plexiform neurofibroma. **A** Large plexiform neurofibroma, involving multiple branches of a nerve. **B** Cape-like massive soft tissue neurofibroma with hyperpigmentation draping shoulder and upper back of a patient with NF1. **C** Sectioned surface of the cut neurofibroma is smooth, glistening, uniformly tan, semitranslucent, and firm.

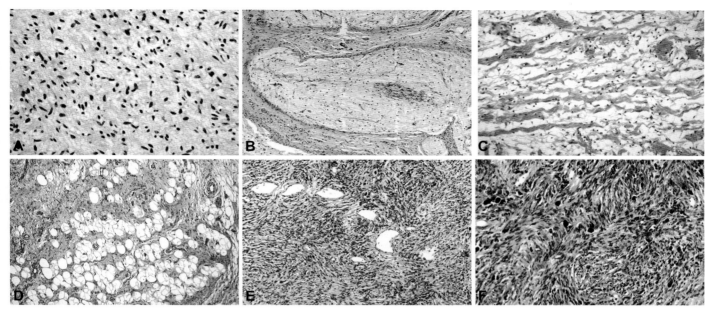

Fig. 11.10 Neurofibroma. **A** Dispersed cells with small, often comma-shaped nuclei without mitotic activity is a typical histological finding. **B** Nerve fascicles of plexiform neurofibroma are expanded by tumour cells and abundant myxoid stroma; note the bundles of nerve fibres at the fascicle's centre. **C** Collection of thick collagen fibres in solitary intraneural neurofibroma. **D** Diffuse neurofibroma showing involvement of fibroadipose tissue. **E** Diffuse neurofibroma showing areas of hypercellularity. **F** Neurofibroma showing patches of melanin-pigmented cells.

Histopathology

In contrast to schwannoma, the cells of a neurofibroma are loosely arranged and diffusely infiltrate the involved nerve. All forms show spindle-shaped cells with a small amount of cytoplasm. They are smaller in size than schwannoma cells, with round, ovoid, and comma-shaped nuclei separated by collagen fibres and myxoid material. Tumour cell processes are not distinguishable on light microscopy from collagen fibres. Most localized and diffuse cutaneous tumours exhibit only this loose arrangement of cells, nerves within the tumour being infrequent and small. In intraneural neurofibromas, solitary or plexiform, nerve fascicles are expanded by dispersed tumour cells enmeshed in abundant myxoid matrix. Loosely clustered variably thick collagen fibres may be present in the solitary form. Both forms of intraneural neurofibroma are encompassed by a prominent perineurium or thickened epineurium. Residual bundles of nerve fibres are often seen at their centres. Massive soft tissue neurofibromas may infiltrate skeletal muscle as well as fibroadipose tissue, and be focally hypercellular. Some show focal dense aggregates of benign small tumour nuclei, an appearance likely due to diminished or absent tumour matrix. Tumours of soft tissue may contain melanin-pigmented cells, arranged in irregular patches or diffusely distributed {837}. Rarely, small unencapsulated monomorphic nodules composed of differentiated Schwann cells, proven by strong staining for S100 protein, are found in plexiform neurofibromas {819,2472}. Onion-bulb-like proliferations of strongly S100-positive Schwann cells can also be seen in plexiform tumours. A perineurial-like cell counterpart is the pseudomeissnerian body, detectable in diffuse and massive soft tissue neurofibromas. Its constituent cells form a spherical structure of circumscribed collections of S100 protein-positive, stacked, thin, lamellar cell processes. The body differs from the Meissner corpuscle in its composition of layered perineurial-like cells instead of layered nerve fibres. Although rarely seen, neurofibromas may also show divergent differentiation. Reported thus far are angiosarcoma and mucin-producing glands with neuroendocrine cells {460}.

Immunophenotype

Staining for S100 protein is always positive, but labels only 40–50% of cells {2932}. Staining for collagen IV is common {1336}. Scattered perineurial cells showing positivity for GLUT1 {1182} or claudin-1 {2276} are seen in some tumours. Neurofibromas contain only limited numbers of EMA-positive cells, most only found in residual perineurium and at the periphery of pseudomeissnerian bodies. Perineurial-like cells are positive for EMA and GLUT1, whereas stromal cells are CD34-positive. Axons in varying numbers, shown by positivity for neurofilament proteins, are present in neurofibroma, particularly plexiform tumours.

Ultrastructure

Electron microscopy shows a mixture of cell types, the two most diagnostically important being the differentiated Schwann cell, with or without axons, and the perineurial-like cell {769}. The perineurial-like cell features long, very thin cell processes, many pinocytotic vesicles, and interrupted basal lamina. In the company of Schwann cells, it is the ultrastructural marker cell for neurofibroma. Fibroblasts are comparatively infrequent.

Genetics

Neurofibromas are monoclonal neoplasms that develop in individuals with NF1 {2579}, or sporadically, most likely due to inactivation of both copies of the *NF1* gene {505, 2446,2512}. Allelic loss of the *NF1* gene region of 17q has been confirmed in Schwann cells. Other chromosomal losses are not common, but have been reported on 19p, 19q, and 22q {1454}.

Localized intraneural and plexiform neurofibromas with focal hypercellularity and enlarged hyperchromatic nuclei frequently

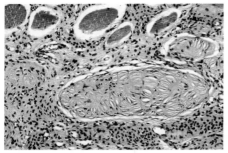

Fig. 11.11 Massive diffuse neurofibroma showing Pseudo-meissnerian bodies.

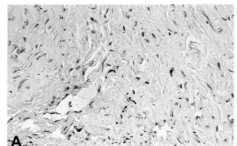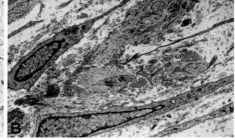

Fig. 11.12 Neurofibroma. **A** Immunoexpression of S100 protein. **B** Perineurial-like cells, the ultrastructural marker cell of neurofibroma, showing very delicate, elongated cell processes.

show deletion of 9p with a minimal region of overlap containing *CDKN2A*, *CDKN2B* and *MTAP* {178}.

Prognostic factors

Localized cutaneous neurofibromas are consistently benign. Plexiform neurofibromas and solitary intraneural neurofibromas arising in sizeable nerves are precursor lesions of a majority of malignant PNST. The lifetime risk for malignant PNST in NF1 patients may be up to 5–10% {777}. Diffuse cutaneous neurofibromas rarely undergo malignant transformation. Massive soft tissue neurofibromas, invariably benign, may overlie an intraneural or plexiform neurofibroma-derived malignant PNST. Hypercellularity of otherwise unremarkable neurofibroma cells, atypical tumour cells with hyperchromatic smudgy nuclei, or mitotic activity, alone or together, do not indicate malignant change ("atypical neurofibroma"). Evidence for this is most commonly a hypercellular area in which the tumour nuclei are at least three times the size of ordinary neurofibroma nuclei and uniformly hyperchromatic.

Perineurioma

J.L. Hornick
C.D.M. Fletcher
J.A. Fletcher

Definition

Perineuriomas of soft tissue are nearly always benign peripheral nerve sheath tumours composed entirely of perineurial cells. Intraneural {744} and mucosal {1218} types also exist.

ICD-O code

Perineurioma   9571/0
Malignant perineurioma   9571/3

Epidemiology

Perineuriomas of soft tissue are rare. About 200 cases have been reported {744,972,1220,1575, 2300,2790}. These tumours are slightly more common in females than males and occur over a wide age range, with a peak in middle-aged adults {1220}. Children are rarely affected. Sclerosing perineuriomas are more common in males and usually affect young adults {838,3013}.

Etiology

Soft tissue perineuriomas are nearly always sporadic tumours. Very rare cases have been reported in patients with neurofibromatosis type 1 or type 2 {119,2251}.

Sites of involvement

These tumours most commonly arise on the lower limbs, followed by the upper limbs and trunk {1220}. The head and neck region, visceral organs, and central body sites are rarely affected. Sclerosing

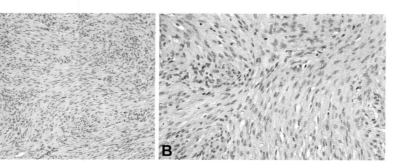

Fig. 11.13 Perineurioma of soft tissue. **A** The tumour shows a storiform growth pattern. **B** The tumour cells contain uniform ovoid to elongated nuclei. Note the fibrillary stroma.

perineuriomas are commonly found on the fingers and palms {838}.

Clinical features
Perineuriomas of soft tissue usually present as painless masses. Subcutaneous tissue is involved more often than deep soft tissue. About 10% of cases are limited to the dermis {1220}.

Macroscopy
Grossly, soft tissue perineuriomas are well-circumscribed but unencapsulated. The cut surface is usually firm or rubbery and yellow, tan, or white. A small subset of tumours shows a gelatinous appearance. Size ranges from < 1 cm to 20 cm in size, although most tumours are between 1.5 and 10 cm in greatest dimension. The mean size for superficial tumours is 3 cm, compared with 7 cm for deep-seated tumours {1220}.

Histopathology
Soft tissue perineuriomas typically show a predominantly storiform growth pattern. Other distinctive architectural features include long fascicles with tumour cells arranged in a lamellar fashion and perivascular whorls. The tumour cells are usually slender spindle cells with wavy or tapering nuclei, indistinct nucleoli, and characteristic delicate bipolar cytoplasmic processes. Some perineuriomas of soft tissue contain shorter, ovoid tumour cells. The stroma is usually collagenous; about 20% of cases contain at least focally myxoid matrix {1220}. Mitotic activity is typically scarce or absent. Occasional soft tissue perineuriomas show degenerative nuclear atypia, including pleomorphic and multinucleate cells, some with nuclear pseudoinclusions {1220}. Plexiform architecture has rarely been reported {1839,3055}. Sclerosing perineuriomas are composed of cords of small epithelioid to spindle cells in a dense collagenous stroma {838}. Reticular perineuriomas are composed of anastomosing cords of elongated spindle cells with a lacy or reticular architecture {1021}. The very rare malignant perineuriomas (perineurial malignant peripheral nerve sheath tumour) show cytoarchitectural features that are similar to those of benign perineuriomas of soft tissue, in addition to hypercellularity, nuclear atypia and hyperchromasia, and a high mitotic rate {1181}.

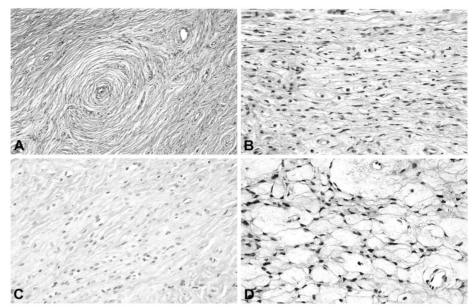

Fig. 11.14 Perineurioma. **A** Perivascular whorls are a typical feature. Note the collagenous stroma. **B** The lesions shows a lamellar arrangement of elongated spindle cells with tapering nuclei in a somewhat myxoid stroma. **C** Sclerosing perineurioma composed of cords of epithelioid cells in a dense collagenous stroma. **D** Reticular perineurioma composed of anastomosing elongated spindle cells with a lacy architecture.

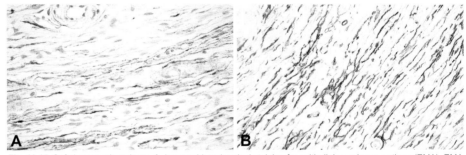

Fig. 11.15 Soft tissue perineurioma **A** Immunohistochemical staining for epithelial membrane antigen (EMA). EMA highlights the delicate bipolar cytoplasmic processes of the tumour cells. **B** Expression of CD34 is often more diffuse than EMA.

Immunophenotype
Like normal perineurial cells, the tumour cells in perineurioma usually (but not always) express EMA {1220}, which ranges from weak and focal to strong and diffuse. Claudin-1 and GLUT1 are also often positive {881,3013}. CD34 is expressed in about 60% of soft tissue perineuriomas {1220}. A small subset of tumours show focal staining for SMA. Staining for S100 protein and GFAP is negative. In addition to EMA, sclerosing perineuriomas may show focal staining for keratins {838}.

Ultrastructure
Soft tissue perineuriomas consist of spindle cells with long tapering nuclei and extremely thin cytoplasmic processes in a collagenous stroma. The cells often contain prominent pinocytotic vesicles and are surrounded by discontinuous external lamina {972,1575,2300}. Frequent tight junctions are another typical feature. Malignant soft tissue perineurioma shows similar ultrastructural features {1181}.

Genetics
Chromosome 22 deletions and monosomies are found in many soft tissue perineuriomas but are not diagnostically specific, being found also in benign schwannomas, among other soft tissue tumours. One apparent target of the chromosome 22 deletions is the *NF2* tumour suppressor gene: *NF2* mutations are found in conventional and sclerosing perineuriomas, and a patient with NF2 had a perineurioma of soft tissue {1556,2251}.

Chromosome arm 10q aberrations, in addition to the 22q deletions, are found in some sclerosing perineuriomas {326, 1850}. No genetic studies of malignant soft tissue perineuriomas have been reported.

Prognostic factors

Conventional perineuriomas of soft tissue (and sclerosing and reticular variants), including those with degenerative nuclear atypia, are benign and recur rarely {838, 1021,1220}. Malignant perineuriomas may sometimes metastasize, but appear to behave in a less aggressive fashion than conventional malignant peripheral nerve sheath tumours {1181}.

Granular cell tumour

A. Lazar

Definition

A benign tumour showing neuroectodermal differentiation and composed of large, oval to round cells with copious eosinophilic, distinctively granular cytoplasm.

ICD-O code   9580/0

Synonyms

Granular cell schwannoma; granular cell nerve sheath tumour; granular cell myoblastoma; Abrikossoff tumour.

Epidemiology

Granular cell tumour (GCT) usually occurs in adults in the fourth to sixth decades of life, but can be encountered at any age. They are more prevalent in males than females (ratio, 2–3 : 1) and in African-Americans {234,1520}.

Etiology

Multiple GCTs may arise in association with Noonan syndrome {1651,2292,2552}.

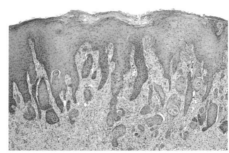

Fig. 11.16 This granular cell tumour of the tongue shows extensive pseudoepitheliomatous hyperplasia that could be interpreted as squamous cell carcinoma in a small biopsy.

Sites of involvement

The head and neck, including tongue, is a common location. The breast and proximal extremities may be involved {13}. GCT usually affects the skin/subcutis or submucosa, but visceral involvement of the gastrointestinal and respiratory tracts is common {2566, 2836}. While most GCTs are solitary, up to 10% are multifocal, and can be regional or involve multiple organ sites {234,1520}.

Clinical features

Usually asymptomatic, GCT can be pruritic to painful in the skin and tongue. Cutaneous lesions are firm, flesh-coloured to reddish-brown and 0.5–3.0 cm in size. Tumour growth is usually indolent.

Macroscopy

GCTs are uninodular, firm masses involving the skin/subcutis or submucosa often with a hyperplastic overlying epidermal surface. On sectioning, the tumour has a yellowish, finely granular texture.

Histopathology

A variety of neoplasms can show granular-cell change. GCT was originally thought to show muscular differentiation, but current evidence suggests neuroectodermal and more specifically peripheral nerve sheath differentiation that is likely Schwannian in type. GCT has ill-defined borders and is composed of nests and trabeculae of large, oval to round cells with intensely eosinophilic, granular cyto-

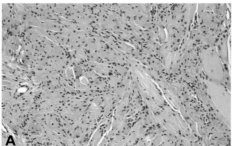
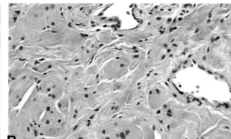
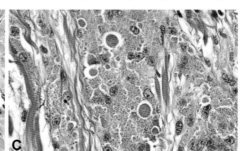

Fig. 11.17 Granular cell tumour. **A** Infiltration of collagenous stroma and skeletal muscle (in the tongue) is common. **B** Lesions are often poorly circumscribed and somewhat infiltrative at their periphery. **C** Large phagolysosomes can be found in virtually every case in varying numbers.

plasm. Cell borders are indistinct, producing a syncytial appearance. Nuclei are usually centrally situated and range from uniformly small, mildly hyperchromatic to larger and vesicular with distinct nucleoli. Mitoses are variable in number, but usually not prominent.

The finely granular appearance of the cytoplasm is due to massive accumulation of lysosomes includinglarger intracytoplasmic granules highlighted by clear halos {763}. Perineural infiltration is common. For cutaneous GCT and GCT arising in sites such as the tongue and oesophagus with overlying squamous epithelium, pseudoepitheliomatous hyperplasia is sometimes seen and when extensive can raise the consideration of squamous cell carcinoma.

Immunophenotype

GCTs are generally reactive for S100 protein, CD68, NKI-C3 (CD63) and NSE, with the latter three likely nonspecific and caused by the cytoplasmic lysosomal content {847}. MITF and TFE3 show diffuse nuclear reactivity in most cases, but HMB45 is uniformly negative and only very rarely is there focal reactivity for Melan-A {993}. Staining for SMA, desmin, neurofilament protein (NFP), GFAP and keratins is negative {1772}.

Prognostic factors

While GCT is benign, local recurrence can sometimes be seen after incomplete excision, perhaps due to complications associated with perineural spread. Malignant granular cell tumours are described in subsequent sections.

Dermal nerve sheath myxoma

J.F. Fetsch
S.M. Dry

Definition

Dermal nerve sheath myxoma is a benign peripheral nerve sheath tumour that typically arises in skin or subcutis and often has a multinodular growth pattern. It features small epithelioid, ring-like and spindled Schwann cells embedded in abundant myxoid matrix.

ICD-O code   9562/0

Synonyms

This tumour has often been referred to as the "classic" or myxoid variant of neurothekeoma. However, there is compelling evidence that true nerve sheath myxomas are clinically and biologically distinct from other recognized subtypes of "neurothekeoma," so this approach cannot be endorsed {831,835,940,1222,1550,2462, 2532}. While some neurothekeomas have abundant myxoid matrix, these tumours share many characteristics with cellular neurothekeoma and lack convincing evidence of schwannian differentiation {831}.

Epidemiology

Dermal nerve sheath myxomas are rare. They have been documented in patients ranging in age from 8 to 84 years (median, 34 years) and are equally frequent in males and females {66,835}. Nerve sheath myxomas are more than five times rarer than so-called neurothekeomas {831,835}. They differ clinically from cellular neurothekeomas by having: (i) a higher median age at onset; (ii) no female predominance; (iii) a substantially different anatomical distribution; and (iv) a higher rate of local recurrence {835,940,1222, 1550}.

Sites of involvement

More than 85% of cases arise in the extremities {835}. The fingers are the most common site, accounting for approximately 36% of cases {259,835}. Other

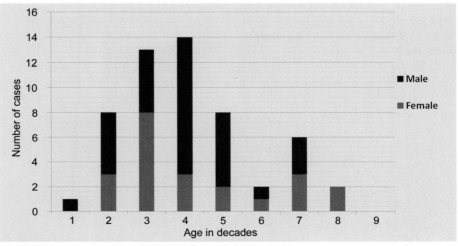
Fig. 11.18 Age distribution of dermal nerve sheath myxoma for 54 patients.

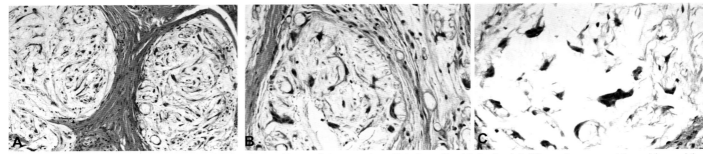

Fig. 11.19 Dermal nerve sheath myxoma. **A**, **B** and **C** show low- and intermediate-power views. Note the multinodularity, the rind of fibrous tissue around the nodules, and the abundant myxoid matrix. The neoplastic Schwann cells are arranged in cords and syncytial-like aggregates. Some have a ring-like appearance and resemble fat cells.

frequently affected sites include the knee, lower leg, ankle and foot.

Clinical features
Dermal nerve sheath myxomas typically present as small, superficial, slowly growing masses. The lesions are often asymptomatic, but pain may be elicited with pressure in some instances.

Macroscopy
Resection specimens are typically small and often include overlying epidermis. The tumours generally range from 0.4 to 4.5 cm in greatest dimension, with most lesions being < 2.5 cm in size {835}. Tissue fragments have a rubbery to firm consistency, and on cut section, the tumours form well-demarcated, glistening, mucoid nodules within skin and subcutis.

Histopathology
Dermal nerve sheath myxoma typically forms a multinodular mass. The tumours have abundant myxoid matrix and are usually bordered by dense fibrous connective tissue. They contain small epithelioid, ring-like, stellate and spindled neoplastic Schwann cells {835}. The epithelioid Schwann cells are arranged in cords, nests and syncytial-like aggregates. Some of the Schwann cells with ring-like morphology may superficially resemble fat cells. Infrequent Schwann cells may be multivacuolated and have spider-like

cytoplasmic processes. Rare examples may show focal nuclear palisading or Verocay body-like structures. There is generally only mild nuclear atypia, and scattered cytoplasmic–nuclear invaginations are often encountered. Mitotic figures are uncommon. Most cases have no discernible mitotic activity, but occasional examples with 3 mitoses per 25 wide HPF have been documented. A small number of delicate intralesional fibroblast-like cells may be evident. Scattered small-calibre vessels are present, but a complex microvascular network is absent.

Immunophenotype
The neoplastic Schwann cells are diffusely immunoreactive for S100 protein and moderately to diffusely reactive for GFAP and CD57 {66,259,835,1550}. Rare Schwann cells may react with the AE1/AE3 keratin cocktail. Strong immunoreactivity for collagen IV is typically present around the tumour cells. Small numbers of EMA-positive perineurial cells can be found in the fibrous capsule, and occasional delicate CD34-positive intraneural fibroblasts may be present. Infrequent cases may have rare detectable neurofilament protein-positive axons.

Ultrastructure
These tumours show true nerve-sheath differentiation by ultrastructural analysis {66,259,2462,3014}.

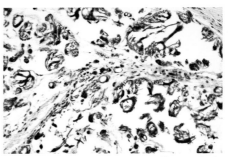

Fig. 11.20 Nerve sheath myxoma. The neoplastic Schwann cells express S100 protein.

Genetics
Microarray-based gene-expression profile analysis has shown nerve sheath myxomas to have a similar molecular genetic signature to dermal schwannomas {2532}. In contrast, cellular neurothekeomas have a genetic signature that more closely resembles cellular fibrous histiocytomas.

Prognostic factors
Dermal nerve sheath myxomas are benign tumours. Incomplete removal is associated with a high rate of local recurrence. In one relatively large study, 47% of patients treated by local excision experienced one or more (with a maximum of five) local recurrences {835}.

Solitary circumscribed neuroma

H. Kutzner

Definition
Solitary circumscribed neuroma (SCN) is a benign peripheral nerve sheath tumour composed of Schwann cells, axons, and perineurial fibroblasts.

ICD-O code
Neuroma   9570/0

Synonym
Palisaded encapsulated neuroma {2311}

Epidemiology
SCN is a relatively common tumour. It affects adults of either sex and may arise at any age, with a peak incidence in the fourth to seventh decades of life. Presentation under the age of 20 years is rare {1469,2311}.

Sites of involvement
The skin of the head and neck and the oral mucosa are the principal sites of involvement {1469,2311}, with < 10% of tumours occurring on trunk, extremities, and glans penis {856,1469,1509,2015, 2311}. The centre of the face is the most common location {856,1509}. SCN is localized in the dermis, and rarely extends into the subcutis.

Clinical features
SCN presents as a small, solitary, painless, skin-coloured, dome-shaped nodule, < 1 cm in diameter. Most tumours have been present for many years. Multifocal tumours are exceedingly rare {1339}. Correct clinical diagnosis of SCN is exceptional: the most common diagnoses include melanocytic naevus and basal cell carcinoma {1509}, reflecting the bland dome-shaped morphology of the tumour.

Macroscopy
These tumours are relatively small. They are localized in the dermis and resemble non-pigmented melanocytic dermal naevi.

Histopathology
SCN is a dermal tumour that presents with a typically lobular growth pattern, with asymmetrical contours and sharply delineated borders. Fungating, plexiform, and multilobular variants may occur {100,102, 1339}. The overlying epidermis and the surrounding connective tissue lack significant changes. SCN is not fully encapsulated: almost all tumours are only partially surrounded by a perineurial capsule consisting of loosely aggregated fibroblasts. In about 50% of cases, the nerve of origin becomes apparent adjacent to the base of the tumour. SCN consists of intersecting cellular Schwann cell fascicles, often with prominent interfascicular clefting {551,856}. Fascicles are composed of densely aggregated isomorphic fusiform Schwann cells with elongated slender cytoplasm and wavy nuclei. In a minority of cases, SCN shows epithelioid, vascular, or myxoid features {100,101,1339,2788}. Palisading is unusual; Verocay bodies are infrequent; there is no Antoni A and Antoni B zonation. Mitoses and significant nuclear pleomorphism are lacking {1469}. In sharp contrast to neurofibroma and schwannoma, SCN is replete with multiple

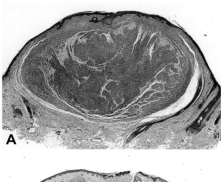

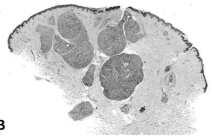

Fig. 11.21 Solitary circumscribed neuroma. **A** Sharply circumscribed dermal tumour composed of Schwann cell fascicles with prominent interfascicular clefting. **B** Plexiform variant.

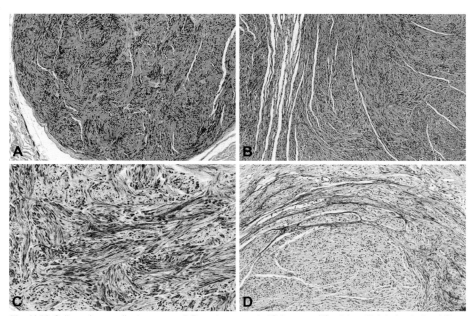

Fig. 11.22 Solitary circumscribed neuroma. **A** Densely aggregated Schwann cell fascicles with interfascicular clefting. This tumour is only partially encapsulated by a thin layer of perineurial fibroblasts. **B** Typical intersecting Schwann cell fascicles with interfascicular clefting. **C** Most tumours are replete with neurofilament-positive axons amidst Schwann cells (neurofilament). **D** Perineurial fibroblasts express EMA .

neurofilament-positive axons amidst the Schwann cells {99}.

Immunophenotype
Schwann cells express S100 protein, and are surrounded by type IV collagen. Axons strongly express neurofilament protein. Endoneurial and perineurial fibroblasts can best be demonstrated with anti-CD34. The incomplete perineurial capsule shows strong positivity for EMA, and to a lesser extent positivity for claudin-1 and GLUT1. SCN is negative for GFAP {99,102,856,1469}.

Prognostic factors
The clinical course of SCN is entirely benign: local excision is curative {1469}. Tumours usually do not recur {1509}. There is no known malignant transformation.

Ectopic meningioma/meningothelial hamartoma

A. Perry

Definition
Ectopic meningioma is a meningothelial neoplasm occurring entirely outside the anatomical regions that normally contain meningothelial (arachnoidal cap) cells, such as intracranial and intraspinal compartments. In contrast, meningothelial hamartoma represents a developmental rest, with collections of non-neoplastic arachnoidal cells found typically on the scalp.

ICD-O code
Ectopic meningioma   9530/0

Synonyms
Extradural, extracranial/extraspinal, extraneuraxial, heterotopic, cutaneous, calvarial, and intraosseous meningiomas; meningothelial choristoma; rudimentary meningocele; sequestrated meningocele

Epidemiology
Ectopic meningiomas are rare. In one review of cases diagnosed within the CT era, they accounted for 1.6% of all resected meningiomas and presented at all ages, with bimodal peaks occurring in the second decade of life and in the fifth to seventh decades {1537,1654}. There was a slight female predominance.
Meningothelial hamartomas are typically found in neonates or infants, with no known sex or racial predisposition {148, 534,2685}.

Etiology
The etiology of ectopic meningiomas is unknown, although four hypotheses have been postulated, with histogenesis resulting from: (i) meningothelial cells carried along nerve sheaths as they exit the skull or vertebral column; (ii) ectopic arachnoidal cap cells; (iii) meningothelial cells displaced during trauma; and (iv) pluripotent mesenchymal cells capable of undergoing meningothelial differentiation or metaplasia.
Meningothelial hamartomas are thought to be pathogenetically related to meningoceles and meningoencephaloceles, which result from neural-tube defects. In contrast, however, no intracranial connection is found in the hamartomas.

Sites of involvement
More than 90% of ectopic meningiomas present in the head and neck region {1654}. While many reports list the orbit as the most common site, only tumours with no connection to the optic nerve's dural sleeve should be considered as ectopic. Other locations include the skull, sinonasal tract, oropharynx, middle ear, scalp, parotid gland, and neck. By definition, an intracranial/spinal component must be carefully excluded. For instance, *en plaque* (carpet-like) meningiomas extensively invade the skull and may be misinterpreted as a purely intraosseous meningioma.
Meningothelial hamartomas typically present as solitary scalp masses, most often in the occiput. By definition, there is no intracranial connection {148,2685}.

Clinical features
Presenting signs and symptoms for ectopic meningiomas vary greatly with site of involvement, although the most common pattern is that of a painless, slowly growing mass. Likewise, meningothelial hamartoma is typically detected as an incidental scalp mass or dimple, sometimes with alopecia; some become tender over time.

Macroscopy
The gross pathology of ectopic meningiomas is similar to that of intracranial examples, except that invasion of surrounding tissues is much more common. Colour and consistency vary with

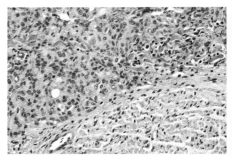

Fig. 11.23 Ectopic (meningothelial) meningioma surrounding and tracking along the paraspinal nerve root. Invasion of adjacent skeletal muscle was seen in other sections.

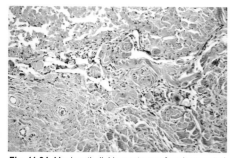

Fig. 11.24 Meningothelial hamartoma of scalp resected from the occiput of a neonate. The lesion involved the dermis and subcutaneous soft tissue. Note the slit-like spaces mimicking vascular channels, in association with occasional more easily recognizable meningothelial clusters and psammoma bodies.

cellularity, collagen deposition, and tumour grade, but a rubbery tan-white mass is most common.

Hamartomas are solitary nodules, plaques, or spongy to cyst-like tan-grey, red, or flesh-coloured lesions in the dermis and/or subcutaneous soft tissue of the scalp.

Histopathology
The same range of histological appearances that are encountered intracranially may be seen in ectopic meningiomas {2223}, although the meningothelial (syncytial) subtype is most frequent. Examples of all WHO grades (I–III) have been reported, with benign tumours most common. Hamartomas most often appear as cutaneous slit-like spaces that may resemble lymphatics or angiosarcoma. However, they are lined by meningothelial, rather than endothelial cells {148, 2685}. Larger meningothelial clusters and psammoma bodies are occasionally encountered.

Immunophenotype
Highly sensitive and specific markers of meningiomas and meningothelial hamartomas are lacking, with coexpression of EMA and vimentin being most consistent. Positivity for progesterone receptor is also common {2753}.

Ultrastructure
Meningiomas and hamartomas contain overlapping cytoplasmic processes likened to the interlocking pieces of a jigsaw puzzle. Desmosomes and other intercellular junctions are common.

Prognostic factors
As with other meningiomas, tumour grade and extent of resection play important prognostic roles. Intraosseous cases involving the skull base have higher rates of recurrence than those of the convexity. Distant metastases have been reported in about 6% of cases, mostly in anaplastic (malignant) examples {1537}. Hamartomas are usually cured by surgery alone, although rare recurrences have been reported.

Nasal glial heterotopia

L.D.R. Thompson

Definition
A mass of mature, heterotopic neuroglial tissue isolated from the cranial cavity, most often presenting in and around the nose.

Synonyms
Nasal glioma (use of this term is discouraged as it implies neoplasm); neuroglial heterotopia; glial choristoma; nasal atretic cephalocele; ectopic glial tissue

Epidemiology
Most patients present as newborns, with > 90% of cases diagnosed by age 2 years {2693}. Rare cases are reported in adults {2215}. These lesions are equally frequent in males and females {2216}.

Etiology
Nasal glial heterotopia (NGH) is a congenital, nonhereditary malformation with anterior displacement of mature cerebral tissue that has lost connection with the intracranial contents {428}.

Sites of involvement
The lesion is situated externally on or near the bridge of the nose (about 60% of cases), within the nasal cavity (30%), or both (10%), where a defect in nasal bones allows for communication {2215,2748}.

Clinical features
Extranasal NGH presents as a smooth noncompressible subcutaneous mass usually over the dorsum of the nose. The intranasal lesions usually present with nasal obstruction or nasal deformity {2215,2748}. Glial heterotopia may occur at other sites (paranasal sinuses, nasopharynx, pharynx, tongue, palate, tonsil, orbit), and is sometimes referred to as "facial glioma" {143}. A helpful clinical sign is absence of expansion or pulsation

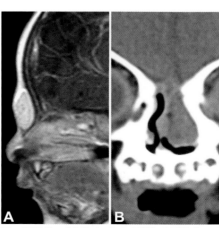

Fig. 11.25 Nasal glial heterotopia (NGH). **A** MRI of nasal bridge NGH. **B** CT shows a mass within the nasal cavity.

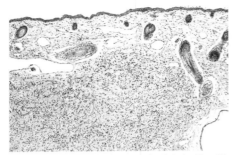

Fig. 11.26 Nasal glial heterotopia. Intact skin with underlying cellular glial tissue.

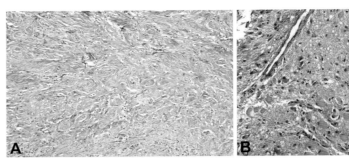

Fig. 11.27 Nasal glial heterotopia. **A** Glial tissue set within fibrosis connective tissue can be difficult to identify. **B** Glial tissue with astrocytes.

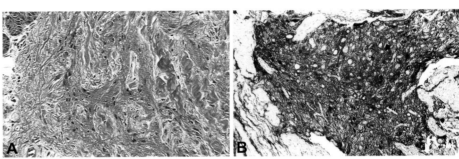

Fig. 11.28 Nasal glial heterotopia. **A** Trichrome stains glial tissue red in a background of "blue" fibrosis. **B** GFAP immunostaining strongly and diffusely highlights the neural tissue.

of the mass following compression of the ipsilateral jugular vein (negative Furstenberg test), due to lack of connection of the mass with the cerebrospinal-fluid system. Importantly, radiographic imaging scans (CT and MRI) reveal a soft-tissue mass without an intracranial component or bony defect. If a defect is identified, then an encephalocele is more likely {2277,3031}.

Macroscopy
The lesion appears as a polypoid, smooth, soft, grey-tan, nontranslucent mass, usually 1–3 cm in diameter {2215}.

Histopathology
The lesion is nonencapsulated, composed of variably sized islands of glial tissue separated by bands of vascularized fibrous connective tissue. The glial tissue may merge with the collagen, sometimes obscuring the diagnosis {3031}. The astrocytes are evenly spaced, with occasional large gemistocytes. Astrocyte enlargement or multinucleation may occasionally

be seen. Neurons are rare or absent. Mitoses are absent {1251,2215, 2748}. Rarely, choroid plexus, ependyma-lined clefts and pigmented retinal epithelium are seen, especially for lesions of the palate and nasopharynx.

NGH should be separated from nasal encephalocele and fibrosed nasal polyp, and has been reported to develop in association with sinonasal undifferentiated carcinoma {2747,3031}.

Immunophenotype
The glial tissue can be confirmed by a trichome stain (glial tissue is blue, while fibrosis is red) or with immunoreactivity for GFAP, NSE or S100 protein {670,1420, 2215,2748}.

Prognostic factors
Excision is curative, but incomplete excision can be accompanied by recurrence (15–30% of cases). There is no locally aggressive behaviour {2215,2693}.

Benign Triton tumour

A. Perry

Definition
An expansile intraneural mass characterized by the intimate interposition of mature skeletal muscle fibres with nerve fibres.

Synonyms
Neuromuscular choristoma; neuromuscular hamartoma; nerve rhabdomyoma

Epidemiology
Benign Triton tumours are extremely rare {1152,1702}. Most present in infancy or childhood, although rare cases in adults have been seen. The sexes are roughly equally represented.

Sites of involvement
Classic cases involve large nerves or plexi, most commonly the sciatic nerve or the brachial plexus.

Clinical features
Patients present with either progressive pain or classic features of peripheral neuropathy/plexopathy.

Macroscopy
Fusiform-nerve enlargement with multifascicular involvement is typical. On cut surface, a subset of nerve fascicles appears beefy red, like skeletal muscle. Intraoperative stimulation of the involved nerve causes contraction of not only the innervated muscle, but also the abnormal nerve.

Histopathology
Haphazardly arranged bundles of mature skeletal muscle with cross-striations are intercalated between clusters of nerve fibres. Reported cases involving cranial nerves also display adipose tissue, although it remains unclear whether this is a different entity.

Prognostic factors
As these lesions typically involve large functional nerves, accurate intraoperative diagnosis is critical to prevent an overly aggressive approach. Although considered benign, a recent study suggests an association with postsurgical fibromatosis (desmoid) {1152}. Rare examples of regression have also been reported. Additional follow-up is needed to establish the long-term prognosis for this lesion.

Hybrid nerve sheath tumours

J.L. Hornick
M. Michal

Definition
Hybrid nerve sheath tumours are benign peripheral nerve sheath tumours with combined features of more than one conventional type (neurofibroma, schwannoma, perineurioma).

ICD-O code
Nerve sheath tumour not otherwise specified (NOS)   9563/0

Epidemiology
Tumours showing hybrid features of more than one type of conventional benign nerve sheath tumour have recently been recognized and are uncommon {819,1214, 1870 ,2527,3051}. The most common example is schwannoma/perineurioma, around 50 cases of which have been reported {16,1214,1389}. About 10 cases of hybrid neurofibroma/schwannoma have been reported {819}. These tumours occur over a wide age range, with a peak in young adults and an equal sex distribution.

Etiology
Hybrid schwannoma/perineurioma occur sporadically {1214,1389,1870}. Hybrid neurofibroma/schwannomas may arise in patients with neurofibromatosis {819,1111}.

Sites of involvement
Hybrid nerve sheath tumours show a wide anatomical distribution in somatic soft tissue {819,1214,1389,2527}. Rare cases arise in the gastrointestinal tract {16,1214}. Most tumours showing hybrid features of

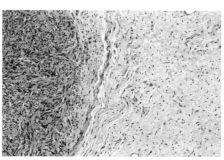

Fig. 11.29 A well-delineated Schwann cell nodule in a plexiform neurofibroma.

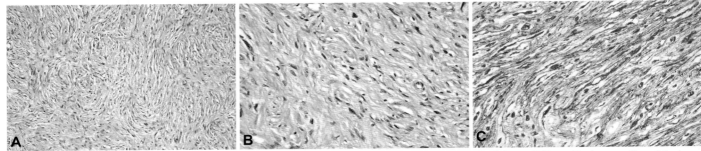

Fig. 11.30 Hybrid schwannoma/perineurioma. **A** The tumour shows a storiform architecture, similar to perineurioma of soft tissue. **B** Many of the tumour cells contain plump, tapering nuclei and eosinophilic cytoplasm, typical of Schwann cells. The perineurial cell component is often inconspicuous. **C** Double immunolabelling for S100 protein (red) and EMA (brown) highlights alternating Schwann cells and perineurial cells, respectively.

schwannoma and reticular perineurioma have been reported on the fingers {1870}.

Clinical features
Hybrid nerve sheath tumours present as painless masses. Most arise in subcutaneous tissue or dermis {819,1214,1870}.

Macroscopy
Grossly, hybrid nerve sheath tumours are well-circumscribed, usually with a firm cut surface. The size range is broad, with most tumours measuring between 1 and 8 cm {1214,1389,1870}.

Histopathology
Hybrid neurofibroma/schwannoma has a biphasic appearance, consisting of hypercellular, schwannomatous nodules within an otherwise typical neurofibroma, which may show a plexiform architecture {819}. Hybrid schwannoma/perineurioma shows a storiform or fascicular growth pattern and is usually composed of an intimate admixture of alternating Schwann cells with plump nuclei and eosinophilic cytoplasm (which usually predominate) and perineurial cells with slender nuclei and delicate elongated cytoplasmic processes {1214}. Mitotic activity is scarce. Degenerative nuclear atypia may be observed. Rare hybrid schwannoma/ perineuriomas show a biphasic appearance and a lobulated growth pattern, either with separate schwannomatous and perineurial nodules or schwannomatous nodules surrounded by a perineurial component with a reticular growth pattern and myxoid stroma {1389,1870}.

Immunophenotype
Staining for S100 protein is positive in the Schwann cells and EMA is positive in the perineurial cells. Hybrid neurofibroma/ schwannoma contains neurofilament protein-positive axons and CD34 is often positive in a subset of cells in the neurofibromatous component, whereas the schwannomatous nodules show strong, diffuse expression of S100 protein {819}. Most hybrid schwannoma/perineuriomas contain alternating S100 protein-positive Schwann cells and EMA-positive perineurial cells {1214}. CD34, claudin-1, and GFAP are usually also positive {1214}.

Genetics
One hybrid nerve sheath tumour with a point mutation in *NF2* has been reported {1389}.

Prognostic factors
Hybrid nerve sheath tumours are benign with rare local recurrence {819,1214,1870}.

Malignant peripheral nerve sheath tumour

G.P. Nielsen
C.R. Antonescu
R.A. Lothe

Definition

A malignant nerve sheath tumour arising from a peripheral nerve, from a pre-existing benign nerve sheath tumour (usually neurofibroma) or in a patient with neurofibromatosis type 1 (NF1). In the absence of these settings, the diagnosis is based on the constellation of histological, immunohistochemical and ultrastructural features suggesting Schwann-cell differentiation.

ICD-O code

Malignant peripheral nerve sheath tumour
(MPNST)   9540/3
Epithelioid MPNST   9542/3
Malignant Triton tumour   9561/3

Synonyms

Malignant schwannoma; neurofibrosarcoma; neurogenic sarcoma

Epidemiology

MPNST is a rare tumour accounting for up to 5% of soft tissue sarcomas {1600}.

Etiology

Up to 50% of MPNSTs arise in patients with the hereditary syndrome NF1, approximately 10% are radiation-induced and the remainder affect individuals without a known genetic predisposition {707}.

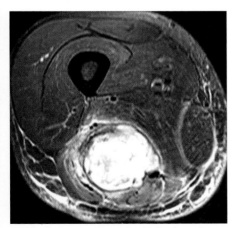

Fig.11.32 An axial T1-weighted MRI of a malignant peripheral nerve sheath tumour arising in the sciatic nerve. The tumour demonstrates homogeneous contrast enhancement, and lacks the zonation phenomenon that is sometimes present in benign nerve sheath tumours.

In patients with NF1, those with plexiform neurofibromas have the highest rate of malignant transformation {2802}. Extremely rarely, MPNST arises from schwannoma {389,1800,2991}, ganglioneuroblastoma/ganglioneuroma {2333} or pheochromocytoma {2410}.

Sites of involvement

MPNST most commonly arises in the extremities, followed by the trunk and the head and neck area {707,2670}. The sciatic nerve is most frequently affected.

Clinical features

MPNSTs are typically seen in patients aged 20–50 years, although they can also arise in children, especially those with NF1 {706}. Patients with NF1 are usually younger at the time of presentation than patients with sporadic tumours {707, 2670}. The presenting symptoms are those of an enlarging painless or painful mass that may be palpable or discovered on imaging studies. When involving a nerve, the patient may present with neuropathic symptoms, such as paraesthesia, motor weakness or radicular pain {2670}. There are no specific radiographical features that distinguish MPNSTs from other high-grade sarcomas, except possible origin from a large nerve. In patients with NF1, FDG-PET imaging technique is sensitive in the detection of MPNSTs {305}.

Macroscopy

There is usually a large fusiform mass involving a major nerve. The tumours are often > 5 cm at the time of diagnosis. In patients with NF1, the sarcoma often arises in association with a plexiform neurofibroma. The tumour has a tan-white, fleshy cut surface with areas of haemorrhage and necrosis.

Histopathology

MPNST has a diverse microscopic appearance. Typical cases are composed of spindle cells showing a fascicular growth pattern, often with a branching haemangioperictyoma-like vascular pattern, as

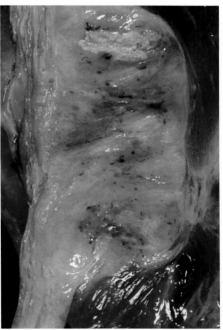

Fig. 11.31 Malignant peripheral nerve sheath tumour of the sciatic nerve. The cut surface is tan, with yellow areas of necrosis. The uninvolved nerve can be seen distally.

well as alternating hypercellular and hypocellular areas. The cells can have a whorling or rarely palisading growth pattern and geographic areas of necrosis. The neoplastic cells are mitotically active, spindle- or serpentine-shaped with hyperchromatic nuclei and pale cytoplasm. MPNST can occasionally show extensive pleomorphism, simulating a high-grade undifferentiated pleomorphic sarcoma; sometimes MPNST has fibroblastic features. The neoplastic cells tend to concentrate around blood vessels; in these areas the cells become plumper and the endothelial cells more epithelioid. Heterologous elements, such as skeletal muscle, bone, cartilage and blood vessels, are present in approximately 15% of tumours. A malignant Triton tumour is an MPNST with skeletal-muscle differentiation. Glandular differentiation with or without mucin production is rarely seen in MPNST (glandular MPNST); almost all of these tumours arise in patients with NF1

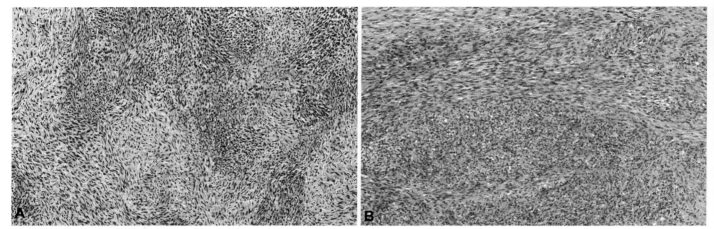

Fig. 11.33 Malignant peripheral nerve sheath tumour. **A** Tumour composed of cellular areas alternating with less cellular areas ("tapestry" appearance or "marble-like" pattern). **B** The tumour is cellular and has a fascicular growth pattern mimicking a fibrosarcoma or a synovial sarcoma.

{2987}. Melanin pigment can be seen rarely, especially in tumours arising from spinal nerves. When MPNST arises in a peripheral nerve, the neoplastic cells tend to track along the nerve bundles, often for a long distance. In this setting it is imperative to examine the nerve margins, preferably at the time of surgery.

In MPNST arising in neurofibroma in patients with NF1, there are occasionally areas that show increased cellularity and nuclear atypia without overt features of malignancy and these regions might represent transition from neurofibroma to MPNST. The distinction between these "atypical" neurofibromas and low-grade MPNST is often problematic, especially on a small biopsy.

Epithelioid MPNST is a rare variant of MPNST (< 5% of cases), which is composed of plump, epithelioid cells with abundant eosinophilic cytoplasm, sometimes embedded in abundant extracellular myxoid matrix and typically showing lobulated growth. Although rare, epithelioid MPNST is the most common MPNST

to arise from a pre-existing benign schwannoma {1800}. Epithelioid MPNST is not associated with NF1.

Immunophenotype

Immunohistochemically, MPNST is positive for S100 protein in < 50% of cases and for GFAP in 20–30% of cases. The staining is usually focal; diffuse staining for S100 protein is rarely compatible with conventional MPNST and should raise the possibility of other tumours, such as cellular schwannoma, melanoma, clear cell sarcoma or interdigitating dendritic cell sarcoma. Epithelioid MPNST, however, is strongly and diffusely positive for S100 protein but lacks staining for melanoma markers and SMARCB1 (INI1) (50%). Epithelioid MPNST can also show keratin positivity. Most MPNSTs are TP53-positive and p16INK4a -negative. The glands in glandular MPNST are positive for keratin and CEA and can show staining for neuroendocrine markers.

Other heterologous components (such as skeletal-muscle differentiation, angiosar-

comatous areas) stain for appropriate markers.

Ultrastructure

MPNST has nonspecific ultrastructural features and is often difficult to diagnose. The features seen in benign tumours such as intertwining cell processes, basal lamina and long spacing collagen are very often absent in MPNST. Rhabdomyoblastic differentiation is seen in malignant Triton tumour and, in glandular MPNST, glandular differentiation with surface microvilli is present; neuroendocrine granules may be seen.

Genetics

Patients with NF1 carry germline alterations in the *NF1* gene (17q11.2), encoding the tumour suppressor protein neurofibromin. Biallelic mutations of *NF1* are found in a significant portion of all MPNSTs {273,1860,2819}. Most MPNSTs exhibit complex karyotypes with multiple structural and numerical changes, often near-triploid {1662,1804,1850,2469}. Metaphase

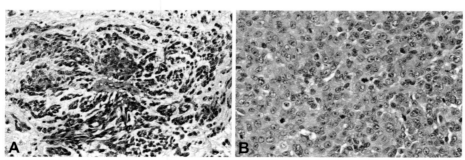

Fig. 11.34 Epithelioid malignant peripheral-nerve sheath tumour. **A** The neoplastic cells are epithelioid and embedded in an extracellular myxoid matrix. **B** The neoplastic cells in this tumour are cohesive. The cells have eosinophilic cytoplasm and nuclei with prominent nucleoli. Several mitoses are present.

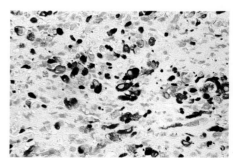

Fig. 11.35 Immunohistochemical staining for desmin in a malignant Triton tumour. The rhabdomyoblastic cells show strong cytoplasmic staining for desmin.

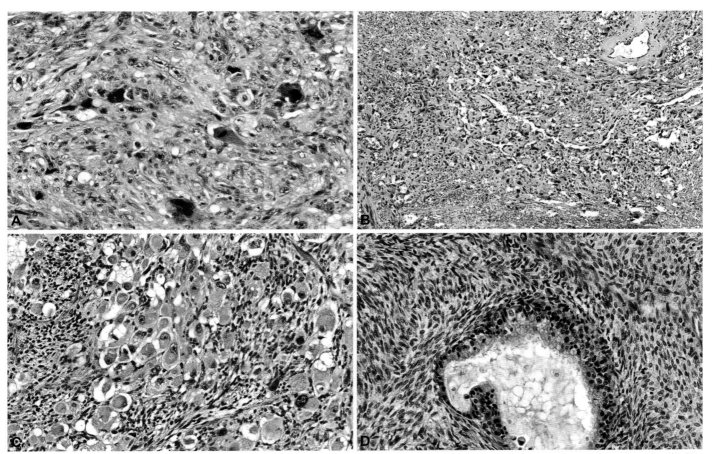

Fig. 11.36 Malignant peripheral nerve sheath tumour (MPNST). **A** This anaplastic tumour that arose in a patient with NF1 shows obvious pleomorphism and may be difficult to distinguish from a pleomorphic undifferentiated sarcoma. **B** The high-grade angiosarcomatous component in an MPNST arising in a patient with NF1. **C** Malignant Triton tumour showing extensive rhabdomyoblastic differentiation; the cells are epithelioid and contain abundant eosinophilic cytoplasm. **D** MPNST showing glandular differentiation containing mucin-secreting glands.

CGH shows that an average of 18 aberrations (range, 2–35) and a ratio of gains versus losses of close to 1 : 1 are present {308}. Common changes to DNA copy number include gains from chromosome arms 7p, 8q and 17q and losses from 9p, 11q, 13q, and 17p {308,1730,3022,3042}. No consistent differences between NF1 and non-NF1-associated MPNSTs have been reported. Gains of 7p and 17q {2469}, the combined profile of 16q gain and loss of 10q and Xq {308} and minimally overlapping regions along chromosome 12 appear to carry prognostic information for patients with MPNST {3042}. *TP53* mutations are relatively rare {1663, 2871}, but nuclear immunohistochemical staining for TP53 has been shown to be a prognostic indicator {307,3042,3074}. Aberrations in 9p21 in MPNST target the *CDKN2A* gene, and homozygous deletions of this locus are common {19, 199,1468,2044}. This gene encodes the two non-homologous isoforms p14ARF and p16INK4a, both with an important impact on cell-cycle progression.

Prognostic factors

Most MPNSTs are aggressive tumours with a poor prognosis. Truncal location, tumour size > 5 cm, local recurrence, and high grade are adverse prognostic factors. Survival of patients with NF1-associated MPNST appears to be lower than that of patients with sporadic MPNST {2670}. Malignant Triton tumours are particularly aggressive.

Malignant granular cell tumour

J.C. Fanburg-Smith

Definition
A rare high-grade sarcoma with a Schwannian phenotype, composed of malignant granular cells with cytoplasmic lysosomal inclusions {810}.

ICD-O code   9580/3

Epidemiology
Malignant granular cell tumour is extremely rare.

Sites of involvement
The most common locations are the soft tissue of the thigh, proximal upper extremity, trunk and then distal extremity. Head and neck and oral locations are less common for malignant tumours {810}.

Clinical features
Malignant granular cell tumours occur with a female predominance and age range of 3–70 years (mean of 40 years) {810}. Despite a Schwannian phenotype, origin from a nerve is generally not identified {810}.

Macroscopy
Tumour sizes range from 1 to 18.2 cm, usually being > 5 cm {810,1267}. Grossly, tumours are pale grey and firm, often deeper (subcutaneous/intramuscular) than their benign counterparts.

Histopathology
Although many cases have high-grade spindle or polygonal cell morphology with eosinophilic, granular cytoplasm, some

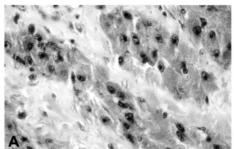

Fig. 11.37 Malignant granular cell tumour (MGCT). **A** Sarcomatoid spindling and loss of benign Zellballen compartmentalization are common features. **B** Cases must have vesicular nuclei with extremely large prominent nucleoli diffusely present to qualify for one of six criteria for malignancy.

cases are morphologically bland and not obviously malignant. Hallmark features include sarcomatoid morphology, vesicular nuclei with prominent nucleoli, increased mitotic activity, > 2 mitoses per 10 HPF in areas of highest mitotic activity, geographical necrosis, marked pleomorphism, and high nuclear to cytoplasmic ratio {810,1267,2893}. Most malignant granular cell tumours have necrosis and/or high mitotic activity {2010}, but these parameters alone may not identify all tumours that metastasize {531}.

Immunophenotype
As with benign lesions, most malignant granular cell tumours demonstrate strong diffuse positivity for S100 protein and CD68 {810,2326}.

Ultrastructure
Malignant granular cell tumours are characterized by abundant cytoplasmic

typical/angulated lysosomes filled with amorphous granular material and focal tubular/mitochondrial/myelin-like remnants, long-spacing collagen, external lamina, and nerve sheath-like interdigitating cytoplasmic extensions {810}.

Genetics
Two of three cases showed loss of distal 5p {660,2011,2166}. Monosomy 22, trisomy 10, and loss of CDKN2A, as detected by FISH, may suggest a relationship with or alternate classification as granular malignant peripheral nerve sheath tumour {660,2166}.

Prognostic factors
Malignant granular cell tumour has a 50% rate of metastasis {810}. Local recurrence, metastasis, larger tumour size, and older patient age are adverse prognostic factors {810}.

Ectomesenchymoma

C.M. Coffin

Definition
Ectomesenchymoma consists of rhabdomyosarcoma with a neuronal or neural component. These lesions are possibly of neural crest origin or may represent a variant of rhabdomyosarcoma.

ICD-O code   8921/3

Synonym
Gangliorhabdomyosarcoma {1199,1451}

Epidemiology
Ectomesenchymoma is very rare, mainly affecting children aged < 5 years {274, 1382,1966}.

Sites of involvement
Paratesticular soft tissue, external genitalia, pelvis, abdomen, and head/neck are principal sites {274,1382,1966}.

Clinical features
Ectomesenchymoma presents as a superficial or deep soft-tissue mass.

Macroscopy
The multilobulated mass is tan, with variable necrosis and haemorrhage, and averages 5 cm in diameter (range, 3–18 cm) {274}.

Histopathology
Rhabdomyosarcoma, typically embryonal or spindle-cell type, intermingles with neuronal or neural components, including ganglion cells, ganglioneuroma, neuroblastoma or malignant peripheral nerve sheath tumour {274,1372,1382,1966}. Histological variants may include alveolar rhabdomyosarcoma or peripheral primitive neuroectodermal tumour. Treated or metastatic rhabdomyosarcoma may contain ganglion cells {724,2502}.

Immunophenotype
The rhabdomyosarcomatous component expresses myogenin, MyoD1, desmin, and MSA; the neuroblastic component reacts for synaptophysin, chromogranin, and NSE; schwannian foci express S100 protein {274,1451,1966}.

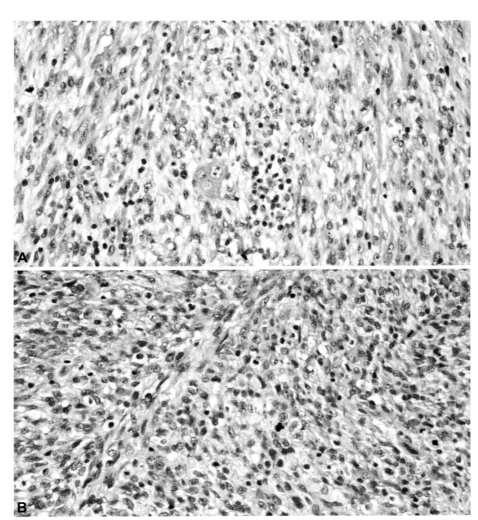

Fig. 11.38 Ectomesenchymoma. **A** A multinucleated ganglion cell is present in the centre, surrounded by primitive rhabdomyoblasts, strap cells, and a patchy lymphocytic infiltrate. **B** A focus of rhabdomyosarcoma in ectomesenchymoma contains primitive round cells, rhabdomyoblasts, and strap cells.

Genetics
Cytogenetic and array CGH features similar to those of embryonal rhabdomyosarcoma have been observed {874, 1235}. Rare tumours with myogenic and neural differentiation with t(11;22) are probably a variant of Ewing sarcoma {2606}. The relationship to intracranial "ectomesenchymoma" is unclear {1437}.

Prognostic factors
With treatment based on rhabdomyosarcoma protocols, the outcome is similar to that of rhabdomyosarcoma {274}. Favourable prognostic factors include size < 10 cm, low stage, superficial location, and absence of alveolar rhabdomyosarcoma.

CHAPTER 12

Tumours of uncertain differentiation

Acral fibromyxoma

Intramuscular myxoma

Juxta-articular myxoma

Deep ("aggressive") angiomyxoma

Pleomorphic hyalinizing angiectatic tumour of soft parts

Ectopic hamartomatous thymoma

Atypical fibroxanthoma

Angiomatoid fibrous histiocytoma

Ossifying fibromyxoid tumour

Myoepithelioma/myoepithelial carcinoma/mixed tumour

Haemosiderotic fibrolipomatous tumour

Phosphaturic mesenchymal tumour

Synovial sarcoma

Epithelioid sarcoma

Alveolar soft part sarcoma

Clear cell sarcoma of soft tissue

Extraskeletal myxoid chondrosarcoma

Malignant mesenchymoma

Desmoplastic small round cell tumour

Extrarenal rhabdoid tumour

PEComa

Intimal sarcoma

Acral fibromyxoma

J.F. Fetsch

Definition
Acral fibromyxoma is a benign fibroblastic neoplasm that is restricted to acral sites and most often involves the periungual region of the digits.

ICD-O code   8811/0

Synonyms
Digital fibromyxoma; cellular digital fibroma

Epidemiology
This entity has been reported in individuals ranging in age from 4 to 86 years, with about 70% of patients aged 40 years or older {27,834,1200,1635,1679,1912,2263, 2721,2859}. Males are more frequently affected than females (ratio, 2 : 1) {27,834, 2263}.

Sites of involvement
Almost all reported cases have involved either the hands or feet {27,834,1200, 2263}. An estimated two thirds or more of cases are ungual or periungual in location, but other acral sites, including the palm and sole, may also be affected {27, 834,2263}. The most frequent site of involvement is the big toe {27,834,2263}.

Clinical features
The lesions typically present as solitary,

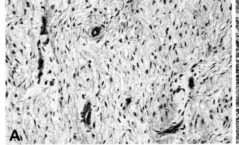
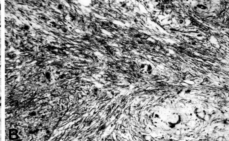

Fig. 12.01 Superficial acral fibromyxoma **A** This lesion from the heel region shows close similarity to the periungual tumour in Fig. 12.02C. **B** Positive immunoreactivity for CD34.

slowly growing masses on a finger or toe. However, 40% of these lesions are painful {1200}. Many examples cause nail deformity, and some tumours may cause scalloping of the underlying bone {834,2859}.

Macroscopy
Gross examination reveals a superficial, dome-shaped, polypoid or verrucoid mass with an intact or ulcerated overlying epidermis. Many resection specimens include portions of the nail or nail bed. Examples have ranged from 0.6 cm to 5 cm in greatest dimension, with a median of 1.5 cm {834}. The process has a soft to firm consistency, and the cut surface ranges from glistening and myxoid to off-white, firm and fibrous.

Histopathology
This is a moderately cellular, dermal-based, proliferation of spindled and stellate-shaped fibroblasts embedded in myxoid or collagenous matrix. The cells have loose fascicular and broad storiform growth patterns. There are often increased vessels and many mast cells in the stroma. Mitotic figures are usually sparse (averaging < 1 per 10 HPF). Occasional multinucleate cells are encountered in approximately half of the cases. Generally, there is minimal nuclear atypia, but rare examples may have scattered cells with moderate atypia and pleomorphism {27,834, 1679,2263}. These latter cases retain a low mitotic rate, and atypical mitotic figures are absent. The lesions may have a lobular or irregular and infiltrative contour.

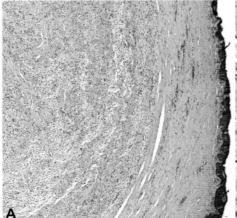
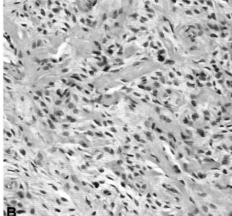
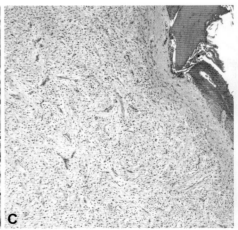

Fig. 12.02 Superficial acral fibromyxoma **A**, **B** and **C** show periungual examples of superficial acral fibromyxoma. Note the uniform spindled cells with loose fascicular, random and broad storiform growth patterns. These lesions have varying amounts of myxoid matrix, and there is mildly accentuated vasculature.

Many specimens contain overlying nail-bed epithelium {27,834, 2263}. Extension into the superficial subcutis is common, and rare larger examples may involve underlying fascia or abut bone.

Immunophenotype
Staining for CD34 is typically positive {27, 834,1635,1679,2263}. EMA expression is variable {27,834,1679,2263,2721}. S100 protein, GFAP, actin, desmin, and keratin are typically negative.

Genetics
Unlike intramuscular or cellular myxomas, *GNAS* mutations are absent {1200}.

Prognostic factors
The rate of recurrence appears to be low, probably in the range of 15–20% {27, 834,1200}. There are no documented instances of metastasis.

Intramuscular myxoma

G.P. Nielsen
P.C.W. Hogendoorn

Definition
Intramuscular myxoma is a benign soft tissue tumour characterized by bland spindle-shaped cells embedded in hypovascular, abundantly myxoid stroma.

ICD-O code   8840/0

Epidemiology
Intramuscular myxoma is more common in females and most patients are aged 40–70 years at the time of diagnosis.

Sites of involvement
The most frequently affected sites are the large muscles of the thigh, shoulder, buttocks and upper arm.

Clinical features
Patients usually complain of a painless soft tissue mass. Mazabraud syndrome is the combination of intramuscular myxoma(s) and skeletal fibrous dysplasia. Angiographic studies reveal a poorly vascularized tumour {1424}. MRI studies show that the tumour is bright on T2-weighted images and has low signal intensity relative to skeletal muscle on T1-weighted images {1477,2483}.

Macroscopy
Grossly, the tumours have a gelatinous, lobulated cut surface. They can measure up to 20 cm {1128}; however, most tumours are between 5 and 10 cm in greatest diameter; larger ones are usually cellular myxomas. Although intramuscular myxomas may appear well-circumscribed,

closer inspection often reveals ill-defined borders where the tumour merges with the surrounding skeletal muscle. Fluid-filled cystic spaces may be present.

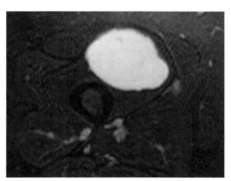

Fig. 12.03 Intramuscular myxoma. T2-weighted MRI shows a well-circumscribed, hyperintense tumour.

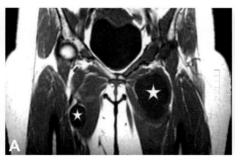
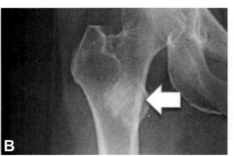

Fig. 12.04 Mazabraud syndrome. **A** Intramuscular myxomas are seen in the proximal muscles of the lower extremities (*). **B** Fibrous dysplasia is present in the proximal femur (arrow).

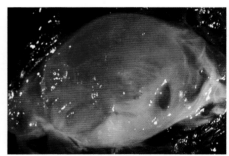

Fig. 12.05 Intramuscular myxoma composed of a gelatinous mass with internal septa. The tumour is well-circumscribed overall, but shows some infiltration of the surrounding skeletal muscle (left of tumour).

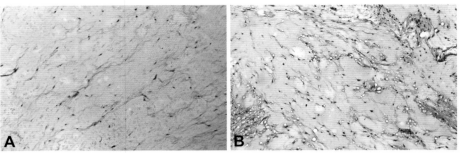

Fig. 12.06 Intramuscular myxoma **A** The tumour is hypocellular, hypovascular and contains abundant extracellular mxoid matrix. **B** In this example, the extracellular matrix shows a prominent frothy appearance, mimicking lipoblasts.

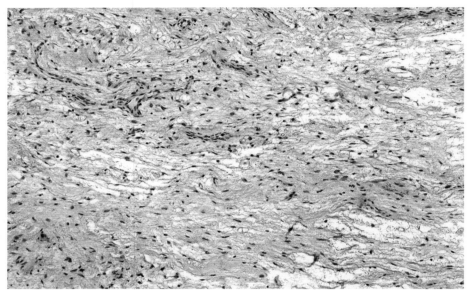

Fig. 12.07 Cellular intramuscular myxoma. The cells within the cellular areas are bland and have no cytological atypia, mitoses or pleomorphism.

Histopathology

Classic intramuscular myxoma is composed of uniform, cytologically bland spindle- and stellate-shaped cells with tapering eosinophilic cytoplasm and small nuclei {750,1884}. The cells are separated by abundant extracellular myxoid stroma containing very sparse capillary-sized blood vessels. This matrix is composed of glycosaminoglycans, comparable to low-grade myxofibrosarcoma {2967}. The stroma may be vacuolated and may show cystic change. Sections from the interface of the tumour and the surrounding skeletal muscle frequently show infiltration between muscle fibres or around individual skeletal muscle cells, which may be atrophic. Areas of increased cellularity are present in many intramuscular myxomas and they can occupy 10–90% of the tumour {2040,2848}. Increased number of cells, more numerous collagen fibres and blood vessels characterize these areas and, if this pattern predominates, then the term "cellular myxoma" may be used {2848}. Mitoses, pleomorphism, hyperchromasia or necrosis are not present even in the most cellular areas {2040,2848}. The vessels in these hypercellular regions are capillary-sized, but occasional thick-walled vessels with smooth muscle in their walls are also present.

Immunophenotype

Immunohistochemically, the cells show variable staining for CD34, desmin and actin. Staining for S100 protein is negative.

Ultrastructure

The tumour cells have the features of fibroblasts or myofibroblasts with prominent secretory activity. The cells contain well-developed dilated rough endoplasmic reticulum, Golgi complexes, free ribosomes, pinocytotic vesicles and occasional filaments. Also seen are more primitive-appearing mesenchymal cells and histiocyte-like cells. Intracytoplasmic lipid droplets can be seen {1128}.

Genetics

No consistent aberrations have been detected among five cases with karyotypic data {1915}. Point mutations of the *GNAS* gene are common in intramuscular myxomas {630,2114}. Mutations in codon 211 (Arg to His, and Arg to Cys) were detected in five of six intramuscular myxomas with and without fibrous dysplasia of bone {2114}. *GNAS* encodes the α-subunit of the guanine nucleotide binding protein, i.e. the G-protein that stimulates the formation of cAMP. *GNAS* mutations are absent in low-grade myxofibrosarcoma, which can be useful in the differential diagnosis with cellular myxoma {2114}.

Prognostic factors

Conventional intramuscular myxoma is a non-recurrent tumour. The cellular variant has a small risk of local non-destructive recurrence {2848}.

Juxta-articular myxoma

G.P. Nielsen
P.C.W. Hogendoorn

Definition
Juxta-articular myxoma is a rare, benign soft tissue tumour that usually arises in the vicinity of a large joint (particularly the knee), and has histological features resembling a cellular myxoma. These lesions are frequently associated with ganglion-like cystic changes, raising the possibility of a reactive/degenerative pathogenesis.

ICD-O code   8840/0

Synonyms
Parameniscal cyst; periarticular myxoma

Epidemiology
In the largest series, the patients ranged in age from 16 to 83 years (median, 43 years) {1813}; a tumour arising in a girl aged 9 years has also been reported {563}.

Sites of involvement
Most lesions (88%) occur in the vicinity of the knee joint. Other locations include the elbow, shoulder, ankle and hip.

Clinical features
The patients present with a swelling or a mass that can be painful or tender. The duration of symptoms ranges from weeks to years. Radiographic studies show a soft tissue mass that has imaging characteristics similar to those of intramuscular myxoma {1425}.

Macroscopy
The tumour is slimy and gelatinous, frequently with cystic areas. The tumours range in size from 0.6 to 12 cm (mean, 3.8 cm; median, 3.5 cm).

Histopathology
Histologically, this tumour is reminiscent of the cellular form of intramuscular myxoma and is composed of bland-appearing spindle cells embedded in a hypovascular myxoid stroma. Although areas of increased cellularity are often present, mitotic figures are absent or very rare. Cystic, ganglion-like spaces, are seen in 89% of cases. These cystic spaces are lined by a layer of delicate fibrin or thicker layer of collagen. The periphery of the tumour is ill defined and infiltrates adjacent tissues. Areas of haemorrhage, haemosiderin deposition, chronic inflammation, organizing fibrin and fibroblastic reaction may be seen, especially in recurrent tumours.

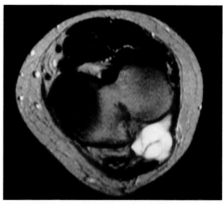

Fig. 12.08 Juxta-articular myxoma. MRI of a tumour located adjacent to the knee joint, showing a homogeneous bright signal, similar to intramuscular myxoma.

Genetics
Clonal chromosomal abnormalities have been reported in a single case of juxta-articular myxoma {2493}. Juxta-articular myxomas lack mutations of the *GNAS* gene, in contrast to intramuscular myxomas {2113}.

Prognostic factors
In the series reported by Meis & Enzinger {1813} 10 of 29 (34%) tumours recurred locally, sometimes more than once.

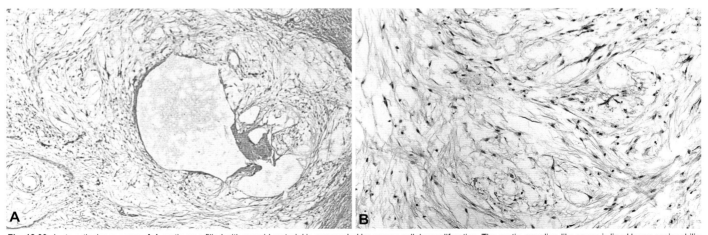

Fig. 12.09 Juxta-articular myxoma **A** A cystic area filled with myxoid material is surrounded by a more cellular proliferation. The cystic, ganglion-like space is lined by an eosinophilic layer of fibrin. **B** Note the bland appearance of the spindle cells.

Deep ("aggressive") angiomyxoma

J.F. Fetsch
J.A. Bridge

Definition

Deep ("aggressive") angiomyxoma (AAM) is a benign mesenchymal neoplasm that arises in deep soft tissue of the pelvicoperineal region. The tumour has abundant myxoedematous matrix and a dominant population of stellate and spindle cells, that often exhibit some myoid differentiation.

ICD-O code   8841/0

Epidemiology

AAM usually affects adult females in the third to seventh decades of life, with a peak in the fourth to fifth decades {421, 832,1027}. Women aged 60 years and older can occasionally be affected. AAM does not occur before puberty. While there are rare legitimate examples of AAM in men {1278,2791}, many tumours that have been classified as such are actually other types of mesenchymal neoplasm.

Sites of involvement

This tumour affects pelvicoperineal, inguino-scrotal and retroperitoneal sites.

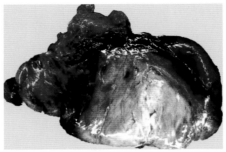

Fig. 12.10 A gross specimen of deep ("aggressive") angiomyxoma. Note the lobular contour of the tumour, adherence to regional structures, and glistening, off-white, cut surface.

Clinical features

Patients often present with a slow-growing mass in the pelvicoperineal region that is either asymptomatic, or associated with vague discomfort, a pressure-like sensation, dull pain or dyspareunia {832}. On physical examination, tumour size may be significantly underestimated, because the bulk of the process is concealed within deep soft tissues {832}. When the true size becomes apparent through imaging, more than half of the lesions are ≥ 10 cm {832}. CT imaging reveals a soft tissue mass that tends to grow around pelvic floor structures without causing significant disruption of the vaginal or rectal musculature {447,2142}.

Macroscopy

Resected tumours are commonly > 10 cm and sometimes > 20 cm in size {832, 2643}. Small tumours of < 5 cm in size are less frequent. The neoplasms often have a lobular contour, but there is adherence to fat, muscle and other regional surfaces. The cut surface is usually glistening or myxoid with a pinkish-tan colour. Haemorrhagic foci and areas with cystic change may be present.

Histopathology

AAMs generally show low to moderate cellularity, with small, stellate and spindled cells embedded in loosely collagenous, myxoedematous matrix containing scattered vessels of varying calibre. The dominant neoplastic element has relatively scant eosinophilic cytoplasm. There is no significant atypia or pleomorphism. While multinucleation can be seen, it is uncommon. Mitotic figures are infrequent. A common additional feature is the presence of scattered larger spindled cells with well-developed myoid (myofibroblastic vs true smooth muscle) features, randomly distributed in small numbers within the tumour or more characteristically zonated around entrapped nerves and vessels {832,1027,2576}. These cells are immunohistochemically distinct from the vascular smooth muscle they often encircle {832}. Aggressive angiomyxomas are typically only weakly positive for mucosubstances, and oedema fluid is a major component of the extracellular matrix {832}.

Immunophenotype

Neoplastic cells often show moderate to diffuse nuclear immunoreactivity for estrogen and progesterone receptor proteins, {231,832,848,1783} and variable reactivity for desmin and actins {832, 1027}. CD34 expression, if present, is only focal. The larger well-developed

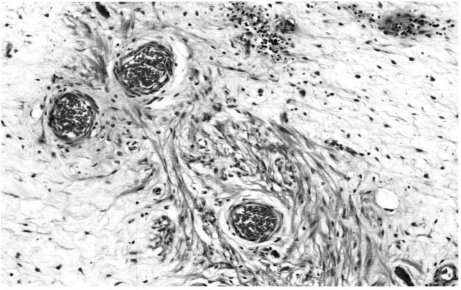

Fig. 12.11 Deep ("aggressive") angiomyxoma. Spindled, well-developed, myoid cells often aggregate around larger nerves and vessels.

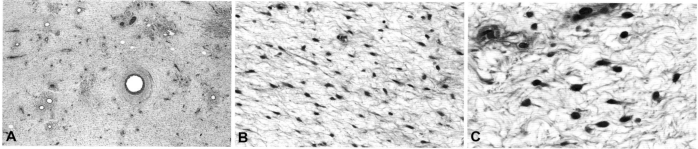

Fig. 12.12 Deep ("aggressive") angiomyxoma. Low- (**A**), intermediate- (**B**) and high-power (**C**) views. Note the uniform, low to moderate cellularity, loose myxoedematous matrix and small, stellate-shaped and spindled neoplastic cells with only mild atypia.

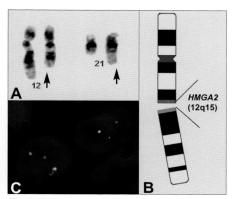

Fig. 12.13 Rearrangements of 12q15, the region in which the *HMGA2* gene is located, are recurrent in deep ("aggressive") angiomyxoma. **A** Partial G-banded karyotype exhibiting a t(12;21)(q15;q21.1). **B, C** Dual-colour FISH with a probe-set flanking *HMGA2* demonstrates the presence of a rearrangement of this locus in tumour interphase nuclei (split red and green signals).

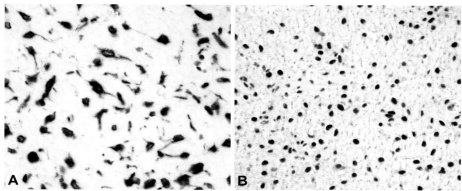

Fig. 12.14 Deep ("aggressive") angiomyxoma. **A** Immunoreactivity for desmin in tumour cells. **B** Immunoreactivity for estrogen receptor protein in tumour cells.

myoid cells that are a focal finding have stronger, more uniform expression of actin and desmin than most lesional cells {832}. Many tumours exhibit aberrant nuclear expression of HMGA2 (HMGIC) protein {231,699,1780,2076}.

Genetics

Karyotypic aberrations involving chromosome region 12q13–15 predominate in the small number of aggressive angiomyxomas that have been characterized {2308,2796}. Rearrangements of the *HMGA2* locus (12q14.3) have correspondingly been demonstrated by interphase FISH with associated *HMGA2* transcriptional upregulation confirmed by RT-PCR in some studies (approximately 35% of tumours analysed) {1806,2308}. Molecular mechanisms for *HGMA2* involvement include either generation of a fusion transcript or expression of the entire gene achieved through alterations affecting the telomeric (3') untranslated region {1390, 1865,2078}.

Prognostic factors

Local recurrence occurs in > 35% of cases {421,832,1027,2643}. More than one recurrence is very uncommon. Complete excision is the preferred management if this can be accomplished without undue morbidity. When the risk of morbidity is high or there is a desire to preserve fertility, lesser intervention is acceptable {421}. Local recurrences may be late in onset {421,832}.

There are several reports documenting a dramatic response to hormonal therapy (gonadotropin-releasing hormone [GnRH] agonist]) {848,1782,2541}.

Pleomorphic hyalinizing angiectatic tumour of soft parts

S.W. Weiss
A.P. Dei Tos

Definition

Pleomorphic hyalinizing angiectatic tumour of soft parts (PHAT) is a rare, locally aggressive tumour consisting of spindled and pleomorphic cells, clusters of ectatic, fibrin-lined vessels, and inflammatory cells.

ICD-O code   8802/1

Sites of involvement

PHATs typically develop in the subcutis of the lower extremity, particularly the ankle and foot, and rarely in deep soft tissue {893,2587}.

Clinical features

PHAT occurs equally in adult men and women {893,2587}. Tumours are slowly growing masses, often of long duration, which are occasionally mistaken for haematoma.

Macroscopy

Tumours are poorly circumscribed, tan to maroon masses.

Histopathology

PHAT is composed of thin-walled ectatic vessels embedded in a spindled stroma. The vessels are lined by fibrin, which leaks into the stroma creating large areas of hyalinization. The cells are spindled to pleomorphic and contain intranuclear inclusions and fine haemosiderin granules. Mitotic activity is low to absent. A variable

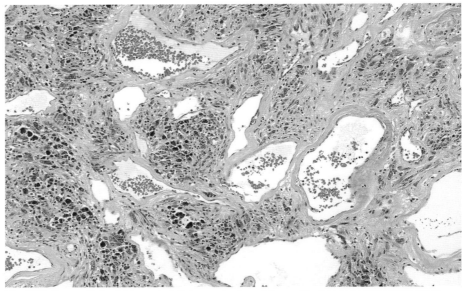

Fig. 12.15 Pleomorphic hyalinizing angiectatic tumour showing ectatic vessels set against a hypocellular stroma.

inflammatory infiltrate, usually mast cells, is present. Many PHATs have a peripheral zone of bland spindled cells, termed "early PHAT," that represents the precursor for classic PHATs. Early PHATs may have features that overlap with haemosiderotic fibrolipomatous tumour (HFLT) {893}.

Immunophenotype

The tumours express CD34 and lack S100 protein.

Genetics

The translocations t(1;3)(p31;q12) and t(1;10)(p31;q25) have been described in one case of PHAT {2917}, but have not been reported by other authors {87}.

Prognostic factors

Between 30% and 50% of PHATs recur locally, but recurrences can usually be controlled by re-excision. Rarely, PHATs recur as a bona fide myxoid pleomorphic sarcoma {893}. Due to limited data, the long-term prognosis is not well-defined.

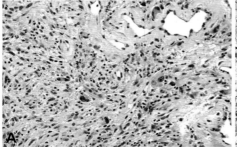
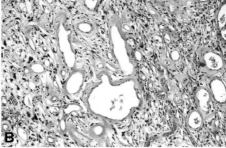
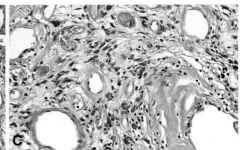

Fig. 12.16 Pleomorphic hyalinizing angiectatic tumour (PHAT). **A** PHAT showing atypia of stromal cells. **B** Perivascular hyalinization in a PHAT. **C** Hyalinizing vessels within PHAT.

Ectopic hamartomatous thymoma

J.K.C. Chan

Definition
Ectopic hamartomatous thymoma is a benign tumour of the lower neck showing an admixture of spindle cells, epithelial islands and adipose cells suggesting branchial origin. Despite use of the term "thymoma" in the nomenclature, this tumour shows no evidence of thymic origin or differentiation.

ICD-O code   8587/0

Synonym
Branchial anlage mixed tumour {105}

Sites of involvement
The tumour occurs exclusively in the superficial or deep soft tissues of the supraclavicular, suprasternal or presternal region {105,419,776,833,844,1161,1873, 2366,2404,3064}. An exceptional case has been reported in the posterior axillary region {1388}.

Clinical features
The tumour affects adults with a median age of 42.5 years and shows a markedly higher incidence in males (male to female ratio, > 10 : 1) {420,833,1161,3064}. Patients present with a long-standing mass lesion.

Macroscopy
This well-circumscribed tumour usually measures a few centimetres in diameter, but some tumours can be much larger (up to 19 cm). It shows grey-white to yellowish solid cut surfaces which may be punctuated by small cysts.

Histopathology
The tumour shows haphazard blending of spindle cells, epithelial islands and adipocytes, which are present in highly variable proportions. Plump spindle cells exhibit fascicular or lattice-like growth, and possess bland-looking elongated nuclei with pointed ends and light-staining cytoplasm; some cells can have a myoid appearance due to the presence of eosinophilic cytoplasm. Delicate spindle cells found between the fascicles have

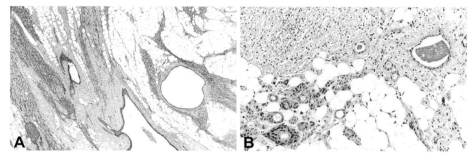

Fig. 12.17 Ectopic hamartomatous thymoma. **A** Haphazard blending of spindle cells, epithelial islands and adipose cells. Some cysts are also seen. **B** The epithelium sometimes takes the form of glandular structures. Note the presence of intermingled adipose cells.

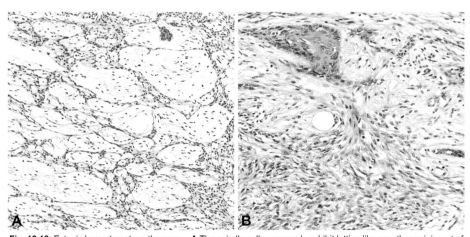

Fig. 12.18 Ectopic hamartomatous thymoma. **A** The spindle cells commonly exhibit lattice-like growth, reminiscent of atrophic thymus. **B** Characteristically elongated strands of epithelium merge into spindle cells. The epithelium commonly shows squamous differentiation.

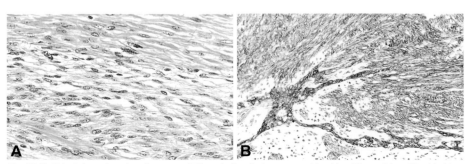

Fig. 12.19 Ectopic hamartomatous thymoma. **A** The spindle cells form compact fascicles. The nuclei are bland-looking, often with pointed ends. Some cells have deeply eosinophilic cytoplasm, suggestive of a myoid phenotype. **B** Immunostaining for keratin highlights the epithelial strands and the spindle cells. The immunonegative smaller stromal cells in between are strongly positive for CD34 (not shown).

smaller nuclei and scanty cytoplasm. The epithelial component takes the form of squamous islands, syringoma-like tubules, anastomosing networks, simple glandular structures and epithelium-lined cysts. The epithelial islands are surrounded by a fibrous sheath or merge imperceptibly into the plump spindle cells.

Immunophenotype

Both the epithelial and plump spindle cell components stain diffusely and strongly for keratin, particularly high-molecular-weight keratin, indicating that the spindle cells are epithelial in nature. The plump spindle cells are often immunoreactive for actin, but not desmin {105,833,1873, 2404,3064}. The delicate spindle cells are usually positive for CD34 but negative for keratin.

Prognostic factors

This benign lesion rarely recurs after complete excision {833}. In the rare examples reported to show malignant change, there has not been recurrence or metastasis {1873}. Such cases focally feature closely packed glands lined by highly atypical cells, but there is no frank invasion beyond the parent tumour.

Atypical fibroxanthoma

J.E. Calonje
T. Brenn
P. Komminoth

Definition

Atypical fibroxanthoma is a benign, dermal-based tumour of uncertain lineage, presenting on sun-damaged skin of the elderly. Despite histological features more typically associated with malignancy, the outcome is favourable with only rare local recurrence. Definitive diagnosis requires complete excision.

ICD-O code   8833/0

Synonyms

Use of the term "superficial malignant fibrous histiocytoma" should be discouraged as it may suggest an aggressive disease course and result in overtreatment.

Epidemiology

Atypical fibroxanthoma is a tumour of the elderly, presenting mainly in the seventh and eighth decades of life {177,1680}. Incidence is much higher in men than women, and Caucasians are almost exclusively affected {177}. Incidence is highest in geographical areas of high annual UV irradiation. Patients with xeroderma pigmentosum are at risk of developing tumours at a young age, including childhood, although this is very rare.

Etiology

There is a close link with exposure to UV irradiation, and UV-signature mutation

can be demonstrated in the *TP53* gene {625,1680,2416}. Presentation in the setting of radiotherapy has been demonstrated and immunosuppression may play an additional pathogenetic role.

Sites of involvement

Presentation is on actinically-damaged skin, commonly the head and neck area, in particular the scalp {1680}. The upper extremities are rarely affected.

Clinical features

Atypical fibroxanthoma presents as a solitary, nodular or polypoid tumour measuring < 2 cm in diameter. A history of short duration and rapid growth is characteristic. The tumours are pink/red or flesh-coloured and ulceration and bleeding is common. Bluish-brown hyperpigmentation due to intratumoral haemorrhage is rare {661}.

Macroscopy

The tumours are well-demarcated with nodular or polypoid outlines. Ulceration is common.

Histopathology

Atypical fibroxanthoma is a dermal-based tumour with a nodular or polypoid configuration. Solar elastosis of the adjacent dermis is typically present and may be marked. The tumours are exophytic and

often ulcerated. Collarette formation of the lateral epidermis is frequently present. The growth pattern is pushing rather than infiltrative, and tumours are largely confined to the dermis with only focal pushing extension into superficial subcutis, typically along pre-existing fibrous septa. The cellular component is arranged in sheets and fascicles of epithelioid cells, spindle cells and multinucleated forms in varying

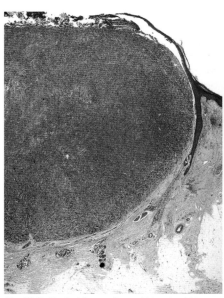

Fig. 12.20 Atypical fibroxanthoma. This polypoid tumour is confined to the dermis and shows epidermal ulceration and collarette formation.

proportions often admixed with lipidized cells and a chronic inflammatory infiltrate. Nuclear pleomorphism is marked, including bizarre cells with hyperchromatic or vesicular chromatin patterns and large and often multiple nucleoli. There is brisk and atypical mitotic activity. A wide morphological spectrum is recognized {177, 1680}. The spindle-cell variant is characterized by atypical but monomorphic spindle cells organized in long, intersecting fascicles {362}. Intratumoral haemorrhage and haemosiderin deposition may be marked, leading to an erroneous impression of angiosarcoma (pseudoangiomatous/haemorrhagic variant). Rare findings include clear or granular cell change, admixed osteoclast-like giant cells, stromal keloidal or myxoid change and a focally storiform growth pattern {528,2345,2390, 2767}. Osteoid and chondroid formation is exceptional {436,2974}. A plaque-like growth pattern within superficial dermis and intratumoral regression have also been recorded {2644}. Most importantly, tumour necrosis, invasion into deep subcutis, underlying skeletal muscle or fascia, lymphovascular invasion and perineurial infiltration are absent and are not compatible with a diagnosis of atypical fibroxanthoma.

Immunophenotype

Atypical fibroxanthoma is largely a diagnosis of exclusion and no positive diagnostic immunohistocemical marker exists. The diagnosis requires extensive immunohistochemical work-up, in particular to exclude melanoma, poorly differentiated carcinoma, angiosarcoma and leiomyosarcoma. By definition, tumour cells lack expression of S100, keratin, CD34, desmin and h-caldesmon; however, careful interpretation is necessary to avoid diagnostic pitfalls. The presence of intratumoral S100-positive dendritic cells may be cause for concern. Nonspecific expression of Melan-A/Mart-1 or HMB45 may rarely be detected, particularly in the multinucleate tumour giant cells {2590, 2754}. Antibodies against high-molecular-weight keratins are particularly useful in the exclusion of squamous cell carcinoma, and multiple different keratin antibodies should be used. Focal staining for EMA and rare expression of p63 has been observed in atypical fibroxanthoma. Although this appears to have no discriminatory value on its own, it raises a

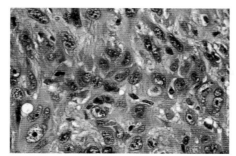

Fig. 12.21 Atypical fibroxanthoma. The cellular component comprises pleomorphic epithelioid cells.

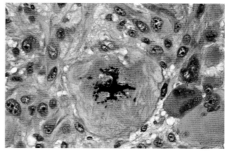

Fig. 12.22 Atypical fibroxanthoma. Mitotic activity is brisk and includes atypical forms.

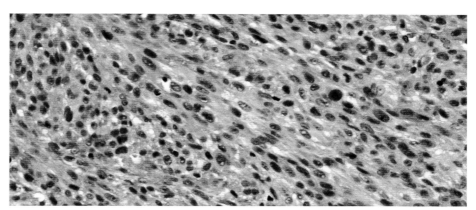

Fig. 12.23 Atypical fibroxanthoma. Spindle cell atypical fibroxanthoma is characterized by atypical but monomorphous spindle cells arranged in intersecting fascicles.

possible relationship of these tumours with poorly differentiated and spindle cell squamous cell carcinoma {988,1367, 1680}. Expression of SMA and calponin is a frequent finding, especially in the spindle cell variant {1652}, but staining for desmin and caldesmon is negative. Nonspecific, granular expression of CD31 may occasionally be seen in atypical fibroxanthomas, with potential for overdiagnosis as cutaneous angiosarcoma {1680}. CD34 and ERG expression is however negative. Identification of better differentiated areas with vasoformative elements is a further clue to the diagnosis of angiosarcoma. Since nonspecific and nondiscriminatory positive staining is often observed for CD10, CD99 and CD68 {599, 1367,2960}, use of these antibodies should be discouraged.

Genetics

Various approaches, e.g. analyses of DNA index and apoptotic regulators and proliferation assays, have failed to elucidate distinct pathogenetic pathways {734,1166,1875,2135,2287,2944,2992}. Only a few chromosomal or mutational

analyses of atypical fibroxanthoma have been reported {625,1900,2414,2416,2417}. CGH analysis identified copy-number changes in 20 of 24 cases with, on average, fewer aberrations per case than in undifferentiated pleomorphic sarcomas; amplification was seen in one case only {1900}. The most common imbalances were deletions of 9p (58%) and 13q (58%).

Prognostic factors

The behaviour of atypical fibroxanthoma is benign in the vast majority of cases, provided that strict diagnostic criteria are applied. Tumours show rare local recurrence, but distant metastasis is exceptional {578}. Tumours with documented metastasis frequently include those reported before the advent of immunohistochemistry. Furthermore, metastatic potential is observed in tumours showing necrosis, invasion into deep subcutis and beyond, as well as lymphovascular invasion and perineurial infiltration {578}. These features are not compatible with a diagnosis of atypical fibroxanthoma in a strict sense and these tumours should be regarded as pleomorphic dermal sarcoma.

Angiomatoid fibrous histiocytoma

C.R. Antonescu
S. Rossi

Definition

Angiomatoid fibrous histiocytoma (AFH) is a rarely metastasizing subcutaneous lesion with distinctive morphological features, having varying proportions of spindled or histiocytoid cells, arranged in a nodular pattern, pseudovascular spaces and prominent lymphoplasmacytic rim. Most of these tumours exhibit an *EWSR1-CREB1* fusion gene.

ICD-O code   8836/1

Synonym

Angiomatoid malignant fibrous histiocytoma

Epidemiology

There is equal sex distribution with a peak incidence in the first two decades of life, although rare cases have been described from birth {103} to age 79 years {76}.

Sites of involvement

Limbs are the most common sites for AFH, followed closely by trunk and head and neck. About two thirds of cases occur in areas where lymph nodes are normally found, e.g. antecubital fossa, popliteal fossa, axilla, inguinal area and neck.

Clinical features

Patients typically present with a painless superficial soft tissue lump, sometimes resembling a haematoma. Occasionally, systemic symptoms, such as severe anaemia and weight loss, have been described and may precede detection of the mass {514,751}.

Macroscopy

Median tumour size is 2.0 cm, with a wide range of 0.7–12 cm {514,751}. It is typically well circumscribed and firm, grossly simulating a lymph node. On cut surface, the lesion shows a multilocular haemorrhagic appearance, simulating a haematoma or intranodal haemorrhage.

Histopathology

There are four key morphological features that can be found in varying proportions: (i) nodules of either spindle or more histiocytoid cells, with a distinctive syncytial growth; (ii) pseudoangiomatous spaces filled with blood and surrounded by tumour cells; (iii) thick fibrous pseudocapsule with prominent haemosiderin deposition; and (iv) pericapsular cuffing of lymphoplasmacytic cells with occasional germinal centres, mimicking a lymph-node metastasis.

A subset of AFH has a predominantly small blue-cell phenotype, which can be confused with high-grade undifferentiated

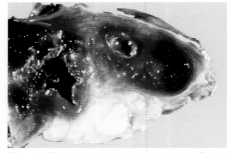

Fig. 12.24 Macroscopically, angiomatoid fibrous histiocytoma resembles haematoma or haemorrhage within a lymph node.

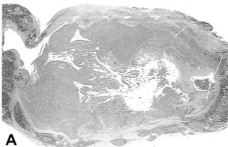
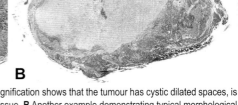

A   B

Fig. 12.25 Angiomatoid fibrous histiocytoma. **A** Low magnification shows that the tumour has cystic dilated spaces, is partially filled with blood and is surrounded by lymphoid tissue. **B** Another example demonstrating typical morphological features: fibrohistiocytic and lymphoid proliferation, angiomatoid blood-filled cystic spaces, and pseudocapsule, all simulating a tumour within a lymph node.

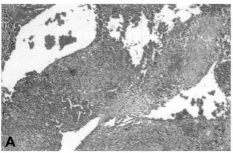
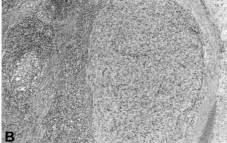
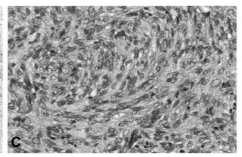

A   B   C

Fig. 12.26 Distinctive histopathological features of angiomatoid fibrous histiocytoma (AFH). **A** Pseudoangiectatic cystic spaces, filled with blood and lined by tumour cells. **B** Lymphocytic cuffing with occasional germinal centres mimicking a true lymph node. **C** AFH with spindle-cell morphology, bland nuclei with open chromatin and arranged in a syncytial growth pattern.

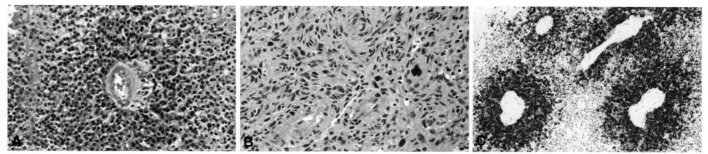

Fig. 12.27 Distinctive histopathological features and immunoprofile of angiomatoid fibrous histiocytoma (AFH). **A** AFH with predominantly small-cell morphology. **B** Rare cases may show nuclear pleomorphism and hyperchromasia. **C** Desmin immunoreactivity.

sarcomas. The small cell component is typically composed of dark, hyperchromatic nuclei, with scant eosinophilic cytoplasm, which can be misdiagnosed as Ewing sarcoma on the basis of various findings, including *EWSR1* rearrangement, CD99 immunoreactivity and the undifferentiated/small cell morphology. The predominantly spindle cell subtype typically shows uniform cytomorphology with eosinophilic or clear cytoplasm, vesicular nuclei and low proliferation activity. More pleomorphic examples with brisk mitotic activity have been described without prognostic implications.

Immunophenotype

Staining for desmin and EMA, as well as CD68 and CD99, is positive in about 50% of AFH cases {813,1123}. Tumours are consistently negative for S100 protein, CD21, CD35, CD34 and keratins.

Genetics

The most common genetic abnormality is a t(2;22) translocation, resulting in *EWSR1-CREB1* fusion in > 90% of cases {76,2376}. Rare cases instead show *FUS-ATF1* {2285, 2909} or *EWSR1-ATF1* {1082,1083,2600}. The transcript structure is consistently composed of exon 7 of *EWSR1* fused to exon 7 of *CREB1*. The predicted protein structure of EWSR1-CREB1 parallels closely that of EWSR1-ATF1 {81}. No obvious correlations between fusion transcript type and clinicopathological findings are noted. Identical fusions involving *ATF1* and *CREB1* are found in both AFH and clear cell sarcoma {81,84,2159}.

Prognostic factors

AFH has overall indolent behaviour with 2–10% local recurrence and < 1% metastasis, usually to the locoregional lymph nodes {813}. Rare deaths attributable to late distant metastases have been reported {514,751,1760,2234}. There are no known clinical or morphological factors that correlate with outcome or predict metastasis.

Ossifying fibromyxoid tumour

M.M. Miettinen
H. Kawashima
S.W. Weiss

Definition
Ossifying fibromyxoid tumour (OFMT) is a rare, usually S100 protein-positive, mesenchymal neoplasm of uncertain lineage, with cords and trabeculae of ovoid cells embedded in a fibromyxoid matrix, often surrounded by a peripheral partial shell of lamellar bone.

ICD-O code
Ossifying fibromyxoid tumour   8842/0
Ossifying fibromyxoid tumour,
  malignant   8842/3

Epidemiology
Lesions occur in adults of all ages, with a median age around 50 years. Considering the long duration before diagnosis (up to 20 years), most patients probably develop tumours when aged < 40 years. This tumour is more common in males (sex ratio, 1.5 : 1).

Sites of involvement
The most common sites are the thigh, head and neck collectively, and the trunk wall; > 40% of cases occur in the lower extremity {757,1882,1965,2752}.

Clinical features
Most patients present with a painless, subcutaneous mass. Radiological studies characteristically, but not invariably, reveal a well-circumscribed, lobulated mass, surrounded by an incomplete ring of calcification {757,2452}. Erosion of underlying bone and periosteal reaction has also been noted in some cases {757,2452}.

Macroscopy
Most lesions range from 3 to 5 cm in greatest dimension, with a median size of about 4 cm. Occasional examples are large, measuring up to 17 cm or more {757}. OFMTs are well circumscribed, nodular or multinodular, and typically covered by a thick fibrous pseudocapsule with or without a shell of bone. On cut section, they are white to tan in colour, and either firm, hard, or rubbery in texture.

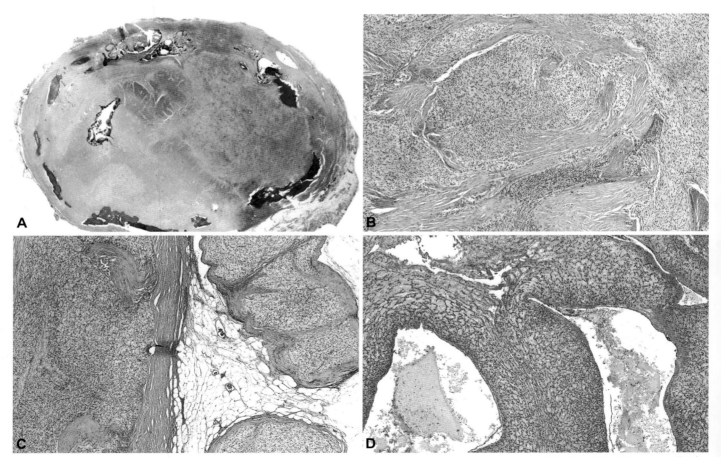

Fig. 12.28 Ossifying fibromyxoid tumour. **A** Low magnification reveals a partial rim of metaplastic bone. **B** Multinodular pattern. **C** Satellite nodules in the surrounding fat. **D** Trabecular architecture with focal cystic change.

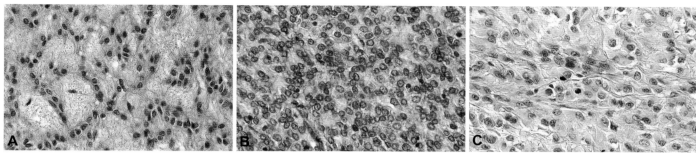

Fig. 12.29 Ossifying fibromyxoid tumour. **A**, **B** and **C** show the characteristic architectural and cytological features of ossifying fibromyxoid tumour. Note the varying trabecular and solid patterns, delicate nucleoli and mitotic figures.

Histopathology

OFMT forms a circumscribed mass that in most cases contains an incomplete peripheral zone of metaplastic bone, often lamellar in quality. Extracapsular satellite nodules may occur in the surrounding fat. The tumour is composed of lobules of uniform, round to spindle-shaped cells often arranged in cords or trabeculae, surrounded by variably fibromyxoid stroma. Focal cystic change and curvilinear small-calibre vessels are variably present {757,1876,1882,2476,2971}. The neoplastic cells are monomorphous with round to ovoid nuclei and delicate nucleoli and a scant amount of pale eosinophilic cytoplasm. Mitotic activity is usually < 1 per 10 HPF, but atypical variants with a higher mitotic count exist. The stroma is quite variable and can be predominantly myxoid (positive with Alcian blue, hyaluronidase-sensitive) or collagenous/hyalinized with a prominent vasculature that can exhibit perivascular hyalinization. Calcifications and/or nodules of metaplastic cartilage are occasionally identified. Malignant variants have been defined by some as those of high nuclear grade or high cellularity and > 2 mitoses per 50 HPFs {892}.

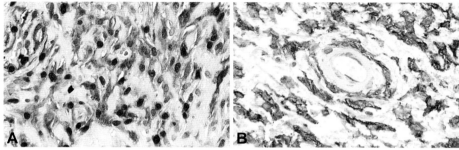

Fig. 12.30 Ossifying fibromyxoid tumour. **A** These tumours typically show both nuclear and cytoplasmic immunopositivity for S100 protein . **B** CD10 immunoreactivity.

Immunophenotype

OFMT is typically positive for S100 protein (> 90% of cases) and desmin (40–50%). The lesions may also express GFAP, keratins, and SMA {757,853,1409,1876, 1882, 2476,2971,3024}.

Genetics

Cytogenic and FISH analyses have shown recurrent rearrangement of the *PHF1* locus at chromosome band 6p21 {956A,1386, 2062,2615}. Involvement of *PHF1* was found in most OFMTs classified as typical or atypical, but only rarely in malignant lesions; the latter instead frequently show loss of chromosome 22 {956A,1024,2062}.

Prognostic factors

Follow-up data indicate that typical OFMT has the potential for recurrence. This is often delayed and occurs 10–20 years or more after the primary excision. A mitotic rate of > 2 per 50 HPFs appears to increase the risk of local recurrence, while satellite nodules and positive margin only weakly correlate with recurrence. There are limited data that phenotypically and immunophenotypically characteristic (S100-positive) examples metastasize. However, some morphologically malignant lesions have metastasized into distant soft tissues and lungs {892}.

Myoepithelioma/myoepithelial carcinoma/mixed tumour

C.D.M. Fletcher
C.R. Antonescu
S. Heim
J.L. Hornick

Definition
Myoepithelial tumours of soft tissue are morphologically and immunophenotypically similar to their counterparts in salivary gland. Myoepithelioma is composed exclusively (or predominantly) of myoepithelial cells. Mixed tumours also show ductal differentiation. Malignant myoepithelial neoplasms are designated myoepithelial carcinomas.

ICD-O code
Myoepithelioma   8982/0
Myoepithelial carcinoma   8982/3
Mixed tumour, not otherwise specified
                              8940/0
Mixed tumour, not otherwise specified,
  malignant   8940/3

Synonyms
Ectomesenchymal chondromyxoid tumour; parachordoma

Epidemiology
Myoepithelial tumours of soft tissue are uncommon {86,989,1216,1409,1871}. They show equal distribution between the sexes and a wide age range, with a peak in young to middle-aged adults (median, 40 years) {1216,1871}. About 20% of tumours affect children; myoepithelial carcinomas predominate in the paediatric population {989}.

Sites of involvement
Most myoepithelial tumours of soft tissue (75%) arise on the limbs and limb girdles (lower > upper); trunk, head and neck are less often affected {86,989,1216}. Rarely, tumours arise in bone or visceral organs {86}.

Clinical features
Most patients present with a palpable mass, usually painless {989,1216,1409}. Subcutaneous tissue is involved somewhat more often than deep soft tissue {1216,1871}. Myoepitheliomas may also arise primarily in the skin {1217,1510}.

Macroscopy
Most myoepithelial tumours of soft tissue are grossly well-circumscribed and nodular; a small subset of cases (mostly carcinomas) shows infiltrative margins. The cut surface ranges from gelatinous and glistening to firm or fleshy. These tumours show a broad size range (1–20 cm in greatest dimension), with a mean size of 4–6 cm {989,1216,1871}.

Histopathology
Myoepithelial tumours show a wide morphological spectrum, similar to their salivary-gland counterparts. Many show a predominantly reticular or trabecular growth pattern with prominent myxoid stroma; focal areas of more nested or solid growth and hyalinized stroma are commonly observed and occasionally predominate {86,989,1216}. Tumour cells range from epithelioid to spindled and typically contain uniform nuclei with eosinophilic to clear cytoplasm. Plasmacytoid cells with hyaline cytoplasmic inclusions may be prominent {830,1216}. Around 10–15% of tumours show osseous or cartilaginous differentiation; squamous or adipocytic metaplasia is more rare {1216}. About 10% of myoepitheliomas contain a minor ductal component, in which case the designation "mixed tumour" may be applied. Tumours with large epithelioid cells showing prominent cytoplasmic vacuolation have been labelled "parachordoma" in the past {538,880}. Myoepithelial carcinomas show similar histological features, in addition to the presence of nuclear atypia, often together with a high mitotic rate and tumour necrosis; some such tumours (especially in children) contain an undifferentiated round cell component {989,1216}.

Immunophenotype
More than 90% of these tumours express broad-spectrum keratins, S100 protein, and calponin {989,1216,1871}. EMA is positive in around two thirds of cases, and GFAP in half of cases {989,1216}. A subset

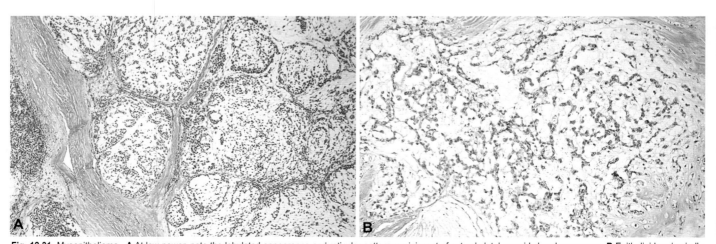

Fig. 12.31 Myoepithelioma. **A** At low power, note the lobulated appearance and reticular pattern reminiscent of extraskeletal myxoid chondrosarcoma. **B** Epithelioid and spindle cells arranged in trabeculae.

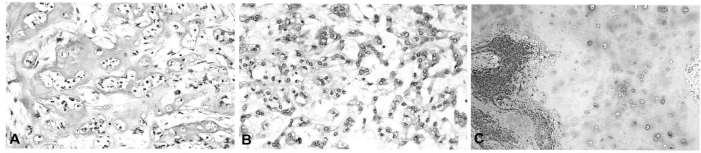

Fig. 12.32 Myoepithelioma. **A** Tumour cells often have clear cytoplasm. When copious and vacuolated, such lesions are sometimes labelled "parachordoma." **B** Ovoid or epithelioid cells with eosinophilic cytoplasm and uniform nuclei. **C** About 10% of cases show cartilaginous or osseous differentiation.

of tumours is positive for SMA and p63 {1216}. Desmin, CD34, and brachyury are consistently negative {989,1216}. Loss of expression of SMARCB1 (INI1) is observed in a subset of myoepithelial carcinomas {989,1215}.

Ultrastructure

Tumour cells often contain actin filaments and desmosome-like junctions and are surrounded by a usually discontinuous external lamina {243}.

Genetics

EWSR1 gene rearrangement is common in myoepithelial tumours arising outside salivary glands, irrespective of anatomical location. In a study of 66 myoepithelial tumours from various sites, *EWSR1* gene rearrangement was identified in 45% of cases, including half the soft tissue lesions tested. *EWSR1* was fused with either *POU5F1* on 6p21 or *PBX1* on 1q23 in 16% of cases each {86}. Most *EWSR1-POU5F*-positive tumours presented in

deep soft tissues of the extremities in young patients, and were composed of nests of epithelioid cells with clear cytoplasm, negative for OCT4 staining. A subset of *EWSR1-PBX1*-positive tumours showed a deceptively bland and sclerotic appearance {86,300}. Only rare cases were reported to harbour t(19;22)(q13;q12), resulting in *EWSR1-ZNF444* {301}, or *FUS* gene rearrangement. The myoepithelial tumours that were negative for *EWSR1* rearrangement were often benign and superficially located and showed ductal differentiation. *PLAG1* gene rearrangement has recently been identified in this subset of benign myoepithelial tumours displaying ductal structures (mixed tumours), which correlates with PLAG1 immunoexpression {138,1087}. These results suggest that soft tissue myoepithelial neoplasms with genuine salivary gland-like morphology are genetically related to their salivary-gland counterparts.

Prognostic factors

Most myoepithelial tumours of soft tissue behave in a benign fashion. The only reliable criterion for malignancy is the presence of moderate to severe nuclear atypia {1216}. Histologically benign tumours recur in 20% of cases and rarely metastasize, whereas myoepithelial carcinomas recur and metastasize in 40–50% of cases {989,1216}. The most common metastatic sites include lungs, lymph nodes, bone, and soft tissue {989,1216}.

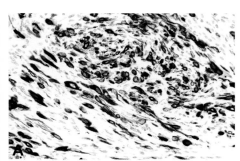
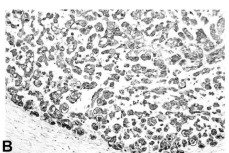

Fig. 12.33 Myoepithelioma. **A** This tumour shows strong immunopositivity for keratin AE1/AE3. **B** S100 protein immunopositivity is seen in the majority of cases.

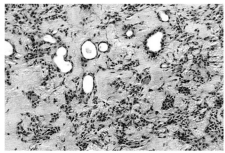
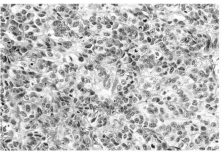

Fig. 12.34 Myoepithelioma/mixed tumour. Around 10% of soft tissue myoepitheliomas show ductal differentiation and are indistinguishable from mixed tumours in salivary gland.

Fig. 12.35 Myoepithelial carcinoma. Nuclear atypia and readily identified nucleoli are the best indicators of malignancy. Also note the frequent mitotic figures.

Haemosiderotic fibrolipomatous tumour

J.C. Fanburg-Smith
C.D.M. Fletcher
F. Mertens

Definition
Haemosiderotic fibrolipomatous tumour (HFLT) is an unencapsulated, locally aggressive neoplasm composed of adipocytes and haemosiderin-laden spindle cells, focally prominent haemosiderin-laden macrophages and scattered chronic inflammatory cells.

ICD-O code   8811/1

Synonym
Haemosiderotic fibrohistiocytic lipomatous lesion

Epidemiology
HFLT occurs most commonly during the fifth and sixth decades in females.

Sites of involvement
The predominant site of involvement is the dorsum of foot, followed by other ankle and foot sites, dorsum of hand, then calf, thigh, and cheek {332,1737,1950}.

Clinical features
HFLT generally presents as a slow-growing, sometimes painful, subcutaneous mass {332,1737,1950}.

Macroscopy
HFLT can reach large sizes, up to 19 cm, with an average of 7.7 cm {332,1737,1950} Grossly, HFLT is a yellow-brown/ dark yellow tumour with occasional haemorrhage.

Histopathology
HFLT consists of fascicles of fibroblastic spindle cells containing haemosiderin, admixed with adipocytes, haemosiderin-laden macrophages, and osteoclast-like giant cells {332,1737}. Occasional larger cells with atypical nuclei are seen in some cases. Mitoses and necrosis are generally absent. Nuclear pseudoinclusions, large ectatic partially-thrombosed vasculature with perivascular hyalinization, and myxoid change are not usual features of this tumour {332,1737}. Lesions may show hybrid features with myxoinflammatory fibroblastic sarcoma.

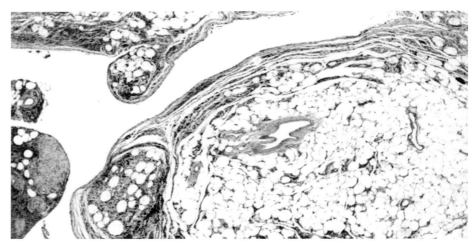

Fig. 12.36 Low-power view of haemosiderotic fibrolipomatous tumour demonstrates mostly adipose tissue with septal, periadipocytic and perilobular bland spindled cells and prominent haemosiderin.

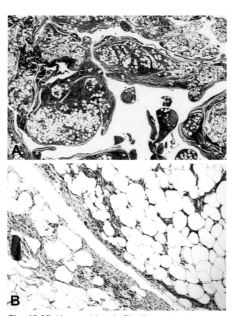

Fig. 12.37 Haemosiderotic fibrolipomatous tumour. **A** Perilobular, septal and periadipocytic spindled cells define this unencapsulated, adipocyte-rich tumour. **B** At higher magnification, the septal, bland spindled fibroblasts can be readily identified.

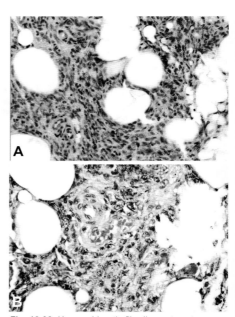

Fig. 12.38 Haemosiderotic fibrolipomatous tumour. **A** Bland spindled cells and haemosiderin pigment are present, largely in macrophages. **B** Other inflammatory cells including histiocytes and scattered mast cells are present.

Immunophenotype
The spindled component of HFLT is mostly positive for CD34 and calponin, and negative for S100 protein, h-caldesmon, desmin and keratins {332, 1737}.

Genetics
All three reported cases of HFLT with abnormal karyotypes shared a near-diploid chromosome number, a balanced or unbalanced t(1;10)(p22–31;q24–25), loss of

material from chromosome arm 3p, and amplification and overexpression of genes, including *VGLL3*, in 3p11–12 {87, 1084,2945}. The breakpoints in the t(1;10) map to *TGFBR3* in 1p22 and in or near *MGEA5* in 10q24 {1084}; the functional outcome of the translocation seems to be transcriptional upregulation of the *FGF8* gene, located close to *MGEA5* on chromosome 10 {1084}. By interphase FISH, 12 of 14 cases had an unbalanced der(10)t(1;10), and 5 of 5 cases showed amplification of *VGLL3* {87}. The same cytogenetic features have been reported in myxoinflammatory fibroblastic sarcoma (MIFS) and tumours showing hybrid HFLT/ MIFS features {87,736,1084}, as well as in a lesion showing mixed features of HFLT and pleomorphic hyalinizing angiectatic tumour {2917}.

Prognostic factors
The rate of local recurrence is 30–50%, especially if initially incompletely excised. After full excision, the local recurrence rate is diminished.

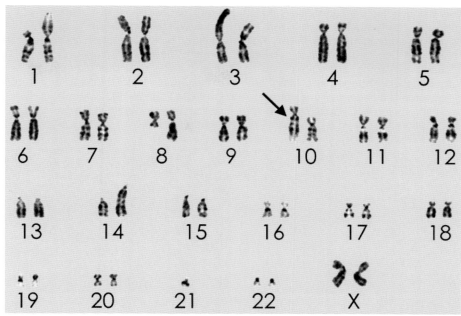

Fig. 12.39 Karyogram of a haemosiderotic fibrolipomatous tumour (HFLT) with the characteristic t(1;10)(p22;q24). The translocation is often, as in the present case, unbalanced, with loss of 10q. The derivative chromosome 10 is indicated by an arrow. The tumour also shows rearrangement of chromosome arm 3p, another frequent aberration in HFLT {1084}.

Phosphaturic mesenchymal tumour

A.L. Folpe

Definition
Phosphaturic mesenchymal tumours are morphologically distinctive neoplasms that produce tumour-induced osteomalacia (TIO) in most affected patients, usually through production of fibroblast growth factor 23 (FGF23).

ICD-O code
Phosphaturic mesenchymal tumour 8990/0
Phosphaturic mesenchymal tumour,
  malignant   8990/3

Synonym
Phosphaturic mesenchymal tumour, mixed connective tissue type

Epidemiology
Phosphaturic mesenchymal tumours are exceptionally rare, with fewer than 250 reported cases {140,245,595,884,1494,2919}. They occur most frequently in middle-aged adults {140,884}, although they have been reported in infants {1352} and the elderly.

Sites of involvement
Phosphaturic mesenchymal tumours may involve essentially any soft-tissue location {140,245,884,2919}. They are extremely rare in the retroperitoneum, viscera and mediastinum {2506,2797}.

Clinical features
Most tumours present as small, inapparent lesions that may require careful clinical examination and radionuclide scans for localization {946,2555}. A long history of osteomalacia is usually, but not always, present. Phosphaturic mesenchymal tumours appear to be responsible for the overwhelming majority of previously reported cases of mesenchymal tumour-associated TIO, although many such cases have been reported with other diagnoses {884}. Some tumours may be identified before osteomalacia becomes clinically evident {140}.

Macroscopy
Most phosphaturic mesenchymal tumours present as nonspecific soft tissue or bone masses, often with a component of fat. Some may be highly calcified.

Histopathology
These tumours are usually composed of

very bland, spindle to stellate cells, which produce an unusual hyalinized to "smudgy"-appearing matrix. A very well-developed capillary network is typically present, with some cases also showing larger vessels arranged in a "staghorn" pericytoma-like pattern, or in a pattern resembling cavernous haemangioma. The matrix of phosphaturic mesenchymal tumour typically calcifies in an unusual "grungy" or flocculent fashion, sometimes forming "flower-like" slate-grey crystals, and, in some instances, may contain foci closely resembling cartilage or osteoid {140,884,2528,2919}. Osteoclasts, fibro-histiocytic spindled cells, haemorrhage, mature adipose tissue and microcystic change may be present. Mitotic activity and necrosis are absent. Malignant phosphaturic mesenchymal tumour most often develops in lesions that have recurred locally, often more than once, and show frankly sarcomatous features {884,2099, 2821}.

Immunophenotype

The phenotype of phosphaturic mesenchymal tumour is nonspecific {442, 884,2528,2659,2774}. The blood vessels within frequently show a lymphatic phenotype {2970}. Expression of FGF23 protein has been documented in some tumours {884}. FGF23 is a phosphaturic hormone that inhibits renal proximal tubule phosphate re-uptake {291,1493,1494,2537, 2538}. Elevated serum levels of FGF23 can be demonstrated in patients with phosphaturic mesenchymal tumour-associated TIO, and tumoral FGF23 expression can be demonstrated by RT-PCR, in cases presenting with or without osteomalacia {140}. Rare phosphaturic mesenchymal tumours with known TIO are FGF23-negative, presumably reflecting production of other phosphaturic hormones.

Genetics

To date, no specific genetic events have been identified. Only two cases have been karyotyped, with no shared aberration {1025}.

Prognostic factors

The overwhelming majority are histologically and clinically benign. Morphologically benign cases frequently recur locally, but are cured with complete excision, with resolution of osteomalacia {595, 884,968,1494}. Malignant tumours may metastasize and cause death from disease.

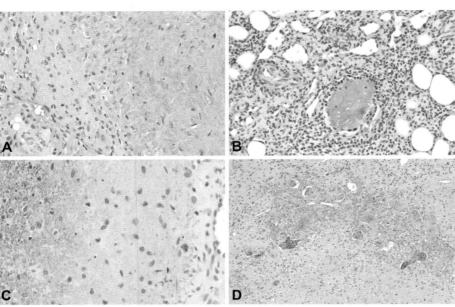

Fig. 12.40 Phosphaturic mesenchymal tumour. A Bland spindled cells and unusual basophilic matrix. B Moderately cellular proliferation of small, bland spindled cells in a highly vascular background. The neoplastic cells produce an unusual smudgy calcified matrix. Mature adipose tissue is also a common finding. C The matrix tends to calcify in a distinctive, "grungy" pattern. D The calcified matrix seen these tumours often incites an osteoclastic giant cell reaction, and may mimic various giant cell-rich tumours of soft tissue and bone.

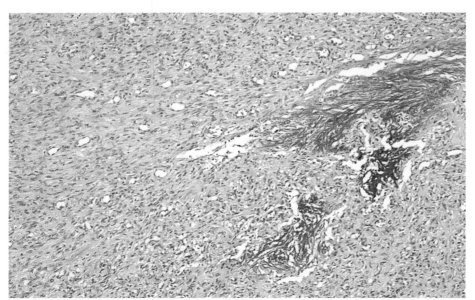

Fig. 12.41 Malignant phosphaturic mesenchymal tumour, showing a fibrosarcoma-like spindle cell sarcoma arising from a pre-existing histologically benign phosphaturic mesenchymal tumour.

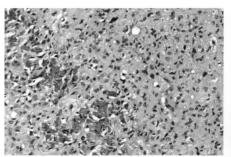

Fig.12.42 Phosphaturic mesenchymal tumour. Myxoid change may be seen in some tumours.

Synovial sarcoma

A.J.H. Suurmeijer
D. de Bruijn
A. Geurts van Kessel
M.M. Miettinen

Definition

Synovial sarcoma is a mesenchymal tumour, which displays a variable degree of epithelial differentiation, including gland formation, and has a specific chromosomal translocation t(X;18)(p11;q11) that leads to formation of a *SS18-SSX* fusion gene.

ICD-O code

Synovial sarcoma,

not otherwise specified	9040/3
spindle cell	9041/3
biphasic	9043/3

Synonyms

Older synonyms, such as tenosynovial sarcoma, synoviosarcoma, synovial cell sarcoma, malignant synovioma, and synovioblastic sarcoma should be abandoned.

Epidemiology

Synovial sarcoma (SS) may occur at any age and is equally distributed between the sexes {2676}. More than half of patients are teenagers and young adults; 58% of cases occur between age 10 and 40 years, and 77% occur before the age of 50 years. In the USA, the age-adjusted incidence is 1.42 per million adults (population-based SEER data) {2676}. The ratio of SS to soft tissue sarcoma is age-dependent, ranging from 15% in patients aged 10–18 years to 1.6% in patients aged > 50 years {2676}.

Sites of involvement

Most tumours (70%) arise in the deep soft tissue of the lower and upper extremities, often in a juxta-articular location. About 15% arise in the trunk and 7% in the head and neck region {2676}. Unusual sites of involvement include male and female external and internal sex organs, kidney, adrenal gland, retroperitoneum, various viscera, mediastinum, bone, CNS, and peripheral nerve {179,852,2460}.

Clinical features

SS usually presents as a mass, which is often painful. Initial growth is often slow and a small circumscribed tumour may misleadingly appear to be a benign lesion by clinical examination and imaging {248}. Delay in diagnosis can also be due to other confusing clinical presentations and imaging features, e.g. pain or joint contracture with no palpable mass, a history of trauma, signs of inflammation {1271}, cystic change, and haematoma formation. Up to one third of synovial sarcomas have radiologically detectable irregular calcification that is occasionally extensive. SS with aggressive growth may erode or invade adjacent bone.

Macroscopy

Grossly, the typical tumour is 3–10 cm in diameter, and usually circumscribed. Minute lesions of < 1 cm occur, especially in hands and feet {1868}. On cut surface, colour and consistency are proportionate to cellularity, collagenization and myxoid change or haemorrhage. Areas may be tan or grey, yellowish or pink, and soft or firm {779}. SS is frequently multinodular, and can be multicystic. Calcification, metaplastic ossification, and necrosis may be present.

Histopathology

Histologically, SS is biphasic or monophasic. In biphasic SS, epithelial and spindle-cell components are present in varying proportions. The epithelial cells are arranged in solid nests or cords or in glands with a tubular or sometimes alveolar or papillary architecture. In glandular areas, epithelial cells are cuboidal or columnar and have ovoid vesicular nuclei and, typically, more abundant and palely eosinophilic cytoplasm than that of the dark blue spindle-cell component. Glandular lumina contain epithelial mucin. Focally, the glandular component can predominate, and may be confused with adenocarcinoma; however, a scant spindle-cell component is virually always found. Rarely, epithelial cells show (keratinizing)

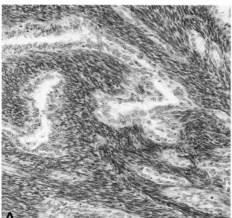
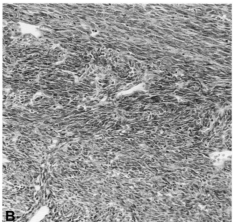
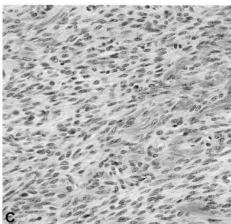

Fig. 12.43 Synovial sarcoma. **A** Biphasic synovial sarcoma with well-formed glandular structures. **B** Monophasic synovial sarcoma with a fascicular architecture and branching vessels. **C** Also note the wiry stromal collagen and mast cells.

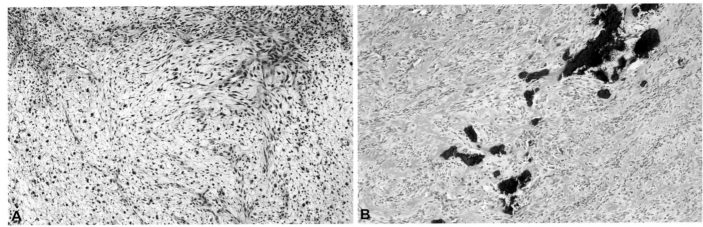

Fig. 12.44 Synovial sarcoma. **A** Monophasic synovial sarcoma with myxoid change. **B** Note the thick hyaline collagen bundles and calcifications.

squamous metaplasia or granular cell change {415}.

The spindle cells in biphasic SS resemble the spindle cells that predominate in monophasic SS. These delicate spindle cells are fairly uniform and relatively small, with sparse cytoplasm and ovoid, bland, but hyperchromatic nuclei with regular granular chromatin and inconspicuous nucleoli. The nuclear to cytoplasmic ratio is high, so that the nuclei appear to overlap. Typically, in both monophasic and biphasic types, the spindle cells are arranged in dense cellular sheets or vague fascicles, with occasional tigroid nuclear palisading or herring-bone pattern. The amount of collagen is variable and usually scant, but the tumour may contain strands of ropy and wiry collagen, bands of hyalinized collagen or foci of dense fibrosis, the latter especially after irradiation. Myxoid change is usually only focally present and rarely predominates, with alternating hypocellular and more cellular areas, and retiform cords or microcysts {1475}. Many SSs focally display a staghorn-shaped vascular pattern, reminiscent of solitary fibrous tumour/so-called haemangiopericytoma. Mast cells can be abundant. In up to one third of SSs, areas with calcification and/or ossification are found, which are sometimes abundant. Most tumours with calcification are biphasic {2855}. In areas with ossification, the osteoid has a lace-like pattern mimicking osteosarcoma, and bone tissue is lamellar and trabecular {1901}. Metaplastic cartilage is rarely seen.

In otherwise typical biphasic or monophasic SS, poorly differentiated areas with rounded or spindled cells showing severe nuclear atypia and high mitotic activity (> 15 per 10 HPFs) may be found. Rarely, SS is entirely poorly differentiated. Poorly differentiated areas are hypercellular areas, in which tumour cells typically show at least two of the following high-grade nuclear features: nuclear crowding, nuclear irregularity, prominent nucleoli or irregular clumping of chromatin {607}. Poorly differentiated areas may be composed of small round hyperchromatic tumour cells (reminiscent of Ewing sarcoma), fascicular spindle cells (reminiscent of MPNST) or epithelioid cells {192}. Compared with typical biphasic and monophasic SS, poorly differentiated areas more often contain areas of necrosis, and thin fibrovascular septa separating groups of tumour cells, whereas mast cells, hyalinized collagen and calcification are less prominent {607}. Poorly differentiated lesions are disproportionately common in elderly patients {415}.

Immunophenotype

Concerning epithelial markers, EMA is expressed more often and more widely than keratins, especially in the monophasic and poorly differentiated subtypes. Epithelial cells in biphasic SS consistently express EMA and keratin, in particular keratins 7, 8, 14, 18, and 19 and may contain almost any keratin, including keratin 20 {1887}. The spindle cells of monophasic SS show (more than) focal expression of EMA in nearly all cases, whereas focal expression of keratins (7, 8, 18, and 19) is found in 70–80% of tumours {1887, 2210}. Poorly differentiated areas of SS nearly always show focal staining for EMA, whereas keratin expression is seen in about 50% of these tumours {1887, 2210}. Focal expression of S100 protein may be detectable in up to 40% of cases {2210}. CD34 immunostaining is very rare in the monophasic subtype {2210}. The large majority of SSs are positive for CD99, which may show membranous staining, mimicking that seen in Ewing sarcoma {2124}. Moderate or strong nuclear staining for the trancriptional corepressor TLE1 is found in 80% of biphasic, monophasic and poorly differentiated tumours {900}. Notably, TLE1 staining is not specific for SS as it may also occur in histological mimics of SS, in particular, MPNST and solitary fibrous tumour {900,2210}.

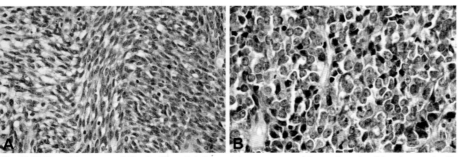

Fig. 12.45 Synovial sarcoma. **A** Poorly differentiated synovial sarcoma resembling malignant peripheral nerve sheath tumour. **B** Poorly differentiated synovial sarcoma resembling Ewing sarcoma.

Ultrastructure

The epithelial component shows luminal microvilli, tonofilaments, cell junctions, and is surrounded by a basement membrane similar to many adenocarcinomas {850}. Monophasic tumours show less specific features, but may contain focal epithelial differentiation as described above.

Genetics

SS is characterized by the t(X;18)(p11;q11) translocation, which is found exclusively in this tumour {1522}. This translocation or complex variants thereof are present in > 95% of all cases, often as the sole abnormality {688}. As a result of the t(X;18) translocation, the *SS18* gene (also known as *SYT* or *SSXT*), on chromosome 18, and one of the *SSX* genes (*SSX1*, *SSX2* or *SSX4*) on the X chromosome are fused {688}. Break-apart FISH and RT-PCR of fusion transcripts have been employed widely to establish an accurate diagnosis {499,1964,2741}. Approximately two thirds of cases carry an *SS18-SSX1* fusion, one third an *SS18-SSX2* fusion, and only a few have been described with an *SS18-SSX4* fusion {55,688}. Most biphasic SSs harbour *SS18-SSX1*, while monophasic lesions may harbour either fusion {1522}.

Prognostic factors

SS has a variable prognosis and favourable and unfavourable histological features have been delineated. Metastatic disease occurs most commonly in lungs and bone. Most distant recurrences develop within a few years after initial diagnosis, but late recurrences do occur, even after 10 years {1487}. Major prognostic determinants are tumour stage at presentation, tumour size, and FNCCLC tumour grade {1058,1487,2740}. Tumours with > 20% poorly differentiated histology show more aggressive behaviour {192, 1689, 2833}. Best outcomes are reported for patients with tumours < 5 cm in diameter, or having < 10 mitoses in 1.7 mm^2, and no necrosis {192}. Minute SSs (< 1 cm) have an excellent prognosis {1868}. Children fare better than adults {2676} and extremity-based SS have a better prognosis than those involving the trunk or head and neck area {374,2676}. The 5- and 10-year disease-specific survival is 83% and 75% in children and adolescents (age < 19 years) and 62% and 52% in adults, respectively {2676}.

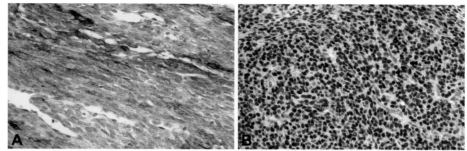

Fig. 12.46 Monophasic synovial sarcoma. **A** Focal immunostaining for EMA in spindle cells. **B** Strong TLE1 immunostaining of cell nuclei.

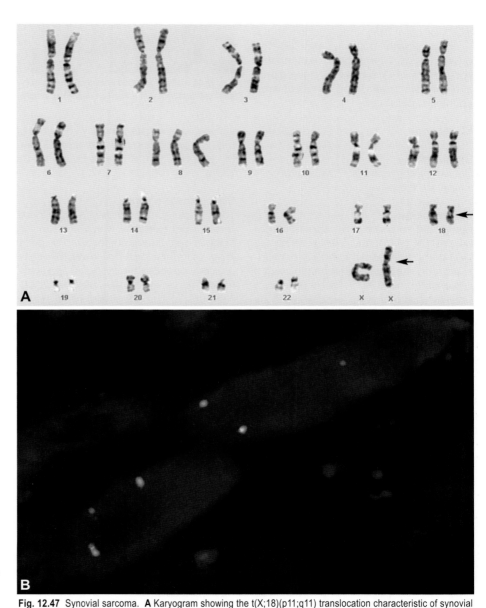

Fig. 12.47 Synovial sarcoma. **A** Karyogram showing the t(X;18)(p11;q11) translocation characteristic of synovial sarcoma (arrows indicate breakpoints). **B** Interphase FISH analysis showing a rearrangement of the *SS18* (18q11) locus in a synovial sarcoma. The red and green signals normally flank the *SS18* locus; splitting of these signals is indicative of a rearrangement.

Epithelioid sarcoma

Y. Oda
P. Dal Cin
W.B. Laskin

Definition

A malignant mesenchymal neoplasm that exhibits epithelioid cytomorphology and a predominantly epithelial phenotype. Two clinicopathological subtypes are recognized: (i) the conventional or classic ("distal") form, characterized by its proclivity for acral sites and pseudogranulomatous growth pattern; and (ii) the proximal-type ("large-cell") variant that arises mainly in proximal/truncal regions, and consists of nests and sheets of large epithelioid cells.

ICD-O code   8804/3

Synonyms

Classic or conventional, "distal" type
Proximal, "large-cell" type

Epidemiology

Epithelioid sarcoma (ES) represents between 0.6% {2374} and 1.0% of sarcomas {1641} and between 4% and 8% of childhood non-rhabdomyosarcomatous soft tissue sarcomas {397}. The classic subtype is reported nearly twice as often as the proximal-type variant {431,2325}. The male to female ratio for the classic subtype is 1.9 : 1 {272,429,789,952,1080, 2261,2325} and 1.6 : 1 for the proximal-type variant {952,1062,1122,2325}. Both tumours affect patients of a wide age range. The classic subtype presents between ages 10 and 40 years (mean/median range, 25.5–33 years) in > 70% of patients {272,429,789,952,1080,2261,2325}. The proximal-type variant tends to affect a

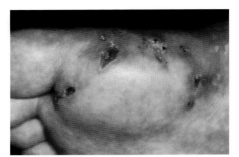
Fig. 12.48 Multiple ulcerating lesions on the sole of the foot in a patient with classic (distal-type) epithelioid sarcoma.

somewhat older population, with > 80% of patients presenting between ages 20 and 65 years (mean, 40 years; median, 38 years) {952,1062,1122,2325}.

Sites of involvement

The classic subtype mostly occurs in the distal upper extremity, with > 60% arising in the fingers and hand, followed by distal lower extremity, proximal lower extremity, proximal upper extremity, trunk, and lastly, head and neck {272,429,789,1080,2261}. Tumours of the foot and hand affect mainly volar surfaces. The proximal-type variant tends to arise in deep soft tissue, and most often affects truncal (pelvoperineal, genital and inguinal) tissue and buttock/hip, followed by thigh, head and neck, distal extremity, and axilla {952, 1062,1122,2325}.

Clinical features

Superficially located examples of classic ES present as solitary or multiple, slowly growing, usually painless, firm nodules. Lesions often result in nonhealing skin ulcers that have a tendency to clinically mimic other ulcerative dermal processes. In comparison, classic and proximal-type tumours located in deep soft tissue are usually larger in size and more infiltrative {1062,1122}. This is one of the few sarcomas that regularly metastasize to lymph nodes. Radiological imaging studies are nonspecific, but occasionally demonstrate a speckled pattern of calcification within the mass.

Macroscopy

The classic subtype usually presents as one or more indurated, ill-defined, dermal or subcutaneous nodules measuring a few millimetres to 5 cm. Deep-seated tumours are multinodular masses that grow up to 15 cm and involve tendons or fascia. The cut surface is glistening with a grey-white or grey-tan colour punctuated by yellow and brown foci representing necrosis and haemorrhage, respectively. The proximal-type variant presents as solitary or multiple whitish nodules ranging from 1 to 20 cm, with areas of haemorrhage and necrosis {1062,1122}.

Histopathology

Classic ES consists of cellular nodules of epithelioid and spindled tumour cells with central degeneration and/or necrosis – a growth pattern that imparts a vaguely granulomatous appearance to the process {1153}. Fusion of necrotizing nodules results in a serpiginous mass

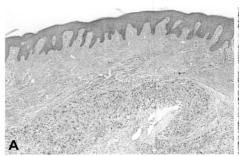
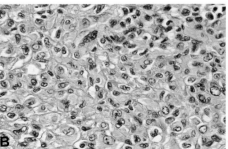
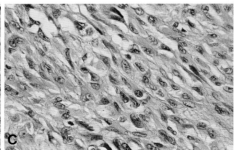
Fig. 12.49 Classic (distal-type) epithelioid sarcoma. **A** Low-power magnification of a nodular lesion centred in the dermis composed of tumour cells surrounding an area of necrosis (pseudogranulomatous growth pattern). **B** Epithelioid tumour cells with abundant eosinophilic cytoplasm. **C** Cells with a plump spindle-shaped morphology.

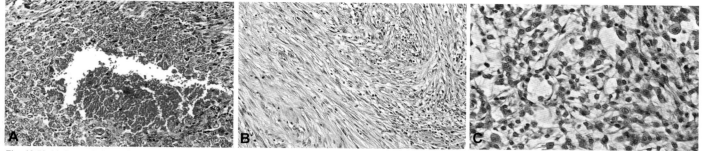

Fig. 12.50 Variants of classic (distal-type) epithelioid sarcoma. **A** Angiomatoid variant with epithelioid cells surrounding a cystic space filled with blood. **B** Fibroma-like variant characterized by a fascicular or whorled arrangement of plump spindle-shaped cells. **C** Myxoid variant showing cord-like or reticular arrangement of epithelioid cells within a mucin-rich stroma.

with central "geographic" necrosis. Deep-situated lesions spread along the fascia as undulating bands of cells punctuated by foci of necrosis. Tumour nodules are composed of large ovoid or polygonal epithelioid cells and plump spindle-shaped cells with deeply eosinophilic cytoplasm and mildly atypical nuclei possessing vesicular chromatin and small nucleoli. The epithelioid cells, which are generally concentrated towards the centre of the nodule, gradually transition with the spindled element. Some cases have predominantly spindled morphology. Mitotic activity is usually low. Dystrophic calcification and metaplastic bone formation are detected in 20% of cases {429}, and aggregates of chronic inflammatory cells are usually present at the periphery of the tumour nodules. Tumours exhibiting loss of cellular cohesion with epithelioid cells surrounding foci of intralesional haemorrhage may simulate angiosarcoma {1878,2885}.

The proximal type is characterized by a multinodular and sheet-like growth of large and sometimes pleomorphic epithelioid (carcinoma-like) cells with enlarged vesicular nuclei and prominent nucleoli {1062,1122,1878}. Spotty foci of tumour necrosis are frequently encountered, but this feature does not generally result in a pseudogranulomatous pattern typical of classic ES. Cells with rhabdoid features occur in both forms, but are more frequently observed in the proximal-type variant where differentiation from extra-renal rhabdoid tumour becomes challenging when the rhabdoid cell is the predominant cell type {1062}. Occasional cases may have a prominent myxoid stroma {876}. Additionally, rare cases of ES demonstrate hybrid histological features of both classic and proximal types.

Immunophenotype
Both classic and proximal-type ES show immunoreactivity for epithelial markers including low- and high-molecular weight keratins and EMA {550,1727,1878,2467}. More specifically, most cases express keratin 8 and 19 {1878}, but are typically negative or only focally positive for keratin 5/6 {1553}. In contrast to carcinoma, CD34 is expressed in > 50% of cases. Loss of nuclear expression of SMARCB1 protein occurs in both types {1215}.

Ultrastructure
Tumour cells of classic ES show a wide spectrum of differentiation from undifferentiated cells to mesenchymal cells exhibiting myofibroblastic and fibroblastic features {851} and epithelial-like cells with well-formed desmosome-like intercellular junctions, surface microvilli, and tonofilaments. The ultrastructural features of proximal-type ES are similar to those of the classic variant. Rhabdoid cells harbour a characteristic tight paranuclear aggregation of intermediate filaments {1062}.

Genetics
Although cytogenetic investigation of primary and metastatic ES has demonstrated complex rearrangements, 22q11 in particular has been implicated in the pathogenesis of these sarcomas {1667}. The involvement of 22q abnormalities also has been supported by loss of heterozygosity analyses {2282}. The genetic alterations of 22q11–12 have included mutation, deletions and other alterations of the tumour suppressor gene *SMARCB1* (*hSNF5*, *INI1*); alterations that have also been observed in paediatric rhabdoid tumours of the kidney and CNS among other neoplastic entities {227,1201}. Although loss of SMARCB1 protein expression has been demonstrated in most examples of ES {1215} and in malignant rhabdoid tumour, the frequency of *SMARCB1* mutations is significantly lower in ES than in malignant rhabdoid tumours {1456,1922}. These findings suggest that

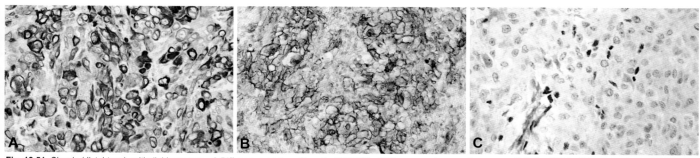

Fig. 12.51 Classic (distal-type) epithelioid sarcoma. **A** Diffuse expression of keratin (CAM5.2). **B** Strong membranous immunopositivity for CD34. **C** Complete loss of SMARCB1 (INI1) protein expression in the tumour cells.

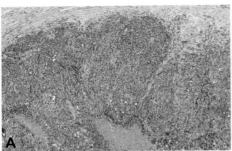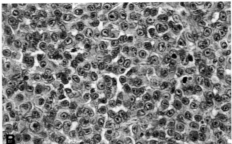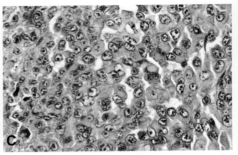

Fig. 12.52 Proximal-type (large-cell) epithelioid sarcoma. **A** Low-power magnification shows a multinodular growth pattern of epithelioid cells with foci of tumour necrosis. **B** Pleomorphic epithelioid tumour cells with abundant, deeply eosinophilic cytoplasm and enlarged vesicular nuclei with prominent nucleoli. **C** Aggregates of rhabdoid cells with glassy intracytoplasmic hyaline inclusions and eccentrically located, vesicular nuclei.

the mechanisms of loss of SMARCB1 protein expression are distinct in these two entities. In addition, chromosome arm 8q gains are frequently observed, particularly as i(8)(q10), in both classic (distal-type) and proximal-type (large-cell) ES.

Prognostic factors

Recent large series have reported 5- and 10-year overall survival rates for all ES of 60–80%, and 42–62%, respectively {151, 358,952,2325,2620}. Metastases develop in 40–50% of patients {151,431,2620}, usually after repeated recurrences, and frequently involve the lung and regional lymph nodes {429,431,2374}. The actuarial 5-year rate of local recurrence is 35% {2620}.

Adverse prognostic factors in both classic and proximal-type ES include male sex, older age, proximal extremity/axial location {431,1304}, involvement of deep soft tissue {1304,2325}, tumour size > 5 cm {431,1304,2325}, tumour multifocality {151, 431}, high mitotic activity {431,1304}, nodal involvement {151}, proximal-type histology with presence of rhabdoid cells {952, 2325}, high FNCLCC histological grade {952}, and extensive necrosis {1304}. The prognosis for patients with proximal-type ES is significantly worse than that for patients with classic ES {397,952,1304, 2325}, but better than that for malignant rhabdoid tumour {1304,1456}. Large size and early tumour metastasis are associated with poor outcome in proximal-type tumours {1122}.

Alveolar soft part sarcoma

N.G. Ordóñez
M. Ladanyi

Definition

Alveolar soft part sarcoma (ASPS) is a rare, distinctive sarcoma composed of large, uniform, epithelioid cells having abundant, eosinophilic, granular cytoplasm, arranged in solid nests and/or alveolar structures. It is characterized by an *ASPSCR1-TFE3* fusion gene.

ICD-O code   9581/3

Epidemiology

ASPS is rare, with a reported frequency of 0.2–0.9% of all soft tissue sarcomas {828,1126,1571}. It can occur at any age, but is most common between ages 15 and 35 years. It is rare before age 5 and after age 50 years. There is a female to male predominance of about 2 : 1 in the first three decades of life; however, this ratio is reversed after age 30 years, when men are slightly more often affected than women {2130,2258}.

Sites of involvement

In adults, ASPS occurs most commonly in the deep soft tissue of the thigh or buttock. In children and infants, the head and neck region, especially the tongue and orbit, is the most common site of origin. Isolated cases have also been reported in a variety of unusual locations, including the lung {2602}, stomach {3028}, liver {2518}, breast {2995}, bone {2188}, larynx {1506}, heart {1677}, urinary bladder {58}, and female genital tract, more often in the uterine cervix {2041,2356}.

Clinical features

ASPS usually presents as a slowly growing, painless mass. Metastasis to the lung or brain is quite often the first manifestation of the disease. Orbital lesions present most commonly with proptosis and lid swelling. Vaginal bleeding is the usual complaint of patients with tumours originating in the female genital tract. Hypervascularity with prominent draining veins can be demonstrated by angiography or contrast-enhanced CT {1660} and high signal intensity on T1–T2-weighted images on MRI are highly suggestive of ASPS {2673}.

Macroscopy

Alveolar soft part sarcomas tend to be poorly circumscribed, pale grey or yellowish in colour, and have a soft consistency. Areas of necrosis and haemorrhage are common, especially in larger tumours.

Histopathology

The distinctively organoid or nesting pattern is best seen at low magnification, but is sometimes absent, especially in children. The nests tend to be uniform, but may vary in size and shape. They are separated by delicate partitions of connective tissue containing sinusoidal vascular channels. Loss of cellular cohesion and necrosis of the centrally located cells in the nests results in the commonly seen pseudoalveolar pattern. In some areas, the pseudoalveolar features may not be easily discerned and the tumour may appear to have a more diffuse growth pattern. The neoplastic cells are generally uniform in size, and round or polygonal with well-defined cell borders, thus, conferring a distinctive epithelioid appearance. The nucleus is usually centrally placed and bland, and contains a prominent nucleolus. Multinucleation and nuclear atypia, although uncommon, can occur. The cytoplasm is abundant, eosinophilic, and somewhat granular, but on occasion, may exhibit clear features that mimics renal cell carcinoma. Mitotic figures are uncommon, but vascular invasion is frequently seen. The cells often contain rhomboid or rod-shaped intracytoplasmic inclusions that may be faintly apparent on H&E, but can be better demonstrated on PAS stains after diastase digestion. On occasion, these inclusions

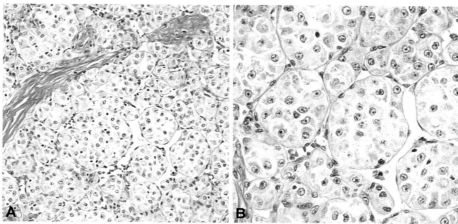

Fig. 12.53 Alveolar soft part sarcoma. A Typical organoid pattern. B The tumour cell nests are outlined by sinusoidal vascular channels.

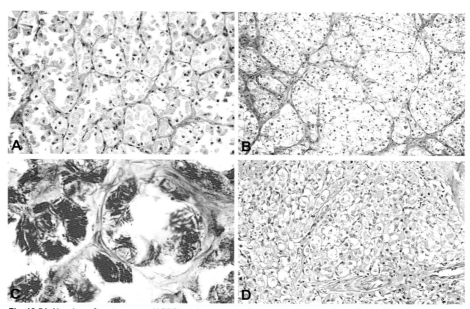

Fig. 12.54 Alveolar soft part sarcoma (ASPS). A Area showing the pseudoalveolar pattern. B Clearing of the cytoplasm, probably caused by degeneration, can mimic renal cell carcinoma. C PAS stain with diastase digestion demonstrates the presence of crystals. D ASPS from the upper limb of an adolescent male. Note the solid growth pattern.

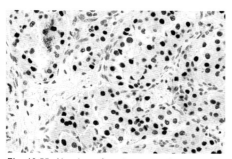

Fig. 12.55 Alveolar soft part sarcoma demonstrating nuclear immunostaining for TFE3.

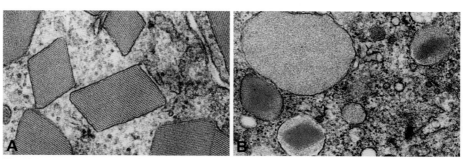

Fig. 12.56 Ultrastructure of alveolar soft part sarcoma. A Membrane-bound, fully developed crystals may adhere to one another, forming a variety of shapes. B Some of the large, membrane-bound secretory granules contain foci of crystallization.

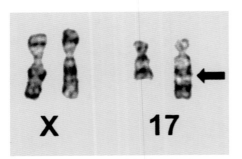

Fig. 12.57 Partial karyotype of alveolar soft part sarcoma showing the characteristic alteration, der(17)t(X;17)(p11.2;q25).

may be numerous; however, they may also be rare or even absent. In addition to the crystals, variable amounts of glycogen and diastase-resistant granules, which probably represent precursors to the crystals, can also be found.

Immunophenotype

The most characteristic finding in ASPS is the consistent demonstration of strong nuclear staining with an antibody that recognizes the carboxy terminal portion of TFE3 retained in the fusion protein, which contrasts with the situation in most normal cells that show only weak or no nuclear reactivity with this antibody {98,2968}. However, prominent nuclear immunoreactivity for TFE3 can also be seen in some granular cell tumours {2795}. About 50% of ASPS tumours express desmin, but the staining is usually focal. Staining for S100 protein can be positive, but in contrast to PEComa, HMB45 is negative. ASPS does not express synaptophysin, chromogranin, neurofilament proteins, keratin, or EMA.

Ultrastructure

By electron microscopy, the nests of the neoplastic cells are surrounded by a dis-continuous basal lamina. The cell membranes are joined by sparse, poorly developed junctions and the cytoplasm contains numerous mitochondria, abundant rough endoplasmic reticulum, and prominent Golgi complexes. The most distinctive feature is the membrane-bound rhomboid or rectangular crystals that are composed of a periodic lattice-work of rigid fibrils with diameters of 5–7 nm and a periodicity of 10 nm {1972, 2130}. Granules containing homogeneous secretory material that on occasion exhibit small foci of crystallization are often seen {2131}. Ultrastructural immunohistochemistry has shown that the granules associated with crystal formation contain aggregates of monocarboxylate transporter protein 1 and its cellular chaperone, CD147 {1521}.

Genetics

Cytogenetically, ASPS is defined by a specific alteration, der(17)t(X;17)(p11;q25) {1348, 2491, 2842}. Because the der(X) resulting from the t(X;17)(p11;q25) is almost always absent, the der(17)t(X;17) may be described in some cases as add(17)(q25), unless the quality of the banding allows for positive identification of the additional material as the short arm of chromosome X. This translocation results in the fusion of the *TFE3* transcription factor gene (from Xp11) with *ASPSCR1* (also known as *ASPL*) at 17q25 {1524}. *ASPSCR1-TFE3* RT-PCR (which identifies two forms of the fusion transcript that differ by the presence or absence of one additional exon of *TFE3*) and FISH for *TFE3* rearrangement are both robust methods for molecular diagnosis {1524,1962,3067}. Although the presence of the *ASPSCR1-TFE3* fusion appears to be highly specific and sensitive for ASPS among sarcomas {1524}, the same gene fusion is also found in a small but unique subset of renal cell carcinomas, often affecting young patients {93,1157}. The ASPSCR1-TFE3 fusion protein localizes to the nucleus where it functions as an aberrant transcription factor, causing activation of MET signalling, rendering ASPS cells sensitive to MET inhibition {2794}.

Prognostic factors

ASPS seldom recurs locally after complete resection, but metastases are common with long-term follow-up. Metastases can occur early in the course of the disease, sometimes before detection of the primary lesion, or much later, even decades after resection of the primary and despite the absence of local recurrence {814,1611,1622}. In a large study, the survival rates for patients with no evidence of metastasis at the time of diagnosis were 60% at 5 years, 38% at 10 years, and 15% at 20 years {1611}. Factors that can influence prognosis are patient age at presentation, tumour size, and the presence of metastases at diagnosis. Another large series found a 5-year disease-free survival of 71% in patients presenting with localized disease, compared with only 20% in patients presenting with metastases {2258}. Histological features have no prognostic significance. It has been reported that there is an increase of metastases with increasing age {1611}. Patients who present with large tumours are most likely to have metastases at the time of diagnosis {780}. The most common sites of metastasis, in decreasing order of frequency, are lung, bone, and brain {1611,2258}. Metastasis to the lymph nodes is uncommon.

Clear cell sarcoma of soft tissue

C.R. Antonescu

Definition

Clear cell sarcoma (CCS) is a malignant neoplasm typically involving deep soft tissue of the extremities, in close proximity to tendons and aponeurotic structures. Distinctive features include nested growth pattern, consistent melanocytic differentiation and a recurrent *EWSR1-ATF1* fusion gene in most cases.

ICD-O code   9044/3

Synonym

Malignant melanoma of soft parts

Epidemiology

These rare tumours mainly affect young adults, with peak incidence in the third and fourth decades of life, and occur equally frequently in males and females.

Sites of involvement

The overwhelming majority of cases occur in the extremity, with the foot/ankle region accounting for 40% of cases. It is typically a deep-seated tumour, often intimately associated with tendons or aponeuroses. The tumour may extend to the subcutis, but the skin is typically uninvolved. The head and neck or trunk region are rarely affected {470,618,721, 748,1671}. Rare examples in the retroperitoneum, viscera or bone have been reported. In the gastrointestinal tract, CCS often arise in the small bowel, with less common gastric and colonic involvement.

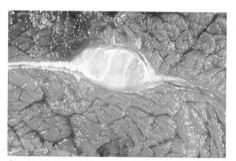

Fig. 12.58 Clear cell sarcoma. This well-circumscribed tumour arose in the plantaris tendon of a woman aged 18 years. Despite the small size of the tumour, she died from disseminated metastases 4 years later.

Clinical features

The tumour usually presents as a slowly growing mass, being present for several weeks to several years. Pain and/or tenderness is present in half of the cases. Lymph-node involvement is frequent.

Macroscopy

Most tumours are relatively small (< 5 cm); however, lesions measuring > 10 cm have been described. The cut surface shows a lobulated grey-white mass with a well-circumscribed, pushing border. Pigmentation, necrosis or cystic changes are rarely encountered.

Histopathology

At low power, CCS shows a characteristic nested growth pattern, with collagenous bands dividing the tumour into distinct compartments. Most CCSs display predominantly epithelioid morphology, but

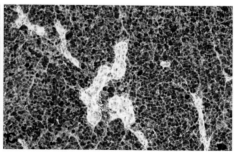

Fig. 12.59 Area from a clear cell sarcoma showing wreath-like giant cells.

not uncommonly areas of spindling are present. Less often the tumours show an alveolar growth or rhabdoid features. Despite its name, CCS cells most often display palely eosinophilic or amphophilic cytoplasm, with true clearing being present only in a minority of neoplastic cells. Although the tumour cells show vesicular nuclei with macronucleoli, nuclear pleomorphism and lower mitotic activity is significantly lower than in metastatic melanoma. Scattered wreath-like multinucleate giant cells are often present and can be a useful diagnostic clue. Melanin is often not detected at the H&E level, but can be highlighted by Fontana stain in two thirds of cases.

Compared with the classic soft tissue lesions, the gastrointestinal CCSs show somewhat distinctive pathological features, with monotonous epithelioid cells arranged in solid, nested or pseudo-papillary patterns.

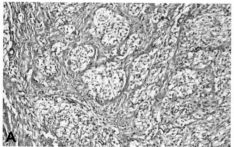
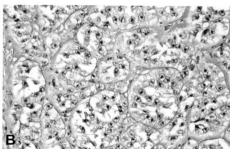

Fig. 12.60 Clear cell sarcoma. **A** Nests of clear polygonal cells separated by fibrous septa. **B** Typical morphological appearance with more granular amphophilic cytoplasm and uniform vesicular nuclei with distinct macronucleoli. **C** There is strong and diffuse immunoreactivity for S100 protein.

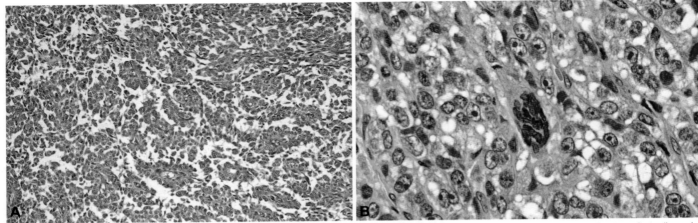

Fig. 12.61 Gastrointestinal clear cell sarcoma. **A** Pseudopapillary growth pattern, which can be mistaken for a papillary carcinoma. **B** Scattered osteoclast-type giant cells can be seen in some but not all cases.

The cells have clear to lightly eosinophilic cytoplasm and inconspicuous nucleoli. Scattered osteoclast-type giant cells are noted in a subset of cases. On the basis of these findings and the less consistent melanocytic differentiation, there is still debate as to whether gastrointestinal CCS represents a pathological entity distinct from the soft-tissue counterpart, despite similar genetic abnormalities.

Immunophenotype
Reactivity for S100 protein, HMB45, MITF and other melanoma antigens is consistently noted with a strong and diffuse staining pattern {1188}. The gastrointestinal CCSs show similar strong reactivity for S100 protein, but less consistent expression of other melanocytic markers {81,506}.

Ultrastructure
Melanosomes in varying stages of development are present in the majority of tumours analysed ultrastructurally {1422,1971}.

Genetics
The genetic hallmark of CCS is the presence of a reciprocal translocation t(12;22)(q13;q12), resulting in the fusion of *EWSR1* with *ATF1* in > 90% of cases {84,3075}. The most common fusion transcript is type 1, with exon 8 of *EWSR1* fused in-frame with *ATF1* codon 65. A related variant translocation, t(2;22)(q32.3;q12),

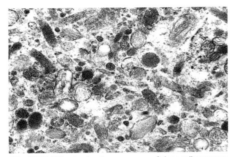

Fig. 12.62 Ultrastructural appearance of clear cell sarcoma from a male aged 23 years, showing a mixture of stage II and III melanosomes.

resulting in an *EWSR-CREB1* fusion, was recently reported in a small subset (6%) of CCS {1188,2904}. No significant association between the transcript type and immunohistochemical profile or patient outcome was found {497,1188}. Like the soft-tissue counterpart, gastrointestinal CCS displays *EWSR1* rearrangements involving either *ATF1* or *CREB1* {81,517, 1681}.

ATF1 and CREB1 are members of the CREB basic leucine-zipper transcription factor family and bind to cAMP inducible promoters. In CCS, the EWSR1-ATF1 fusion protein targets the melanocyte-specific *MITF* promoter, required for cell proliferation as well as triggering ectopic melanocytic differentiation {582}.

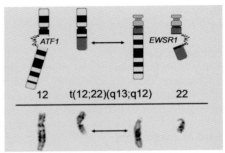

Fig. 12.63 Schematic and partial G-banded karyotype of the 12;22 translocation in clear cell sarcoma.

Prognostic factors
Despite an often prolonged clinical course, CCS is associated with poor prognosis, with survival rates at 5, 10 and 20 years, respectively, of 67%, 33% and 10% {1188,1671}. Nodal metastasis develops in half of patients. The lung and bone are the other frequent sites of metastasis. The 5-year survival rate overestimates long-term survival, since many patients develop recurrences and metastases, sometimes > 10 years after diagnosis. Tumour size (> 5 cm), necrosis and local recurrence are unfavourable prognostic markers {2440}. The gastrointestinal CCSs are highly aggressive tumours with early spread to locoregional lymph nodes, peritoneum and liver metastasis.

Extraskeletal myxoid chondrosarcoma

D.R. Lucas
G. Stenman

Definition

Extraskeletal myxoid chondrosarcoma (EMC) is a malignant mesenchymal neoplasm of uncertain differentiation characterized by abundant myxoid matrix, multilobular architecture and uniform cells arranged in cords, clusters and fine networks. Despite the name, there is no convincing evidence of cartilaginous differentiation. These tumours are characterized by *NR4A3* rearrangement.

ICD-O code   9231/3

Synonym

Chordoid sarcoma

Epidemiology

EMC is rare, accounting for < 3% of soft tissue sarcomas {2799}. It usually occurs in adults with a median age of 50 years {701,1816}. Only rare cases in childhood or adolescence have been reported {1073}. The male to female ratio is 2 : 1.

Sites of involvement

Most EMCs arise in the deep soft tissues of the proximal extremities and limb girdles; thigh being the most common site {754,1816}. Less common sites include the trunk, head and neck, paraspinal soft tissue, abdomen, pelvis and foot. Rare tumours have also been reported in the finger {2112}, cranium {2444}, retroperitoneum {919}, pleura {997} and bone {1410}.

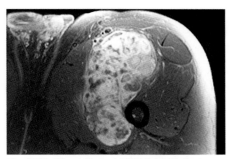

Fig. 12.64 T2-weighted axial MRI highlights the hyperintense signalling and pronounced lobular architecture in an extraskeletal myxoid chondrosarcoma of the thigh.

Clinical features

Patients most often present with an enlarging, deep-seated soft tissue mass, often accompanied by pain and tenderness. Some may mimic a haematoma. Tumours around joints can restrict range of motion.

Macroscopy

EMCs form large, well-demarcated tumours contained within a pseudocapsule. Median size is 7 cm; however, the range is highly variable and includes very large tumours of up to 30 cm {1816}. On cut surface, EMC has a well-defined multinodular architecture comprised of glistening, gelatinous areas separated by fibrous septa. Intratumoral haemorrhage, cystic cavities and geographic areas of necrosis are common. Highly cellular tumours are fleshy.

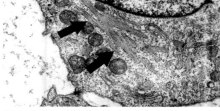

Fig. 12.65 Ultrastructurally, extraskeletal myxoid chondrosarcoma often has parallel bundles of microtubules located within cisternal spaces as indicated (arrows). These structures, although highly characteristic, are detected in fewer than half of tumours.

Histopathology

EMC has a multinodular architecture defined by fibrous septa that divide the tumour into hypocellular lobules with abundant pale blue myxoid or chondromyxoid matrix that is rich in sulfated proteoglycans. Well-formed hyaline cartilage is virtually never seen. The stroma is strikingly hypovascular. The cells characteristically interconnect with one another to form cords, small clusters and complex, trabecular or cribriform arrays. The cells have a modest amount of deeply eosinophilic, finely granular to vacuolated cytoplasm and uniform round to oval nuclei. The chromatin is evenly distributed often with a small, inconspicuous nucleolus. Mitotic activity is usually low. Some tumours have prominent rhabdoid cytoplasmic inclusions. Rare cases are hypercellular

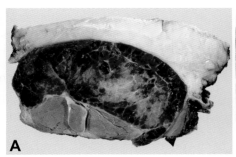 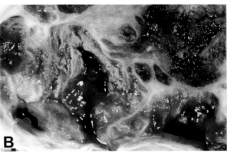

Fig. 12.66 Extraskeletal myxoid chondrosarcoma. **A** Grossly, these tumours are well-demarcated, contained by a pseudocapsule and have a lobular architecture defined by fibrous septa. **B** Cystic cavities, haemorrhage and necrosis are often found on the cut surface. Note the well-defined lobular architecture and thick fibrous septa.

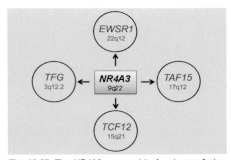

Fig. 12.67 The *NR4A3* gene and its four known fusion partner genes in extraskeletal myxoid chondrosarcoma. The chromosomal localization of the genes is indicated.

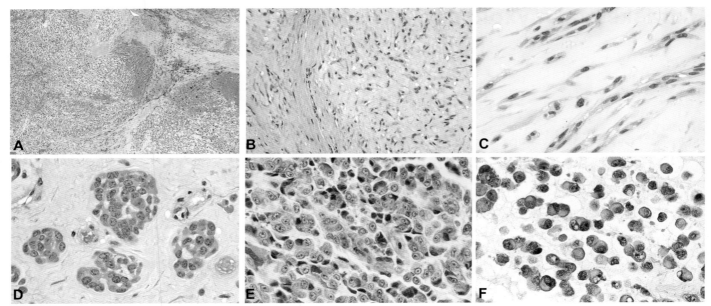

Fig. 12.68 Extraskeletal myxoid chondrosarcoma (EMC). **A** Lobular architecture, thick fibrous bands and areas of acute haemorrhage, haemosiderosis and scarring. **B** EMCs are characterized by abundant myxoid matrix and interconnecting cords of uniform cells. **C** Spindle-cell differentiation is common and when present can be either focal or diffuse. Note the interconnecting growth pattern. **D** The cells sometimes form cohesive clusters mimicking an epithelial neoplasm. **E** Cellular EMC is characterized by sheets and cords of cells with little intervening myxoid matrix. The cells frequently have an epithelioid morphology and large vesicular nuclei with prominent nucleoli and brisk mitotic activity. **F** Rhabdoid cells with eccentric eosinophilic cytoplasm and perinuclear hyaline globules are seen in some EMCs. These cells are frequently negative for SMARCB1 (INI1) by immunohistochemistry.

and have higher grade, often epithelioid cytomorphology.

Immunophenotype

S100 protein is positive in up to 20% of cases, and CD117 (KIT) is positive in up to 30%. Expression of synaptophysin and NSE have been demonstrated in some tumours {1115,2112,2122}. Tumours with rhabdoid features are often negative for SMARCB1 (INI1).

Ultrastructure

Dilations within the rough endoplastic reticulum filled with granular amorphous material identical to the extracellular matrix and ruffled cytoplasmic borders are common findings. Intracisternal microtubules are very characteristic of EMC, but are present in fewer than half of tumours {75,1816,2161}. Dense-core neurosecretory granules have also been reported {1115}.

Genetics

Cytogenetically, EMC is characterized by a t(9;22)(q22;q12) translocation or less frequently a t(9;17)(q22;q11) or t(9;15)(q22;q21) translocation {118, 2158, 2492, 2572, 2573, 2575, 2649}. Although the t(9;22) has been found as the sole anomaly, most

cases also show secondary chromosome changes, including trisomy for 1q25-qter, 7, 8, 12, and 19 {2161, 2573}.

Molecular characterization of the t(9;22) and subsequently also of the t(9;17) variant translocation has shown that they result in gene fusions in which the *NR4A3* gene in 9q22 is fused to either *EWSR1* in 22q12 or *TAF15* in 17q12 {118,1519, 2158,2572}. *NR4A3* (also known as *TEC*, *CHN*, and *NOR1*) encodes an orphan nuclear receptor belonging to the steroid/thyroid receptor gene family, whereas *EWSR1* and *TAF15* (also known as *TAF2N*, *RBP56*, and *TAF(II)68*) belong to the TET family of multifunctional proteins that bind both RNA and DNA. Two additional gene fusions, *TCF12-NR4A3* and *TFG-NR4A3*, have also been identified in single cases of EMC {1187,2575}. The *NR4A3*-fusions, which are present in > 90% of EMCs {1185,2161,2573}, have not been found in any other sarcoma and may therefore be considered as a hallmark of this disease.

The molecular consequences of the NR4A3 fusions in EMC have only partly been elucidated. The EWSR1-NR4A3 and TAF15-NR4A3 fusion proteins are strong transcriptional activators {1415,1518}. There is evidence suggesting that coexpression

of native NR4A3 and its coactivator SIX3 may be an alternative mechanism to gene fusion {1191}.

Prognostic factors

EMC is an aggressive malignant neoplasm. Although often associated with prolonged survival, it has high rates of local and distant recurrence and disease-associated death {701,1816,2425}. Local recurrence ranges from 37% to 48%, while metastases occur in approximately half the cases {701,1816}. Metastases are usually pulmonary; however, extrapulmonary and disseminated metastases also occur {2425}. Interestingly, prolonged survival even in the face of metastatic disease is not uncommon. Two large retrospective series {701,1816} report 5-, 10- and 15-year overall survival rates of 82–90%, 65–70%, and 58–60%, respectively. Older age, large tumour size (especially tumours > 10 cm) and proximal location are adverse prognostic factors {1816,2122}. Some studies suggest that tumours with increased cellularity and atypia are more aggressive {75,1669, 2122}. Others suggest that the presence of rhabdoid cells represents an adverse histological finding {2122,2136}.

Malignant mesenchymoma

H.L. Evans

The term "malignant mesenchymoma" has been applied in the past to sarcomas that exhibit two or more lines of specialized differentiation. However, it has become apparent that this group does not form a clinicopathological entity, and that potential candidates for the designation can be more appropriately classified in other ways. Among those with a fatty component are myxoid liposarcomas with cartilaginous metaplasia, atypical lipomatous tumours (well-differentiated liposarcomas) with osseous, cartilaginous, smooth muscle, or skeletal muscle elements, dedifferentiated liposarcomas with the same elements in the dedifferentiated component, and pleomorphic liposarcomas with osteogenic areas. Nonfatty neoplasms meeting the definition include malignant peripheral nerve sheath tumours with heterologous elements (as seen in about 15% of cases), the rare leiomyosarcomas that have osteosarcoma-like or rhabdomyosarcomatous zones and the occasional embryonal rhabdomyosarcomas that demonstrate focal cartilage. Obviously all of these are different neoplasms, and "lumping" them together under one heading is misleading, and this diagnosis is therefore discouraged.

Desmoplastic small round cell tumour

C.R. Antonescu
M. Ladanyi

Definition
Desmoplastic small round cell tumour (DSRCT) is a malignant mesenchymal neoplasm composed of small round tumour cells associated with prominent stromal desmoplasia and polyphenotypic differentiation. It has a consistent *EWSR1-WT1* gene fusion.

ICD-O code
8806/3

Synonyms
Intra-abdominal desmoplastic round cell tumour; intra-abdominal desmoplastic small cell tumour with divergent differentiation; polyphenotypic small round cell tumour

Epidemiology
DSRCT primarily affects children and young adults, who usually present with widespread abdominal serosal involvement {963}. There is a striking predominance in males, with peak incidence in the third decade of life, although it occurs over a wide range (first to fifth decades).

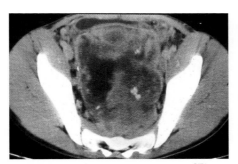
Fig. 12.69 Desmoplastic small round cell tumour. CT image of a large pelvic desmoplastic small round cell tumour.

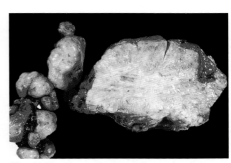
Fig. 12.70 Desmoplastic small round cell tumour presenting as one dominant tumour mass and multiple smaller tumour nodules. The cross-section shows a solid white-tan cut surface, with foci of necrosis.

Sites of involvement
The vast majority of patients develop tumours in the abdominal cavity, frequently located in the retroperitoneum, pelvis, omentum and mesentery. Multiple serosal implants are common. Clinical presentation outside the abdominal cavity is rare and is mainly restricted to the thoracic cavity and paratesticular location {532}. Less common presentations occur in the limbs, head and neck, kidney, and brain {2898}.

Clinical features
Presenting symptoms are usually related to the primary site, such as pain, abdominal distention, palpable mass, acute abdomen, ascites, and organ obstruction.

Macroscopy
The typical gross appearance consists of multiple tumour nodules studding the peritoneal surface. Often there is a dominant tumour mass accompanied by

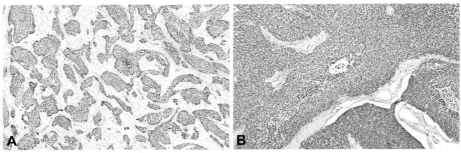

Fig. 12.71 Desmoplastic small round cell tumour. **A** Characteristic morphology with variably sized nests in a desmoplastic stroma. **B** Solid growth pattern with large confluent nests.

smaller satellite nodules. The cut surface is firm, grey-white, with foci of haemorrhage and necrosis.

Histopathology

DSRCT is characterized by variably sized and shaped, sharply outlined nests of small neoplastic cells, usually surrounded by a prominent desmoplastic stroma. Central necrosis is common and cystic degeneration can also be seen. Some tumours focally exhibit epithelial differentiation, with glands or a rosette pattern. The tumour cells are typically uniform with small hyperchromatic nuclei, scant cytoplasm and indistinct cytoplasmic borders. In a subset of cases, tumour cells can show intracytoplasmic eosinophilic rhabdoid inclusions. Some tumours have larger cells with greater pleomorphism. Mitoses are frequent and individual cell necrosis is common. The desmoplastic stroma is composed of fibroblasts or myofibroblasts embedded in a loose extracellular material or collagen. Prominent stromal vascularity is also present, ranging from complex capillary tufts to larger vessels with eccentric thickened walls.

Immunophenotype

DSRCT shows a distinctive and complex pattern of multi-phenotypic differentiation, expressing proteins associated with epithelial, muscular and neural differentiation. Most cases are immunoreactive for keratins, EMA, vimentin, desmin and NSE. Distinctive dot-like staining is seen with desmin and occasionally with other intermediate filaments. Myogenin and MyoD1 are consistently negative. Nuclear expression of WT1 (using antibodies to the

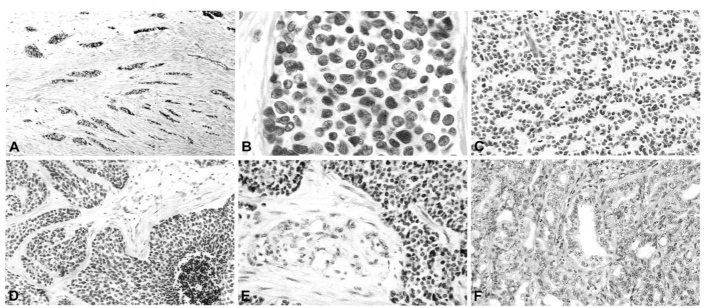

Fig. 12.72 Desmoplastic small round cell tumour. **A** Infiltrative growth pattern and "indian-file" appearance. **B** Small round cells with minimal nuclear pleomorphism. **C** Rosette formation. **D** Focal necrosis. **E** Glomeruloid vascular proliferation. **F** Epithelial features with gland formation.

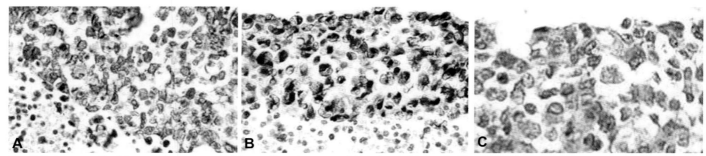

Fig. 12.73 Immunoprofile of desmoplastic small round cell tumour. Strong immunoreactivity for keratin (**A**), desmin (**B**) and NSE (**C**).

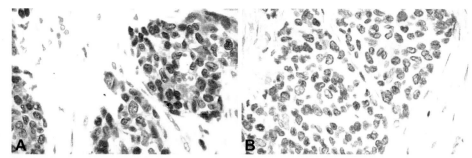

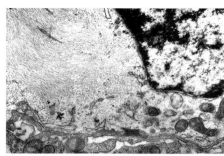

Fig. 12.74 Immunodetection of EWSR1-WT1 chimeric protein in desmoplastic small round cell tumour. **A** Strong nuclear reactivity with the WT1 (C19) antibody directed to the carboxy terminus of WT1. **B** No reactivity with the WT1 antibody directed to the amino terminus of WT1.

Fig. 12.75 Ultrastructure of desmoplastic small round cell tumour demonstrates neoplastic cells with typical whorls of intermediate filaments and well-formed desmosome junctional structures.

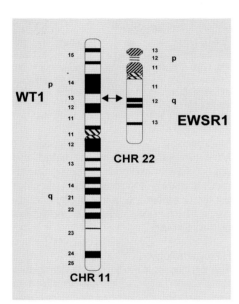

Fig. 12.76 Diagrammatic representation of chromosomal breakpoints in desmoplastic small round cell tumour with t(11;22)(p13;q12) translocation.

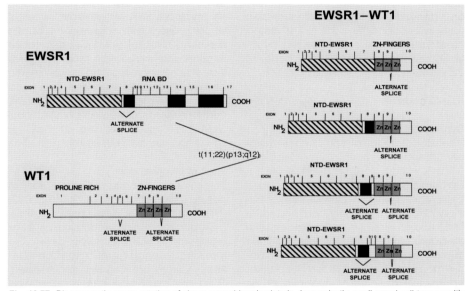

Fig. 12.77 Diagrammatic representation of chromosomal breakpoints in desmoplastic small round cell tumour with *EWSR1-WT1* fusion transcripts. All chromosome 11 breakpoints involve intron 7 of *WT1*, suggesting that the preservation of the last three zinc-finger motifs of *WT1* is crucial to sarcomagenesis. The majority of chromosome 22 breakpoints involve intron 7 of *EWSR1* and, infrequently, introns 8 and 9.

carboxy-terminus but not the amino-terminus) is usually seen {152,1176}. The stromal component is positive for SMA, suggesting myofibroblastic origin.

Ultrastructure
Most cells have a primitive/undifferentiated appearance with small amounts of cytoplasm and scant organelles. A notable feature is the presence of paranuclear aggregates and whorls of intermediate filaments. Rare dense-core granules can be seen occasionally. Few cells are connected by cell junction complexes, including well-formed desmosomes.

Genetics
DSRCT is characterized by a recurrent chromosomal translocation t(11;22)(p13;q12) {225,2353,2451}, resulting in the fusion of the *EWSR1* gene in 22q12 and the Wilms tumour gene, *WT1*, in 11p13 {587,964, 1523}. The most common chimeric transcript comprises an in-frame fusion of the first 7 exons of *EWSR1*, encoding the potential transcription modulating domain, and exons 8–10 of *WT1*, encoding the last three zinc fingers of the DNA-binding domain. Rare variants including additional exons of *EWSR1* can also occur {80}. Detection of the *EWSR1-WT1* gene fusion can be especially useful in cases with unusual clinical or histological features {962}.

Studies of the EWSR1-WT1 aberrant transcription factor have revealed deregulation of several target genes {961}.
Interestingly, the serosal lining of body cavities, the most common site of DSRCT, has high transient fetal expression of the *WT1* gene. EWSR1-WT1 is expressed in tissues derived from the intermediate mesoderm, primarily those undergoing transition from mesenchyme to epithelium {2272,2291}. This pattern recapitulates the epithelial differentiation noted in DSRCT.

Prognostic factors
Overall survival is poor, despite multimodality therapy {1530,2239}.

Extrarenal rhabdoid tumour

Y. Oda
J.A. Biegel

Definition
A highly malignant soft tissue tumour, mainly affecting infants and children, which consists of characteristic rounded or polygonal neoplastic cells with glassy eosinophilic cytoplasm containing hyaline-like inclusion bodies, eccentric nuclei and macronucleoli. Morphologically and genetically identical tumours also arise in the kidney and brain. The majority of tumours are characterized by alterations of the *SMARCB1* gene in 22q11.2.

ICD-O code   8963/3

Synonyms
Rhabdoid tumour of soft tissue; malignant rhabdoid tumour

Epidemiology
Extrarenal rhabdoid tumour is exceedingly rare, and is largely confined to infants and children since the diagnosis of rhabdoid tumour requires the exclusion of other overlapping entities with rhabdoid morphology {1452,2092}. Like other aggressive paediatric tumours such as rhabdomyosarcoma and neuroblastoma, congenital disseminated tumours with a rapid and fatal clinical course have been reported {2949}. Among fetal and neonatal rhabdoid tumours, the extrarenal rhabdoid tumour is more common than those in kidney or brain {1288}.

Etiology
There are no specific predisposing factors for sporadic tumours. Familial cases are typically associated with germline mutations in the *SMARCB1* gene (*INI1, hSNF5* or *BAF47*) in 22q11.2 {228,277, 719,2516,2876}. Germline mutations or deletions in *SMARCB1* may be present in as many as 35% of patients, most of whom present with apparently sporadic disease {277,719}. All newly diagnosed patients with rhabdoid tumours, regardless of anatomical location or age, should be offered genetic testing to rule out a germline *SMARCB1* mutation or deletion. Furthermore, families with constitutional *SMARCB1* mutations are at risk for schwannomatosis {389,2692}.

Sites of involvement
This tumour seems to arise frequently in deep, axial locations {809,1452,2093, 2798} such as the neck, paraspinal region, perineal region, abdominal cavity or retroperitoneum, and pelvic cavity. Extremities, especially the thigh, or cutaneous lesions are also well-documented. This tumour also often affects visceral organs such as the liver, thymus, genitourinary tracts and gastrointestinal system. The liver appears to be the most common visceral location {276}.

Clinical features
Most present as a rapidly enlarging soft tissue mass {1236}. Occasional cases present with multiple cutaneous nodules.

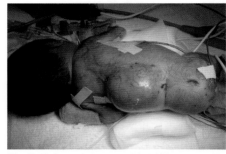

Fig. 12.78 Congenital extrarenal rhabdoid tumour. In this neonatal patient, a huge paravertebral and retroperitoneal tumour is evident. Multiple metastatic lesions were also identified at birth.

Macroscopy
Most tumours are unencapsulated and are > 5 cm in maximum diameter. The tumour is usually soft, grey to tan in colour on its cut surface, and frequently accompanied by foci of coagulative and haemorrhagic necrosis.

Histopathology
The tumour is characterized by "rhabdoid cells" with large, vesicular, rounded to bean-shaped nuclei, prominent nucleoli, and abundant cytoplasm, arranged in sheets or in a solid trabecular pattern. Many tumour cells have juxtanuclear eosinophilic, PAS-positive, diastase-resistant hyaline inclusions or globules. At the periphery, tumour cells infiltrate surrounding tissue. Nuclear pleomorphism is not evident, while mitotic figures are frequently observed. The tumour often

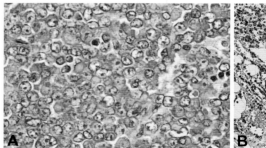
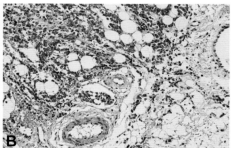

Fig. 12.79 Extrarenal rhabdoid tumour. **A** Characteristic rhabdoid cells with eosinophilic cytoplasm containing glassy inclusion-like bodies, eccentric vesicular nuclei, and prominent nucleoli. **B** Tumour cells are infiltrating the surrounding fibro-adipose tissue.

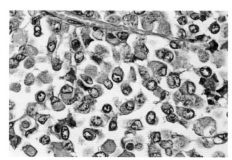

Fig. 12.80 Extrarenal rhabdoid tumour. Rhabdoid cells with abundant eosinophilic cytoplasm show a discohesive growth pattern.

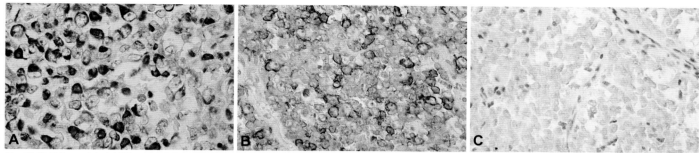

Fig. 12.81 Extrarenal rhabdoid tumour. **A** Strong positive cytoplasmic immunoreactivity for keratin CAM5.2, which is confined to the inclusions. **B** Focal membranous positivity for EMA. **C** Positive nuclear expression of SMARCB1 (INI1) protein is observed in the vascular endothelial cells and inflammatory cells, but completely absent in the tumour cells.

shows loss of cellular cohesion. Some cases demonstrate predominant proliferation of undifferentiated small round cells with only a small number of typical rhabdoid cells. These rhabdoid cells are also focally or diffusely observed in some carcinomas, sarcomas, meningiomas, melanomas, and mesotheliomas {2093}. The proximal-type epithelioid sarcoma is an especially important differential diagnosis, because both tumours have similar morphology, immunohistochemical features, and SMARCB1 gene deletions {1062,1456,1922}. Therefore, ancillary techniques such as immunohistochemistry, ultrastructural studies, and molecular genetic analysis are required to exclude the possibility of other malignant neoplasms with rhabdoid features.

Immunophenotype
Most of these tumours show coexpression of vimentin and epithelial markers such as keratins and EMA {2093}. The expression of neural or neuroectodermal markers such as CD99 and synaptophysin is also frequently observed in soft tissue tumours. Less commonly, the cells express MSA and focal S100 protein. The signifance of these results is uncertain. Extrarenal rhabdoid tumours are characterized by loss of SMARCB1 expression {1201,1208}.

Ultrastructure
The tumour cells show characteristic paranuclear bundles of cytoplasmic filaments. These filaments are approximately 10 nm in diameter and represent intermediate filaments, predominantly composed of keratin (8 and 18), while the filamentous network throughout the cytoplasm is made up of vimentin {1291}. Large globular tangles of intermediate filaments contain

entrapped rough endoplasmic reticulum, mitochondria, and lipid droplets {1452, 2798}.

Genetics
Extrarenal rhabdoid tumours arise as a consequence of homozygous inactivation of the SMARCB1 gene in chromosome band 22q11.2 {228,2876}. Approximately 98% of extrarenal rhabdoid tumours, malignant rhabdoid tumour of kidney (MRTK), and atypical teratoid/rhabdoid tumour (AT/RT) demonstrate genomic alterations of both copies of the gene, including coding-sequence mutations, partial or whole gene deletions, and copy-neutral loss of heterozygosity events that unmask a recessive allele on the remaining homologue {1305}. Extrarenal rhabdoid tumours have a particularly high incidence of homozygous deletions of the SMARCB1 gene. This is often a consequence of a chromosomal translocation between chromosome band 22q11.2 and a variety of different partner chromosomes. FISH, high-resolution genomic microarray or MLPA assays may be used to show that

the translocation is unbalanced at the molecular level, resulting in deletion of SMARCB1. The second allele is usually lost as a result of an interstitial 22q11.2 deletion. Consistent with its function as a classic tumour suppressor gene, initiating germline mutations or deletions in SMARCB1 function as the "first hit" in patients who have a genetic predisposition to the development of rhabdoid tumours. Such patients are also at risk for MRTK and AT/RT. In rare rhabdoid tumours with retained SMARCB1 expression, mutation and/or loss of the SMARCA4 (BRG1) gene in 19p13.2 {2471} has been reported.

Prognostic factors
Regardless of location, patient outcome is dismal. Because of its rare incidence, there are no large studies of survival analysis in uniformly treated patients with extrarenal tumours. A recent study described the clinical presentation and treatment for 26 patients. The median age was 28 months, and overall 5-year survival was < 15% {276}. Many patients have metastases at presentation.

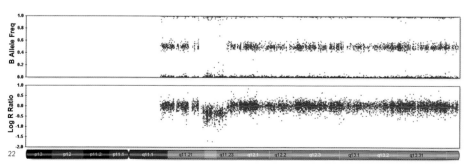

Fig. 12.82 Extrarenal rhabdoid tumour. Single nucleotide polymorphism array analysis (Illumina 610K Beadchip) showing a deletion in 22q11.23 in a patient with a rhabdoid tumour.

PEComa

J.L. Hornick
C.-C. Pan

Definition

Neoplasms with perivascular epithelioid-cell differentiation (PEComas) are mesenchymal tumours composed of distinctive cells that show a focal association with blood vessel walls and usually express melanocytic and smooth-muscle markers. The PEComa family includes angiomyolipoma (AML), clear cell "sugar" tumour of the lung (CCST), lymphangioleiomyomatosis (LAM), and a group of histologically and immunophenotypically similar tumours arising at a variety of soft-tissue and visceral sites {887,1221,1740}.

ICD-O codes

PEComa	8714/0
Malignant PEComa	8714/3

Synonyms

Clear cell myomelanocytic tumour; monotypic epithelioid angiomyolipoma

Epidemiology

PEComas other than AML and LAM are rare, with about 200 reported cases {267, 886,890,2204,2738}. PEComas are markedly more frequent in females than males (female to male ratio, 6 : 1), with a wide age range and a peak in young to middle-aged adults (mean age, 45 years) {887, 890,1221}.

Etiology

Most PEComas other than AML and LAM are sporadic; a small subset is associated with the tuberous sclerosis complex (TSC) {267,890,1223}.

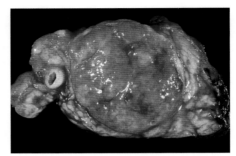

Fig. 12.83 PEComa. This pancreatic tumour is grossly well circumscribed with a fleshy cut surface.

Sites of involvement

PEComas show a wide anatomical distribution, but most often arise in the retroperitoneum, abdominopelvic region, uterus, and gastrointestinal tract {886, 890,2853}. Sclerosing PEComas arise most frequently in the retroperitoneum {1223}. PEComas may also arise in somatic soft tissue, skin, and bone {1616, 1842,3016}.

Clinical features

PEComas usually present as painless masses. Uterine PEComas may present with vaginal bleeding {890,2853}. Gastrointestinal PEComas may present with haematochezia or abdominal pain.

Macroscopy

PEComas are grossly well-circumscribed with a firm and fibrous or fleshy cut surface. Tumours show a wide size range, with a mean of 5–8 cm {890,1223}.

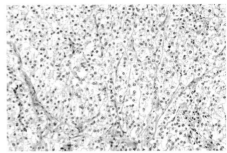

Fig. 12.84 PEComa. Note the typical nested architecture.

Histopathology

PEComas typically show a nested architecture and are usually composed of uniform epithelioid cells with abundant granular eosinophilic or clear cytoplasm and round nuclei with small nucleoli. The nests or trabeculae are typically surrounded by thin-walled capillary vessels. A small subset of tumours is dominated by spindle cells {886}. Focal association with blood vessel walls, with a radial arrangement of tumour cells and subendothelial growth, is a typical feature. Uterine PEComas may show an infiltrative growth pattern {2853}. About 15% of PEComas are composed of cords of cells in a densely collagenous stroma (sclerosing PEComas) {1223}. Otherwise typical PEComas may contain occasional multinucleate cells and show limited pleomorphism, but mitotic figures are usually scarce or absent {890}.
Malignant PEComas are characterized by mitotic activity, necrosis, marked nuclear atypia, and pleomorphism {267,890,1221}.

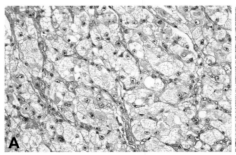

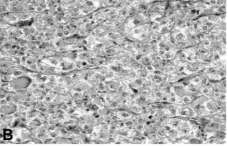

Fig. 12.85 PEComa. **A** The epithelioid tumour cells contain abundant clear cytoplasm. **B** Some tumours are composed of cells with granular eosinophilic cytoplasm. Note the trabecular architecture and prominent thin-walled vessels.

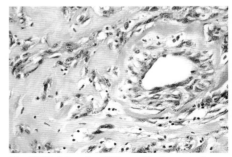

Fig. 12.86 Sclerosing PEComa. The tumour cells are focally situated within the wall of a dilated blood vessel.

Immunophenotype

PEComas typically express melanocytic markers, such as HMB45 (the most sensitive), Melan-A, and MITF, and muscle markers, such as SMA and calponin {887, 890,1221}. Desmin and h-caldesmon are less often extensively positive {1221, 1223}. Some tumours lack expression of muscle markers {887}. About 10% of tumours show focal expression of S100 protein. About 10% of cases show strong nuclear staining for TFE3 {94,890}.

Ultrastructure

Tumour cells contain abundant cytoplasmic glycogen; pre-melanosomes, thin filaments with occasional dense bodies, hemidesmosomes, and poorly formed intercellular junctions may also be detected {886,2738}.

Genetics

A CGH study of nine renal and extrarenal PEComas showed a variety of losses and gains {2154}. LOH was found in 11 PEComas and involved the *TSC2* locus in 7 cases {2153}. Deletion of 16p, the location of the *TSC2* gene, indicates the oncogenetic relationship of PEComas with AML as a *TSC2*-linked neoplasm. A subset of PEComas harbours a *TFE3* gene fusion {94}, which correlates with strong nuclear immunoreactivity. One case arising in the colon showed a *SFPQ-TFE3* gene fusion {2714}. The presence of a t(3;10)(?p13;?q13) has been reported in one cytogenetically analysed case {886}.

Prognostic factors

Owing to their rarity, firm minimal criteria for malignancy in PEComas have not been established. Clinically malignant PEComas are typically large, usually show marked nuclear atypia, pleomorphism, readily identified mitoses, necrosis, and infiltrative margins, and often pursue an aggressive clinical course {887,890, 1221}. PEComas lacking these features only rarely metastasize. The most common metastatic sites are the liver, lymph nodes, lungs, and bone.

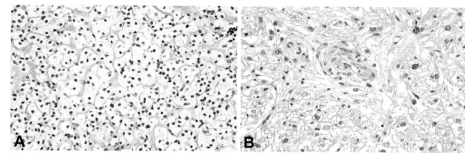

Fig. 12.87 PEComa. **A** This tumour is composed of small nests of clear cells with small round nuclei and sharply defined cell borders ("sugar" tumour). **B** A tumour with a sheet-like growth pattern. Note the granular to clear cytoplasm and uniform nuclear morphology.

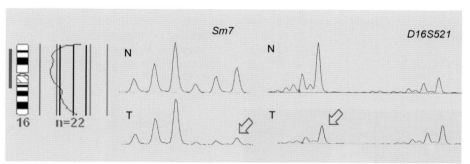

Fig. 12.88 Loss of chromosome arm 16p demonstrated by CGH and loss of heterozygosity analysis using microsatellite markers *Sm7* and *D16S521*, which flank the locus of the *TSC2* gene.

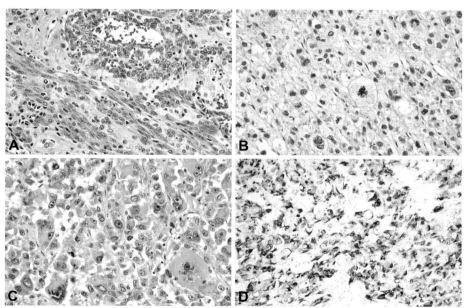

Fig. 12.89 PEComa. **A** Some tumours show spindle cell morphology. **B** Malignant PEComa composed of epithelioid tumour cells with clear cytoplasm, nuclear atypia, and mitotic activity. Note the trabecular architecture. **C** A malignant PEComa with marked nuclear atypia and pleomorphism. Note the abundant granular eosinophilic cytoplasm. **D** Expression of HMB45 is a characteristic feature.

Intimal sarcoma

B. Bode-Lesniewska
M. Debiec-Rychter

Definition

Intimal sarcomas are malignant mesenchymal tumours arising in large blood vessels of the systemic and pulmonary circulation. The defining feature is predominantly intraluminal growth with obstruction of the lumen of the vessel of origin and the seeding of emboli to peripheral organs.

ICD-O code   9137/3

Epidemiology

Intimal sarcomas are very rare tumours, pulmonary intimal sarcomas being almost twice as common as tumours of aortic origin {261,346,652,2212,2500}. Pulmonary intimal sarcomas are slightly more common in females (sex ratio, 1.3), while aortic tumours occur equally frequently in males and females. Mean age at time of diagnosis is 48 years for pulmonary tumours and 62 years for aortic intimal sarcomas {346}.

Sites of involvement

Intimal sarcomas of the pulmonary circulation mainly involve the proximal vessels and are frequently located in the pulmonary trunk (80%), right or left main pulmonary arteries (50–70%), or both (40%) {346,347,2070}. Some tumours also involve the pulmonary valve or extend into the right ventricular outflow tract. Direct infiltration or lung metastases are observed in 40% of patients, while extrathoracic spread occurs in 20% of cases, involving lungs, kidneys, lymph nodes, brain and skin {346,347}. Aortic intimal sarcomas mostly arise in the abdominal aorta between the celiac artery and the iliac bifurcation and approximately 30% are located in the descending thoracic aorta {346,2439,2500}.

Clinical features

The clinical presentation is often nonspecific and related to tumour emboli {920, 2457,3079}. Proper diagnosis is often delayed or made post mortem. In pulmonary intimal sarcomas, recurrent pulmonary embolic disease is the most common primary diagnosis. Intimal sarcomas of the aorta commonly present with consequences of emboli (claudication, absent pulses, back pain, abdominal angina, malignant hypertension, rupture of aneurysm formed by the tumour) {2012,2056}. Conventional imaging methods are often disappointingly nonspecific, but the neoplastic nature of the tissue occluding the lumen can be suspected in modern diagnostic procedures (CT, MRI, PET) {2139, 2478,2755,2976}.

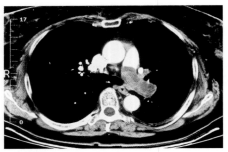

Fig. 12.90 Intimal sarcoma. Chest CT of a patient with an intimal sarcoma of the left pulmonary artery.

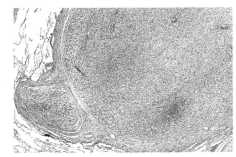

Fig. 12.91 Intimal sarcoma. Spreading of the tumour along the intrapulmonary branches of the pulmonary artery {261}.

Macroscopy

Intimal sarcomas by definition are mostly intravascular polypoid masses attached to the vessel wall, grossly resembling thrombi and extending distally along the branches of the involved vessels. Occasionally a mucoid lumen cast can be recovered intraoperatively or harder, bony areas corresponding to osteosarcomatous differentiation are found. Some of the aortic tumours may cause thinning and aneurysmal dilatation of the vessel wall

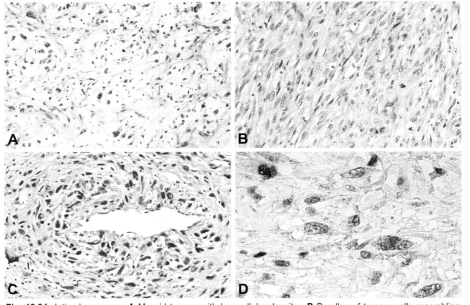

Fig. 12.94 Intimal sarcoma. A Myxoid tumour with low cellular density. B Bundles of tumour cells resembling leiomyosarcoma. C An endothelially lined vascular cleft surrounded by pleomorphic tumour cells. D Nuclear immunoexpression of MDM2 protein in numerous tumour cells.

with adherent thrombotic material suggesting atherosclerotic changes, particularly in the abdominal aorta.

Histopathology

Intimal sarcomas are usually poorly differentiated mesenchymal malignant tumours, consisting of mildly to severely atypical spindle cells with varying degrees of mitotic activity, necrosis and nuclear polymorphism. Some tumours show large myxoid areas or epithelioid morphology {1002,2500}. Prominent spindling and bundling may resemble leiomyosarcoma. Rare cases may contain areas of rhabdomyo- or osteosarcomatous differentiation {346,347,1002,1231,2070}.

Immunophenotype

Variable positivity for SMA has been observed and some tumours exhibit positive staining for desmin. Nuclear expression of MDM2 can be observed in up to 70% of cases {261,652}. In a typical case of intimal sarcoma, endothelial markers are negative {1231,2439,2500}.

Genetics

Using CGH and microarray-based CGH, gain or amplification of the 12q12–15 region (containing the *CDK4*, *TSPAN31*, *MDM2*, and *GLI* genes) and 4q12 were reported as the most constant genetic aberrations {261,3059,3065}. Interphase FISH analysis revealed amplification of *PDGFRA* and *KIT (CD117)* and amplification/polysomy of *EGFR* in all and six out of eight tumours, respectively {2709}. In a recent high-resolution CGH array study, six of eight tumours showed 4q12 amplification, with the common region containing only *PDGFRA*. Other, less consistent alterations were gains/amplifications in 7p14–22, 8q11–23, 12p11, 12q13–15 (containing *GLI*, *CDK4*, *DDIT3*, *HMGA2*, *BEST3* and *MDM2*) and losses in 3q12–21, 9p21 (homozygous loss of *CDKN2A/CDKN2B* in three tumours), 10q22, 12q12 and 12q23. Frequent high-level (co)amplifications or gains of the *PDGFRA* (in 81%), *EGFR* (in 76%), and/or *MDM2* (in 65%) genes were confirmed in 21 tumours by FISH analysis {652}.

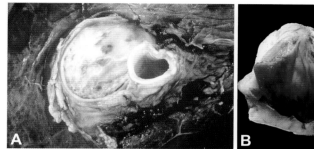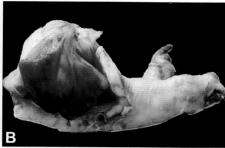

Fig. 12.93 Intimal sarcoma. **A** View of the hilum of the resected lung of a patient with obstruction of the lumen of the pulmonary artery by tumour tissue. **B** Endarterectomy specimen of another patient with intimal sarcoma of the pulmonary artery.

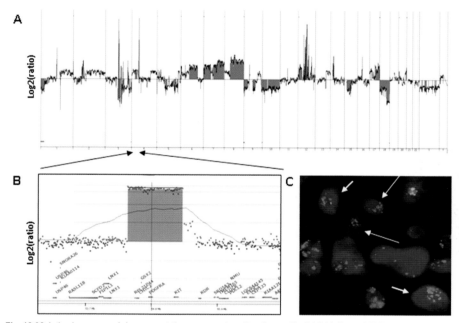

Fig. 12.92 Intimal sarcoma. **A** A representative copy number alteration profile (244K Agilent aCGH), showing high-level amplification of *PDGFRA*/4q12 and *MDM2*/12q14–15 regions, gain of 6q, 7, 8q, 12p and 17q, and partial/total losses of 1p, 3q, 5q, 9p, 10, 15q, 18 and X. The individual probes are arranged according to their genomic location (*x* axis) and their respective tumour/reference log2 ratios (*y* axis). **B** aCGH profile of a selected region of chromosome band 4q12, showing high-level amplification of genes *CHIC2*, *PDGFRA* and *KIT*. **C** Representative example of dual-colour interphase FISH images of intimal sarcoma, showing exclusive high-level amplification of *PDGFRA* (red signals; long arrows) or *MDM2* (green signals; short arrows), intermingled with cells showing separate amplicons for both genes.

Prognostic factors

The prognosis for patients with intimal sarcomas is poor, with mean survival of about 5–9 months in patients with aortic sarcomas and 13–18 months in patients with pulmonary sarcomas {261,346,2070, 2212,2503}.

CHAPTER 13

Undifferentiated/unclassified sarcomas

Undifferentiated/unclassified sarcomas

C.D.M. Fletcher
F. Chibon
F. Mertens

Definition
A soft tissue sarcoma showing no identifiable line of differentiation when analysed by presently available technology. At present, this is a heterogeneous group and a diagnosis of exclusion, although genetic subgroups are emerging. Not included are dedifferentiated types of specific soft tissue sarcoma, in which the dedifferentiated component is commonly undifferentiated.

ICD-O codes
Undifferentiated round cell sarcoma   8803/3
Undifferentiated spindle cell sarcoma   8801/3
Undifferentiated pleomorphic sarcoma 8802/3
Undifferentiated epithelioid sarcoma   8804/3
Undifferentiated sarcoma,
   not otherwise specified   8805/3

Epidemiology
Undifferentiated soft tissue sarcomas (USTS) are uncommon mesenchymal neoplasms that are anatomically ubiquitous and occur at all ages with no difference between the sexes. USTS account for up to 20% of all soft tissue sarcomas. Those with round cell morphology are most frequent in young patients and may ultimately prove to be specific entities; those that are pleomorphic (often known as pleomorphic malignant fibrous histiocytoma in the past) occur mostly in older adults.

Etiology
The etiology of most USTS is unknown. However, at least 25% of radiation-associated soft tissue sarcomas are undifferentiated {987,1555}.

Sites of involvement
USTS may be found at any location. Published data are limited but, overall, it seems that these lesions are most common in somatic soft tissue.

Clinical features
USTS has no characteristic clinical features that would distinguish it from other types of sarcoma, other than a frequently rapid growth rate.

Macroscopy
USTSs are a heterogenous group and thus have no distinctive macroscopic features, other than the frequent presence of necrosis.

Histopathology
USTS may be broadly divided into pleomorphic, spindle cell, round cell and epithelioid subsets, but none have specific defining features other than their lack of an identifiable line of differentiation {861}. Pleomorphic USTS closely resembles other specific types of pleomorphic sarcoma and is often patternless, with frequent bizarre multinucleate tumour giant cells.

Spindle cell USTS most often shows a fascicular architecture with variably amphophilic or palely eosinophilic cytoplasm and tapering nuclei. Round cell USTS consist of relatively uniform rounded or ovoid cells with a high nuclear to cytoplasmic ratio and most often closely resembles other specific types of round cell sarcoma, especially Ewing sarcoma. USTS with epithelioid morphology has been little studied as yet {2421}, but is probably not rare. Morphologically these lesions closely resemble metastatic carcinoma or melanoma, but generally lack nesting and have amphophilic or palely eosinophilic cytoplasm and large vesicular nuclei. Importantly, genomic profiling may reveal that some seemingly undifferentiated sarcomas can be classified more specifically {379,496,498,1904}.

Immunophenotype
As defined, USTS shows no reproducible immunophenotype, nor any pattern of protein expression that would allow more specific subclassification. However, USTS may often show small numbers of cells that may express keratin, actin, desmin or EMA and there may be patchy positivity for CD99 in round cell neoplasms. Vimentin and CD34 may be positive, but have no discriminatory value.

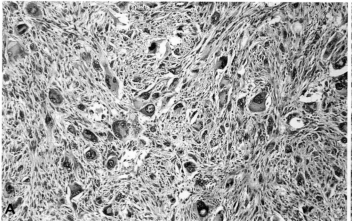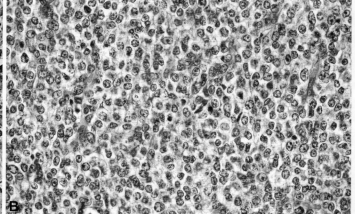

Fig. 13.1 Undifferentiated sarcoma. **A** Pleomorphic morphology. **B** Round cell morphology.

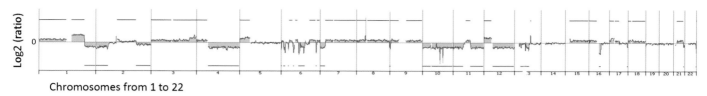

Fig. 13.2 Array-based CGH profile of an undifferentiated pleomorphic sarcoma. Gains and losses of genetic material are over and below the baseline (Log2 [ratio] = 0), respectively.

Ultrastructure

As defined, USTS shows no evidence of any specific line of differentiation by electron microscopy.

Genetics

Undifferentiated round cell and spindle cell sarcomas

Small round cell sarcomas in which *EWSR1* is involved in non-ETS fusions with genes such as *PATZ1*, *POU5F1*, *SMARCA5*, *NFATC2* or *SP3* are often simply classified as undifferentiated or poorly differentiated round cell sarcoma (round cell USTS) rather than Ewing sarcoma {638,1915,2894}. The number of cases with such fusions is, however, still small and it remains to be seen whether they represent one or more separate entities, or whether they are better classified as variants of Ewing sarcoma. *CIC-DUX4* is another recurrent gene fusion, resulting from a t(4;19)(q35;q13) or a t(10;19)(q26;q13), associated with paediatric round cell USTS {1299,1383, 2335, 3039}. Although the genes involved in the fusion are different from those in Ewing sarcoma, the chimeric *CIC-DUX4* protein has been shown to upregulate genes of the PEA3 subclass of the ETS family of genes, thus providing a molecular link between Ewing sarcoma and round cell USTS showing *EWSR1-ETV1* and *EWSR1-*

ETV4 fusions {1383}. In contrast, there are strong arguments, e.g. from gene-expression profiling, to suggest that Ewing-like sarcomas with the *BCOR-CCNB3* fusion, arising from an inversion of the X-chromosome, represent a separate and distinct entity {2243}. Most cases described above are presently treated in the same way as Ewing sarcoma. A number of other so-far non-recurrent and molecularly uncharacterized balanced chromosome aberrations, as well as numerical changes, have been detected in paediatric round cell USTS or spindle cell USTS {30,34,1483,2508,2682}.

Undifferentiated pleomorphic sarcomas

The genetic aspects of undifferentiated pleomorphic soft tissue sarcoma (pleomorphic USTS) are difficult to evaluate because of the shifting diagnostic criteria used throughout the years. Bearing these shortcomings in mind, cytogenetic aberrations have been detected in more than 70 cases published as storiform or pleomorphic malignant fibrous histiocytoma (MFH), MFH of no specified type (NST), pleomorphic sarcoma, or undifferentiated pleomorphic sarcoma {1915}. In general, the karyotypes tend to be highly complex, and complete descriptions of all aberrations are rare. Extensive intercellular

variation, frequent telomeric associations and coexistence of several ploidy levels show that these tumours are genetically highly unstable and no specific recurrent aberration has been identified {864,1915, 2132}. All chromosomes are involved in structural rearrangements, particularly chromosomes 1, 3, 5, 7, 9, 11, and 12. Cytogenetic signs of gene amplification are seen in close to 30% of the cases, ring chromosomes and double minutes being equally common. It should be noted that undifferentiated sarcomas with 12q14–15 amplification including *MDM2* and *CDK4* are now classified as dedifferentiated liposarcomas {443,498}.

Data obtained from chromosome- and array-based CGH analyses reinforce the concept that pleomorphic USTS is characterized by complex combinations of chromosomal gains and losses, and have refined the mapping of imbalances. Practically all chromosome arms are affected by imbalances, with losses clustering to 1q, 2p, 2q, 8p, 9p, 10q, 11q, 13q, and 16q, and gains to 1p, 1q, 5p, 7p, 7q, 9q, 14q, 17p, 19q, and 20q {379,444,1485, 2561}. Further studies, using directed gene- and protein-level analyses as well as global gene expression profiling, have shown that potential target genes in frequently deleted regions include *RB1* on

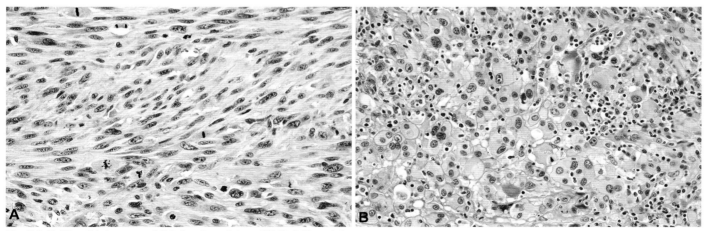

Fig. 13.3 Undifferentiated sarcoma. **A** Spindle cell morphology. **B** Epithelioid morphology.

13q, *TP53* on 17p, *CDKN2A* and *CDKN2B* on 9p, and *PTEN* on 10q; the TP53 and RB1 pathways are inactivated in virtually all pleomorphic USTS {444,975,2221}. The chromosomal complexity characterizing these sarcomas is associated with over-expression of a limited number of genes involved in the control of mitosis and chromosome integrity, as well as tumour aggressiveness {443}.

Prognostic factors

Because of the lack of substantive studies, data are limited. The majority of USTSs are morphologically high grade. Among pleomorphic sarcomas in adults, those that are undifferentiated and arise in limbs or trunk have a reported 5-year metastasis-free survival rate of 83% {866}. USTS with epithelioid morphology seems to be more aggressive {2421}. Reported survival for USTS, whether of round cell or spindle cell/pleomorphic type, in children, is 70–75% {33,2203,2598}.

WHO Classification of
Tumours of Bone

WHO classification of tumours of bone[a,b]

CHONDROGENIC TUMOURS

Benign
Osteochondroma	9210/0
Chondroma	9220/0
Enchondroma	9220/0
Periosteal chondroma	9221/0
Osteochondromyxoma	9211/0*
Subungual exostosis	9213/0*
Bizarre parosteal osteochondromatous proliferation	9212/0*
Synovial chondromatosis	9220/0

Intermediate (locally aggressive)
Chondromyxoid fibroma	9241/0
Atypical cartilaginous tumour/ Chondrosarcoma grade I	9222/1*

Intermediate (rarely metastasizing)
Chondroblastoma	9230/1*

Malignant
Chondrosarcoma	
Grade II, grade III	9220/3
Dedifferentiated chondrosarcoma	9243/3
Mesenchymal chondrosarcoma	9240/3
Clear cell chondrosarcoma	9242/3

OSTEOGENIC TUMOURS

Benign
Osteoma	9180/0
Osteoid osteoma	9191/0

Intermediate (locally aggressive)
Osteoblastoma	9200/0

Malignant
Low-grade central osteosarcoma	9187/3
Conventional osteosarcoma	9180/3
Chondroblastic osteosarcoma	9181/3
Fibroblastic osteosarcoma	9182/3
Osteoblastic osteosarcoma	9180/3
Telangiectatic osteosarcoma	9183/3
Small cell osteosarcoma	9185/3
Secondary osteosarcoma	9184/3
Parosteal osteosarcoma	9192/3
Periosteal osteosarcoma	9193/3
High-grade surface osteosarcoma	9194/3

FIBROGENIC TUMOURS

Intermediate (locally aggressive)
Desmoplastic fibroma of bone	8823/1*

Malignant
Fibrosarcoma of bone	8810/3

FIBROHISTIOCYTIC TUMOURS

Benign fibrous histiocytoma/ Non-ossifying fibroma	8830/0

HAEMATOPOIETIC NEOPLASMS

Malignant
Plasma cell myeloma	9732/3
Solitary plasmacytoma of bone	9731/3
Primary non-Hodgkin lymphoma of bone	9591/3

OSTEOCLASTIC GIANT CELL RICH TUMOURS

Benign
Giant cell lesion of the small bones	

Intermediate (locally aggressive, rarely metastasizing)
Giant cell tumour of bone	9250/1

Malignant
Malignancy in giant cell tumour of bone	9250/3

NOTOCHORDAL TUMOURS

Benign
Benign notochordal tumour	9370/0*

Malignant
Chordoma	9370/3

VASCULAR TUMOURS

Benign
Haemangioma	9120/0

Intermediate (locally aggressive, rarely metastasizing)
Epithelioid haemangioma	9125/0

Malignant
Epithelioid haemangioendothelioma	9133/3
Angiosarcoma	9120/3

MYOGENIC TUMOURS

Benign
Leiomyoma of bone   8890/0

Malignant
Leiomyosarcoma of bone   8890/3

LIPOGENIC TUMOURS

Benign
Lipoma of bone   8850/0

Malignant
Liposarcoma of bone   8850/3

TUMOURS OF UNDEFINED NEOPLASTIC NATURE

Benign
Simple bone cyst
Fibrous dyplasia   8818/0*
Osteofibrous dysplasia
Chondromesenchymal hamartoma
Rosai-Dorfman disease

Intermediate (locally aggressive)
Aneurysmal bone cyst   9260/0*
Langerhans cell histiocytosis
   Monostotic   9752/1*
   Polystotic   9753/1*
Erdheim-Chester disease   9750/1*

MISCELLANEOUS TUMOURS

Ewing sarcoma   9364/3
Adamantinoma   9261/3
Undifferentiated high-grade pleomorphic
  sarcoma of bone   8830/3

ª The morphology codes are from the International Classification of Diseases for Oncology (ICD-O) {916A}. Behaviour is coded /0 for benign tumours, /1 for un-specified, borderline or uncertain behaviour, /2 for carcinoma in situ and grade III intraepithelial neoplasia, and /3 for malignant tumours; ᵇ The classification is modified from the previous WHO histological classification of tumours {870A} taking into account changes in our understanding of these lesions. * These new codes were approved by the IARC/WHO Committee for ICD-O in 2012.

TNM classification of bone sarcomas

T – Primary tumour

TX	Primary tumour cannot be assessed
T0	No evidence of primary tumour
T1	Tumour 8 cm or less in greatest dimension
T2	Tumour more than 8 cm in greatest dimension
T3	Discontinuous tumours in the primary bone site

N – Regional lymph nodes

NX	Regional lymph nodes cannot be assessed
N0	No regional lymph-node metastasis
N1	Regional lymph-node metastasis

M – Distant metastasis

M0	No distant metastasis
M1	Distant metastasis
	M1a Lung
	M1b Other distant sites

G – Histopathological grading

Translation table for three- and four-grade systems to a two-grade (low grade vs high grade) system

TNM Two-grade system	Three-grade systems	Four-grade systems
Low grade	Grade I	Grade I
		Grade II
High grade	Grade II	Grade III
	Grade III	Grade IV

Note: If grade cannot be assessed, Ewing sarcoma is classified as high grade. If grade cannot be assessed, classify as low grade.

Stage grouping

Stage IA	T1	N0	M0	Low grade
Stage IB	T2–3	N0	M0	Low grade
Stage IIA	T1	N0	M0	High grade
Stage IIB	T2	N0	M0	High grade
Stage III	T3	N0	M0	High grade
Stage IVA	Any T	N0	M1a	Any grade
Stage IVB	Any T	N1	Any M	Any grade
	Any T	Any N	M1b	Any grade

Note: Use N0 for NX. For T1 and T2, use low grade if no grade is stated.

A help-desk for specific questions about the TNM classification is available at http://www.uicc.org.

References

1. American Joint Committee on Cancer (AJCC) Cancer Staging Manual 7th ed. Edge SB, Byrd DR, Compton CC, Fritz AG, Greene FL, Trotti III H. eds. New York: Springer. 2010
2. International Union against Cancer (UICC): TNM classification of malignant tumors 7th ed. Sobin LH, Gospodarowicz MK, Wittekind Ch. eds. Wiley-Blackwell. Oxford. 2010

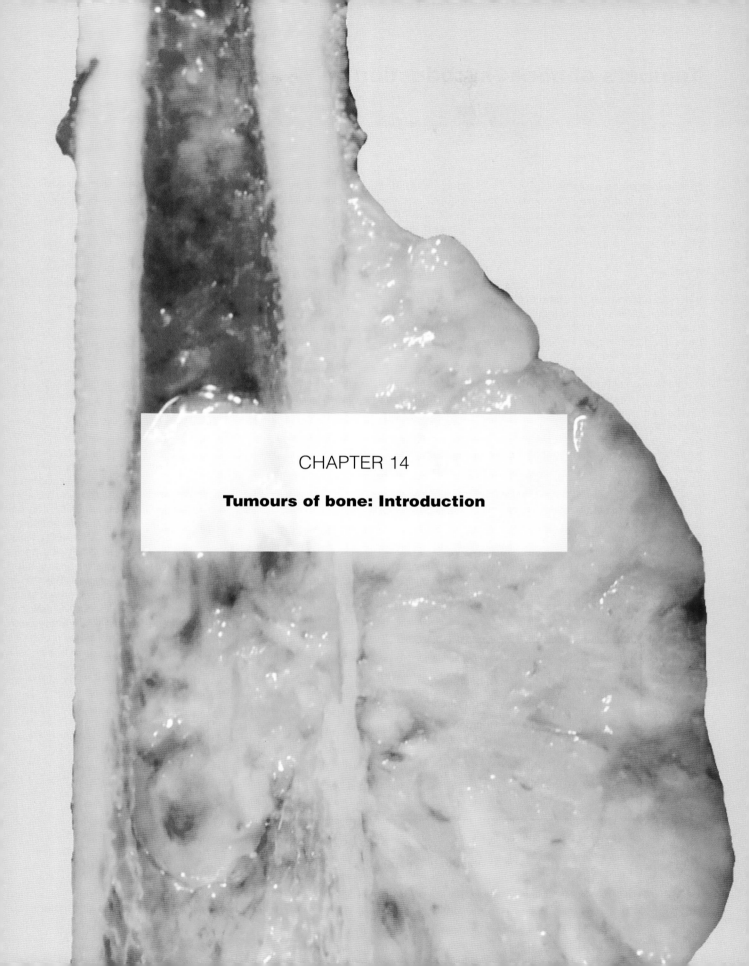

CHAPTER 14

Tumours of bone: Introduction

Tumours of bone: Introduction

R.J. Grimer
P.C.W. Hogendoorn
D. Vanel

Epidemiology and etiology

Among the wide array of human neoplasms, primary tumours of bone are relatively common; however, clinically significant bone neoplasms are infrequent.

Incidence

The true incidence of benign bone tumours is unknown, although older radiographical studies have suggested that a substantial proportion of the population has an indolent lesion. In contrast, bone sarcomas are rare and account for only 0.2% of all neoplasms for which data were obtained in one large series {2020}. Comparison of the incidence rate of bone sarcomas with that of the closely related group of soft tissue sarcomas indicates that osseous neoplasms occur at a rate approximately one tenth that of their soft-tissue counterparts. The overall annual incidence rate for bone sarcomas in North America and Europe is 0.8 per 100 000 population. Somewhat higher incidence rates were reported in Argentina and Brazil (1.5–2) and Israel (1.4) {2190}.
The incidence rates of specific bone sarcomas are age-related and as a group, have a bimodal distribution. The first well-defined peak occurs during the second decade of life, while the second occurs in people aged > 60 years. The risk of development of bone sarcomas during the second decade of life is close to that of the > 60 years population, but in absolute numbers more cases develop in the second decade.

Predisposing lesions

Although the majority of primary bone malignancies appear to arise de novo, it is increasingly apparent that some develop in association with recognizable precursors (Table 14.01). Paget disease, radiation injury, bone infarction, chronic osteomyelitis and certain pre-existing benign tumours are the most clearly established precancerous conditions {23,502,986,1077,1259, 2953,157,916,941,1908,2771}. Recently, attention has been focused on a small number of reported cases of bone sarcoma arising in association with implanted metallic hardware, joint prostheses and bone grafts, but a causal association has not been proven {978,1090,1392,2213, 1270,1392}.

Genetic predisposition

Osteosarcoma, the most frequent primary malignancy of bone, can develop in associ-

Table 14.01 Predispositions for bone tumours

Ollier disease (enchondromatosis) and Maffucci syndrome
Familial retinoblastoma syndrome
Li-Fraumeni syndrome
Rothmund-Thomson syndrome
Multiple osteochondromas
Paget disease
Radiation
Fibrous dysplasia
Bone infarction
Chronic osteomyelitis
Metallic and polyethylene implants
Osteogenesis imperfecta
Giant cell tumour of bone

ation with retinoblastoma, Li-Fraumeni, and Rothmund-Thomson syndromes, among others (Table 27.01). The most frequent familial form of osteosarcoma occurs in the autosomal dominant retinoblastoma syndrome {746,1701,463, 1653, 2025,1102}. Affected family members carry a germline alteration inactivating one of the RB1 gene alleles. The role of the TP53 gene in the development of osteosarcoma is exemplified by its association with the Li-Fraumeni syndrome characterized by TP53 germline mutations {1606,1607,1713,1008}. An increased risk for the development of osteosarcoma has also been identified in families with Rothmund-Thomson syndrome; RECQL4 mutations have been identified in approximately two thirds of Rothmund-Thomson syndrome patients {1430,2896,2897}.

Clinical features

Bone tumours present in a number of different ways:
- Pain
- Swelling
- Pathological fracture
- Loss of use/neurological changes
- Incidental finding.

The most common presentation of a symptomatic benign tumour is an aching pain that is frequently intermittent, but

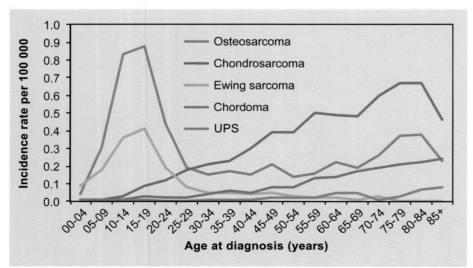

Fig. 14.01 Age-specific incidence rates by histological subtype, all races, both sexes {1973}. UPS, undifferentiated pleomorphic sacoma.

many present for the first time with a pathological fracture in a previously asymptomatic individual (e.g. a fractured humerus through a simple bone cyst). Osteoid osteomas typically present with night pain in the middle of a long bone that is relieved by simple analgesics or anti-inflammatories. Osteochondromas typically present as a painless lump, whilst chondroblastomas typically present with pain and stiffness of the affected joint.

Clinical findings with bone tumours are often very non specific. Swelling and tenderness over the affected bone are the most common findings, but there will be limitation of joint movements if there is either irritation of the joint by the tumour or frank growth of tumour into the joint. Systemic findings are rare in primary bone tumours unless there is disseminated disease, or an associated condition such as multiple osteochondromas, Ollier disease or neurofibromatosis {458}.

Malignant tumours typically present with pain that gradually gets worse and is non-mechanical in nature {2957}. By the time of diagnosis, many patients will be suffering with night pain that will be waking them from sleep. As most bone tumours start inside the bone, swelling only becomes apparent once the cortex is breached and the tumour starts to expand either under or through the periosteum. Swelling is thus a later presentation of bone tumours. The presence of swelling in a limb associated with pain, particularly night pain, should always lead to further investigation. There is clearly a wide differential diagnosis for patients presenting in this manner with the most common diagnoses being:

- Metastases
- Malignant bone tumour
- Benign bone tumour
- Infection
- Haematological disorder.

Obtaining a diagnosis for a symptomatic patient as quickly as possible is essential but delays in diagnosis are frequent {2585}. A simple algorithm based on the most likely diagnosis for a patient of a particular age has been advocated {1038}. This is based on the fact that under the age of 35 years, metastatic carcinoma is uncommon, whilst over that age the likelihood of a bone tumour being a metastasis from a known or undiagnosed carcinoma increases {1712}.

Up to 43% of malignant bone tumours will arise around the knee, but under the age of 20 years this rises to 56% (Table 14.02). Any child or adolescent therefore, with pain and/or swelling around the knee that does not settle, should have the possibility of a bone tumour included in the diagnosis and be investigated.

The second most common site is the pelvis—which is numerically the most common site of presentation for both Ewing sarcoma and chondrosarcoma. Delays in diagnosis here are frequent with symptoms being very non-specific and often long-lasting {2998}. Referred pain to the leg or knee is not infrequent and many patients will have been investigated prior to diagnosis without the possibility of a bone tumour being considered. Night pain again is often the key that should alert the clinician to the possibility of a bone tumour being present.

Pathological fractures in bone tumours are often associated with pre-existing

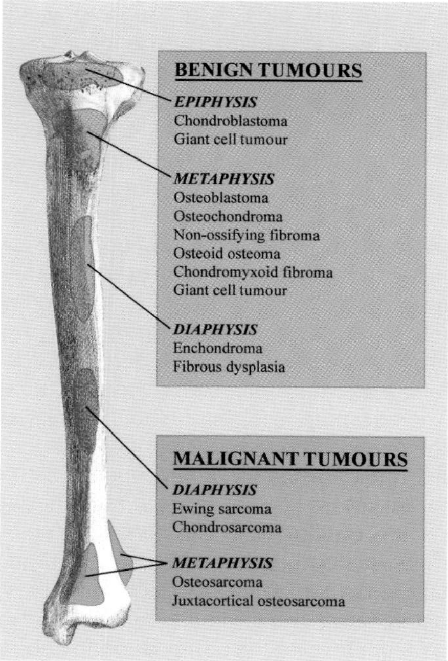

Fig. 14.02 Common spatial distribution in the long bones of benign and malignant primary bone tumours.

symptoms of pain or discomfort in the limb and often minimal force causes the fracture. Awareness of the possibility of a pathological cause for the fracture is essential to prevent inadvertent internal fixation {11}. Usually the history combined with the imaging manifestations are sufficient.

Blood tests are not usually helpful in diagnosing bone tumours, with certain exceptions. The alkaline phosphatase level is raised in around 46% of patients with osteosarcoma (and is a poor prognostic sign) {132}, whilst LDH, ESR and CRP may be raised in Ewing sarcoma and again this is a poor prognostic indicator {130}.

Imaging
Diagnosis
A radiographical differential remains the first step in imaging of bone tumours. In case of diagnostic problems, the next step is CT. MRI is the main imaging modality for local staging, treatment evaluation and detection of recurrences. PET is still under evaluation. Important parameters in imaging evaluation include tumour location, size, margins, type of matrix, and periosteal reaction. Certain tumours are more common in particular bones. Adamantinoma, usually found in adults, selectively involves the anterior cortex of the shaft of the tibia. The most common epiphyseal tumour in childhood is chondroblastoma,

Table 14.02 Most common locations of presentation for primary malignant bone tumours and overall risk of a pathological fracture at time of diagnosis*

	Knee[a] (%)	Hip and pelvis[b] (%)	Shoulder girdle[c] (%)	Lower leg (%)	Upper limb (%)	Trunk[d] (%)	Risk of pathological fracture (%)
Osteosarcoma	66	15	10	5	3	1	9
Chondrosarcoma	17	48	15	4	9	7	12
Ewing sarcoma	22	44	11	13	7	3	6
Undifferentiated pleomorphic sarcoma	41	29	9	5	14	2	16
All diagnoses	43	31	11	7	5	3	10

*Data from 3000 primary malignant bone tumours seen at Royal Orthopaedic Hospital, Birmingham.

[a] Knee tumours include distal femur, proximal tibia and proximal fibula.
[b] Hip and pelvis tumours include pelvis and proximal femur locations.
[c] Shoulder girdle tumours include proximal humerus, scapula and clavicle.
[d] Trunk includes spine, ribs etc.

and after the closure of the epiphyseal plate, giant cell tumour is the most common. Tumour size may provide some insight as to the anticipated behaviour of the lesion. A tumour < 6 cm in greatest dimension is likely to be benign whereas one >6 cm may be benign or malignant. The axis of the lesion is also useful to determine. Tumours are rarely centrally located, such as simple bone cyst. They are most often excentric. A cortical location is necessary to diagnose a non-ossifying fibroma. Finally, the tumour can be a surface lesion e.g. parosteal osteosarcoma. The next step is to determine the limits of the tumour. The patterns of bone destruction indicate the aggressiveness of the lesion. Most lesions appear radiolucent on the radiographs, but some are sclerotic. Arciform calcifications suggest cartilaginous tumours. The pattern of periosteal new bone formation reacting to the tumour crossing the cortex depends upon the progression of the tumour. When the tumour grows slowly, the periosteum has enough time to build a thick layer of bone. When multiple layers of periosteal formation are present, there is probably a succession of fast and slow growth phases of progression. Perpendicular periosteal formations are a very useful radiological sign, strongly suggesting malignancy. The Codman triangle indicates an elevated pe-

Table 14.03. Grading of bone sarcoma {2385}

Grade	Sarcoma type
Grade I	Parosteal osteosarcoma
	Grade I chondrosarcoma
	Clear cell chondrosarcoma
	Low-grade intramedullary osteosarcoma
Grade II	Periosteal osteosarcoma
	Grade II chondrosarcoma
	Classic adamantinoma
	Chordoma
Grade III	Osteosarcoma (conventional, telangiectatic, small cell, secondary, high-grade surface)
	Undifferentiated high-grade pleomorphic sarcoma
	Ewing sarcoma
	Grade III chondrosarcoma
	Dedifferentiated chondrosarcoma
	Mesenchymal chondrosarcoma
	Dedifferentiated chordoma
	Malignancy in giant cell tumour of bone

riosteal reaction, broken by the growth of the tumour. It can be seen in both benign and malignant processes. Cortical disruption and soft-tissue involvement usually indicate aggressiveness. A thin layer of new bone formation, ossified around the tumour, suggests a slow evolution and therefor a benign process, even if the cortex is destroyed. On the contrary, tumour on both sides of a not yet destroyed cortex indicates a very aggressive lesion {328}.

Multiple lesions are seen in chondromas, osteochondromas, Langerhans cell histiocytosis, metastases, vascular tumours, and more rarely in multifocal osteosarcomas and metastatic Ewing sarcoma.

On the basis of clinical and radiological signs, one should first diagnose benign lesions for which a subsequent biopsy may not be necessary: > metaphyseal fibrous defect > fibrous dysplasia > osteochondroma > enchondroma > simple bone cyst > vertebral haemangioma. Radiography is always the starting point. CT provides additional information and is the examination of choice when the tumour is arising in flat bones or axial skeleton. It is the best technique to guide diagnostic needle biopsies and perform radiofrequency ablations {2342,2343}. Small lucency of the cortex, localized involvement of the soft tissues, and thin peripheral periosteal reaction can be seen. CT also allows measurement of the cartilage cap thickness in osteochondroma: the cuff is thin in benign lesions and thick (> 1.5–2 cm in adults) in peripheral chondrosarcomas {1400}. MRI is rarely useful in the diagnosis, but can display fluid levels in blood-filled cavities, especially aneurysmal bone cysts, more accurately than CT {2784}. It can also help diagnose the low signal of fibrous tissue, the high, lobulated signal of cartilage on T2-weighted sequences and the inflammatory reaction around some benign (osteoid osteoma, osteoblastoma, chondroblastoma) and vascular tumours {331}. MRI diffusion, perfusion and spectroscopy have limited diagnostic value {3060}.

Radiographical staging

Focal extent and staging is based on MRI {770}. Bone metastases are best detected on radionuclide bone scans or whole body MRI. Pulmonary metastases are evaluated on chest CT. Its sensitivity is quite good, but specificity remains poor {2241}.

Effectiveness and follow-up of treatment

Some primary malignant tumours are treated with preoperative chemotherapy before removal. MRI provides an accurate study of the tumour volume. Signal decrease on T2-weighted sequences indicates increased ossification or more fibrous tissue in the tumour {1204}. Lack of increase in signal intensity of the lesion after injection of the contrast agent suggests necrosis. MRI with dynamic contrast enhancement may be useful for differentiating post-chemotherapeutic change from viable tumour {593,2837, 2877}, but results are only reliable immediately before surgery, and not after a single cycle of chemotherapy, which would detect changes attributable to treatment {1203}.

Grading and staging
Grading

Bone tumours vary widely in their biological behaviour. Histological grading is an attempt to predict the behaviour of a malignant tumour based on histological features. There is no generally accepted grading system for bone sarcomas and the FNCLCC grading system used in soft tissue sarcomas has never been validated in bone tumours. In bone sarcomas, the histological subtype often determines grade. For instance, Ewing sarcoma, mesenchymal chondrosarcoma and dedifferentiated chondrosarcoma are always considered high grade, and parosteal osteosarcoma is considered low grade. In conventional chondrosarcoma, the grading system as proposed by Evans et al {788} is widely used. Comparable to the system proposed in the Third Edition of the WHO Classification of tumours of soft tissue and bone, a grouping into:
- Benign
- Locally aggressive or rarely metastasizing
- Malignant

is proposed. Definitions of these categories are as follows along the lines of the soft-tissue tumour counterparts:

Benign

Most benign bone tumours have a limited capacity for local recurrence. Those that do recur do so in a non-destructive fashion and are almost always readily cured by complete local excision/curretage.

Intermediate (locally aggressive)

Bone tumours in this category often recur locally and are associated with an infiltrative and locally destructive growth pattern. Lesions in this category do not have any evident potential to metastasize but typically require wide excision with a margin of normal tissue, or application of a local adjuvant in order to ensure local control. The prototypical lesion in this category is grade I chondrosarcoma.

Intermediate (rarely metastasizing)
Bone tumours in this category are often locally aggressive (see above) but, in addition, show the well-documented ability to give rise to distant metastases in occasional cases. The risk of such metastases appears to be < 2% and is not reliably predictable on the basis of histomorphology. Metastasis in such lesions is usually to the lung. Prototypical examples in this category include giant cell tumour of bone.

Malignant
In addition to the potential for locally destructive growth and recurrence, malignant bone tumours (known as bone sarcomas) have a significant risk of distant metastasis, ranging in most instances from 20% to almost 100%, depending upon histological type and grade. Some (but not all) histologically low-grade sarcomas have a metastatic risk of only 2–10%, but such lesions may advance in grade in a local recurrence, and thereby acquire a higher risk of distant spread

(e.g. chondrosarcoma, periostal osteosarcoma). It is important to note, that in this new grouping, the intermediate categories do not correspond to histologically determined intermediate grade in a bone sarcoma (see below), nor do they correspond to the ICD-O /1 category described as uncertain whether benign or malignant. The locally aggressive subset with no metastatic potential, as defined above, are generally given ICD-O /1 codes, while the rarely metastasizing lesions are given ICD-O /3 codes. This categorization is especially useful for categorizing rarely metastasizing tumours, which in essence are considered benign, such as giant cell tumour of bone, and sarcomas, which in practice do not metastasize like atypical cartilaginous tumour/chondrosarcoma grade I. When osteosarcoma, leiomyosarcoma and so-called fibrosarcoma of bone need to be graded, cellularity, i.e. the relative proportion of cells to matrix, and nuclear features of the tumour cells are the most important criteria used for grading. Generally, the higher the grade, the more cellular the tumour. Irregularity of the nuclear contours, enlargement and hyperchromasia of the nuclei are correlated with grade. Mitotic figures and necrosis are additional features useful in grading {788}. While a number of grading systems are used worldwide, a three-tier grading system seems to be most widely used. The sig-

nificance of histological grading is limited by interobserver variability and the fact that the majority of tumours fall into the intermediate range. This resulted in a two-tier system simply designating a tumour as low grade (low and intermediate grade in three-tier system) or high grade (grade 3 and 4 in four-tier system). In general, low-grade lesions have a < 25% risk of metastasis. High-grade lesions have a great risk of local recurrence and > 25% risk of distant spread. Guidelines for reporting and grading of bone tumours are available both from USA as well as European perspectives {2385,1197,1724A, 1270}.

Staging
In bone tumours, TNM staging includes histological subtype, size, continuity, grade, as well as the local and distant spread, in order to estimate the prognosis of the patient. Lymph-node metastases in bone sarcomas are rare. The special staging system adopted by the musculoskeletal society first described by Enneking and co-authors has gained acceptance {2985}. Although staging systems have been described for both benign and malignant bone tumours, the usefulness is primarily in the description of malignant bone tumours {62,2196}.

CHAPTER 15

Chondrogenic tumours

Osteochondroma

Chondromas: enchondroma, periosteal chondroma

Chondromyxoid fibroma

Osteochondromyxoma

Subungual exostosis and bizarre parosteal osteochondromatous proliferation

Synovial chondromatosis

Chondroblastoma

Chondrosarcoma (grades I–III) including primary and secondary variants, and periosteal chondrosarcoma

Dedifferentiated chondrosarcoma

Mesenchymal chondrosarcoma

Clear cell chondrosarcoma

Osteochondroma

J.V.M.G. Bovée
D. Heymann
W. Wuyts

Definition
A benign cartilaginous neoplasm consisting of a cartilage-capped bony projection on the surface of bone, containing a marrow cavity that is continuous with that of the underlying bone.

ICD-O code   9210/0

Synonym
(Osteo)cartilaginous exostosis

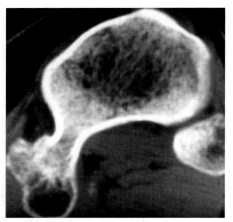

Fig. 15.01 Axial CT of an osteochondroma demonstrating continuity of both the stalk and centre of the lesion with the tibial cortex and medullary cavity, respectively.

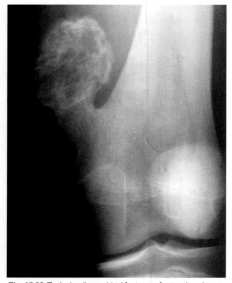

Fig. 15.02 Typical radiographical features of osteochondroma.

Epidemiology
Osteochondroma is one of the most common benign bone tumours {1258,2815}. The reported incidence; 35% of benign and 8% of all surgically removed bone tumours, may be an underestimation as many osteochondromas are asymptomatic and not detected or resected {2815}. Most cases present in the first three decades of life, with males affected slightly more frequently than females. Approximately 15% of presenting patients have multiple lesions characteristic of the autosomal dominant hereditary multiple osteochondromas syndrome (see Chapter 27).

Etiology
Biallelic inactivation of the *EXT1* or *EXT2* gene within the cartilage cap of the majority of sporadic and hereditary osteochondromas supports the neoplastic nature of these lesions. The cell of origin is likely to be a proliferating chondrocyte of the growth plate {1343}. The *EXT* gene products, exostosin-1 and -2, are glycosyl-transferases involved in heparan sulfate (HS) biosynthesis. The cartilage cap of osteochondroma is composed of a mixture of wildtype and mutated (HS-deficient) cells {589,1343,1757}. HS proteoglycans are key modulators of endochondral ossification, forming an osmotic gradient around chondrocytes and controlling signal transduction {1074}. Loss of HS may give the mutated chondrocyte a proliferative advantage, leading to loss of polarity {478,591}. HS is also involved in hedgehog signalling {1472}, and perturbed signalling is thought to cause a defect in formation of the bony collar. As a result, *EXT*-mutated cells may grow out of the bone and recruit normal cells to form an osteochondroma.

Sites of involvement
Osteochondromas arise in bones preformed by endochondral ossification, explaining in part their localization; the most common sites of involvement are the metaphyseal region of the distal femur, upper humerus, proximal tibia and fibula {2815}. Involvement of flat bones is less common.

Clinical and imaging features
Many osteochondromas are asymptomatic and found incidentally. Symptoms often relate to the size and location of the lesion. The most common presentation is a hard mass of long-standing duration. Secondary complications include fracture, bursa formation, arthritis and impingement on adjacent tendons, nerves, vessels or spinal cord {2955}. Increasing pain and/or a growing mass in an adult patient may be a manifestation of malignant transformation to secondary peripheral chondrosarcoma.

Solitary osteochondromas are located at the diaphysis or metaphysis of the bone. Characteristically, the cortex is continuous with the bony stalk and shows normal central trabeculation. Large tumours with thick (> 1.5–2 cm in an adult), unmineralized, cartilaginous caps should raise the suspicion of malignant transformation. The size of the cartilaginous cap is best estimated using T2-weighted MRI {198,957}.

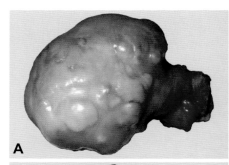

A

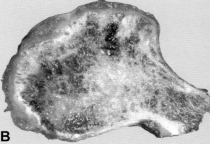

B

Fig. 15.03 Osteochondroma. **A** Macroscopic view showing the external cartilage cap. **B** Cut section revealing the continuity of the cortex and marrow cavity with that of the underlying bone.

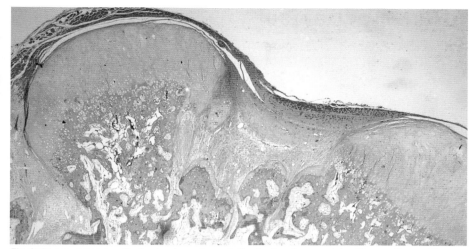

Fig. 15.04 Low-power view of osteochondroma demonstrating the three layers: perichondrium, cartilage and bone.

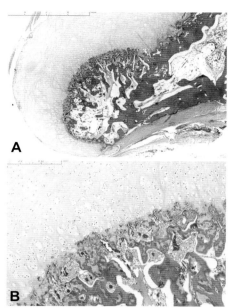

Fig. 15.05 Osteochondroma. **A** The cartilage cap centred by trabecular bone. **B** Endochondral ossification occurs at the bone–cartilage interface. Columns of proliferative chondrocytes surrounded by cartilaginous hyaline matrix, resembling the normal growth plate.

Macroscopy

Osteochondromas may be sessile or pedunculated. The cortex and medullary cavity are continuous with the bony stalk and the centre of the lesion, respectively. The cartilage cap is usually thin (and thickness decreases with age).

Histopathology

The lesion has three layers: perichondrium, cartilage and bone. The outer layer is a non-neoplastic, fibrous perichondrium that is continuous with the periosteum of the underlying bone. Below this is a hyaline cartilage cap that mimics disorganized growth plate-like cartilage, and undergoes enchondral ossification. Secondary changes may include irregular calcification and myxoid degeneration. The distinction between osteochondroma and low-grade secondary peripheral chondrosarcoma is histologically difficult and should be made in a multidisciplinary team {588}. Large peripheral nodules, separated by wide fibrous bands composed of hypercellular cartilage with chondrocyte atypia should raise the suspicion of malignancy. Fractures within a stalk may elicit a focal fibroblastic response. In very rare instances, osteosarcomas, spindle cell sarcomas or dedifferentiated chondrosarcomas can develop in osteochondroma {285,1535,2633}.

Genetics

Cytogenetic aberrations involving 8q22–24.1, the location of the *EXT1* gene, are found in a subset of sporadic and hereditary osteochondromas {321,821,1856}. Most mutations found in *EXT1* or *EXT2* in patients with hereditary multiple osteochondroma are predicted to result in a truncated or non-functional protein {1326}. Germline mutations in *EXT1* combined with loss of the remaining wildtype allele have been demonstrated in a subset of hereditary osteochondromas {197,283, 2317,3077}. In approximately 80% of solitary osteochondromas, homozygous deletions of *EXT1* can be found within the cartilage cap {1095,3077}. Mouse models involving conditional mutations also indicate that biallelic inactivation of *EXT1* is required for osteochondroma formation {1343,1757}. However, due to the mosaic composition of the cartilaginous cap, the detection of such a second hit depends on the ratio of wildtype versus mutated cells in the examined specimen. Mutations in *IDH1* or *IDH2* are absent in osteochondromas {54,2165}.

Prognostic factors

Excision of osteochondroma is usually curative and recurrence is seen with incomplete removal. Multiple recurrences should raise the suspicion of malignancy. The risk of malignant transformation to secondary peripheral chondrosarcoma is estimated at about 1% for solitary and up to 5% for multiple osteochondromas {1592,2466,2955}.

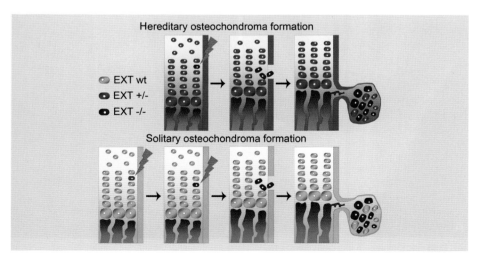

Fig. 15.06 Osteochondroma formation. A second hit in *EXT* in a proliferating cell of the growth plate near the bony collar underlies osteochondroma formation in multiple osteochondromas patients. The cells lose polarity and grow out of the bone through a defective bony collar due to disturbed hedgehog signalling. In the cartilaginous cap, *EXT* -/- cells are intermingled with *EXT* +/- cells (mosaicism). In solitary osteochondromas, two somatic hits are required in a single chondrocyte {280A}.

Chondromas: enchondroma, periosteal chondroma

D.R. Lucas
J.A. Bridge

A group of benign bone tumours of hyaline cartilage sharing many histological features. However, they differ with respect to location and clinical features. Enchondroma and periosteal chondroma are sporadic and usually solitary.

Enchondroma

Definition
Enchondroma is a benign hyaline cartilage neoplasm that arises within the medullary cavity of bone. Most tumours are solitary; however, they occasionally involve more than one bone, or site in a single bone.

ICD-O code
Enchondroma   9220/0

Synonym
Central chondroma

Epidemiology
Enchondromas are relatively common, accounting for 10–25% of all surgically removed benign bone tumours {2816}. The true incidence is actually much higher since many tumours are incidental radiographic findings and never biopsied. The age distribution is wide, ranging from 5 to 80 years. However, the majority of patients present within the second to fifth decades of life. Both sexes are equally affected.

Sites of involvement
The short tubular bones of the hand are most commonly affected (approximately 40% of cases). The long tubular bones, especially proximal humerus, distal tibia, and proximal and distal femur, are next in frequency {2816}. Enchondromas are very uncommon in flat bones such as the pelvis, ribs, scapula, sternum or vertebrae, and are exceedingly rare in the craniofacial bones.

Clinical and imaging features
Enchondromas in the short tubular bones of the hands and feet may present as palpable swellings, with or without pain, and pathological fractures. Long bone tumours are more often asymptomatic, unless aggravated by mechanical stress. Many are detected incidentally in radiographs, MRI or bone scans. Enchondromas are usually "hot" on bone scan. Radiographically, enchondromas form well-marginated tumours that vary from radiolucent to heavily mineralized. When present, the mineralization pattern is highly characteristic; consisting of punctate, flocculent, or ring and arc patterns. Long bone tumours are usually centrally located within the metaphysis. Enchondromas in the small tubular bones can be centrally or eccentrically located, and larger tumours can completely replace the medullary cavity {2706}. In small and medium-sized tubular bones and in thin flat bones, enchondromas are frequently expansile (enchondroma protuberans) {352}. In the large long bones, such as the femur, tibia or humerus, endosteal erosion or scallop-

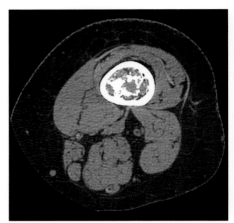

Fig. 15.07 CT image of a femoral enchondroma illustrates the dense, solid calcifications.

ing may be present; however cortical thickening and/or bone expansion should raise the suspicion of chondrosarcoma {341}.

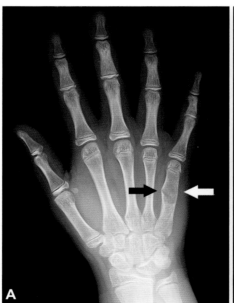 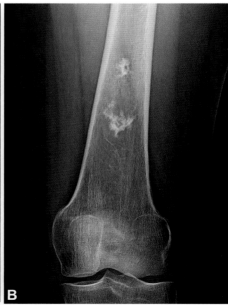

Fig. 15.08 Enchondroma. **A** Enchondromas in small tubular bones frequently present with pathological fractures. Note cortical attenuation (white arrow) and incomplete or "greenstick" fracture (black arrow). Characteristic small punctate calcifications are evident. **B** This femoral diaphyseal tumour shows a characteristic mineralization pattern consisting of trabecular, ring and arc-like calcifications. Enchondromas involving large long bones are non-expansile with no or only minimal endosteal erosion or "scalloping" of the cortex.

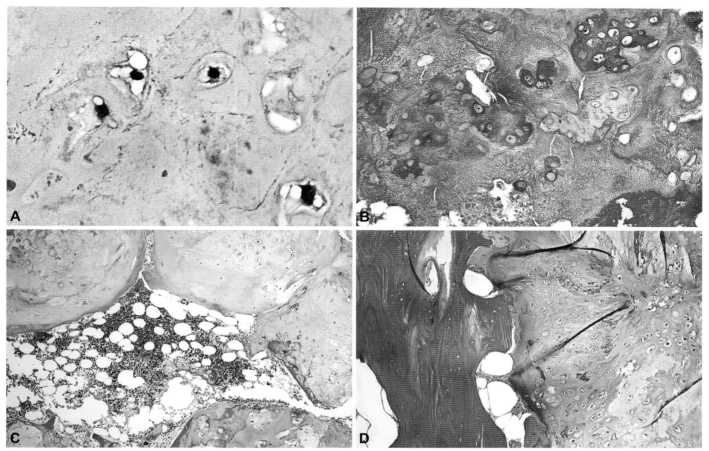

Fig. 15.09 Enchondroma. **A** The chondrocytes are typically situated within sharp-edged lacunar spaces. The cytoplasm is frequently retracted to form vacuoles and spider-like eosinophilic extensions. Nuclei are small, round and hyperchromatic, although larger, vesicular nuclei can also be present. Mitotic figures are usually nonexistent and binucleation is uncommon. Finely stippled calcifications within the hyaline matrix are common. **B** Some enchondromas become heavily calcified, as shown by densely stippled and solid areas of deeply basophilic staining. The chondrocytes are often necrotic in these areas; reduced to eosinophilic bodies within lacunae. **C** Enchondromas commonly have a multinodular architectural pattern characterized by islands of cartilage encased by thin mantles of bone that are often separated by marrow. This pattern is more common in larger tumours. Enchondromas in small tubular bones tend to have a more confluent architecture. **D** Although enchondromas can erode the endosteal surface of the cortex, they do not invade the Haversian system or destroy bone.

Macroscopy

Most enchondromas are < 5 cm in size. Because most tumours are treated by curettage, the specimen is usually received in fragments. The tissue is grey-white and opalescent. Gritty, yellow and red foci represent areas of calcification and ossification, respectively. In the intact state, enchondromas are well-marginated. They frequently have a multinodular architecture, comprising nodules of cartilage separated by bone marrow. This multinodular pattern is more common in long bones compared to small tubular bones, where enchondromas usually have a confluent growth pattern.

Histopathology

In general, enchondromas are hypocellular, avascular tumours with abundant hyaline cartilage matrix. They typically stain pale blue with H&E due to their high content of matrix proteoglycans. The chondrocytes are situated within sharp-edged lacunar spaces, and have finely granular eosinophillic cytoplasm that is often vacuolated. The nuclei are typically small and round with condensed chromatin. Slightly larger nuclei with open chromatin and small nucleoli are common. The cells can be evenly distributed or arranged in small clusters. More than one cell per lacuna, as well as occasional binucleated cells, can be present. Mitotic activity is absent. Chondrocytes, not confined to lacunae, assume bipolar or stellate shapes. Myxoid matrix rarely accounts for more than a minor component of a tumour. The architecture of enchondroma varies from multinodular to confluent. Delicate fibrous septa or thin mantles of lamellar bone surround the nodules. Normal marrow elements are often present between nodules. Although endosteal erosion is present in some cases, enchondromas do not invade the Haversian system, entrap pre-existing bone trabuculae or invade adjacent soft tissue. The degree of mineralization is variable. This is due to basophilic-stippled and solid calcification, as well as endochondral ossification. Areas of ischaemic necrosis are common, especially in heavily calcified tumours. Here, the chondrocytes are reduced to eosinophilic bodies. Enchondromas in the small bones of the hands and feet can be more cellular and cytologically atypical than in long-bone tumours. Without proper radiographic correlation, such lesions can be mistaken for chondrosarcomas. Criteria in the context of enchondromatosis are less well defined.

Genetics
Genomic imbalances are rare in enchondromas, with nearly all tumours exhibiting a diploid or near-diploid complement {2145,2383}. Although a tumour-specific anomaly has not been identified for this entity, aberrations of chromosome 6 often resulting in loss of material and re-arrangements of 12q13–15 are frequent {340,2411}. Truncated or full-length *HMGA2* (12q15) transcripts have been noted in two enchondromas with and without karyotypic anomalies of this locus respectively {546}. In enchondromas, PTHLH signalling is active, but independent of Indian hedgehog (IHH) signalling, irrespective of the presence or absence of enchondromatosis (Ollier disease/Maffucci syndrome) {2381}. Heterozygous somatic *IDH1/IDH2* mutations have been detected in at least 50% of solitary enchondromas and approximately 90% of enchondromas from patients with enchondromatosis {54}. Importantly, these *IDH1/IDH2* mutations appear to be confined to enchondromas, periosteal chondromas and central/periosteal chondrosarcomas, and are absent in other mesenchymal neoplasms, including other cartilaginous tumour subtypes {54,564}.

Prognostic factors
Enchondromas requiring treatment are usually successfully treated by curettage, and local recurrences are uncommon. Occasionally, an enchondroma will recur many years later, and rarely recur as an atypical cartilaginous tumour/low-grade chondrosarcoma {531A}.

Periosteal chondroma

Definition
Periosteal chondroma is a benign hyaline cartilage neoplasm of bone surface that arises beneath the periosteum.

ICD-O code 9221/0

Synonyms
Juxtacortical chondroma, parosteal chondroma

Epidemiology
Periosteal chondromas are much less common than enchondromas, account-

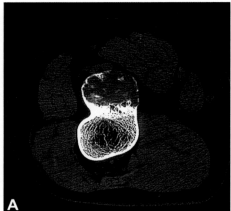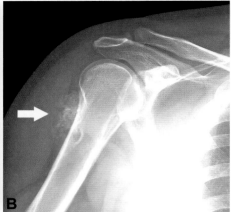

Fig. 15.10 Periosteal chondroma. **A** CT image of a periosteal chondroma of the posterior femur illustrates characteristic radiographic findings. The tumour is well demarcated, partially mineralized and contained by a discontinuous thin layer of periosteal bone. The underlying cortex is thickened and sclerotic and there is peripheral buttressing around the base of the tumour. **B** This radiograph depicts a mineralized tumour (arrow) with underlying cortical sclerosis.

ing for < 2% of chondromas {323,2816}. They occur in children and adults, with males outnumbering females by three to two {167,1602,2816}.

Sites of involvement
Periosteal chondromas occur most commonly in the long bones. The proximal humerus is a characteristic location {323,2816}. The small tubular bones are also common sites {167,323, 1602}.

Clinical features and imaging
Periosteal chondromas present as palpable, often painful, masses {167,323}. Radiographically, they appear as radiolucent or mineralized bone-surface tumours that form sharply-marginated erosions (or "saucerization") of the cortex. Typically, the underlying cortex is scalloped, and the tumour is bordered by solid periosteal buttressing. Tumours are < 5 cm in greatest diameter {167,1602,2816}.

Macroscopy
Periosteal chondromas form well-marginated bone-surface tumours. The cortex underlying the tumour is usually indented and thickened. Solid periosteal buttressing encloses the tumour on its sides.

Histopathology
Periosteal chondromas have a sharp margin with the underlying thickened cortex. Although they sometimes erode and scallop the cortex, they do not penetrate into cancellous bone. The degree of cellularity and the cytological features are similar to other chondromas; however, occasionally

periosteal chondromas are more cellular and show greater nuclear pleomorphism and more binucleation.

Genetics
Like enchondroma, periosteal chondroma also frequently harbours heterozygous mutations in *IDH* genes. Specifically, six of eight periosteal chondromas analysed had *IDH1* mutations {54}. Clonal chromosomal abnormalities have been described in seven cases of periosteal chondroma; loss of chromosome 6 material and rearrangements of 2q37, 4q21–25, and 11q13–15 have been detected in two cases each {340,2411}.

Prognostic factors
Periosteal chondromas have been treated with intralesional, marginal, and en-bloc excisions, and the recurrence rate is low regardless of type of surgery {167,1602}.

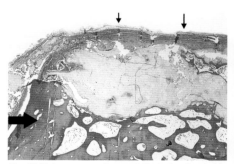

Fig. 15.11 Low-power micrograph illustrating the classic features of periosteal chondroma. The tumour is situated beneath the periosteum (small arrows) and erodes the underlying sclerotic cortex. Thick periosteal buttressing is present at the periphery (large arrow).

Chondromyxoid fibroma

S. Romeo
T. Aigner
J.A. Bridge

-Definition

A benign cartilaginous neoplasm, composed of lobules formed by spindle-shaped cells with myofibroblastic features at the periphery, and stellate and chondrocyte-like cells towards the centre. The extracellular matrix of the lobules is fibrous at the periphery and myxoid and chondroid towards the centre.

ICD-O code   9241/0

Epidemiology

Chondromyxoid fibroma is a very rare tumour {2361,2835}. Although it may affect a wide age range (first to seventh decades of life), it occurs more often in the second and third decades of life and more frequently in males {965,2994}.

Sites of involvement

Chondromyxoid fibroma can occur at almost any osseous site. It is most frequent in the long bones, most often the proximal tibia and the distal femur. Approximately 25% of cases occur in the flat bones, mainly the ilium. The bones of the feet are also involved, especially the metatarsals. Other sites of involvement include the ribs, vertebrae, skull and facial bones, and tubular bones of the hand.

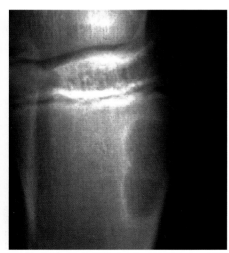

Fig. 15.12 Proximal tibial chondromyxoid fibroma. This lytic lesion exhibits sharply circumscribed and sclerotic borders with scalloping.

Clinical and imaging features

Pain is the most common symptom, usually mild and sometimes present for several years {2994}. Swelling is noted infrequently, more often in tumours of the bones of the hands and feet.

Radiographically, chondromyxoid fibroma in a long bone is typically a metaphyseal, eccentric, sharply marginated, oval zone of rarefaction, with attenuation and expansion of one cortex. Lesions of the rib or ilium may be discovered as incidental radiological findings {2994}. Less frequently the tumour is juxtacortical {144}. The longitudinal axis of the lesion corresponds to that of the involved bone, and the size ranges from 1 to 10 cm (average, 3 cm). In the small bones, fusiform expansion of the entire bone is typical. Most lesions are entirely lucent; approximately 10% may show focal calcified matrix, more often detectable with CT scans. There may be cortical destruction, but it is contained by the periosteum {2361,2994}. Rarely, contiguous bones are affected {334}.

Macroscopy

Gross features of chondromyxoid fibroma include well-defined margins, bluish-grey or white tumour, lack of obvious necrosis, cystic change, and liquefaction. The tumour is multilobulated and well demarcated from the surrounding bone. Typically there are scalloped margins.

Histopathology

Typically, chondromyxoid fibroma is sharply demarcated from the surrounding bone. Rarely, there is entrapment of surrounding bone trabeculae by tumour. Lobules of tumour may be separate from the main lesion. A lobular pattern with stellate or spindle-shaped cells in a myxoid background is evident {2361}. Lobules demonstrate hypocellular centres with hyper cellular peripheries. The centre of the lobules show morphological features more similar to hyaline cartilage, in terms of both extracellular matrix and cell composition {2357,2593}. Microscopic, cystic or liquefactive change is uncommon and usually focal when present. Hyaline cartilage is

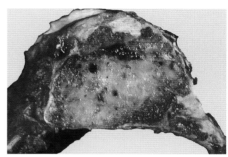

Fig. 15.13 Chondromyxoid fibroma of the ilium. Note the yellow-grey relatively uniform lesion, with sharply demarcated borders and expansion of the bone.

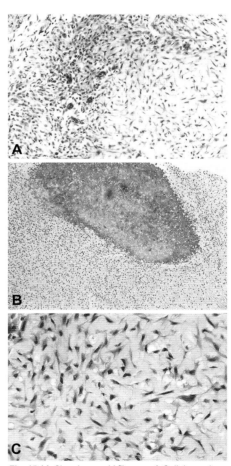

Fig. 15.14 Chondromyxoid fibroma. **A** Cellular regions with multinucleated giant cells are present peripheral to the lobules. **B** Focal coarse calcification. Note that these elements surround hyaline cartilage. **C** Moderate nuclear enlargement is present in these cells, and the eosinophillic cytoplasmic processes are prominent.

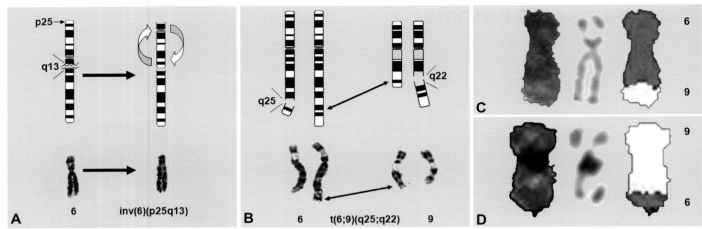

Fig. 15.15 Partial G-banded karyotypes and schematics of two recurrent events in chondromyxoid fibroma: the pericentric inversion, inv(6)(p25q13) **(A)** and the 6;9 translocation, t(6;9)(q25;q22) **(B)**, respectively. **C** and **D** Spectral karyotypic image of the derivative chromosomes in the translocation presented in part B.

present in 19% of cases {2994}. Calcification, when present, is usually coarse, and occurs more frequently in older patients and in flat-bone tumours {3007}. Individual cells within lobules have oval to spindled nuclei and indistinct to densely eosinophillic cytoplasm. Cytoplasmic extensions, often bipolar or multipolar, are frequent. Enlarged, hyperchromatic and pleomorphic nuclei are noted in 20–30% of cases. Mitoses are uncommon, although atypical mitoses have been noted {2994}. Because of these features, differential diagnosis with high-grade central chondrosarcoma is considered. However clinicoradiological features and histology are quite distinct; chondrosar-

comas more often affect older patients and the diaphysis of long bones with more frank atypia and mitoses are often present. Osteoclast-like giant cells are often present at the lobular peripheries. There may also be haemosiderin deposition and inflammatory cells, usually lymphocytes. Areas of aneurysmal bone cyst are noted in approximately 10% of long- and flat-bone lesions {2994}.

Immunophenotype

The cartilaginous nature of this tumour is reflected by immunopositivity for S100 protein {255,565,1461, 3071}.The extracellular matrix is immunopositive for collagen II and SOX9, mainly in the centre of

the lobules {2593}. Immunoreactivity for SMA and MSA has been noted in regions peripheral to the lobules {2360}.

Ultrastructure

Ultrastructurally, the stellate cells have irregular cell processes, scalloped cell membranes, cytoplasmic fibrils and glycogen, features of both chondroblastic and fibroblastic differentiation {2036, 2360}. Cells with the classic features of chondrocytes, those with myofibroblastic features, and intermediate forms have been described in chondromyxoid fibroma {2036,2360}.

Genetics

Chromosome 6 aberrations are frequent but heterogeneous; regions commonly involved include 6p23–25, 6q12–15, and 6q23–27 {2359}. Two rearrangements, inv(6)(p25q13) and t(6;9)(q25;q22), are frequent either as the sole anomaly or accompanied by other karyotypic abnormalities {2574,3027}. Rearrangement of 6q13 has also been identified in a juvenile juxtacortical chondromyxoid fibroma {1332}. Molecular characterization of three loci (6q13, 6q23.3 and 6q24) has revealed a hemizygous deletion of 6q24 as well as balanced and unbalanced rearrangements of 6q13 and 6q23.3 as recurrent events {2359}. Examination of the matrix composition and gene-expression pattern in chondromyxoid fibroma has shown a cartilaginous "profile" {2362, 2593,3080}.

Prognostic factors

The prognosis is excellent, even for recurrent tumours. Recurrence occurs in approximately 15% of cases treated with curettage and bone grafting.

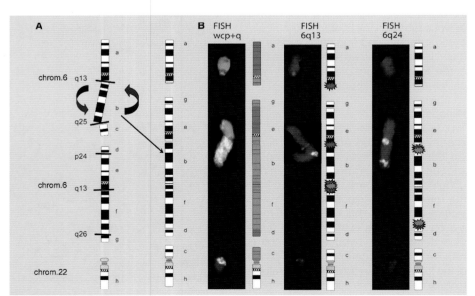

Fig. 15.16 Chondromyxoid fibroma. Complex rearrangements affecting both homologues of chromosomes 6 are frequent in chondromyxoid fibroma. **A** Left, ideogram of normal chromosomes 6 and 22; identified breakpoints are indicated by lines. Right, ideograms of the observed rearrangements. Involved chromosome segments are annotated from a to h. **B** Representative metaphase FISH experiments..

Osteochondromyxoma

J.A. Carney
C.A. Stratakis

Definition
A rare, benign, sometimes locally aggressive, chondroid and osteoid matrix-producing tumour, with extensive myxoid changes. It has occurred in patients with or suspected of having Carney complex, an autosomal dominant neoplasia-predisposing syndrome.

ICD-O code   9211/0

Epidemiology
Osteochondromyxoma is rare, occurring in about 1% of patients with Carney complex {383,384, 2665}. The tumour can occur at a wide age range and the lesion is congenital in some cases {382}.

Etiology
The etiology is unknown, but osteochondromyxoma is presumed to be the morphological expression of a Carney complex-type myxoma occurring in bone.

Sites of involvement
Cases have been reported in the ethmoid bone, nasal conchae, and tibia.

Clinical and imaging features
Patients present with a painless mass, usually found upon screening for skeletal involvement in cases of Carney complex. The lesion can grow destructively, and symptoms and prognosis depend on the site involved. Radiologically, osteochondromyxomas have a benign appearance and a variable interface with the surrounding host bone, but locally aggressive features with soft-tissue extension have also been reported.

Macroscopy
The lesions are circumscribed and unencapsulated and show a lobulated growth pattern with a white and light-yellow gelatinous, cartilaginous, and haemorrhagic gross appearance. Usually there is erosion of the cortex without penetration.

Histopathology
The tumours are generally hypocellular due to separation of the cells by abundant intercellular ground substance. Exceptional foci are cellular. The cells form sheets, with or without a poorly or well-defined microlobular or macrolobular pattern. This architecture results from accumulation of clear and basophilic myxoid matrix in a moderately to hypocellular, loose mesenchyme. The cells are polygonal, stellate, round, and bipolar in shape; a minority are spindle shaped. In limited areas, the cells are packed together, occasionally resembling chondroblasts or histiocytes. The nuclei are medium-sized, pale and vesicular, with a small nucleolus. They have a uniform and bland appearance. There are occasional mitotic figures. Binucleation is very rare. The cell cytoplasm stains PAS-positive; the staining is abolished by diastase predigestion. Positivity is strongest where there is little intercellular matrix. Both cytoplasm and intercellular matrix stain positive for colloidal iron. The staining is reduced by hyaluronidase predigestion. The cell products include: (i) mucopolysaccharide

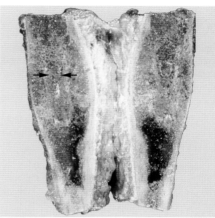

Fig. 15.17 Tibial osteochondromyxoma. The longitudinally sectioned tibia showed a heterogeneous, elongated, oval tumour. Inferiorly, the lesion was demarcated by a zone of haemorrhage (probably biopsy-related.) Superiorly, the lesion was poorly delineated. A vague cylindrical zone (arrows) had a cartilaginous appearance and contained a small cyst with mucoid content.

ground substance that varies between virtually transparent, acidophilic, basophilic, gel-like or solid (cartilage); (ii) osteoid and bone; and (iii) acidophilic hyaline fibrous nodules and bands. The proportion of these components determines the appearance of the tumour, which varies considerably. Where more matrix is present, the cells are separated into small, irregularly shaped groups and into strands and cords. In these areas, polygonal cells are less common than fusiform, stellate, and bipolar cells; cellularity is decreased; and eosinophilic-staining intercellular tissue is less common than basophilic tissue. The

Table 15.01 Selected clinical features of patients with osteochondromyxoma of bone {382}

Patient (n = 4)	Sex	Age at biopsy	Site	Presentation	Radiographical interpretation	Treatment	Follow-up (years)	Other conditions in patient
1	Male	13 months	Ethmoid	Painless proptosis	Benign neoplasm	Orbital exenteration, ethmoidectomy, sphenoidectomy, chemotherapy	Dead; local recurrence (3)	None; mother had Carney complex
2	Female	14 months	Tibia	Painless mass	Benign neoplasm or infection	Block resection	Alive and well (19)	Lentigines, skin myxomas, Cushing syndrome
3	Male	2 months	Nasal concha	Painless mass, nasal obstruction	Benign neoplasm	Subtotal resection; subsequent resection for tumour persistence	Alive and well (11)	Lentigines, eye and oral pigmented spots, large-cell calcifying Sertoli cell tumour
4	Male	8 days	Radius	Painless mass	Malignant neoplasm or infection	Biopsy only	Alive and well (12)	Pigmented skin lesions; father had Carney complex

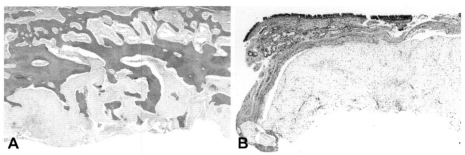

Fig. 15.18 Osteochondromyxoma. **A** A sheet of tumour cells with overall clear appearance and vague lobular pattern (right) erodes the bony cortex of the tibial lesion. The hypocellular tumour with dilated sinusoids penetrates between narrow reactive bony trabeculae just beneath the periosteum (top). **B** The circumscribed but unencapsulated hypocellular myxochondroid tumour abuts the nasal submucosa.

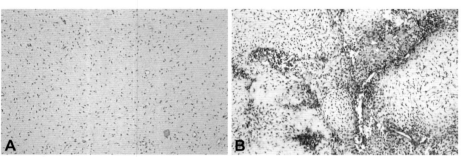

Fig. 15.19 Osteochondromyxoma. **A** The tumour is composed of a patternless sheet of cells separated by abundant basophilic mucopolysaccharide ground substance. **B** Polygonal, elongated, and stellate-shaped cells are arranged in moderate-sized lobules.

matrix varies from stringy, clear, and lightly basophilic, to gel-like, solid and cartilage-like. These zones blend with areas of mature cartilage, where well-outlined round cells occupy evenly disposed spaces. Occasionally, these cells are arranged in pairs, small groupings, or linear arrays, resembling epiphyseal plate cartilage.

Elsewhere, hyaline fibrous bands coalesce, trap cells, become calcified, and form osteoid and bone. Some of the mature bony trabeculae are bordered by plump osteoblasts.

Genetics

Four cases of osteochondromyxoma arising in patients with Carney complex or with a family history of Carney complex were karyotypically normal {382}. Carney complex is a genetically heterogeneous disorder with two genetic loci (*CNC1* and *CNC2*) being implicated {1427,2665}. *CNC1* results from inactivating mutations of the tumour suppressor gene *PRKAR1A*; to date more than 120 *PRKAR1A* mutations have been reported in patients with Carney complex {1227}. *PRKAR1A* encodes the protein kinase A (PKA) regulatory subunit type IA, an important regulator of cAMP signalling. *Prkar1a* (+/-) mice develop bone tumours with a high frequency {2202}. The gene for *CNC2* remains to be identified.

Prognostic factors

The rate of local recurrence rate appears to correlate with sites that may be difficult to access and consequently limit the extent of surgical resection and achievement of clear margins. Deaths have been reported in cases where the tumours are inaccessible by surgery. No metastases have been reported.

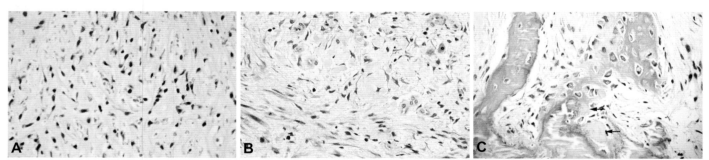

Fig. 15.20 Osteochondromyxoma. **A** Polygonal and bipolar tumour cells in a barely perceptible, weakly basophilic matrix. Nuclei are hyperchromatic as a result of decalcification. **B** Spindle cells and polygonal cells in a loose matrix with round eosinophilic hyaline areas. **C** Osteoid formation present in an area of polygonal cells with lightly eosinophilic cytoplasm. The nuclei are round and regular with occasional lobulation and grooving.

Subungual exostosis and bizarre parosteal osteochondromatous proliferation

R. Sciot
N. Mandahl

Subungual exostosis

Definition
A benign osteochondromatous proliferation involving the distal phalanx.

ICD-O code
9213/0

Synonym
Dupuytren exostosis.

Epidemiology
Subungual exostosis has a peak incidence in the second and third decades, with a male predominance {1903}.

Sites of involvement
The great toe is the most frequent location; other toes and fingers are rarely affected.

Clinical features
Swelling and pain are typical, sometimes associated with ulceration. Radiographs show an outgrowth of trabeculated bone. Importantly, the cortex and medulla of the underlying bone are not continuous with the lesion {1587}.

Macroscopy
The lesion consists of a cartilage cap and a bony stalk.

Histopathology
There is a gradual maturation from a peripheral spindle cell proliferation to hyaline cartilage to trabecular bone. Loosely arranged spindle cells are present in the intertrabecular spaces.

Genetics
All seven cytogenetically analysed cases of subungual exostosis have featured a t(X;6)(q24–26;q15–25), often as the sole anomaly {555,2661,3048}. Both breakpoint regions harbour collagen genes; *COL12A1* at 6q13–14 and *COL4A5* at Xq22. *IRS4* is located less than 100 kb from the Xq22 breakpoint. No fusion transcripts between *IRS4* and *COL12A1* or *COL4A5* and *COL12A1* have been identified in subungual exostosis; however, increased expression of IRS4 has been

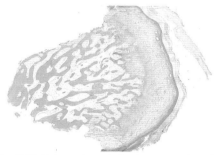

Fig. 15.21 Subungual exostosis. Low-power view of subungual exostosis, showing the osteochondroma like architecture.

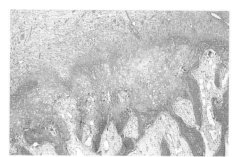

Fig. 15.22 Subungual exostosis. High-power view highlighting the transition of a peripheral spindle-cell proliferation to hyaline cartilage to trabecular bone.

shown {1853}. The exact mechanism conferring transcriptional deregulation of *IRS4* is unknown.

Prognostic factors
Simple excision is usually curative and recurrences are rare.

Bizarre parosteal osteochondromatous proliferation

Definition
An osteochondromatous proliferation involving the surface of bone, usually affecting the proximal small bones of the hands or feet.

ICD-O code
9212/0

Synonym
Nora's lesion

Epidemiology
Bizarre parosteal osteochondromatous proliferation (BPOP) has a peak incidence in the third and fourth decades of life {1826}.

Sites of involvement
The small bones of the hands or feet are most commonly involved; approximately 25% of lesions occur in long bones.

Clinical and imaging features
Swelling with or without complaints of pain is the typical clinical presentation. A well-marginated, heterotopic, mineralized mass

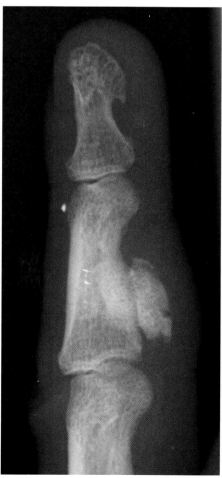

Fig. 15.23 BPOP of the middle phalanx of the ring finger, clearly depicting the parosteal location of the osteochondromatous proliferation.

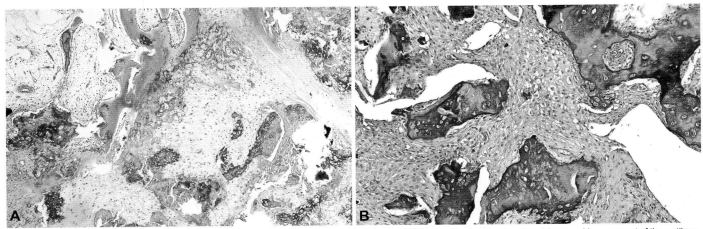

Fig. 15.24 BPOP A BPOP with a more disorganized mixture of mainly bone and cartilage. B Detail of BPOP, showing the "blue bone" and the more bizarre aspect of the cartilage.

attached to the cortex is seen on radiographs. In contrast to osteochondroma, the lesion is not contiguous with the underlying cortex and spongiosa of the involved bone {1053}.

Macroscopy
The lesion is composed of an often abundant and lobulated cartilage cap and a bony stalk.

Histopathology
As in subungual exostosis, cartilage, bone and spindle cells are present, but often in a more disorganized fashion. In addition, the cartilage is hypercellular with enlarged chondrocytes ("bizarre") and shows a peculiar purplish blue mineralization ("blue bone").

Genetics
Of four cases of BPOP with clonal chromosome aberrations, two showed a similar translocation, t(1;17)(q32–42;q21–23), as the sole anomaly {745,2051}, one displayed supernumerary ring chromosomes containing chromosome 12 sequences {3048}, and one exhibited a paracentric inversion of 7q {2415}. Interphase FISH analyses of four additional BPOPs revealed breakpoints in 1q32 in four cases and in 17q21 in three cases {2051}. These data indicate that most BPOPs are characterized by a t(1;17) or variant thereof. BPOP lacks IRS4 expression {1853} and thus, appears to be genetically distinct from subungual exostosis.

Prognostic factors
Following excision, recurrences may present in about half of cases {191}.

Synovial chondromatosis

R. Sciot
J.A. Bridge

Definition
A benign neoplasm presenting as multiple hyaline cartilage nodules, typically present in the subsynovial tissue.

ICD-O code   9220/0

Synonym
Synovial osteochondro(mato)sis

Epidemiology
Synovial chondromatosis typically occurs in the third to fifth decades of life and is twice as common in males as females.

Sites of involvement
Two thirds of cases involve the knee joint, but any joint can be affected, including the temporomandibular joint {1056}. Some cases are entirely extra-articular and are termed tenosynovial chondromatosis {843}.

Clinical and imaging features
Pain, swelling, palpable nodules, joint clicking, locking or movement restriction, as well as secondary osteoarthritis are common signs. On radiograph and CT, small masses, round and calcified at the periphery, are visible inside the joint. When not calcified, they appear in the joint effusion as round small masses on MRI.

Macroscopy
Multiple grey-white, cobblestone-like, often similarly sized nodules are seen, all or not attached to synovial tissue. There may be multiple loose bodies.

Histopathology
Nodules consist of hyaline cartilage, in which the chondrocytes are clustered. Nodules are often surrounded by synovial tissue. Calcification and/or ossification occur. This entity needs to be distinguished from multiple osteochondral loose bodies in osteoarthritis. Nuclear enlargement, binucleation, pleomorphism and myxoid degeneration are characteristic, but sheets of atypical chondrocytes, necrosis, mitotic figures, and crowding and spindling of peripheral nuclei suggest transformation to conventional chondrosarcoma {366,583,2979}. Malignant transformation is extremely rare.

Genetics
Clonal karyotypic abnormalities have been detected in eight cases of synovial chondromatosis; all have exhibited diploid or near-diploid complements with chromosome 6 anomalies, rearrangements of 1p22, 1p13, and extra copies of chromosome 5 in order of frequency {339}. A predisposition to synovial chondromatosis development has been observed in mice deficient in Gli3, a hedgehog signalling pathway suppressor protein. Correspondingly in humans, expression levels of the hedgehog target genes *PTCH1* and *GLI1* are substantially higher in synovial chondromatosis than in normal synovial tissues {1211}. *IDH1* and *IDH2* mutations are absent {54}.

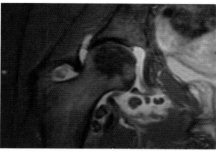

Fig. 15.25 Synovial chondromatosis of the hip. Extensive joint effusion with multiple loose bodies (MRI).

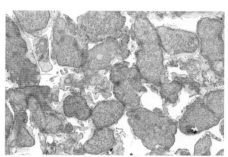

Fig. 15.26 Synovial chondromatosis. Multiple hyaline cartilage nodules characterize synovial chondromatosis. Some mineralization can be appreciated.

Prognostic factors
Recurrence is found in 15–20% of cases, with higher rates in tenosynovial cases {843}. Malignant transformation is extremely rare, usually in longstanding cases with multiple recurrences, leading to bone invasion, but metastases are only seen in 29% of cases {366}.

Chondroblastoma

S.E. Kilpatrick
S. Romeo

Definition
A benign, chondroid-producing neoplasm composed of chondroblasts. It usually arises in the epiphyses or apophysis of skeletally immature patients.

ICD-O code   9230/1

Epidemiology
Chondroblastomas account for < 1% of all bone tumours. Most patients are aged between 10 and 25 years at diagnosis, and there is a male predominance. Patients with skull and temporal bone involvement tend to present at an older age (40–50 years) {2805}.

Sites of involvement
More than 75% of cases involve the long bones; the most common anatomical sites are the epiphyseal regions of the distal and proximal femur, proximal tibia, and proximal humerus {257,2805}. Equivalent sites within flat bones such as the acetabulum and ilium are not uncommon. Other classic sites of involvement include the talus, calcaneus, and patella. Within the craniofacial region, the temporal bone is most frequently affected. Chondroblastomas almost invariably involve a single bone.

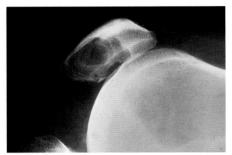

Fig. 15.27 Chondroblastoma. Plain film radiograph illustrating a multicystic, well-circumscribed lesion involving the patella.

Clinical and imaging features
The vast majority of patients complain of localized pain, often mild, but sometimes of many years duration. Soft-tissue swelling, joint stiffness and limitation, and limp are reported less commonly. A minority of patients may develop joint effusions, especially around the knee. Temporal bone involvement may be associated with hearing loss, tinnitus, and/or vertigo {214,2805}.
Radiologically, chondroblastomas are typically lytic, centrally or eccentrically placed, relatively small lesions (3–6 cm), occupying less than half of the epiphysis and are sharply demarcated, with or without a thin sclerotic border. There is generally no expansion of the bone. Periosteal reaction is frequent and sometimes distant from the primary lesion. On MRI, extensive oedema can be seen. Limited involvement of the metaphysis may be present {257,2805}. Matrix calcifications are only visible in about one third of patients {2805}.

Macroscopy
The majority of chondroblastomas are curetted, appearing as multiple pinkish-tan soft-tissue fragments which may exhibit areas of calcification, haemorrhage, or cystic changes.

Histopathology
Histologically, the characteristic cells are uniform, round to polygonal with well-defined cytoplasmic borders, clear to slightly basophilic cytoplasm, and a round to ovoid nucleus (chondroblasts), often growing in cellular sheets. They often exhibit longitudinal grooves and one or more small or inconspicuous nucleoli. Randomly distributed osteoclast-type giant cells are almost always present. Variably-sized nodules of amorphous, amphophilic to eosinophilic material (chondroid) accompanies the

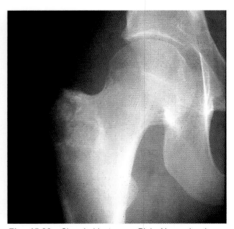

Fig. 15.28 Chondroblastoma. Plain X-ray showing a multiloculated, circumscribed lytic defect with a sclerotic rim involving the greater trochanter. Involvement of the apophysis, such as the greater trochanter, is considered analogous to epiphyseal involvement of a long bone and not uncommon in chondroblastoma.

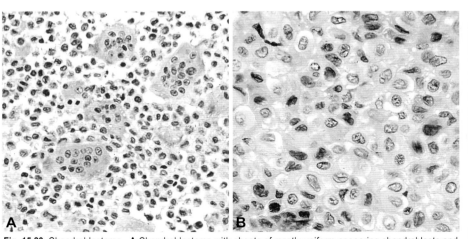

Fig. 15.29 Chondroblastoma. **A** Chondroblastoma with sheets of mostly uniform-appearing chondroblasts and numerous randomly-distributed osteoclast type giant cells. **B** Cytologically, the individual chondroblasts are round to polygonal with sharply defined cytoplasmic borders, round to ovoid nuclei, and occasional small nucleoli. Nuclear grooves and indentations are frequently seen.

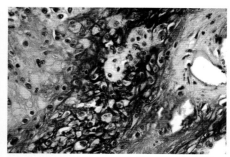

Fig. 15.30 Chondroblastoma. In the appropriate clinical setting, pericellular "chicken wire" calcifications are virtually pathognomonic of chondroblastoma.

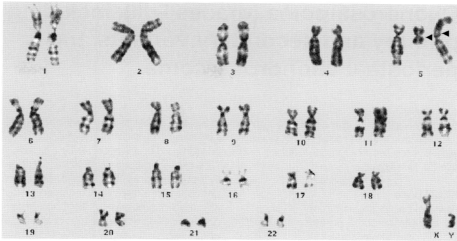

Fig. 15.31 Chondroblastoma. G-banded karyotype of a chondroblastoma with the following complement: 47,XY,+5,t(5;5)(p10;p10).

chondroblasts {1262,2805}. Mature hyaline cartilage is relatively uncommon. A fine network of pericellular "chicken wire" calcifications, is characteristic. Individual chondroblasts may exhibit cytological atypia, represented by large, hyperchromatic nuclei; nevertheless, such features do not adversely affect prognosis {2455,2622}. Mitoses can be frequent, but atypical forms are never seen. Aneurysmal bone cyst-like changes are found in up to one third of cases {2805}.

Immunophenotype

The chondroblasts generally express S100 protein and SOX9 {1461,1930}. Positivity for keratins, especially 8, 18 and 19, and p63 is frequently observed {280,1193, 2509}. Immunohistochemical stains are rarely needed to establish the diagnosis.

Ultrastructure

Ultrastructural studies reveal deep indentations of the nuclear membrane and features, such as abundant rough endoplasmic reticulum and long cytoplasmic processes, typical of fetal chondroblasts {2646}.

Genetics

Flow cytometric studies reveal that most chondroblastomas are diploid with low proliferation fractions {733,2726}. Clonal abnormalities have been described in 14 chondroblastomas {1735,2363,2574, 2689,2708,2850}. Heterogeneous rearrangements of chromosomes 5 and 8, both balanced and unbalanced, appear to be the most common. However, no diagnostically relevant genetic alterations have been found. *IDH1* and *IDH2* mutations are absent {54}.

Prognostic factors

Between 80 and 90% of chondroblastomas are successfully treated by simple curettage with bone grafting. Local recurrence rates range between 14 and 18% {257,2455, 2622,2805}. Temporal bone lesions recur in up to 50% of cases and are probably related to anatomical localization and difficulties of surgical extirpation {214}. Rarely, pulmonary metastases may develop from histologically benign chondroblastomas {1029,2336,2977}. However, these metastases are clinically nonprogressive and often satisfactorily treated by surgical resection and/or simple observation {2336}. There are no reliable histological parameters capable of predicting more aggressive behaviour.

Chondrosarcoma (grades I–III), including primary and secondary variants and periosteal chondrosarcoma

P.C.W. Hogendoorn
J.V.M.G. Bovée
G.P. Nielsen

A locally aggressive or malignant group of cartilaginous matrix-producing neoplasms with diverse morphological features and clinical behaviour.

ICD-O code

Atypical cartilaginous tumour/ chondrosarcoma grade I	9220/1
Chondrosarcoma grade II/III	9220/3

Primary central chondrosarcoma

Definition
A primary chondrosarcoma arising centrally in bone without a benign precursor.

Epidemiology
Primary central chondrosarcoma accounts for about 20% of malignant bone tumours {2815}. It is the third most common primary malignancy of bone after myeloma and osteosarcoma. Approximately 85% of chondrosarcomas are primary and of the conventional type. Primary chondrosarcoma is a tumour of adulthood and older age. Most patients are aged >50 years. The peak incidence is in the fifth to seventh decades of life. There is a slight male predominance.

Sites of involvement
This lesion can arise in any bone derived from enchondral ossification. The most common skeletal sites are the bones of the pelvis (most frequently the ilium) followed by the proximal femur, proximal humerus, distal femur and ribs. About 75% of the tumours occur in the trunk, femur and humerus. The small bones of the hands and feet are rarely involved (1% of all chondrosarcomas) {289}. Chondrosarcoma is rare in the spine and craniofacial bones, where it usually involves the base of the skull.

Clinical and imaging features
Local swelling and/or pain are the most common presenting symptoms. The symptoms are usually of long duration (months to years). Tumours located in the skull base can cause neurological symptoms. In the long bones, primary chondrosarcomas usually occur in the metaphysis or diaphysis where they produce fusiform expansion with cortical thickening. They are radiolucent with variably distributed punctate or ring-like opacities (mineralization). Cortical erosion or destruction is usually present. The cortex is often thickened but periosteal reaction is scant or absent. CT scans aid in demonstrating matrix calcifications. MRI can be helpful in delineating the extent of the tumour and establishing the presence of soft-tissue extension. Dynamic contrast–enhanced MRI is particularly helpful in identifying low-grade malignancy or areas of progression towards higher grade {957}. Imaging approaches to detect the abnormal metabolite produced by mutant *IDH* are being developed, and may become useful in the near future {64,1357}. Primary central chondrosarcomas have been found to occur in association with the development of estrogen receptor-positive breast cancer at a relative early age {480,2095}.

Macroscopy
Chondrosarcomas have a translucent, lobular, blue-grey or white cut surface corresponding to the presence of hyaline cartilage. There may be areas containing myxoid or mucoid material and cystic changes. Yellow-white, chalky areas of calcium deposit are commonly present

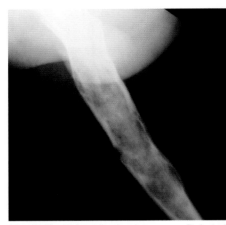

Fig. 15.32 High-grade chondrosarcoma. Endosteal scalloping of a mixed lesion with "popcorn-like" calcifications indicating cartilaginous matrix.

(mineralization). Erosion and destruction of the cortex with extension into soft tissue may be seen.

Histopathology
At low magnification, chondrosarcomas show abundant blue-grey cartilage matrix production. Irregularly shaped lobules of cartilage varying in size and shape are present. These lobules may be separated by fibrous bands or permeate bony trabeculae. Calcified areas suggesting the presence of a pre-existing enchondroma can often be found.

The distinction between enchondroma and

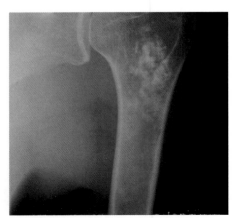

Fig. 15.33 Plain radiograph of a low-grade chondrosarcoma in a long bone demonstrating "popcorn-like" calcifications.

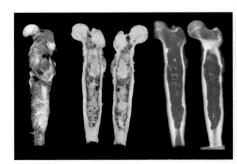

Fig. 15.34 Primary central chondrosarcoma grade III. The proximal femur and the femoral shaft with bulging in the proximal shaft. Side by side: bisected tumour and X-ray of surgical specimen. The lesion has thickened the cortex or irregularly eroded it. Discrete punctate opacities are present.

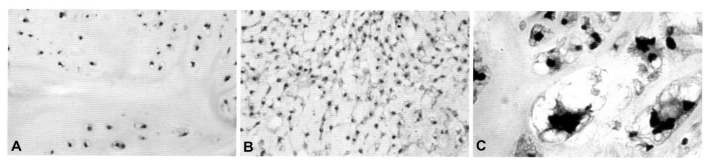

Fig. 15.35 Grade I chondrosarcoma. **A** Few cells with no variation in size and shape (the cytology is indistinguishable from that of enchondroma). **B** Grade 2 chondrosarcoma is characterized by hypercellularity. The cells show variation in size and shape with extensive myxoid matrix component. **C** Grade 3 chondrosarcoma: High cellularity, with prominent pleomorphic appearance and atypia. Mitotic figures are present.

atypical cartilaginous tumour/grade I chondrosarcoma can be difficult and is subjected to a high inter-observer variability {725,2578}. High cellularity, presence of host bone entrapment (permeation of cortical and/or medullary bone), absence of host bone encasement, open chromatin, mucoid matrix quality and an age >45 years favour chondrosarcoma {725,1909}. The chondrocytes are atypical, varying in size and shape and contain enlarged, hyperchromatic nuclei. The extent of atypia is usually mild to moderate. Binucleation is frequently seen. Myxoid changes or chondroid matrix liquefaction is a common feature of chondrosarcomas. Necrosis and mitoses can be seen.

The histological criteria used for a diagnosis of chondrosarcoma in the phalangeal bones are different. Increased cellularity, binucleated cells, hyperchromasia, myxoid change may all be present in enchondroma in this location. A diagnosis of phalangeal chondrosarcoma is made based on the presence of cortical destruction or soft-tissue extension or the presence of mitoses {289}.

Grading is important in chondrosarcoma. Several studies have confirmed its usefulness in predicting histological behaviour and prognosis. Chondrosarcomas are graded on a scale of I to III. The grading is based primarily on nuclear size, nuclear staining (hyperchromasia), cellularity and mitoses {788}. Atypical cartilaginous tumour/grade I tumours are moderately cellular and contain hyperchromatic, plump nuclei of uniform size. Occasionally binucleated cells are present. Mitoses are absent. Grade II tumours are more cellular and contain a greater degree of nuclear atypia, hyperchromasia and nuclear size. Mitoses can be found. Grade III lesions are more cellular and pleomorphic and atypical than grade II. Mitoses are more easily detected. The cells at the periphery of the lobules are less differentiated and become spindled. In a large series of 338 patients, 61% were grade I, 36% were grade II, and 3% were grade III {250}.

Immunophenotype
Only a small percentage of the *IDH1* mutations (approximately 20%) can be identified using the specific IDH1 R132H antibody {54,2165}.

Prognostic factors
Histological grade is the single most important predictor of local recurrence and metastasis {250,959}. Atypical cartilaginous tumour/grade I chondrosarcomas be-

have as locally aggressive lesions, and only metastasize in exceptional cases. Their 5-year survival is 83% and patients die from locally recurrent tumour that is difficult to manage surgically (e.g. pelvis or skull) {788,959}. Atypical cartilaginous tumour/grade I chondrosarcomas in the long bones can be treated with curettage and local adjuvants and have a good prognosis {959}. Approximately 10% of tumours that recur show an increase in the degree of malignancy. Grade II and III chondrosarcomas have a worse prognosis; these combined groups have a 5-year survival of 53%, and patients should be treated with en-bloc resection {959}. Occasionally in chondrosarcomas there is coexistence of various histological grades in the same tumour; areas with the highest histological grade predict prognosis.

Secondary central chondrosarcoma

Definition
A central chondrosarcoma arising in a pre-existing enchondroma.

Epidemiology
Secondary chondrosarcoma frequently develops in solitary enchondroma, although there are no data available detailing the associated risk. Patients with Ollier disease and Maffucci syndrome have a markedly increased risk of developing secondary chondrosarcomas, around 40% and 53%, respectively {1638, 2453,2484,2870}, which is dependent on the location of the tumours (see Chapter 27) {2870}. Patients with secondary chondrosarcoma are generally younger than patients with primary chondrosarcoma.

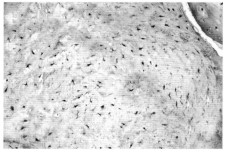

Fig. 15.36 Chondrosarcoma showing entrapment of pre-existing host lamellar bone.

Fig. 15.37 Chondrosarcoma. Myxoid changes can be prominent.

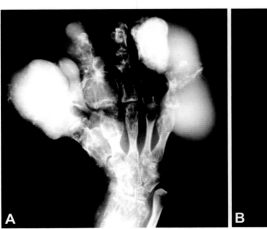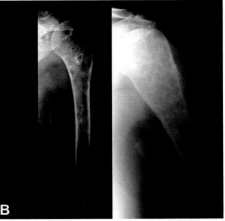

Fig. 15.38 Secondary central chondrosarcoma arising in a patient with Maffucci syndrome. **A** Multiple cartilaginous masses involve bones of the hand and are associated with soft-tissue angioma. **B** In the proximal humerus, the enchondroma enlarged in size and had the radiographical features of chondrosarcoma.

Clinical and imaging features

Continued growth of known enchondromas in adults should raise the suspicion of malignant transformation. Radiographically, cortical destruction and soft-tissue extension of pre-existing enchondromas are signs indicating the development of secondary central chondrosarcoma.

Macroscopy

Gross appearance is similar to primary central chondrosarcoma.

Histology

Histological features are similar to those of primary central chondrosarcoma, although criteria to distinguish them from enchondroma are different in the context of Ollier disease and Maffucci syndrome, in which enchondromas display increased cellularity and nuclear atypia (see Chapter 27). As a result, the differential diagnosis between enchondroma and atypical cartilaginous tumour/grade I secondary central chondrosarcoma is difficult and is based on the presence of an infiltrative growth pattern in conjunction with the radiographic and clinical features.

Immunophenotype

The immunophenotype is similar to that of primary central chondrosarcoma.

Prognostic factors

The prognosis as chondrosarcoma in enchondromatosis is the same as for conventional chondrosarcoma and depends on the site and grade of the tumour.

Secondary peripheral chondrosarcoma

Definition

Secondary peripheral chondrosarcoma is a chondrosarcoma juxtaposed to the cartilaginous cap of an osteochondroma.

Epidemiology

The risk of malignant transformation to secondary peripheral chondrosarcoma is estimated around 1% for solitary and up to 5% for multiple osteochondromas {1592, 2466,2955}.

Sites of involvement

Any portion of the skeleton may be involved. However, the pelvic and shoulder girdle bones are most frequently affected.

Clinical and imaging features

A change in clinical symptoms in a patient with a known precursor lesion might indicate the development of a chondrosarcoma. Sudden pain or increased swelling is a frequent complaint. In osteochondromas, plain X-rays show irregular mineralization. The size of the cartilaginous cap can be well established with T2-weighted MRI {198,957}. A cartilage cap > 1.5–2 cm should raise the suspicion of malignant transformation.

Macroscopy

Chondrosarcomas secondary to osteochondroma show a thick (> 1.5–2 cm) lobulated cartilage cap. The cartilage usually shows cystic cavities.

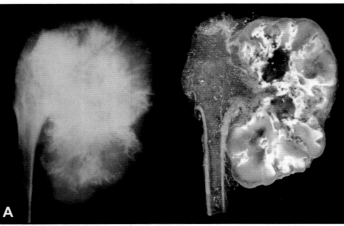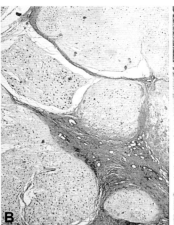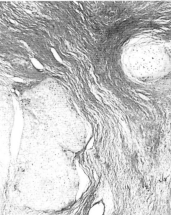

Fig. 15.39 Secondary peripheral chondrosarcoma arising in a patient with multiple osteochondromas. **A** Plain X-ray and surgical specimen of a tumour of the right proximal fibula: note the thickness of the cartilaginous cap and flaring of the cortex (macro) and the fuzzy indistinct margins with irregular mineralization visible on X-ray. **B** Discrete peripheral nodules of cartilage are embedded in the soft tissue at the periphery of the lesion. These features explain the irregular margins and the possibility of local recurrence when the lesion is resected with inadequate surgical margins.

Histopathology

Secondary peripheral chondrosarcomas are generally low-grade tumours. Criteria for histological grading are similar to those for central chondrosarcoma {788}. The formation of nodules, mitosis, myxoid change and cystic cavities can be seen, although objective histological parameters to identify malignant transformation of an osteochondroma are lacking {588}. There is increased vascularization as compared to osteochondroma {592}. Clinical features and radiographical evaluation combined with the thickness of the cartilaginous cap are crucial to establish a diagnosis of low-grade secondary peripheral chondrosarcoma.

Prognostic factors

Patients with secondary peripheral chondrosarcomas show a diverse clinical course, ranging from slow insidious tumour growth to rapid neoplastic progression, depending on the location (the pelvis, shoulder and hip bear a worse prognosis) and histological grade {365}.

Periosteal chondrosarcoma

Definition

A malignant hyaline cartilage neoplasm, which occurs on the surface of bone and originates from the periosteum.

Synonym

Juxtacortical chondrosarcoma

Epidemiology

In the SEER data, only 3 of 667 chondrosarcoma were classified as periosteal {683}. The tumour occurs in adults, primarily in the second to fourth decades of life, with a slight male predominance {412, 2069}

Sites of involvement

The most frequent sites of involvement are the metaphysis of long bones, most commonly the distal femur and the humerus.

Clinical features and imaging

Patients present with pain, with or without swelling. Radiologically the tumour presents as a large lobular mass (often > 5 cm) localized on the cortex, which can be either thickened or thinned. Marrow involvement is very rare. Typical cartilaginous calcifications are seen. A calcified shell can be present. The lesions are well delineated towards the soft tissue {2069, 2851}.

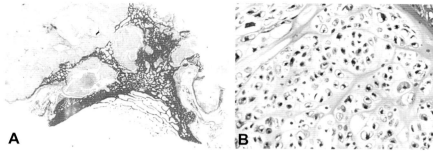

Fig. 15.40 Periosteal chondrosarcoma. **A** At low power, the cartilage lesion is pasted on the cortex. **B** High-power view shows highly cellular and pleomorphic cartilaginous cells.

Macroscopy

A large (usually > 5 cm) lobulated mass is attached to the surface of the bone {2069}. On cut section the tumour is grey-glistening and is often associated with gritty white areas of enchondral ossification and calcification {412}. The tumour erodes the underlying cortex; the medullary canal is usually not involved {2069}.

Histopathology

Histologically, a cartilage producing malignant tumour is seen on the external surface of the bone, marked by well-differentiated lobular cartilage with extensive areas of secondary calcifications and endochondral ossification {412}. Osteoid or bone directly formed by the tumour cells is absent although metaplastic bone formation can be found, often on the edges of the cartilage lobules. The microscopic image resembles that of a grade I or II primary central chondrosarcoma {412,2069}. The significance of histological grading is uncertain. Only rarely is bone marrow invasion observed {412,2069}. The demarcation with the soft tissue is not sharp,

occasionally with splitting growth into the soft tissues {412,2069}. The distinction between periosteal chondroma and chondrosarcoma is based on cortical invasion or invasion of the soft tissue, and the often larger tumour diameter (> 5 cm) in the case of a periosteal chondrosarcoma {1257}.

Prognosis

The reported incidence of local recurrence varies from 13 to 28% and depends on the type of surgical treatment {2170}. Metastases seem rare but are reported {208,2170}

Genetics

IDH1 and *IDH2* mutations are found in primary (38–70%) and secondary (86%) central chondrosarcomas in addition to periosteal chondrosarcomas (4/4 cases, 100%) {54,56,2165}. These mutations are early events since they occur in enchondromas (sporadic as well as associated with Ollier disease and Maffucci syndrome; see Chapter 27) {56,2165}. The genetic events causing malignant transformation of enchondroma are unknown.

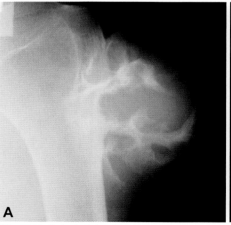
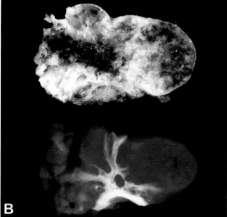

Fig. 15.41 Periosteal chondrosarcoma. **A** X-ray shows the lesion arising on the bone surface with multilobular appearance. **B** Gross features and the X-ray of the surgical specimen from the partial cortex resection of the lesion.

For osteochondroma formation, inactivation of the *EXT1* or *EXT2* gene is required. In contrast, most secondary peripheral chondrosarcomas arising in osteochondroma are wildtype *EXT* indicating that *EXT* is not important for chondrosarcomagenesis and that the non-mutated cells in osteochondroma are more vulnerable for as yet unknown (epi-)genetic changes promoting their malignant transformation {590}.

Cytogenetically, chondrosarcomas are heterogeneous, with karyotypic complexity ranging from single numerical or structural chromosomal aberrations to heavily rearranged karyotypes {312,1719,2708}. Aneuploidy is found with increasing histological grade. Polyploidization of an initially hyperhaploid/hypodiploid cell population is a common mechanism of progression in a subset of central, as well as peripheral chondrosarcomas {290,1085, 2126}. Rare recurrent aberrations include loss of 9p {286,1092, 1546} and 13q {1719}, and gain at 8q24 {1545,1954} and 12q13 {2383}. Primary central and secondary peripheral chondrosarcomas may differ in their genetic makeup, as reflected by differences in LOH pattern and incidence, DNA ploidy status and cytogenetic aberrations {281,286}. Cytogenetic data on periosteal chondrosarcoma are limited; no shared breakpoints have been identified {286}.

Several active signalling pathways have been identified in central chondrosarcoma {284}. The *RB1* pathway is affected in 86% of high-grade chondrosarcomas {2477, 2831} and includes loss of *CDKN2A* and

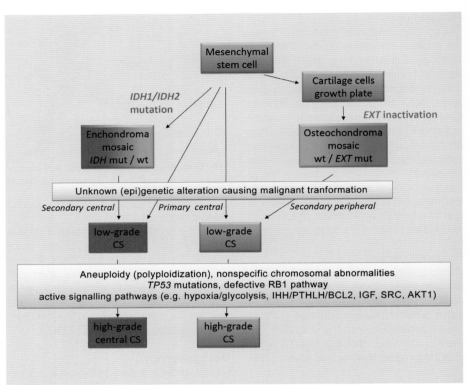

Fig. 15.42 Approximately 50% of solitary enchondromas and chondrosarcomas (CS) harbour *IDH1* or *IDH2* mutations. Enchondromas that carry *IDH1* or *IDH2* mutations (red boxes) as well as osteochondromas with *EXT1* inactivation (green boxes) are composed of intermingled mutated and wildtype cells (intraneoplastic mosaicism). For osteochondroma, it has been shown that the wildtype cells (blue) are prone to progress to malignancy, since the majority of peripheral CS are *EXT* wildtype. Malignant transformation is caused by as yet unknown (epi)genetic alterations. Progression to high grade chondrosarcoma is characterized by aneuploidy, defective cell cycle regulation, and activity of several signalling pathways as shown (mut, mutated; wt, wildtype).

overexpression and/or amplification of *CDK4* {115,2477}. Mutations in *CDKN2A* are absent {115,281}. IHH/PTHLH signalling, which is involved in normal growth-plate signalling, is active in both central and peripheral chondrosarcoma {287,1094,2381,2757} although activity seems to decrease in high-grade peripheral chondrosarcoma {1094}.

Dedifferentiated chondrosarcoma

C. Inwards
P.C.W. Hogendoorn

Definition
A highly malignant variant of chondrosarcoma, characterized by a bimorphic histological appearance with distinct and abruptly separated areas of low-grade chondrosarcoma juxtaposed to a high-grade, non-cartilaginous sarcoma.

ICD-O code   9243/3

Epidemiology
Dedifferentiation develops in 10–15% of central chondrosarcomas {908,2631}. On very rare occasions, dedifferentiation of peripheral chondrosarcoma has been reported {2380}. The median age of patients with dedifferentiated chondrosarcoma is 59 years (range, 15–89 years), and there is a slight male predominance {1039}.

Sites of involvement
The most common sites of involvement are the femur, pelvis, and humerus. In dedifferentiated peripheral chondrosarcoma, the preferred site of involvement follows that of the primary tumour i.e. pelvis, scapula and ribs {2380,2633}.

Clinical and imaging features
The most common clinical presentations include pain, a palpable mass and pathological fracture. Imaging findings are usually indicative of an aggressive, destructive cartilage tumour, with a heterogeneous radiological presentation of both conventional chondrosarcoma—the presence of ring-like densities—as well as lytic, permeable, destructive areas. Bimorphic features, suggesting dedifferentiation, are seen in approximately 50% of CT scans and 30% of MRI and radiographs of histologically proven cases. These include a dominant lytic area within, or adjacent to, a mineralized tumour on radiographs and a large unmineralized soft-tissue mass associated with an intra-osseous chondroid tumour on CT or MRI {1637}. Dedifferentiated areas can be accurately identified using dynamic MRI.

Macroscopy
Typically, the cartilaginous and non-cartilaginous components of the tumour are grossly evident in varying proportions. The blue-grey, lobulated cartilage component is usually located centrally, whereas the fleshy, pale-yellow or tan-brown high-grade sarcoma component is predominantly extra-osseous, or at the site of the pathological fracture.

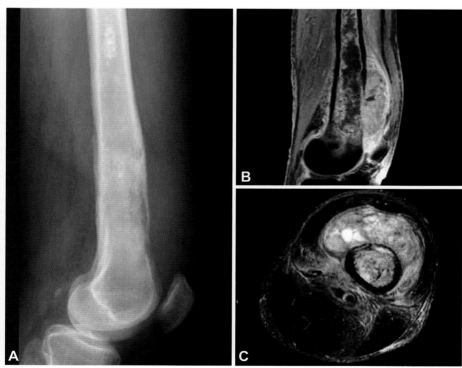

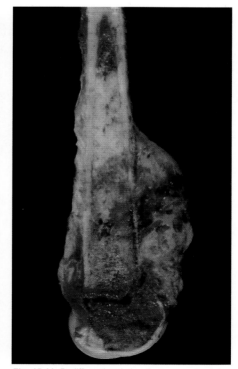

Fig. 15.43 Dedifferentiated chondrosarcoma. **A** Lateral radiograph of the distal femur shows a destructive lesion involving a long segment of the diaphysis and metaphysis with associated cortical thickening, indolent periosteal reaction and chondroid matrix, classic findings for chondrosarcoma. There is less mineral in the distal portion of the lesion along with a large anteriorly associated soft-tissue mass. **B** The sagittal T1-weighted MRI with gadolinium shows extensive myxoid change in the mid anddistal portion of the intramedullary portion of the lesion. **C** The axial T2-weighted MRI clearly delineates the large soft-tissue mass.

Fig. 15.44 Dedifferentiated chondrosarcoma involving the proximal femur. The medullary portion of the tumour has the typical grey-blue appearance of hyaline cartilage. The high-grade sarcoma component corresponds to the yellow-tan and red-brown extra-osseous part of the tumour.

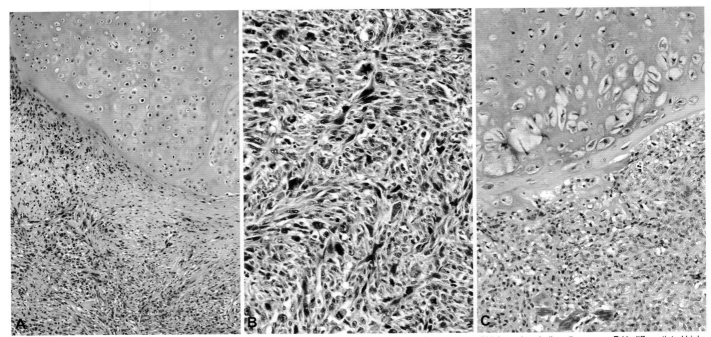

Fig. 15.45 Dedifferentiated chondrosarcoma. **A** There is an abrupt transition between the low-grade chondrosarcoma and high-grade spindle cell sarcoma. **B** Undifferentiated high-grade pleomorphic sarcoma represents the high-grade component of this dedifferentiated chondrosarcoma. **C** Low-grade chondrosarcoma juxtaposed to high-grade osteosarcoma.

Histopathology

There is an abrupt transition between the low-grade hyaline cartilage and high-grade sarcoma components of dedifferentiated chondrosarcoma {548}. The cartilaginous portion can range from enchondroma-like appearance to grade I or grade II chondrosarcoma. The high-grade dedifferentiated component has the appearance of a high-grade undifferentiated sarcoma or osteosarcoma. Less common examples of high-grade angiosarcoma, leiomyosarcoma, rhabdomyosarcoma and giant cell-rich tumours have been reported. Dedifferentiated chondrosarcomas usually show a poor histological response to preoperative chemotherapy.

Immunophenotype

Only a small percentage of the *IDH1* mutations (< 20%) can be identified using the specific IDH1 R132H antibody {54, 2165}. The immunophenotype of the non-cartilaginous component follows its histological line of differentiation, and keratin and desmin expression can be observed.

Genetics

Heterozygous mutations of the isocitrate dehydrogenase 1 and 2 genes (*IDH1* and *IDH2*) are found in approximately 50% of dedifferentiated chondrosarcomas, and have been found in both components {54}. Available cytogenetic data do not indicate any particular chromosomal aberration associated with progression to dedifferentiated chondrosarcoma {286,313, 1719,2087,2146,2450,2688,2727,3047}. Structural and numerical aberrations are most frequently reported for chromosomes 1 and 9, and amplification of the 8q24.12–24.13 region, including the *MYC* gene, occurs in approximately 20% of cases {1954}. The finding of identical *TP53* and *IDH1* mutations in both differentiated and dedifferentiated components is indicative of a common origin, while the extensive genetic differences at other loci suggest an early division of the two cell clones {54,282}. Additional support for a common origin concept comes from combined cytogenetic and immunophenotypical analyses, showing numerical aberrations of chromosome 7 in both components {313}. In dedifferentiated peripheral chondrosarcoma, TGF-β signalling is active in the low-grade component, whereas down regulated PTHLH signalling and different splicing of CD44v3 seem to be operative in the dedifferentiation process {2380}.

Prognostic factors

Patients with dedifferentiated chondrosarcoma have a dismal prognosis, most often as a result of widespread lung metastases. Overall 5-year survival rates ranging from 7% to 24% have been reported {665,908,1039}. Treatment consists of surgery with wide or radical margins {1913}. Chemotherapy and radiation therapy have not been shown to improve prognosis {665,1039,2071}. Poor prognostic factors include presence of a pathological fracture, metastatic disease at diagnosis, pelvic location, and increasing age {1039}.

Mesenchymal chondrosarcoma

Y. Nakashima
G. de Pinieux
M. Ladanyi

Definition

A rare malignant neoplasm characterized by a bimorphic pattern that is composed of poorly differentiated small round cells and islands of well-differentiated hyaline cartilage.

ICD-O code   9240/3

Epidemiology

Mesenchymal chondrosarcomas account for < 3% of all primary chondrosarcomas. Although occurring at any age, the peak incidence is in the second and the third decades of life. Males and females are affected equally {395,409,539, 567,805, 806,1194,1263,1996}.

Sites of involvement

These tumours show a widespread distribution. The craniofacial bones (especially the jawbones) {1446,2867}, the ribs, the ilium, and the vertebrae are the most common sites {211,409,805,806,1117,1996}. Additionally one fifth to one third of the lesions primarily affect the somatic soft tissues {211,409,567,805,1057,1117,1307, 1996} and the meninges are one of the most common sites of extraskeletal involvement {805,806,2391,2461}. Rare visceral involvement can occur {1,567,1004, 1241,1364}.

Clinical and imaging features

The cardinal symptoms are pain and swelling, ranging from a few days to several years {211,1057,1996}. Oncogenic osteomalacia, secondary to mesenchymal chondrosarcoma, has been reported {3078}.

Radiologically, skeletal lesions are primarily lytic and destructive with poor margins, not significantly differing from conventional chondrosarcoma in most cases {1985,1996,3019}. Mottled calcification is sometimes prominent. Some have well-defined margins with a sclerotic rim. Expansion of the bone is frequent, and cortical destruction or cortical breakthrough with extra-osseous extension into the soft tissue is common. Bony sclerosis, cortical thickening, and superficial involvement of

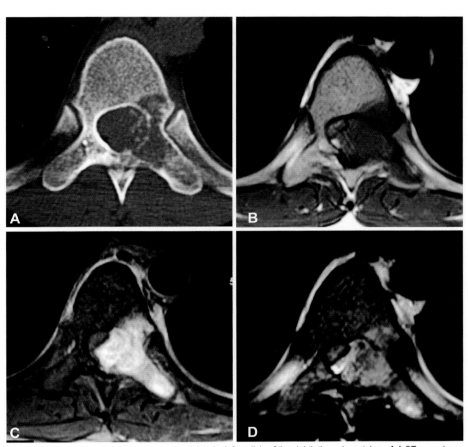

Fig. 15.46 Mesenchymal chondrosarcoma involving the left pedicle of the eighth thoracic vertebra. **A** A CT scan showing an osteolytic and destructive lesion with irregular calcification accompanied by extra-osseous extension into the soft tissue in the vertebral foramen and spinal canal. **B** T1-weighted MRI. **C** T1-weighted MRI with gadolinium enhancement. **D** T2-weighted MRI.

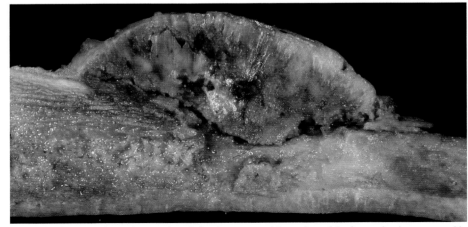

Fig. 15.47 Gross specimen of mesenchymal chondrosarcoma of the surface of the femur, showing a reasonably well-demarcated lesion involving the cortex and soft tissues.

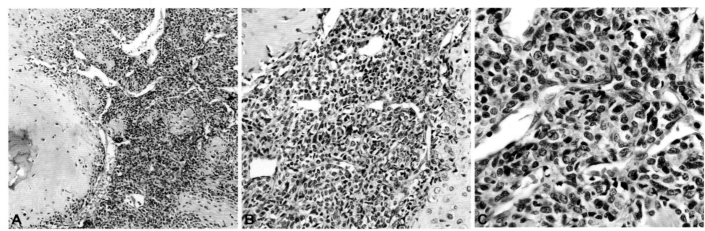

Fig. 15.48 Mesenchymal chondrosarcoma. **A** Combination of cartilaginous islands and highly cellular proliferation with numerous vascular clefts. **B** An abrupt transition between Ewing sarcoma-like high-grade small cell malignancy and low-grade cartilaginous proliferation with calcification. **C** High-power appearance of the small cell proliferation with a myopericytomatous pattern.

the bone surface are also seen. Imaging features of extra-skeletal tumours are also nonspecific, showing chondroid-type calcifications and foci of low signal intensity within enhancing lobules {1130,2522}. The tumour takes up contrast medium on CT or MRI.

Macroscopy

The tumours are grey-white to grey-pink, firm to soft, and usually well-defined, circumscribed masses varying from 3 to 30 cm in maximum diameter {1263,1996}. Lobulation is rare. Most lesions contain hard, mineralized deposits that vary from dispersed foci to prominent areas. Some tumours show a clearly cartilaginous appearance, even in a small section. Foci of necrosis and haemorrhage may be prominent.

Histopathology

The typical biphasic pattern is composed of poorly differentiated small round to oval cells with scant cytoplasm admixed with islands of hyaline cartilage {1263,1996}. The amount of cartilage is highly variable. The cartilage may be distinct from the undifferentiated component or blend gradually with it. In the poorly differentiated areas, the small round cells typically simulate Ewing sarcoma, and a myopericytoma-like

vascular pattern is common. The small cells may be spindle-shaped to some extent. Osteoclast-like multinucleated giant cells may occasionally be seen, and osteoid-like matrix may be present {1996}.

Immunophenotype

Positivity for SOX9 {805,2912} with negative staining for FLI-1 {1583} in the small cell component, may be helpful in distinguishing mesenchymal chondrosarcoma from Ewing sarcoma. The small cell component of mesenchymal chondrosarcomas was also described as positive in varying proportions for CD99 {329, 1028,1194} and desmin {806,960,1194}, while CD45 is negative.

Genetics

A recurrent *HEY1-NCOA2* fusion has been identified in mesenchymal chondrosarcomas, representing an in-frame fusion of *HEY1* exon 4 to *NCOA2* exon 13 at the mRNA level {2895}. This fusion is detected in all well-characterized mesenchymal chondrosarcomas tested, and is absent in other subtypes of chondrosarcomas {2895}. Given that *HEY1* and *NCOA2* are only about 10 Mb apart on chromosome 8, mapping to 8q21.1 and 8q13.3 respectively, and both are in the same orientation, this fusion could arise most sim-

ply from a small interstitial deletion, del(8)(q13.3q21.1), which would be difficult to detect in most conventional banding preparations. Indeed, there are no cytogenetic reports of this deletion in mesenchymal chondrosarcoma, although various abnormalities of chromosome 8 were described in earlier reports {954,2014}. The consistent molecular detection of the *HEY1-NCOA2* fusion in this sarcoma establishes it as a marker of potential clinical utility. Notably, *IDH1* or *IDH2* point mutations are absent {54,564,2165}.

Prognostic factors

Mesenchymal chondrosarcoma is an aggressive neoplasm. Distant metastases are observed even after a delay of > 20 years {1996}. The clinical course is frequently protracted and relentless, making long-term follow up mandatory. There is no correlation of prognosis with the histological features of the neoplastic small cell areas or the expression of tumour differentiation genes {1996,2082}. Children, adolescents, and young adults tend to have a slightly better outcome {567}. Mesenchymal chondrosarcoma of the jaw bones appears to have a more indolent course than at other anatomical sites {2867}.

Clear cell chondrosarcoma

E.F. McCarthy
P.C.W. Hogendoorn

Definition
A rare variant of chondrosarcoma, characterized by a proliferation of tumour cells with clear cytoplasm. It occurs most commonly at the ends of long bones.

ICD-O code   9242/3

Epidemiology
Clear cell chondrosarcoma comprises approximately 2% of all chondrosarcomas {2264}. Men are almost three times more likely to develop clear cell chondrosarcoma than women. The reported age range is 12–84 years {251,1290}. However, most patients are aged between 25 and 50 years.

Sites of involvement
Clear cell chondrosarcoma has been reported in most bones in the skeleton, including skull, spine, hands, and feet. However, approximately two thirds of lesions occur in the humeral or femoral head.

Clinical and imaging features
Pain is the most common presenting symptom; 55% of patients had pain for > 1 year, while 18% had symptoms for > 5 years {251}. Radiographically, clear cell chondrosarcoma usually presents as a well-defined, lytic lesion in the epiphysis of a long bone. Occasionally, a sclerotic rim may be present. Some lesions may contain stippled radio-densities, characteristic of cartilage.

Macroscopy
Lesions range from 2 to 13 cm in maximum diameter. They contain soft but gritty material, sometimes with cystic areas. Gross features characteristic of cartilage are not usually present.

Histopathology
The neoplasm consists of sheets of cells with large, round nuclei with central nucleoli. The cells have pale, clear or slightly eosinophilic cytoplasm with distinct cytoplasmic membranes. Osteoclast-like giant cells are frequently present. Mitotic figures are rare. Many lesions also contain zones of conventional low-grade chondrosarcoma with hyaline cartilage and minimally atypical nuclei. This cartilage may be focally calcified or ossified. Woven bone is frequently observed and may form directly in the stroma. Areas of cystic degeneration resembling aneurysmal bone cyst are often present. The clear cells contain glycogen.

Immunophenotype
The clear cells and chondroblastoma-like cells are strongly positive for S100 protein and type II and X collagen {22}.

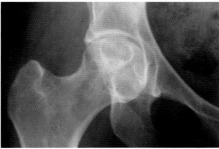

Fig. 15.49 Clear cell chondrosarcoma. X-ray showing a well-defined lytic lesion in the femoral head. There is a thin sclerotic rim. The radiographic image is strongly suggestive of chondroblastoma.

Genetics
Cytogenetic analyses have revealed clonal abnormalities in seven of eight cases with diploid or near-diploid complements predominating, and loss or structural aberrations of chromosome 9 and gain of chromosome 20 recurrent in a small subset {1719,2064,2146,2574, 2629}. CDKN2A alterations appear to be infrequent although all clear cell chondrosarcomas examined lacked expression of CDKN2A {1810,2185}. TP53 overexpression is frequently found in the absence of detectable mutations {2186}. Neither IDH1 nor IDH2 mutations are present {54}.

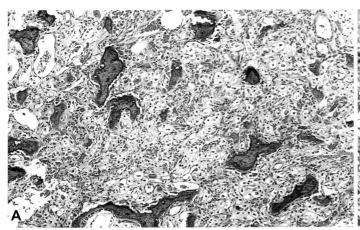
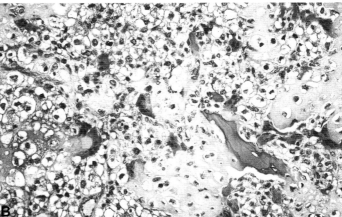

Fig. 15.50 Clear cell chondrosarcoma. **A** Low-power photomicrograph showing sheets of clear cell admixed with seams of woven bone. **B** Sheets of clear cells with areas of mature hyaline cartilage.

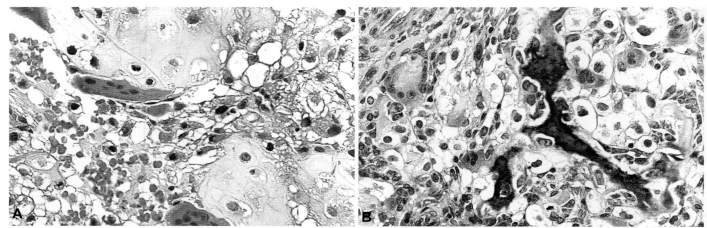

Fig. 15.51 Clear cell chondrosarcoma. **A** Photomicrograph showing multinucleated giant cells associated with chondroid nodules. **B** High-power photomicrograph of typical clear cells. A few osteoclast-like giant cells are present.

Prognostic factors

En-bloc excision with clear margins is usually curative. Marginal excision or curettage results in a recurrence rate of 86% {251,2264}. Metastases, usually to the lungs and other skeletal sites, may develop, and the overall mortality rate in these cases is 15% {1292}. Dedifferentiation to high-grade sarcoma has been reported in three cases {1356}.

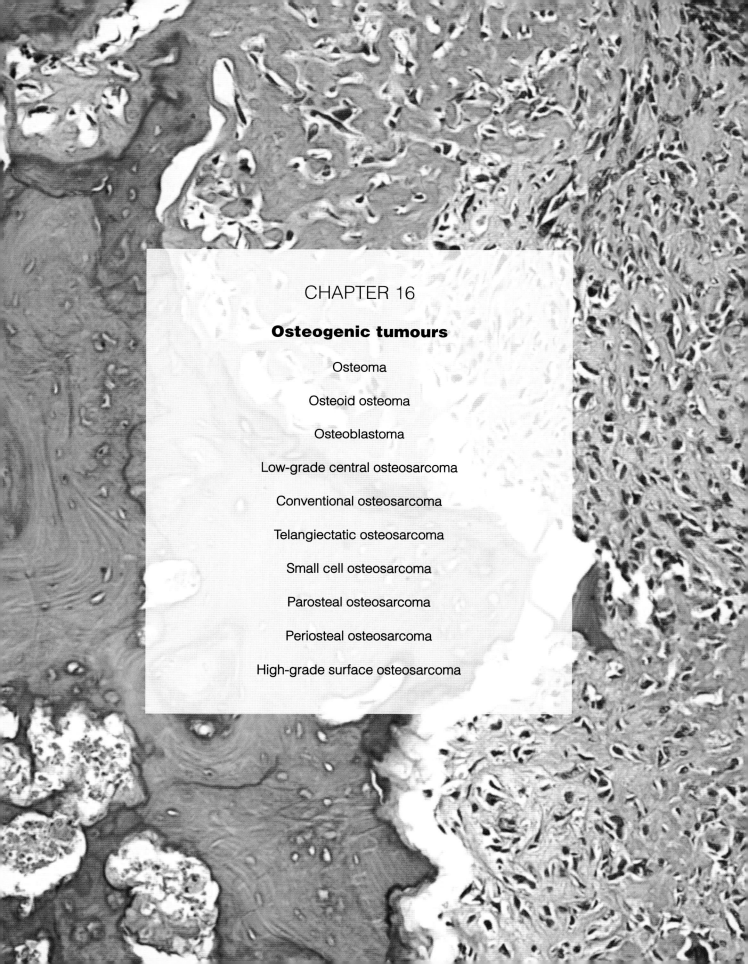

CHAPTER 16

Osteogenic tumours

Osteoma

D. Baumhoer
J. Bras

Definition
A benign tumour composed of compact bone arising on the surface of the bone and, when developing in the medullary cavity, known as enostosis.

ICD-O code   9180/0

Synonyms
Osteoma: ivory exostosis
Enostosis: bone island

Epidemiology
Osteomas affect men and women equally whereas enostoses seem to be more common in males. Since osteomas are commonly incidental findings, their actual prevalence is difficult to determine.

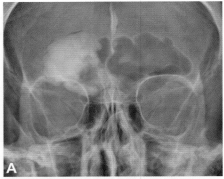

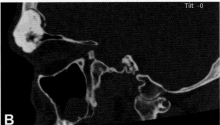

Fig. 16.01 Parosteal osteoma of the right frontal sinus. **A** Computed radiography. **B** CT scan (sagittal multiplanar reconstruction).

Etiology
Multiple osteomas can occur in the autosomal dominantly inherited Gardner syndrome, a variant of familial adenomatous polyposis (FAP), together with supernumerary impacted teeth, and skin and soft tissue tumours {1042}. The etiology of sporadic cases is unknown. Multiple enostoses are observed in Buschke-Ollendorff syndrome (osteopoikilosis) {345}. However, most cases of enostosis seem to represent hamartomatous lesions.

Sites of involvement
Osteomas predominantly affect bone formed by membranous ossification, i.e. calvarial, facial and jaw bones {1547}. They only rarely occur outside the skull {215}. Intramedullary lesions generally originate in the epi- and metaphyses of long bones, the pelvic bones and vertebral bodies.

Clinical and imaging features
Osteomas are usually asymptomatic, but can provoke obstruction of the paranasal sinuses or lead to local swellings {1547}. Osteomas are homogenously ossified, well-limited masses. Enostoses are usually small, spiculated, ossified masses.

Macroscopy
Osteomas are typically well-circumscribed tumours with a broad attachment to the underlying bone. Bone islands are intramedullary foci of compact bone. Most osteomas are < 2 cm in diameter.

Histopathology
Osteomas are predominantly composed of lamellar bone and can be divided histologically into compact, spongious and mixed subtypes. In cancellous areas, the bone is lined by active and inactive osteo-

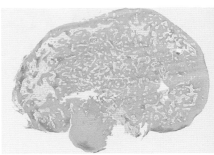

Fig. 16.02 Parosteal osteoma. Low-power image.

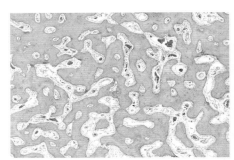

Fig. 16.03 Parosteal osteoma with areas of mature compact and spongious bone.

blasts within a well-vascularized and moderately cellular and fibrous stroma. Especially in the fronto-ethmoid region, active osteoblastic and osteoclastic remodelling may occasionally mimic osteoblastoma {1791}.

Prognostic factors
Asymptomatic cases generally do not require treatment and follow an indolent clinical course.

Osteoid osteoma

A. Horvai
M. Klein

Definition
A benign bone-forming tumour characterized by small size (< 2 cm), limited growth potential and disproportionate pain, usually responsive to non steroidal anti-inflammatory drugs.

ICD-O code   9191/0

Epidemiology
Osteoid osteoma usually affects children and adolescents, although it is occasionally seen in older individuals. It is more common in males.

Sites of involvement
Osteoid osteoma has been reported in virtually every bone, but it is most common in the long bones, particularly in the proximal femur.

Clinical and imaging features
The usual presenting complaint is pain. The pain, at first intermittent and mild with nocturnal exacerbation, eventually becomes relentless to the point of interfering with sleep. On the other hand, it is characteristic for nonsteroidal anti-inflammatory drugs, even in small doses, to completely relieve the pain for hours at a time. About 80% of patients report this characteristic feature {1151}. On physical examination, there is often an area of exquisite, localized tenderness associated with the lesion, and there may be redness and localized swelling. There are sometimes unusual clinical manifestations that are site-dependent. When lesions are located at the very end of a long bone, patients may present with swelling and effusion of the nearest joint, resembling monoarticular arthritis. When osteoid osteoma arises in the spine, it usually affects the neural arch, and patients may present with painful scoliosis due to spasm of the spinal muscles {1428}. When the tumour occurs in the fingers, the persistent soft tissue swelling and periosteal reactions may result in functional loss that leads to numerous surgeries, large en-bloc excisions {2596} and even rare amputations. Osteoid osteoma near or within joints may cause a reactive and inflammatory arthritis that can result in secondary osteoarthritis and ectopic ossification {2073}.

Imaging
On plain films, the lesion is characterized by dense cortical sclerosis surrounding a radiolucent nidus. The cortical sclerosis may be so pronounced that the dense bone obscures the nidus. In those uncommon cases in which the centre of the lesion has ossified, the lesion can appear like a target, demonstrating central sclerosis within an area of circumscribed radiolucency. When plain radiographs demonstrate dense cortical sclerosis, particularly if it is eccentric and fusiform, osteoid osteoma should be suspected. The area containing the actual tumour may be visualized with a Technetium-99 bone scan if it can not be seen on a plain radiograph. Atypical and even misleading radiographic findings may be associated with osteoid osteomas in certain locations. Subperiosteal osteoid osteoma may produce a misleading degree of periostitis, while surface osteoid osteomas arising within joints may be virtually invisible on plain radiographs. The best imaging study to demonstrate osteoid osteoma is a CT

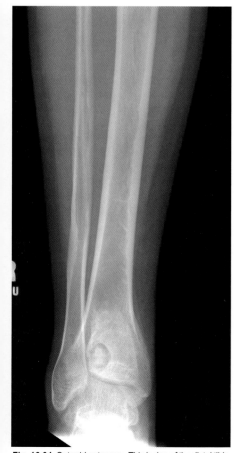

Fig. 16.04 Osteoid osteoma. This lesion of the distal tibia has a targetoid appearance with a radio-opaque centre, a surrounding ring of lucency and a peripheral region of sclerosis.

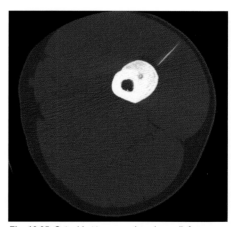

Fig. 16.05 Osteoid osteoma undergoing radiofrequency ablation. An axial CT scan of the thigh shows the introduction of a radiofrequency needle into an osteoid osteoma of the femur. Note the central lucent nidus in the centre of an area of sclerosis.

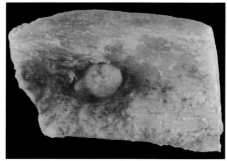

Fig. 16.06 Osteoid osteoma. Grossly, the nidus is 5 mm in diameter and has a hypervascular zone within the surrounding sclerotic cortex.

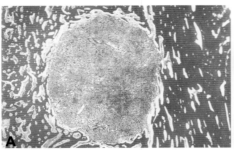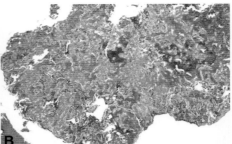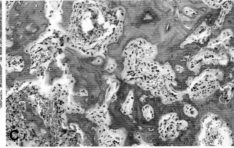

Fig. 16.07 Osteoid osteoma. **A** Very sharp circumscription of nidus near the cortical surface showing dense cortex to the right and reactive neocortex to the left of the lesion. **B** The central nidus of osteoid osteoma demonstrates interconnected, delicate trabeculae of woven bone. Native lamellar bone is present in the left lower corner. **C** Trabeculae are thin and inter-anastomosing with abundant cement lines and a single layer of osteoblasts. The intertrabecular space is filled with fibrovascular stroma.

scan {116}, which should be evaluated at 1mm intervals. MRI is not as sensitive as CT for detecting the nidus, but demonstrates abundant peritumoral oedema {2621}.

Macroscopy

Osteoid osteoma is a small, round, often cortically based, red, gritty or granular lesion surrounded by (and sharply circumscribed from) ivory white sclerotic bone. The lesion seldom exceeds 1cm in greatest diameter.

Histopathology

The essential feature in the central portion of the lesion (nidus) is the presence of differentiated osteoblastic activity {1312}. There is vascularized connective tissue, within which differentiating osteoblasts are engaged in the production of osteoid and sometimes bone. The osteoid may be microscopically disposed in a sheet-like configuration, but very often it is organized into microtrabecular arrays that are lined by a single layer of plump appositional osteoblasts. Osteoclasts may also be seen engaged in remodelling. Significant nuclear pleomorphism is absent in osteoid osteoma and cartilage is also usually absent. Surrounding the tumour, there is almost always an area of hypervascular sclerotic bone. This osteosclerosis tends to be more pronounced as lesions be-

come closer to the bone surface and less pronounced in medullary lesions. The interface between osteoid osteoma and the surrounding reactive bone is very abrupt and circumscribed. When it can be demonstrated histologically, this interface provides very strong histological evidence of indolent local behaviour. Even when the interface between tumour and reactive bone is not demonstrable in sections, the diagnosis becomes apparent by correlating the histological findings with imaging studies.

The pathological evaluation of osteoid osteoma has undergone changes because of the increasing use of minimally invasive techniques to ablate the tumour. If a diagnosis of osteoid osteoma can be made clinically and radiographically, it is sometimes ablated without prior biopsy. In other cases, a core biopsy is obtained prior to ablation. In others cases, fragments obtained from a drill procedure are sent for histological opinion. The yield of diagnostic tissue in these cases is not only lower than with traditional surgery, but the tissue findings are often obscured by heat or crush artefacts {24}.

Immunophenotype

Strong nuclear staining for the regulatory transcription factors Runx2 and Osterix has been described in osteoid osteoma,

providing indirect evidence that it shares common genetic pathways with normal skeletal development {565}.

Genetics

Only three cases of osteoid osteoma have shown clonal chromosome aberrations. Structural alterations involving 22q13.1 were found in two of these cases {163,561}.

Prognostic factors

The prognosis is excellent. Recurrences are uncommon. Some lesions have been reported to disappear without surgical therapy {947}. While traditional surgical excision is curative, it is sometimes challenging to resect small lesions, particularly when there is a great deal of reactive sclerosis. Consequently, less invasive techniques, including CT-guided core drill excision, percutaneous radiofrequency ablation with CT guidance, cryoablation, and laser photocoagulation have been developed {375,947,1991}. There are many advantages to using minimally invasive techniques and the success rate of radiofrequency ablation is about the same as with traditional surgery {593A,2247A}.

Osteoblastoma

C.E. de Andrea
J.A. Bridge
A. Schiller

Definition

A benign bone-forming neoplasm, > 2 cm, which produces woven bone spicules, which are bordered by prominent osteoblasts.

ICD-O code

9200/0

Epidemiology

Osteoblastoma is rare, accounting for about 1% of all bone tumours and is more common in males (2.5 : 1) and affects patients in the age range of 10–30 years, with extremes of 5 and 70 years.

Sites of involvement

Osteoblastoma commonly arises in the posterior elements of the spine and the sacrum (40–55% of cases). In the appendicular sites, the proximal femur, distal femur and proximal tibia are the most frequent. Osteoblastoma less commonly involves the tarsal bones (talus and calcaneous). The vast majority of cases are intraosseous (medullary) but a small percentage can occur on the surface of the bone in a periosteal (peripheral) site.

Clinical and imaging features

Osteoblastomas of the spine have similar symptoms to that of osteoid osteoma; namely back pain, scoliosis and nerve root compression {2023}. The appendicular tumours also produce pain and/or swelling, but these symptoms may be mild enough to last for months before the patient will see a clinician. Non-steroidal anti-inflammatory drugs do not relieve the pain after prolonged therapy. Toxic osteoblastoma is a very rare variant of osteoblastoma associated with systemic symptoms, including fever, anorexia, and weight loss. Osteoblastoma is generally a lytic, well-circumscribed, oval or round defect, almost always confined by a periosteal shell of reactive bone. Limb tumours are metaphyseal, lytic defects with a thin periosteal bone shell. Large tumours also produce aneurysmal bone cyst (ABC)-like changes. Some tumours may arise in a subperiosteal location but are still confined by a thin reactive bone shell. Most osteoblastomas

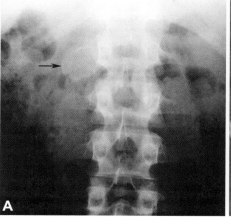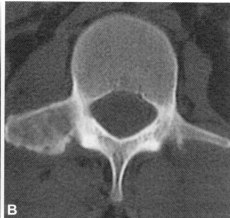

Fig. 16.08 Osteoblastoma. **A** The plain film has an enlarged well-defined lytic lesion of the right transverse process of L1 (see arrow). Although the tumour is large it is still confined by a thin periosteal shell of reactive bone. **B** A CT scan of the same case with a striking increase in size of the right transverse process of L1. The tumour is lytic and expansile, but there is no soft-tissue invasion. Despite the tumour's large size, it is totally surrounded by periosteal new bone.

are totally lytic and < 30% may have focal areas of calcification indicative of tumour bone mineralisation {1672}.

The size of osteoblastomas varies from small (2–3 cm) to enormous (15 cm or more). Most are in the 3–10 cm range. In those cases with secondary ABC changes, the tumours are generally larger. In cases with multiple, fluid-filled cavities, the fluid levels, calcification, and solid component of the lesion suggest the diagnosis of osteoblastoma with ABC-like changes.

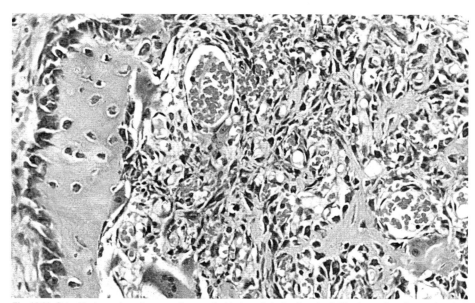

Fig. 16.09 Osteoblastoma. Irregular woven bone, osteoblasts and giant cells, ectactic blood vessels and a reactive shell of periosteal new bone.

Macroscopy

Osteoblastoma has an extremely rich vascular supply and therefore appears red or red-brown, often with a gritty or sandpaper consistency. The tumour is usually round to oval with a thinned cortex and always with a thin periosteal reactive bone shell if the cortex is destroyed. In cystic lesions, blood-filled spaces simulating ABC are prominent. The border between the tumour and medullary cavity is sharp, often with some reactive bone. The tumour has a "pushing" border rather than a permeative or infiltrative border against the endosteal cortical surface and trabecular bone of the marrow.

Histopathology

Osteoblastoma has identical histological features to osteoid osteoma {909,1306}. The tumour is composed of woven bone spicules or trabeculae. These spicules are haphazardly arranged and are lined with a single layer of osteoblasts. The vascularity is rich, often with extravasated erythrocytes. Osteoblasts may have mitoses but they are not atypical. Diffusely scattered osteoclast-type, multinucleated giant cells are often present. Extraordinary hyaline cartilage may be present and may represent microcallus formation. Sometimes the woven bone may be in aggregates or nodules and in such cases must be carefully scrutinised to exclude osteosarcoma. Osteoblastomas do not infiltrate or isolate pre-existing lamellar bone structures as do osteosarcomas, so special attention should be given to the border between pre-existing cortex or marrow trabeculae. The term epithelioid osteoblastoma, previously known as aggressive osteoblastoma, has been used for cases of osteoblastoma with large, plump osteoblasts with a prominent nucleus and nucleoli, sometimes with mitoses {685, 1397}. There is no evidence that epithelioid osteoblastoma has a worse prognosis than the standard type of osteoblastoma. The pseudomalignant variant contains osteoblasts with degenerative nuclear atypia in the absence of mitoses. In some cases osteoblastoma may have ABC-like foci. These areas may overshadow the underlying osteoblastoma.

Genetics

Cytogenetic studies of osteoblastoma are few with characterization of only six cases. These analyses have demonstrated near-diploid complements with unrelated rearrangements {971}.

Prognostic factors

Osteoblastoma is often treated by curettage. Large lesions may have to be excised. The prognosis is excellent and recurrences are unusual, but more likely in cases that were curetted from a bone with difficult surgical access.

Low-grade central osteosarcoma

C. Inwards
J. Squire

Definition

A low-grade malignant bone-forming neoplasm, that arises within the medullary cavity of bone.

ICD-O code   9187/3

Synonym

Low-grade intramedullary osteosarcoma

Epidemiology

Low-grade central osteosarcoma accounts for 1–2% of all osteosarcomas {1501}. The peak incidence is in the third decade of life, and there is a slight female predominance {205,2479}.

Sites of involvement

Approximately 80% of low-grade central osteosarcomas are located in the long bones, predominately in the distal femur and proximal tibia {205,1501, 2479}. Flat bones and small bones of the hands and feet are uncommonly affected {634}.

Clinical and imaging features

Pain and/or swelling are the usual presenting symptoms. The duration of pain may be many months or several years. Radiologically, these tumours are usually large, lytic, coarsely trabeculated, and have focal aggressive features {1501}. They tend to be metaphyseal or diametaphyseal, and often extend to the end of the affected bone. The majority of low-grade central osteosarcomas exhibit some degree of cortical disruption, the most convincing feature of malignancy, and/or periosteal reaction and soft-tissue extension. However, up to one third may show intermediate or well-defined margins suggesting an indolent or benign lesion. CT and MRI are very helpful in delineating the extent of the tumour and identifying cortical abnormalities that may not be evident on radiographs {63}.

Macroscopy

The cut surface of a low-grade central osteosarcoma shows a grey-white tumour with a firm and gritty texture, arising from within the intramedullary cavity. Cortical destruction with or without a soft-tissue mass may also be seen.

Histopathology

Low-grade central osteosarcoma is composed of a hypocellular to moderately cellular fibroblastic proliferation with variable amounts of osteoid production {2817}. The spindle-shaped tumour cells are arranged in fascicles or interlacing bundles that permeate surrounding cortical and/or cancellous bone. They are characterized by minimal cytological atypia and relatively few mitotic figures. The pattern of bone production is variable. Some tumours contain irregular anastomosing, branching, and curved bone trabeculae, simulating the appearance of woven bone in fibrous dysplasia {205}. Others contain moderate to heavy amounts of bone present as long longitudinal seams of lamellar-like bone resembling parosteal osteosarcoma. Small scattered foci of atypical cartilage are occasionally seen. In addition, benign multinucleated giant cells have been reported in up to 36% of low-grade central osteosarcomas {1501}.

The most helpful histological features that support a diagnosis of low-grade central osteosarcoma over fibrous dysplasia include permeation of pre-existing bone and soft-tissue extension.

Immunophenotype

Immunohistochemical detection of MDM2 and CDK4 may provide a useful diagnostic tool. Expression of these proteins was found in all low-grade central osteosarcomas examined in two separate studies {710,3037}. Benign fibro-osseous lesions are negative for these markers.

Genetics

Gain or amplification of *MDM2* (to include involvement of the 12q13–15 region) is frequent in low-grade central osteosarcoma {2182,710,2722}. This feature, combined with the overall lack of complex chromosomal aberrations and the low frequency of *TP53* mutations, differentiates this osteosarcoma subtype from the more complicated pattern of genetic changes

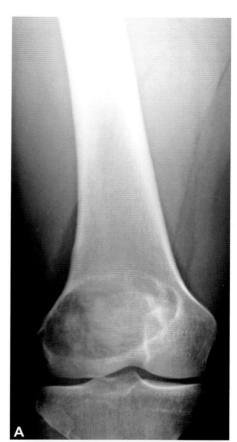

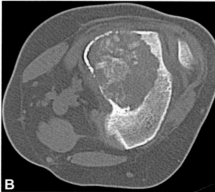

Fig. 16.10 Low-grade central osteosarcoma. **A** X-ray and **B** Axial CT of the distal femur show a well-circumscribed, predominantly lytic lesion in the distal femur with a partial peripheral rim of sclerosis. The CT shows that it contains osteoid matrix and is associated with mild expansion of the bone and subtle cortical permeation. The imaging features favour an indolent growth pattern that would be compatible with a low-grade central osteosarcoma.

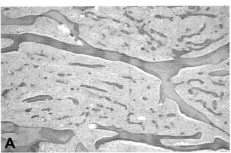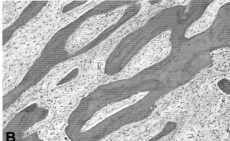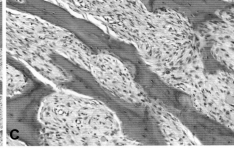

Fig. 16.11 Low-grade central osteosarcoma. **A** Irregularly shaped seams of bone resembling fibrous dysplasia. The tumour has a permeative growth pattern with entrapment of host bone. **B** Bland fibrous stroma surround the bone trabeculae. **C** Higher magnification showing plump spindle cells in a collagenous background.

seen in conventional high-grade osteosarcoma.

Prognostic factors

The prognosis for this tumour is excellent, with 90% overall survival at 5 years {455,2479}. Treatment is surgical removal with a wide margin. High grade dedifferentiation can be seen in the primary tumour, but more commonly in recurrences. Reported rates of progression to high-grade osteosarcoma range from 10% to 36% {455,1501,2479}. Chemotherapy is reserved for cases with progression {455,2479}.

Conventional osteosarcoma

A.E. Rosenberg
A-M. Cleton-Jansen
G. de Pinieux
A.T. Deyrup
E. Hauben
J. Squire

Definition

A high-grade, intra-osseous, malignant neoplasm in which the neoplastic cells produce bone. The tumour is primary when the underlying bone is normal and secondary when the bone is altered by conditions such as previous radiation, co-existing Paget disease, infarction, and rarely, other disorders.

ICD-O code

Osteosarcoma, not otherwise specified	9180/3
Chondroblastic osteosarcoma	9181/3
Fibroblastic osteosarcoma	9182/3
Osteoblastic osteosarcoma	9180/3

Epidemiology

Osteosarcoma is the most common primary high-grade sarcoma of the skeleton. It has a bimodal age distribution with most cases developing between the ages of 10–14 years and a second smaller peak in older adults (30% occur in individuals aged > 40 years) {2140,2445}. The annual incidence rate is approximately 4.4 per 10^6 for people aged 0–24 years, 1.7 per 10^6 people aged 25–59 years and 4.2 per 10^6 in people aged ≥ 60 years {68}. Males are affected more frequently (1.35:1) {2140}.

The incidence of osteosarcomatous transformation in Paget disease is estimated at approximately 1% and is most common in patients with polyostotic disease (approximately 70% of cases), with a peak incidence in the seventh decade and male predominance {656,1077,1259,2456,2953}. Paget osteosarcoma accounts for half of cases of osteosarcoma in patients aged > 60 years.

Osteosarcoma is the most common radiation-induced sarcoma, and represents 2.7–5.5% of all osteosarcomas. Radiation-associated osteosarcoma typically affects older patients (> 40 years) {295,549,2962}.

Osteosarcoma is rarely associated with a variety of other conditions, of which the most important are bone infarction, benign tumours (fibrous dysplasia, simple cyst, liposclerosing myxofibrous tumour etc) and metal prosthetic joints and hardware. Affected patients are usually aged > 40–50 years {523,1229,1333,1478}.

Etiology

Although the etiology is unknown, there is an increased incidence of primary osteosarcoma associated with several genetic syndromes (e.g. Li-Fraumeni {1713,2098}, hereditary retinoblastoma {697}, and Rothmund-Thomson {2557}); in older adults it is often secondary.

The etiology of sarcomatous transformation in Paget disease is not clearly defined. Somatic mutation of the *SQSTM1* locus has been suggested as a potential factor {1103,1846}.

The risk of developing post-radiation

osteosarcoma correlates with radiation dose and use of electrophilic chemotherapeutic agents {1264,1578,2801}. Most patients have received > 20 Gy (mean, approximately 50 Gy) {1097,1578,2519}. An etiological relationship has not been proven in prosthesis and metal hardware-associated osteosarcomas {2883}.

Sites of involvement
Primary osteosarcoma arises in any bone, but the vast majority originate in the long bones of the extremities, especially the distal femur (30%), followed by the proximal tibia (15%) and proximal humerus (15%) i.e. sites containing the most proliferative growth plates. In long bones, the tumour is usually cantered in the metaphysis (90%), infrequently in the diaphysis (9%), and rarely in the epiphysis. Tumours developing in the jaw, pelvis, and spine tend to occur in older individuals {2445}. Involvement of the small bones of the extremities is rare.

Sarcomatous transformation can occur in any Pagetic bone and is most common in the pelvis, humerus, skull and femur. Lesions of the appendicular skeleton are typically metaphyseal–diaphyseal. Compared with the distribution of Paget disease in the skeleton, Paget osteosarcoma occurs at a disproportionately high frequency in the humerus and low frequency in the spine. Multifocal disease occurs in 15–20% of cases and typically involves Pagetic bone; it is uncertain whether this represents metastatic disease or independent primaries {2456,2586,2953}.

Post-radiation osteosarcoma can develop in any irradiated bone, but the most common locations are the pelvis and the shoulder region {1264}.

Other secondary osteosarcomas are located in the affected bone and most often are the long bones of the lower extremities.

Clinical and imaging features
The tumour presents as an enlarging painful mass that may be palpable. The pain is deep-seated, progressive, and noted weeks to several months before diagnosis. The overlying skin may be warm, erythematous, oedematous, and cartographed by prominent engorged veins. Large tumours may restrict range of motion, decrease musculoskeletal function, cause joint effusions and, in advanced cases, result in weight loss and cachexia. In 5–10% of cases, the heralding event is a sudden, devastating, pathological fracture through the destructive mass.

The radiographical appearance of osteosarcoma is extremely variable; it typically presents as a large, destructive, poorly-defined, mixed lytic and blastic mass that transgresses the cortex and forms a large soft tissue component. The periphery of the tumour is the least mineralized and soft-tissue components may have a fine "cloud-like" pattern of radiodensity. It has avid uptake on technetium scans and is heterogeneous on CT and MRI.

Osteosarcoma developing in Pagetic bone is typically heralded by pain, swelling and a palpable mass. Pathological fracture is common in femoral lesions. Imaging studies frequently show a Pagetic bone within which is a lytic (approximately 60% of cases) destructive mass that often transgresses the cortex and extends into the soft tissues.

Radiation osteosarcoma usually has a latency period of at least two years and

is often longer (median, 11–15 years). Symptoms and imaging findings are similar to conventional osteosarcoma. Findings of radiation osteitis (trabecular coarsening and cortical lysis) are present in half of cases. Tumours are rarely multifocal.

Macroscopy
Conventional osteosarcoma usually presents as a large (> 5–10 cm), metaphyseal, intramedullary, tan–grey-white, gritty mass. Heavily mineralized tumours are tan-white and hard, whereas non-mineralized cartilaginous components are glistening, grey and may be mucinous if the matrix is myxoid, or more rubbery if hyaline in nature. Areas of haemorrhage and cystic change are common. Intramedullary

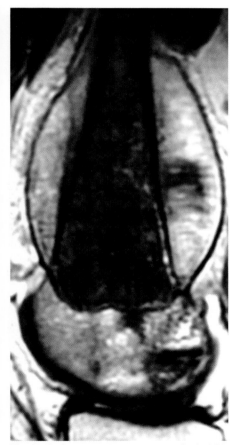

Fig. 16.12 Conventional osteosarcoma. Sagittal T1-weighted MRI revealing a large osteosarcoma of the distal femoral metaphysis. The intra-osseous component has slow signal intensity and the extra-osseous component is heterogeneous.

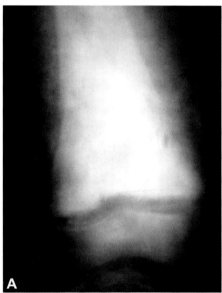

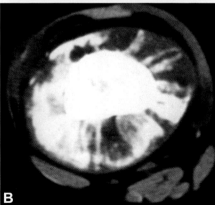

Fig. 16.13 Conventional osteosarcoma. **A** X-ray of osteoblastic osteosarcoma showing a large poorly defined blastic tumour centred in the metaphysis and extending into the soft tissues. **B** Axial CT of osteoblastic osteosarcoma transgressing the cortex and forming a circumferential soft-tissue mass.

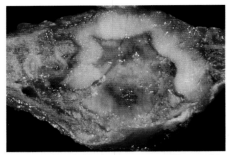

Fig. 16.14 Chondroblastic osteosarcoma of the mandible extending into the soft tissues. The glistening grey-white areas represent the chondroblastic component.

involvement is often considerable, and the tumour usually forms an eccentric or circumferential soft tissue component that displaces the periosteum peripherally.

Secondary osteosarcomas demonstrate the usual gross features of conventional osteosarcoma. The affected bone displays the findings characteristic of the underlying disease process.

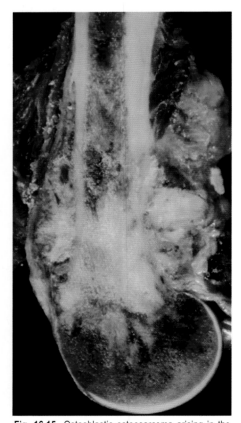

Fig. 16.15 Osteoblastic osteosarcoma arising in the medullary cavity of the metaphysis. The hard tan-white tumour destroys the cortex, extends into the soft tissues, and proximally displaces the periosteum producing Codman's triangle.

Histopathology

Conventional osteosarcoma has a broad spectrum of morphology. The tumour grows with a permeative pattern, replacing the marrow space, surrounding and eroding pre-existing trabeculae, and fills and expands Haversian systems. The neoplastic cells typically demonstrate severe anaplasia and pleomorphism, and may be epithelioid, plasmacytoid, fusiform, small and round or spindled. The cytoplasm is most often eosinophilic, but may be clear. The neoplastic cells often become small and "normalized" in appearance when surrounded by matrix.

Essential to the diagnosis of osteosarcoma is the identification of neoplastic bone; no minimal quantity is required as any amount is sufficient to render a diagnosis. Characteristically, the bone is intimately associated with the tumour cells, varies in quantity, is woven in architecture, and is deposited as primitive, disorganized trabeculae that may produce filigree and coarse lace-like patterns or broad, large sheets formed by coalescing trabeculae. The bone is eosinophilic when unmineralized and basophilic/purple if mineralized, and may have a Pagetoid appearance caused by haphazardly deposited cement lines. Distinguishing unmineralized matrix (osteoid) from other eosinophilic extracellular materials, especially collagen, may be difficult and subjective. Collagen tends to be more fibrillar, lies compressed between the cells, and is frequently deposited in broad aggregates.

Conventional osteosarcoma is subclassified according to specific histological features (Table 16.01). Currently, however, there is no relationship between subtype and treatment and prognosis {1138}. Conventional osteosarcoma commonly contains varying amounts of neoplastic cartilage and/or fibroblastic components, and based on the predominant matrix they are subdivided into osteoblastic (76–80%), chondroblastic (10–13%) and fibroblastic (10%) variants {134,1138}. In osteoblastic osteosarcoma the neoplastic bone is the principal matrix, and varies from thin, lace-like trabeculae to compact bone. When the latter is extensive, the tumour is designated the sclerosing type. In chondroblastic osteosarcoma the neoplastic cartilage is usually hyaline and high-grade, but may be myxoid, particularly in tumours arising in jaw bones. The neoplastic cells displaying a chondrocytic phenotype

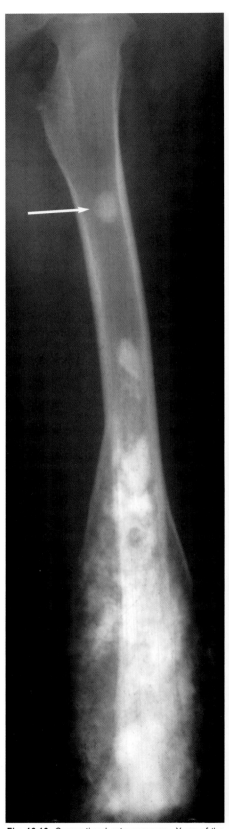

Fig. 16.16 Conventional osteosarcoma. X-ray of the femur with a large osteoblastic osteosarcoma with a proximal skip metastasis.

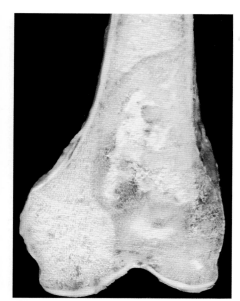

Fig. 16.17 Conventional osteosarcoma. Treated osteosarcoma with good response. The soft-tissue mass has receded and the portions containing foamy macrophages are bright yellow and the area previously occupied by tumour and replaced by fibrous tissue is tan-white.

demonstrate severe cytological atypia and reside in lacunar spaces in hyaline matrix, and demonstrate lesser degrees of atypia and float singly or in cords in myxoid matrix. The cartilage may form a large dominant component or be scattered throughout the tumour, merging with areas containing neoplastic bone. In the proper context, a biopsy containing only high-grade malignant cartilage should strongly raise the suspicion of chondroblastic osteosarcoma. In fibroblastic osteosarcoma, the malignant cells are usually spindled, less frequently epithelioid, and often, but not al-

ways demonstrate severe cytological atypia. The tumour cells are associated with extracellular collagen, which can be extensive, and often arranged in a storiform pattern (previously known as malignant fibrous histiocytoma-like variant). Cells with fibrillar eosinophilic cytoplasm are myofibroblastic in differentiation. Nonneoplastic, osteoclast-type giant cells scattered throughout the tumour are the hallmark of the giant-cell-rich variant {206}, while large polyhedral tumour cells characterize the epithelioid variant {1474}. In the osteoblastoma-like variant, the tumour cells may rim the neoplastic bony trabeculae in a fashion that mimics osteoblastoma. Features that permit its distinction are the permeative growth pattern, cells that are cytologically atypical and cellular intertrabecular regions {204}.The chondroblastoma-like variant resembles its benign counterpart but grows with an infiltrative pattern and demonstrates greater cytological atypia {129}.

Paget osteosarcomas are high-grade osteosarcomas that may show osteo-blastic, fibroblastic or chondroblastic morphology, in decreasing order of frequency. Telangiectatic and small cell variants have also been described.

In radiation-induced osteosarcoma, the histological changes of radiation osteitis may be present.

High-grade osteosarcoma is usually treated with preoperative chemotherapy and the accurate assessment of the chemotherapy response is critical—it is one of the most important prognosticators of overall and disease-free survival {68, 535}. A good response is defined as > 90% necrosis.

Table 16.01 Histological subtypes of osteosarcoma

Osteoblastic (including sclerosing)
Chondroblastic
Fibroblastic
Giant cell rich
Osteoblastoma-like
Epithelioid
Clear cell
Chondroblastoma-like

Immunophenotype

Osteosarcoma, whether primary or secondary, has a broad immunoprofile that lacks diagnostic specificity. Commonly expressed antigens include osteocalcin, osteonectin, S100 protein, actin, SMA NSE, and CD99 {804,1118}. Importantly, as it is a diagnostic pitfall, these tumours may also express keratin and EMA {1573,2109}. It is noteworthy that osteosarcoma is negative with antibodies to Factor VIII, CD31, and CD45.

Ultrastructure

Osteosarcoma cells have the features of mesenchymal cells with abundant dilated rough endoplasmic reticulum. The nuclei may be eccentric and the Golgi apparatus prominent. The matrix contains collagen fibres, which may show calcium hydroxyapatite crystal deposition. These findings can be helpful in excluding Ewing sarcoma/primitive neuroectodermal tumour, metastatic carcinoma and melanoma as well as lymphoma.

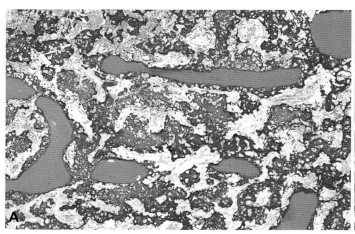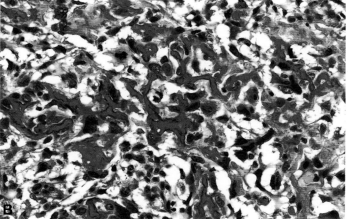

Fig. 16.18 Conventional osteosarcoma. **A** Osteoblastic osteosarcoma infiltrating medullary cavity and encasing pre-existing cancellous bone. **B** Osteoblastic osteosarcoma with pleomorphic malignant tumour cells producing coarse lace-like neoplastic bone.

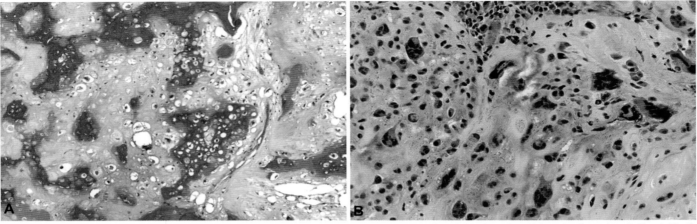

Fig. 16.19 Conventional osteosarcoma. **A** Chondroblastic osteosarcoma with areas of chondrosarcomatous differentiation alternating with bone-forming regions. **B** Chondroblastic osteosarcoma with high-grade cartilaginous component and adjacent neoplastic bone.

Genetics

Cytogenetic studies and genomic profiling
Conventional osteosarcoma has complex highly aneuploid karyotypes with multiple numerical and structural chromosomal aberrations. This unusually high level of chromosomal instability is thought to cause both intra- and intertumoral cytogenetic heterogeneity {2507}. Genomic profiling of tumour DNA using high-resolution array gene copy-number maps has been instrumental in providing detailed findings of the conventional osteosarcoma genome {117,1559,1646,1715,2581,2626, 3070}. Recurrent amplification and DNA copy number gains have been detected at several distinct chromosomal regions: 1p36, 1q21–22, 6p12–21, 8q21–24, 12q11–14, 17p11–13, and 19q12–13. Fewer regions are consistently involved in loss, with 3q13, 8p21, 9p13 and 13q14 being the most frequently reported. A subset of these genomic alterations has been reported to be more common in metastatic osteosarcomas than in primary tumours {3030}. Collectively within these regions of copy-number change, there are multiple candidate genes, some of which have compelling biological evidence for a direct role in osteosarcomagenesis. Mutations of isocitrate dehydrogenase 1 (*IDH1*) and *IDH2* may be helpful in distinguishing between chondroblastic osteosarcoma and chondrosarcoma. Somatic mutations of *IDH1* and *IDH2* were absent in all 222 osteosarcomas examined {54}.

Deletion and LOH of 3q13 in osteosarcoma
Deletion or LOH at 3q13 includes the *LSAMP* gene {1486, 2192, 3030}. *LSAMP* loss appears to correlate with disease progression and poor survival {2192, 3030}.

Amplification of 6p12–21 in osteosarcoma
The chromosomal region 6p12–21 is commonly amplified and DNA gains occur in 40–50% of tumours {1559,1666,1743, 2626}. A candidate gene in this amplified region is the *RUNX2* gene, which promotes terminal osteoblast differentiation {1744}. Elevated *RUNX2* levels have also been reported in conventional osteosarcoma using integrative genomic approaches {2403}, and high levels of *RUNX2* gene expression were found to be associated with poorer responses to chemotherapy {2402}. The *VEGFA* gene also maps to 6p12–21, and it is focally amplified and overexpressed, presumably promoting angiogenesis {3021}. Other potential amplified genes include *E2F3* and *CDC5* {1666}.

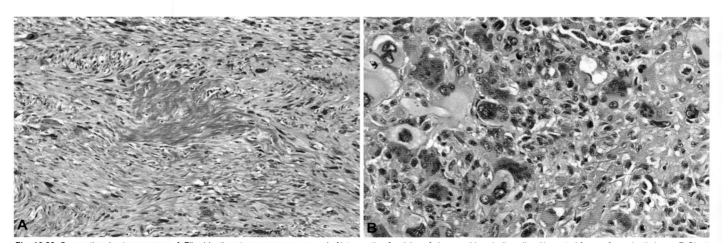

Fig. 16.20 Conventional osteosarcoma. **A** Fibroblastic osteosarcoma composed of intersecting fascicles of pleomorphic spindle cells with central focus of neoplastic bone. **B** Giant cell-rich osteosarcoma with numerous non-neoplastic osteoclast-type giant cells admixed with malignant tumour giant cells and filigree-pattern neoplastic bone.

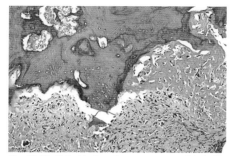

Fig. 16.21 Osteoblastic osteosarcoma associated with Paget disease of the femur.

Amplification and gain of 8q in osteosarcoma
DNA copy-number gain of chromosome region 8q21–24 is widely reported. The *MYC* oncogene (at 8q24.21) is the most frequently amplified, observed in 45–55% of tumours {168,1486,2581,2626,2656, 2723}.

Chromothripsis in osteosarcoma
A novel genetic mechanism referred to as chromothripsis has been postulated by genome sequencing data and appears to be involved in the development of a subset of sporadic de novo osteosarcomas (and chordomas) {1863,2651}. This phenomenon is thought to result from a single cataclysmic event resulting in tens to hundreds of genomic rearrangements.

Genetic predisposition, loss of cell-cycle control and genome stability in osteosarcoma
Patients with hereditary retinoblastoma have a high risk of developing osteosarcoma {697}. The retinoblastoma gene, *RB1* at 13q14 {846,1159}, is one of the most commonly inactivated genes in sporadic osteosarcoma (35% of tumours). The inactivation results from mutations in

the coding and promoter regions, as well as LOH and genomic deletion {91}. Recent extensive studies of LOH in the *RB1* region have failed to confirm it as a prognostic factor {1159}. Inactivation of the *TP53* gene secondary to mutations or LOH/deletions occurs in individuals with Li-Fraumeni syndrome who have an increased incidence of osteosarcoma {1713,2098}. Sporadic tumours have LOH or deletions of the 17p13.1 locus in ~40% of cases {1559,2098,2793}, and amplification of the TP53 antagonist *MDM2* in ~10% {1823}. Individuals with the autosomal recessive familial Rothmund-Thomson and related repair syndromes with loss of *RECQL4* gene (8q24.4) function via truncating mutations are at higher risk of developing osteosarcoma {2557}. Although the rate of *RECQL4* mutation in sporadic osteosarcomas is < 5% {2058}, increased copy number and elevated expression of *RECQL4* is a frequent event, and is implicated in the underlying chromosomal instability of the tumours {1706}.

Deregulation of other cell-cycle genes in osteosarcoma
Amplification of the cyclin dependent kinase gene, *CDK4* (located at 12q13–14), has been detected in approximately 10% of tumours {1823,2581}. Similarly, amplification and overexpression of cyclin E (*CCNE1*) has been reported in osteosarcoma {1646}. Deletion of 9p21 and the *CDKN2A* gene is reported in approximately 15% of osteosarcomas {1659,1924,1925}. Loss of *CDKN2A* is associated with reduced survival and has been implicated in osteosarcoma development from a mesenchymal progenitor {1924}.

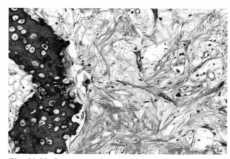

Fig. 16.22 Conventional osteosarcoma. Chemotherapy-induced necrosis in osteosarcoma. The neoplastic woven bone is acellular and the area previously inhabited by tumour cells is composed of reactive fibrous tissue.

Genetic changes in Paget osteosarcoma
Potential susceptibility loci for Paget disease have been linked to multiple chromosomes. {35,573,1011}. *TNFRSF11A* (18q22.1) encodes the receptor activator of NFKβ (RANK), the receptor for RANK ligand, which is critical in osteoclastogenesis; mutations of *TNFRSF11A* are found in a minority of patients with Paget disease and result in an internal duplication, conferring gain of function {1246,3002}.
Downstream in the molecular pathway of RANK is *SQSTM1* (5p35) which encodes p62, an ubiquitin-binding protein. Germline and somatic mutations in *SQSTM1* have been described in familial and sporadic Paget disease respectively {1011, 1846}; moreover, somatic *SQSTM1* mutations have been described in Paget osteosarcoma {1846}. Mutations affect the ubiquitin-binding domain, rendering the p62 protein refractory to degradation, which results in a hyper-responsive RANK-ligand signal {1566}.

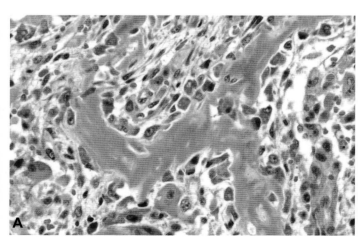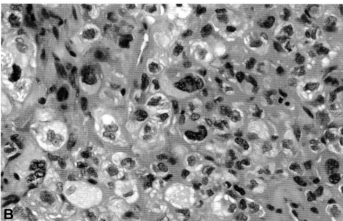

Fig. 16.23 Conventional osteosarcoma. **A** Osteoblastoma-like osteosarcoma with trabeculae of neoplastic woven bone lined by tumour cells mimicking osteoblastoma. **B** Epithelioid osteosarcoma composed of malignant polyhedral cells surrounded by tumour bone.

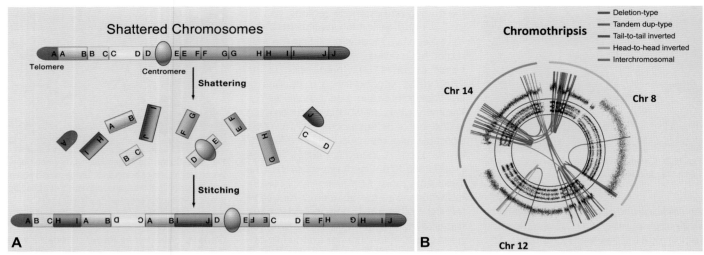

Fig. 16.24 Chromothripsis is proposed to involve the shattering of small groups of chromosomes and their random assembly by non-homologous end-joining as a single event involved in the development of de novo osteosarcomas and chordomas. **A** Stitching together shattered chromosomes by chromothripsis. **B** Genome sequencing of osteosarcoma shows 88 rearrangements involving chromosomes 8, 12, and 14. Modified from {1899A} and {2651}.

A mutation in *VCP* (9p13), encoding Valosin-containing protein, has been described in the rare syndrome of inclusion body myopathy, Paget disease and frontotemporal dementia (IBMPFD) {2910}. Furthermore, high expression of VCP has been described in osteosarcoma {1566}.

Genetic changes in radiation-associated osteosarcoma

Radiation osteosarcomas have complex karyotypes; aCGH analysis reveals that losses are more common than gains. Loss at 1p is much more common than in primary osteosarcoma (57% versus 3%) {2728}. The risk for developing radiation osteosarcoma is higher in patients with bilateral retinoblastoma, which is linked to germline mutations of the tumour suppressor gene *RB1*; more than half of these patients also display somatic inactivating mutations of *TP53* {1006,1007}.

Prognostic factors

Aggressive local growth and rapid haematogenous systemic dissemination characterizes the clinical course of conventional osteosarcoma. Pulmonary metastases followed by skeletal deposits are the most frequent sites of systemic disease. The goal of therapy is to eradicate the primary tumour and eliminate metastases. Local therapy is usually limb salvage wide resection {1724}, and radiation is utilized for unresectable tumours {2346}.

Multiagent chemotherapy for high-grade osteosarcoma has had a dramatic impact on outcome {68,535}. In the pre-chemotherapy era, 80% of patients treated with surgery alone died of disease, whereas 70% of patients are currently long-term survivors {68,535,2346}. Unfortunately, patients presenting with metastatic or recurrent disease have a survival rate of < 20% {456}.

The prognosis of osteosarcoma is influenced by patient age, sex, tumour size/volume, location, surgical margins, and stage {229}. Localized distal disease,

> 90% chemotherapy-induced tumour necrosis, and complete resection are positive prognostic factors associated with a 5-year survival rate of > 80% {829}. Predictors of poor outcome include proximal extremity or axial skeleton involvement, large size/volume, detectable metastases at diagnosis, and poor response to preoperative chemotherapy.

Paget osteosarcoma has a dismal prognosis with a median survival of 8–21 months and a 5-year survival of approximately 10% {656,1259,2526}. Recent data suggest that tumour site, stage and type of therapy are not significant indicators of prognosis {656}.

The prognosis of radiation osteosarcoma is comparable to that of conventional primary high-grade osteosarcoma, with a 5-year disease-free survival rate of 42–58% {133,1466,2519}. Prognosis is worse for pelvic, vertebral and shoulder girdle locations. Histological response to neoadjuvant therapy does not correlate with prognosis {1603}.

Telangiectatic osteosarcoma

A.M. Oliveira
K. Okada
J. Squire

Definition

A high-grade malignant bone-forming neoplasm, characterized by large spaces filled with blood, often with septations.

ICD-O code   9183/3

Epidemiology

Telangiectatic osteosarcoma is a rare subtype, accounting for less than 4% of all osteosarcomas. It most frequently occurs in the second decade of life and has a male predominance (1.5 : 1 male:female ratio) {2818}.

Sites of involvement

Most tumours occur in the metaphyseal region of long tubular bones. The distal femoral metaphysis is the single most common anatomical site (42%), followed by the upper tibia (17%), proximal humerus (9%) and proximal femur (8%) {2818}.

Clinical and imaging features

Clinical presentation is similar to that of conventional osteosarcoma. Pathological fracture is seen in 25% of cases {1858}. Massive bone destruction may explain the high rate of pathological fracture.

Radiographically, the tumour is purely lytic with extensive bone destruction and often soft-tissue extension. Most lesions are located in the metaphysis, and usually extend into the epiphysis. The tumours often expand the cortex of bone and/or disrupt the cortex. Periosteal reactions including Codman's triangle and onion skin are frequent. The finding of significant sclerosis within the lesion militates against the diag-

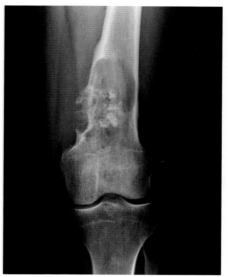

Fig. 16.25 A plain radiograph showing the lytic and destructive nature of telangiectatic osteosarcoma.

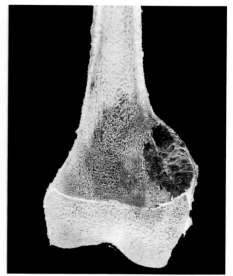

Fig. 16.26 Gross appearance of telangiectatic osteosarcoma with dominant cystic architecture, incompletely filled with blood clots (a bag of blood). There is no fleshy or sclerotic tumour bone formation. The tumour permeates the surrounding medullary canal.

nosis of telangiectatic osteosarcoma. In general, matrix mineralization is sparse, but subtle changes are best seen with CT {1986}. T1-weighted MRI shows heterogeneous low signal intensity, and T2-weighted images show high signal intensity with several cystic foci, fluid levels and an extraskeletal extension of the tumour, similar to aneurysmal bone cyst, but with irregular walls, septae, and nodular and solid components {1986}.

Macroscopy

Macroscopic examination shows a haemorrhagic multicystic lesion filled with blood clots, classically described as a "bag of

blood" {1762}. Fleshy or sclerotic areas are usually not seen. Extensive cortical erosion or destruction associated with nearby soft-tissue involvement may be seen.

Histopathology

The tumour is composed of blood-filled or empty cystic spaces closely simulating aneurysmal bone cyst. The septa show variable thickness and are populated by pleomorphic cells showing significant nuclear hyperchromasia. Some malignant cells can be seen floating in the

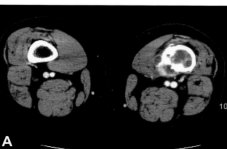
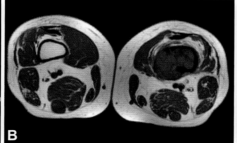
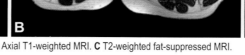

Fig. 16.27 Telangiectatic osteosarcoma. **A** CT image **B** Axial T1-weighted MRI. **C** T2-weighted fat-suppressed MRI.

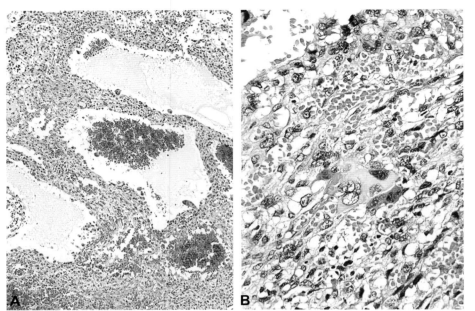

Fig. 16.28 Telangiectatic osteosarcoma. A Low-power microscopy reveals blood-filled or spaces separated by thin septa simulating aneurysmal bone cyst. B The cystic spaces show no endothelial lining. The septae are cellular and contain atypical mononuclear tumour cells.

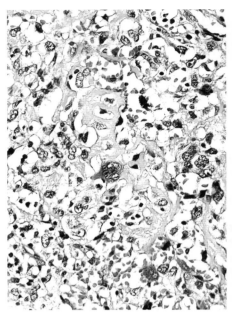

Fig. 16.29 Telangiectatic osteosarcoma. Highly malignant tumour cells produce minimal amounts of fine, lace-like osteoid.

haemorrhagic areas. Atypical mitoses are easily identified. Osteoid formation is usually focal and confluent, but may be absent in a biopsy. The septae also contain osteoclast-type giant cells and, at the edges of the lesion, tumour permeation into pre-existing bone trabeculae is often observed.

Genetics

Genetic studies have only been conducted on seven cases of telangiectatic osteosarcoma to date. Cytogenetic analysis identified trisomy 3 in one case {320}, and in three other tumours, more complex chromosomal changes were reported {871,1207}. Metaphase CGH identified an average of 2.5 aberrations in two telangiectatic osteosarcomas {2144}, and array CGH identified only three regional gains at 1q21–23.2, 1q25.2–31.1, and 7q21.13–21.2 in one tumour {3070}. This suggests that telangiectatic tumours are genetically less complex than conventional osteosarcoma.

Prognostic factors

The overall survival for patients is similar to that for patients with other osteosarcoma subtypes {131,2922}. Telangiectatic osteosarcoma is exquisitely sensitive to modern chemotherapy {2818}.

Small cell osteosarcoma

R.K. Kalil
J. Squire

Definition
A high-grade malignant neoplasm composed of small cells with variable degree of osteoid production.

ICD-O code   9185/3

Epidemiology
Small cell osteosarcoma comprises 1.5% of osteosarcomas {124,212,1994}. Patients range in age from 5 to 83 years, although most are in the second decade of life. There is a slight predominance of females, 1.1 to 1 {124,212,1745,1994}.

Sites of involvement
More than half of the tumours occur in the metaphysis of long bones {124}.

Clinical and imaging features
The clinical and radiographical presentation is similar to that of conventional osteosarcoma {1994}.

Macroscopy
The gross features of small cell osteosarcoma are indistinguishable from those of conventional osteosarcoma.

Histopathology
Small cell osteosarcoma is composed of small cells with scanty cytoplasm, associated with osteoid production. Nuclei are round to oval and the chromatin may be fine to coarse. Mitoses range from 3–5 per HPF. In the less frequent spindle cell type, nuclei are short, oval to spindle, have granular chromatin and inconspicuous nucleoli. A focal haemangiopericytoma-like pattern may be seen. Lace-like osteoid production is always present. Particular care must be taken to distinguish osteoid from fibrin deposits that may be seen among Ewing sarcoma cells.

Immunophenotype
There is no specific immunophenotype for small cell osteosarcoma. Tumour cells may be positive for CD99, osteocalcin, SMA and CD34 {647,651,1687}. Small cell osteosarcoma is negative for FLI1, a feature that may distinguish it from other

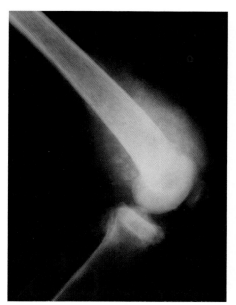

Fig. 16.30 Small cell osteosarcoma. Aggressive process with destruction of the cortex, with lytic and radiodense components admixed. Mineralized tissue in soft-tissue tumour extension strongly suggests osteosarcoma.

small round cell tumours, especially Ewing sarcoma {1583}.

Ultrastructure
The cytoplasm is poorly differentiated and contains microfilaments, ribosomes, mitochondria and rough endoplasmic reticulin in variable amounts. Glycogen is present in 30% of cases. Small junctions are seen in closely apposed cells {663}. The matrix shows flocculent dense material in close apposition to tumour cell membranes, with subplasmalemmal densities in the adjacent cells, possibly a pre-mineralization stage of the matrix. These findings may also be seen in mesenchymal chondrosarcoma, but never in Ewing sarcoma {2168}.

Genetics
Only four molecular cytogenetic studies have been reported {117,168,2061,2574}, and no recurrent chromosomal rearrangement was detected. Molecular studies have been used to exclude the existence of specific sarcoma-associated

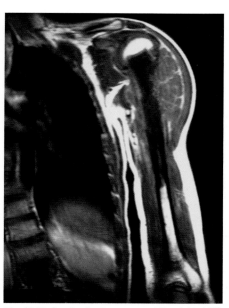

Fig. 16.31 Small cell osteosarcoma. T1-weighted MR image. Although not distinctive, the diagnosis may be suggested when an osteoblastic tumour extends well down into the shaft of the bone with a permeative pattern.

translocations, such as the *EWSR1-FLI1* fusion gene {979,1687}. Another study showed complex structural rearrangements of chromosomes 6, 16, and 17, and monoallelic deletion of *TP53* {2061}.

Prognostic factors
Small cell osteosarcoma itself has a slightly worse prognosis than conventional osteosarcoma, but there are no particular histological, imaging or genetic findings related to prognosis to date {124,1994}.

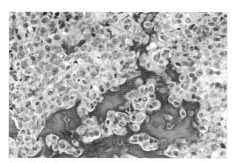

Fig. 16.32 Small cell osteosarcoma. High-power image.

Parosteal osteosarcoma

A. Lazar
F. Mertens

Definition
A low-grade, malignant, bone-forming neoplasm that arises on the surface of bone.

ICD-O code   9192/3

Synonym
Juxtacortical osteosarcoma

Epidemiology
Although rare, parosteal osteosarcoma is the most common type of osteosarcoma of the surface of bone. It accounts for about 4% of all osteosarcomas. There is a slight female predominance and most patients are young adults, with around one third of cases occurring in the third decade of life {632,669,2108}.

Sites of involvement
Around 70% of parosteal osteosarcomas involve the surface of the distal posterior femur. The proximal portions of the tibia and humerus are also relatively common sites. Flat bones are uncommonly affected.

Clinical and imaging features
Patients generally complain of a painless swelling; inability to flex the knee may be the initial symptom. Painful swelling is

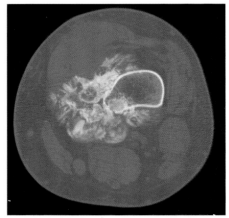

Fig. 16.33 A CT scan of a parosteal osteosarcoma.

sometimes reported. Roentgenograms show a heavily mineralized mass attached to the cortex with a broad base. The tumour has a tendency to wrap around the involved bone. CT and MRI are useful in evaluating the extent of medullary involvement and for selecting areas of possible dedifferentiation for biopsy {679}. The outermost portions of the tumour are usually less mineralized {213}. In some cases there may be an incomplete lucency between the tumour and the underlying bone.

Macroscopy
Parosteal osteosarcoma presents as a hard, lobulated mass, affixed to the underlying cortex. Nodules of cartilage may be present. Occasionally, the cartilage will be incomplete cap-like, covering the surface and causing confusion with osteochondroma. The periphery may be softer and seen to invade skeletal muscle. Focal invasion of the cortex and the medullary cavity may be seen. Soft, fleshy areas, if present, suggest progression (dedifferentiation) to high-grade osteosarcoma.

Histopathology
The tumour consists of spindle cells with minimal atypia, forming well-formed, bony trabeculae that are arranged in a parallel manner. The trabeculae may or may not show osteoblastic rimming. The tumour tends to be hypocellular, although in about 20% of the cases, it is hypercellular and the spindle cells show moderate atypia. About 50% of the tumours will show cartilaginous differentiation. This may be in the form of hypercellular nodules of cartilage within the substance of the neoplasm or as a cap on the surface. When present, the cartilage cap is mildly hypercellular, and the cells show mild cytological atypia and lack the "columnar" arrangement

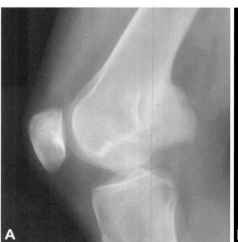
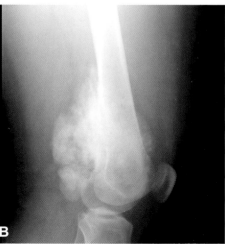
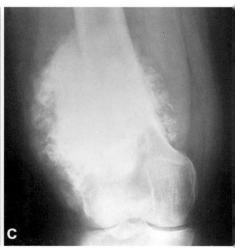

Fig. 16.34 Parosteal osteosarcoma. **A** Plain X-ray shows a heavily mineralized mass attached to the posterior aspect of the distal femur. **B** Extensive surface involvement is typical, with tumour wrapping from posterior to anterior cortical surfaces. **C** The formation of large, heavily mineralized masses surrounding the involved bone is common.

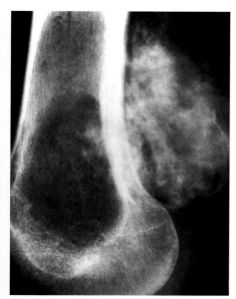

Fig. 16.35 Dedifferentiated parosteal osteosarcoma. The appearance of the lesion on the surface is that of a heavily mineralized mass, typical of parosteal osteosarcoma. There is a very destructive-appearing lesion within the medullary cavity, which was the dedifferentiated component.

seen in osteochondromas. Around 15–25% of the tumours will show high-grade spindle cell areas, indicating progression to high-grade sarcoma (dedifferentiation). This may be seen at the time of the original diagnosis or, more often, at the time of

recurrence {207,2984}. The areas of progression (dedifferentiation) may resemble conventional osteosarcoma or high-grade spindle cell sarcoma (similar to undifferentiated pleomorphic sarcoma).

Immunophenotype

It has recently been suggested that immunohistochemistry for nuclear MDM2 and CDK4 may be helpful to distinguish this tumour from potential fibro-osseous mimics, particularly in small biopsies {709, 710,3037}.

Genetics

Parosteal osteosarcomas are cytogenetically characterized by one or more supernumerary ring chromosomes, often as the sole aberration. The chromosome number is typically near diploid, and the tumours do not show the extensive instability and massive chromosomal rearrangements associated with high-grade osteosarcomas {1915}. The ring chromosomes always contain amplified material from chromosomal region 12q13–15 {985, 1156,2698}. Potential target genes in these amplicons include *CDK4* and *MDM2* which are amplified in more than 85% of the cases {709,710,1156,1823, 2997}. The same genes may be amplified in high-grade osteosarcomas with ring chromosomes, but the overall fre-

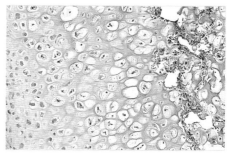

Fig. 16.36 Parosteal osteosarcoma. Extensive cartilaginous differentiation is not uncommon.

quency of amplification in conventional high-grade osteosarcomas is around 10% {1823}. Gene amplification is usually accompanied by increased expression of *MDM2* and *CDK4* at the RNA and protein levels {709,710, 1823}.

Prognostic factors

Prognosis is excellent, with 91% overall survival at 5 years {2108}. Marrow invasion and moderate cytological atypia do not predict a worse prognosis. Incompletely excised, the tumour may recur and progress to high-grade sarcoma. The presence of such areas is associated with a prognosis similar to that of conventional osteosarcoma, but better than dedifferentiation in chondrosarcoma {207}.

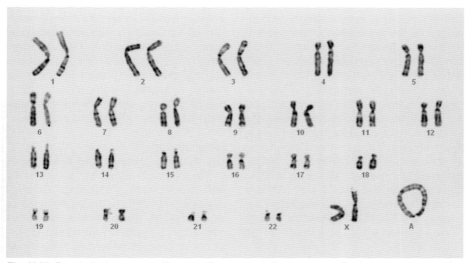

Fig. 16.37 Parosteal osteosarcoma. Karyogram from a parosteal osteosarcoma showing a supernumerary ring chromosome as the sole cytogenetic aberration.

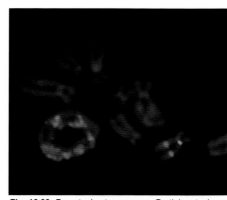

Fig. 16.38 Parosteal osteosarcoma. Partial metaphase spread from a parosteal osteosarcoma. FISH analysis using a centromere-specific probe for chromosome 12 (green) and a locus-specific probe for the *MDM2* locus (red) shows that the ring chromosome contains extra copies of *MDM2*.

Periosteal osteosarcoma

A.G. Montag
J. Squire

Definition
An intermediate-grade, malignant, cartilage and bone forming neoplasm arising on the surface of bone.

ICD-O code   9193/3

Synonym
Juxtacortical chondroblastic osteosarcoma

Epidemiology
Periosteal osteosarcoma accounts for <2% of all osteosarcomas and is about one third as common as parosteal osteosarcoma {2816,2818}. The peak incidence is in the second and third decades of life, although in larger series around 10% of cases are over 50 years old {1037}. There is a slight male predominance in most series, although the largest inter-institutional

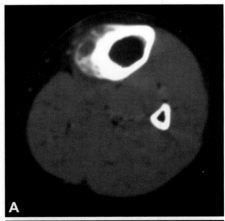

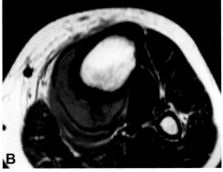

Fig. 16.39 Periosteal osteosarcoma. **A** CT scan. **B** Axial T1-weighted MRI.

series shows a slight female predominance {408,1037}.

Sites of involvement
In contrast to the metaphyseal location of parosteal osteosarcoma, periosteal osteosarcoma is predominantly diaphyseal or diaphyseal/metaphyseal in location, usually presenting as a sessile, anterior, medial lesion, which may almost wrap around the circumference of the bone {1981}. The distal femur and proximal tibia account for nearly 80% of cases, followed by the humerus, fibula, ulna and pelvis {408, 1037,2816}. Less frequent sites include the clavicle, ribs, cranium and the jaw {2816,2818}.

Clinical and imaging features
Limb swelling, mass and/or pain are the most common presenting symptoms, usually for a duration of < 1 year and in half of cases <6 months {408,1037}. Radiographically, a soft-tissue mass is detected on the cortex. Cortical thickening and extrinsic cortical scalloping are present in 82% and 92% of cases, respectively {1981,3026}. Periosteal reaction perpendicular to the bone's long axis and extending into the tumour mass, often with a sunburst or "hair on end" pattern, is present in 95%, while the classic Codman triangle is seen less frequently. In the majority of cases, other foci of mineralization are seen in the soft-tissue component. On CT the non-calcified component has a lower attenuation than the surrounding muscle, with high signal intensity on T2-weighted MR images, consistent with the cartilage matrix. Both CT and MRI are useful for defining margins, medullary extension, and the relationship of the tumour to major vessels and peripheral nerves {1981}.

Macroscopy
The tumour arises from the cortical surface, is broad-based, and may involve nearly the entire circumference {2816, 2818}. Cortical thickening is conspicuous, and secondary scalloping of the thickened or native cortex is seen in most

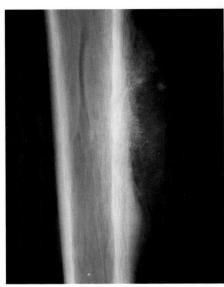

Fig. 16.40 Periosteal osteosarcoma. Plain radiograph of the specimen.

cases. Extension of tumour into the medullary canal has been reported but is rare. The gross appearance is dominated by glistening grey cartilaginous matrix, while the base of the tumour may be heavily ossified. Calcified spicules extend perpendicularly from the cortex into the overlying mass, gradually tapering into the cartilaginous matrix. The advancing outer margin is generally well delineated by a pseudocapsule derived from the thickened periosteum and fibrous reaction.

Histopathology
The features show a predominance of varying atypical cartilage, occasionally with myxoid matrix {2818,2816}. Osteoid-producing areas have the appearance of an intermediate grade osteosarcoma intermixed with cartilaginous elements. Occasional fibroblastic areas may simulate an intermediate grade fibroblastic osteosarcoma. Large areas of conventional osteoblastic osteosarcoma are not seen. The differential diagnosis of periosteal chondrosarcoma or central chondroblastic osteosarcoma with soft-tissue extension may arise.

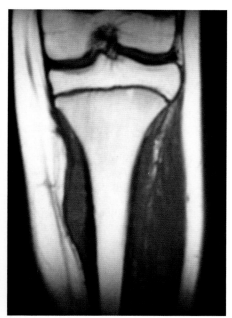

Fig. 16.41 Periosteal osteosarcoma. Coronal T1-weighted MRI.

Genetics

The genetic alterations observed in this subtype of osteosarcoma have been largely inconsistent, but suggest that genomic alterations are less complex than conventional osteosarcoma, with gain of 8q, loss of 6q, and amplification of 8q11–24 and 12q11–15 identified in more than one case {117,320, 2144,2723}. Some cases have exhibited complex chromosomal alterations {984, 1207}. Point mutations in *TP53* are seen in 40% of periosteal osteosarcomas, similar to the frequency in high grade central osteosarcoma {2286}.

Prognostic factors

Periosteal osteosarcoma has a relatively good prognosis with an overall 5- and 10-year survival of 89% and 83% respectively, with approximately 15% of patients developing metastases {408,1037,2368}. Surgical excision is the primary therapeutic modality, with most cases amenable to limb salvage. There is no evidence that

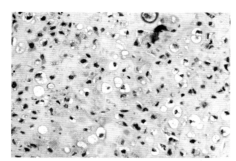

Fig. 16.42 Periosteal osteosarcoma. Areas of cartilaginous matrix with atypical chondrocytes transition to areas of osteoid formation.

chemotherapy provides survival benefit, and post-chemotherapy necrosis in the excision specimen is non-predictive {408,1037,2368}. Age, size, and adequacy of margins are not predictive of long term survival; however, local recurrence is highly associated with an increased risk of metastasis {1037}.

High-grade surface osteosarcoma

L.E. Wold
E.F. McCarthy
J. Squire

Definition

A high-grade, malignant, bone-forming neoplasm which arises on the surface of the bone.

ICD-O code   9194/3

Epidemiology

High-grade surface osteosarcoma comprises <1% of all osteosarcomas. The peak incidence is in the second decade and the age distribution of patients at the time of diagnosis is similar to conventional osteosarcoma. There is a male predominance (male:female ratio approximately 2 : 1) {2110}.

Sites of involvement

The femur is the most commonly affected bone (approximately 50% of cases), followed in frequency by the tibia (approxi-

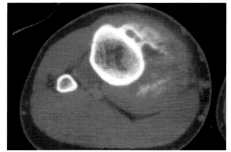

Fig. 16.43 High-grade surface osteosarcoma. CT showing focal mineralization and a large unmineralized soft-tissue component.

mately 20% of cases) and humerus (approximately 10% of cases).

Clinical and imaging features

The most common presenting complaint is a mass (approximately 70%) and many patients have associated pain (approxi-

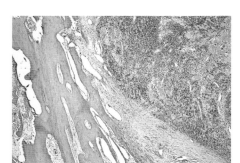

Fig. 16.44 This high-grade surface osteosarcoma shows erosion into the cortex of the underlying femoral shaft and a more fibroblastic histological appearance.

mately 66%). In general, patients present with a short duration of symptoms. Radiographically, high-grade surface osteosarcomas present as a partially mineralized mass on the surface of the affected bone which extends into the adjacent soft tissues. The degree of mineralization of

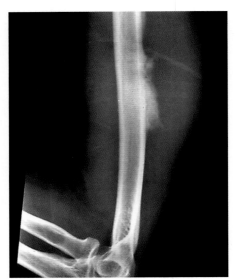

Fig. 16.45 High-grade surface osteosarcoma in the middle portion of the humerus. The lesion is mineralized where it is attached to the bone but there is also a large unmineralized soft-tissue mass.

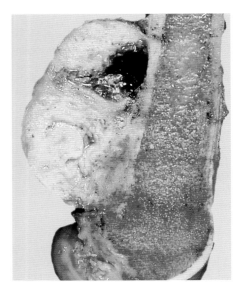

Fig. 16.46 High-grade surface osteosarcoma involving the distal femur. The tumour is soft and fleshy.

these tumours can be variable, but commonly shows the "fluffy" or "cloud-like" appearance associated with conventional osteosarcoma. The tumours are broadly attached to the bony cortex, which is often partially destroyed. Periosteal new bone formation is common at the periphery of the tumour. The radiolucent zone which commonly exists between the heavily min-eralized parosteal osteosarcoma and the underlying cortex is not seen in high-grade surface osteosarcoma.

Macroscopy
The tumour is situated on the cortical surface of the affected bone and generally erodes the cortex. The dominant component of the tumour is outside the bone. Tu-mours vary in consistency depending upon whether they are predominantly osteoblas-tic, fibroblastic or chondroblastic. The tumour extends into the adjacent soft tissues and generally forms a well-circumscribed, lobulated mass.

Histopathology
High-grade surface osteosarcoma shows the same spectrum of histological features as seen in conventional osteosarcoma {2632}. The degree of cytological atypia is greater in high-grade surface osteosarcoma than in periosteal osteosarcoma and the tumour generally shows larger regions of spindle cell differentiation.

Genetics
Amplification of the *TSPAN31* (formerly known as *SAS*) gene localized to 12q13-14 has been reported in a single case of high-grade surface osteosarcoma {2067A}. There are no published observations of cytogenetic aberrations in prechemotherapy biopsies of high-grade surface osteosarcoma.

Prognostic factors
The prognosis is similar to conventional osteosarcoma. A recent study suggests that, in contrast to conventional osteosarcoma, response to preoperative chemotherapy is not a prognostic factor.

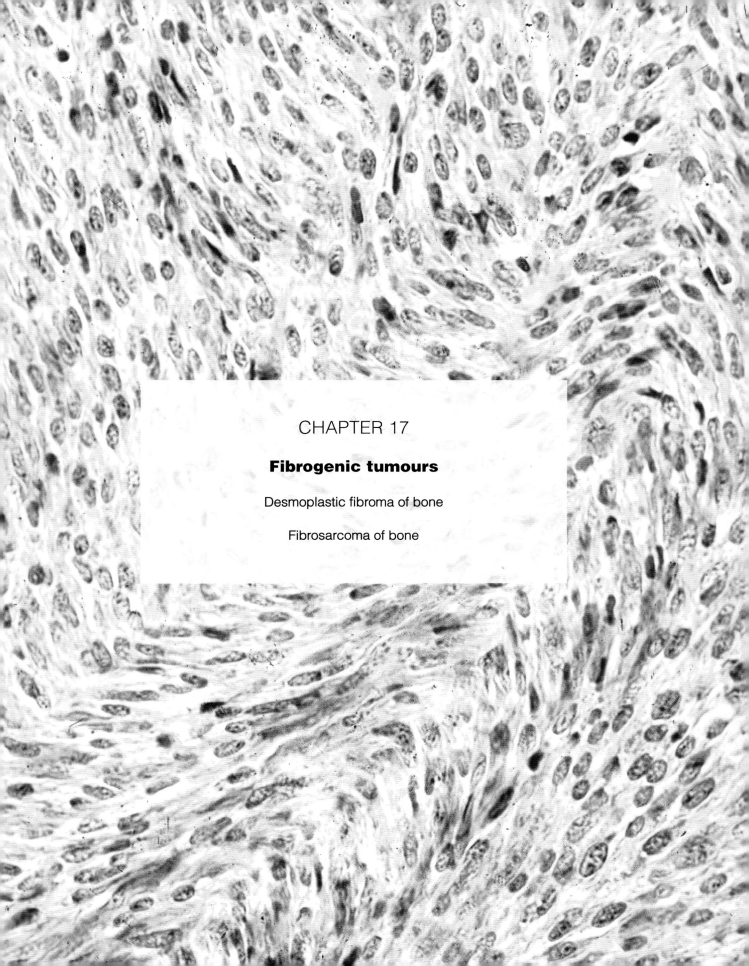

CHAPTER 17

Fibrogenic tumours

Desmoplastic fibroma of bone

Fibrosarcoma of bone

Desmoplastic fibroma of bone

E. Hauben
A-M. Cleton-Jansen

Definition

A rare, benign, locally aggressive neoplasm of bone composed of bland spindle cells and abundant collagen.

ICD-O code   8823/1

Synonym

Desmoid tumour of bone

Epidemiology

Incidence is < 0.1% of all primary bone tumours. Desmoplastic fibroma is most frequent in adolescents and young adults.

Sites of involvement

Desmoplastic fibroma may involve any bone. It is most frequent in the mandible, followed by the meta-epiphyseal region of the femur, tibia, radius, humerus and pelvis.

Clinical features and imaging

The principal symptoms are local swelling or pain. Pathological fracture is the presenting symptom in 12% of cases. Some patients are asymptomatic and the tumour is found incidentally. On radiographs, the lesion is lytic, sometimes poorly limited, and has a low signal on T2-weighted MRI.

Macroscopy

The lesion is firm, tan-white, with a whorled

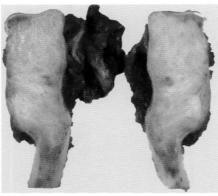

Fig. 17.01 Desmoplastic fibroma. Macroscopy shows an expansive creamy-white fibrous tumour in the proximal tibia.

pattern and circumscribed with scalloped margins.

Histopathology

The tumour is composed of slender, spindle to stellate cells, set in an abundant collagenous matrix. The cells are arranged in long fascicles or whorls. Cellularity is variable as is the density of the collagen. Cellular pleomorphism and atypia is minimal or absent. Mitoses are rare. Mast cells can be present. The lesion is moderately vascular with capillaries and small- to medium-sized, well-developed arterioles regularly dispersed throughout. Morpho-

logically it mimics desmoid-type fibromatosis. Cartilaginous metaplasia is rarely seen {357}.

Immunophenotype

The tumour cells are immunoreactive for SMA, and can be positive for actin and desmin. Nuclear β-catenin is occasionally present, but this is generally in < 10% of the cells {1137}. Immunoexpression of MDM2 and CDK4 is also negative, in contrast to low-grade central osteosarcoma {3037}.

Genetics

Reports on genomic alterations in desmoplastic fibroma are scarce. CGH analysis using a BAC array in a case of desmoplastic fibroma with malignant transformation identified various losses and gains {1905}. In contrast to desmoid-type fibromatosis of soft tissue, no mutations were found in exon 3 of CTNNB1, encoding β-catenin, in a series of 13 desmoplastic fibromas {1137}; thus, genetically there is no evidence to consider desmoplastic fibroma as the intra-osseous counterpart of desmoid-type fibromatosis.

Prognostic factors

Desmoplastic fibroma is locally aggressive. Recurrence is 17% or 55–72% with or without resection, respectively {262}.

Fibrosarcoma of bone

A. Lazar
C. Inwards
S. Knuutila
V.J. Vigorita

Definition
An intermediate- to high-grade, spindle cell, malignant neoplasm of bone, devoid of significant pleomorphism and lacking any line of differentiation other than fibroblastic.

ICD-O code   8810/3

Epidemiology
Historically, "fibrosarcoma of bone" has been applied to primary malignant spindle cell neoplasms of bone in which the tumour cells are typically organized in a fascicular or "herringbone" pattern. A variety of primary bone tumours occupying other specific diagnostic categories may show this histological pattern and thus there are no properties distinctive of, or specific for "fibrosarcoma of bone." This entity is much less commonly used as a specific diagnostic category today, particularly due to the advent of ancillary techniques and evolving classification schemes. Therefore, the incidence is likely much less than reported rates of up to 5% of all primary malignant bone tumours. Tumours with a predominance of this fibrosarcomatous pattern, but likely representing a variety of tumour types, have been described with equal sex distribution and relatively uniform incidence over the second to sixth decades of life with occasional occurrence in infants {195,547, 1261,1548,2358A}. Historically, most studies were likely to be confounded with tumours that would fall under other categories today. Fibrosarcoma of bone, if it does exist on rare occasion, is a diagnosis of exclusion. More casual use of this term outside of this restricted context is discouraged.

Sites of involvement
The distal femur is the most common site (21–47%) with the proximal femur (16%), distal humerus (14%) and proximal tibia (11%) also involved {1261,2701}.

Clinical and imaging features
Local pain, swelling, limitation of motion, and pathological fracture are the most common clinical signs and symptoms. Typical imaging findings include eccentrically located,

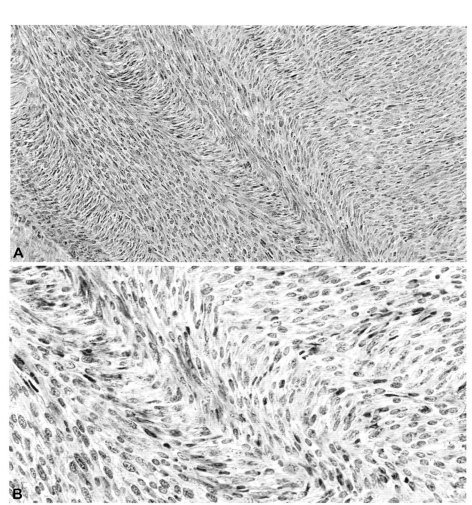

Fig. 17.02 Fibrosarcomatous differentiation in a malignant bone tumour. **A** and **B** show bone lesions with fibrosarcomatous pattern. This "herringbone" or fibrosarcomatous architecture can be encountered in a variety of bone tumours and is no longer considered to specifically indicate a diagnosis of fibrosarcoma of bone.

lytic lesions with a geographical, "moth-eaten", or permeative pattern of destruction, and extension into adjacent soft tissues.

Macroscopy
Grossly, fibrosarcomas are collagenous, resulting in a firm consistency with a trabeculated, white cut surface and circumscribed margins.

Histopathology
The histological features are predominantly a uniformly cellular population of spindle shaped cells arranged in a fasci-

cular or "herringbone" pattern with a variable amount of collagen production. Given that these fibrosarcomatous features can be seen in a wide variety of bone tumours, the great majority of tumours previously considered to reside in this category are probably better placed in other categories. Thus, fibrosarcoma is a diagnosis of exclusion that cannot be made using a limited amount of tissue. The tumour should be devoid of malignant osteoid and cartilage in order to rule out osteosarcoma and dedifferentiated chondrosarcoma. Immunohistochemical stains, including desmin and

SMA, are necessary to rule out leiomyosarcoma. Epithelial markers and molecular studies separate fibrosarcoma from synovial sarcoma. Several historical series allowed for marked cytology pleomorphism resulting in confusing terminology usage for fibrosarcoma and undifferentiated pleomorphic sarcoma. In order to keep classic fibrosarcoma as a separate histological entity, tumours with marked cytological atypia and storiform growth pattern are best classified as undifferentiated pleomorphic sarcomas.

Immunophenotype
Tumour cells lack immunoreactivity for smooth muscle, endothelial, and epithelial markers.

Genetics
There is little information in the literature regarding genetic changes in tumours with fibrosarcomatous differentiation {1081,1135, 2049}. Both chromosomal and aCGH studies show a large number of genomic imbalances. The average number of imbalances, detected by high resolution aCGH, is as high as 43 per tumour {2049}. The most common losses, observed by aCGH, are 6q, 8p, 9p, 10, 13 and 20p, while the most common gains are 1q, 4q, 5p, 8q, 12p, 15, 16q, 17q, 20q, 22, and Xp {2049}. *CDKN2A* in 9p is homozygously deleted in > 60% of 17 cases and *STARD13* in 13q is hetero- or homozygously deleted in 45% of cases {2049}. These studies do not distinguish these tumours from other karyotypically complex bone sarcomas.

Prognostic factors
Five- and ten-year survival rates are as poor as 34% and 28% depending on patient age, grade, site and stage, with metastases to the lungs and other bones commonly noted {210,1261,2169,2701}.

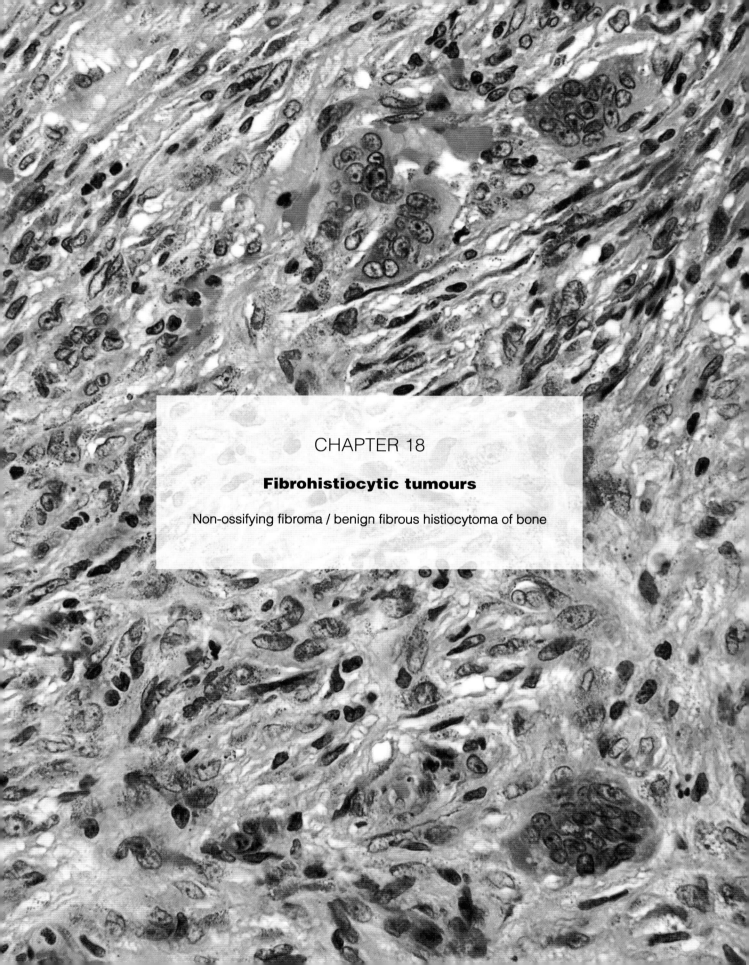

CHAPTER 18

Fibrohistiocytic tumours

Non-ossifying fibroma / benign fibrous histiocytoma of bone

Non-ossifying fibroma/ benign fibrous histiocytoma of bone

G.P. Nielsen
M. Kyriakos

Definition

A benign fibroblastic proliferation admixed with osteoclast-type giant cells. The term "fibrous cortical defect" is used when the tumour is confined to the cortex. The term "non-ossifying fibroma" (NOF) is used for larger tumours that extend into the medullary cavity.

Benign fibrous histiocytoma (BFH) has the same histological features as non-ossifying fibroma, but the clinicoradiological presentation is different; benign fibrous histiocytoma usually involves non metaphyseal region of long bones or the pelvis.

ICD-O code   8830/0

Epidemiology

The incidence of NOF is unknown, as most lesions are asymptomatic and undergo spontaneous resolution. It has been estimated that approximately 30–40% of children have one or more occult lesions {1714}. Radiographical studies have shown that 54% of boys and 22% of girls have fibrous cortical defect at the age of 4 years {1313,2603}.

In contrast, BFH of bone is very rare, with < 100 reported cases {1044,2845}. Although patients range in age from 5 to 75 years at the time of diagnosis {209,2845}, most patients with BFH are older than 20 years of age {1044}.

Sites of involvement

The vast majority of NOFs arise in the metaphysis of long bones of the lower extremities, especially the distal femur and proximal and distal tibia. Multifocal occurrence is not uncommon.

Although 40% of tumours that have been diagnosed as BFH also involve long bones, they are distinguished from NOF by their non-metaphyseal location. Additionally approximately 25% of BFH involve the pelvic bones, especially the ilium {127,356,476,477,637,646,913,948,1089, 1276,1707,1931}.

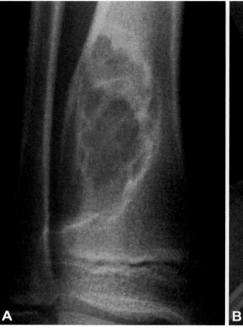
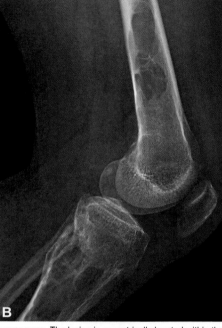

Fig. 18.01 Non-ossifying fibroma. A Typical radiographic appearance. The lesion is eccentrically located within the diametaphysis of the distal tibia. It is lobulated and well-demarcated with a sclerotic rim. B Multiple, large non-ossifying fibromas in a patient with neurofibromatosis type 1. The lesions are lytic, circumscribed, and involve the distal femur and proximal tibia.

Clinical and imaging features

NOF arises in skeletally immature individuals with a peak incidence in the second decade of life. NOF is usually asymptomatic and is often discovered incidentally. Large lesions may be painful and cause pathological fracture {92,2419}. Radio-graphically, NOF is radiolucent and centred in the cortex, usually in the distal metaphysis of a long bone. The cortex is thin, with sclerotic and scalloped borders. They can be uniloculated or multiloculated. The longitudinal axis tends to be parallel to the long axis of the involved

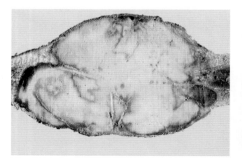

Fig. 18.02 Benign fibrous histiocytoma. The resection specimen shows a pale, cream-yellow cut surface with focal rust-brown areas along its periphery. Marked cortical thinning and endosteal scalloping are evident.

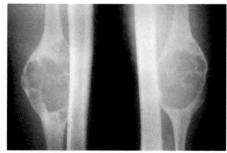

Fig. 18.03 Benign fibrous histiocytoma. A well-defined lytic lesion involving the mid-diaphysis of the fibula with expansion and scalloping of the bone.

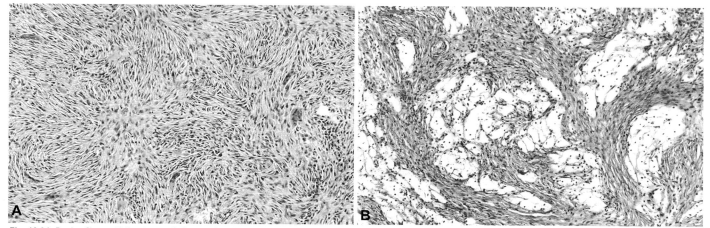

Fig. 18.04 Benign fibrous histiocytoma. **A** Centre of storiform focus shows spindle cells, whose nuclei are elongated or oval with a fine chromatin pattern. Note intracytoplasmic haemosiderin. **B** Clusters of foam cells with pale cytoplasm and small, dark nuclei are seen interspersed among whorled spindle cells. Such foam cells may be absent or so extensive as to dominate the lesion.

bone. CT scan shows a lytic, well-demarcated lesion. MRI shows low T1-weighted and T2-weighted signal intensity. Multiple NOFs can be seen in patients with neurofibromatosis type 1, and in patients with Jaffe-Campanacci syndrome {370,1910, 1958}. The lesions are thought to spontaneously regress over time, as they are rarely seen in adults {92}.

The clinical presentation for BFH is similar to NOF {209,477,637,1044,1906,2818}. Radiographically, BFH is a well-defined, benign looking, radiolucent medullary lesion without matrix formation. Internal trabeculation or pseudoseptations may be evident {477,1044}. Approximately two thirds of the lesions have sclerotic margins, best seen by CT {209,913,1089}. The lesion may thin and expand the cortex with destruction; however, a periosteal reaction is lacking in the absence of fracture {209, 637, 948,1044}. Soft-tissue extension has only rarely been described {104,2047}. At the end of a long bone, BFH may be central or eccentrically located and be indistinguishable from a giant cell tumour of bone (GCT) {2152, 2454}. Scintographic studies usually, but not always, show increased radionuclide uptake in the lesion, as well as gadolinium enhancement on MRI {637,1044,1276, 2845}.

Macroscopy

Grossly, NOF and BFH are similar. They are well circumscribed, red brown with areas of yellow discoloration and contain sclerotic borders. Cystic changes may be present, and haemorrhage and necrosis can be seen in tumours that have undergone a pathological fracture.

Histopathology

NOF and BFH are indistinguishable microscopically and can only be distinguished on the basis of clinical and radiographical features {1044,2640,2845,2454}. The tumours consist of bland, spindle-shaped fibroblasts that are arranged in a storiform growth pattern. Osteoclast-type giant cells are scattered throughout the lesion. Secondary features include haemosiderin deposition within the stromal cells and collection of foamy histiocytes. Cystic changes may be present and areas of necrosis can be seen in the presence of a pathological fracture.

Genetics

Three cases of NOF with chromosome aberrations have been reported, all with near-diploid karyotypes and different structural rearrangements {303,2022,2723}.

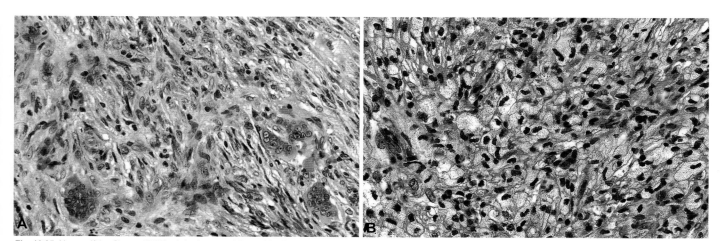

Fig. 18.05 Non-ossifying fibroma (NOF). **A** Lesion containing golden-brown haemosiderin deposition within the stromal cells that are arranged in a vague storiform growth pattern. Scattered osteoclast-type giant cells are also present. **B** Area within a NOF containing numerous foamy histiocytes.

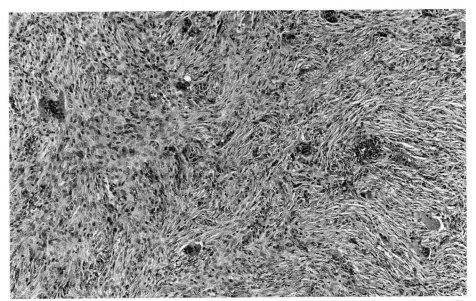

Fig. 18.06 Typical non-ossifying fibroma composed of spindle-shaped cells arranged in a storiform growth pattern with scattered osteoclast-type giant cells. Scattered inflammatory cells and extravasated erythrocytes are present.

Prognostic factors

The prognosis for both non-ossifying fibroma and benign fibrous histiocytoma is excellent. Asymptomatic lesions do not need to be treated. Larger lesions requiring treatment can be curetted. Local recurrences are rare {477,1504,2640,2818}. Rare instances of pulmonary metastasis {2818} or malignant transformation of BFH have been reported {2715}. However, these latter cases are either not well documented or open to question about the original diagnosis.

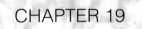

CHAPTER 19

Ewing sarcoma

Ewing sarcoma

E. de Alava
S.L. Lessnick
P.H. Sorensen

Definition

A small, round cell sarcoma showing pathognomonic molecular findings, and varying degrees of neuroectodermal differentiation by light- or electron microscopy, or immunohistochemistry. Ewing sarcoma is characterized by recurrent balanced translocations involving, in almost all cases, the *EWSR1* gene on chromosome 22 and a member of the *ETS* family of transcription factors; this leads to the formation of novel fusion oncogenes that are the key to its pathogenesis.

ICD-O code

Ewing sarcoma   9260/3

Synonym

Askin tumour (for tumours arising in the chest wall)

Epidemiology

Ewing sarcoma is relatively uncommon, accounting for 6–8% of primary malignant bone tumours. However, it is the second most common sarcoma of bone in children and young adults, after osteosarcoma {1068}. Ewing sarcoma shows a slight male predominance, with a sex ratio of 1.4 : 1.

Nearly 80% of patients are younger than 20 years, and the peak age of incidence is during the second decade of life. Patients older than 30 years of age are uncommon, but do occur and are characterized by a similar spectrum of *EWSR1-ETS* gene fusions as seen in childhood forms of the disease {1569}. These tumours are noticeably more common in Caucasians than other ethnic groups.

Etiology

Ewing sarcoma pathogenesis is driven by pathognomonic and etiological *EWSR1-ETS* gene fusions that, as described below, encode chimeric transcription factors that are expressed in these tumours. EWSR1-ETS fusion proteins activate or repress specific sets of target genes that, together with the right timing and cellular context, give rise to the transformed phenotype of Ewing sarcoma. Recent data point to either mesenchymal stem cells {2761} or neural crest-derived stem cells {2886} as the cell of origin of Ewing sarcoma.

Sites of involvement

The most prevalent sites are, in descending order: (i) the diaphysis or metaphy-

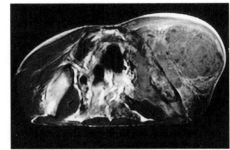

Fig. 19.02 Ewing sarcoma. MRI (T1-weighted image) of pelvic tumour showing a huge soft-tissue mass outside and inside the iliac wing, with modest bone involvement, and compared with the volume of the mass, only little bone destruction.

seal-diaphyseal portion of long bones (femur, tibia, humerus); (ii) the pelvis and ribs, (iii) other bones such as the skull, vertebra, scapula, and short tubular bones of hands and feet. About 10–20% of cases are extraskeletal.

Clinical and imaging features

Pain, severe enough to wake patients (96%), with or without a mass in the involved area (61%), is the most common clinical symptom. Intermittent fever (21%) and anaemia are often seen. Pathological fracture (16%) at diagnosis is uncommon. Radiographically, an ill-defined, most often osteolytic, but sometimes sclerotic (on CT) lesion involving the diaphysis of a long tubular bone, is the most common feature. Permeative or "moth-eaten" bone destruction often associated with "onion-skin"-like multilayered periosteal reaction is characteristic. A large, ill-defined soft-tissue mass is a frequent association. MRI studies help demonstrate the extent of the tumour in the bone and soft tissue.

Macroscopy

Grossly, bone and soft tissue Ewing sarcoma is typically tan-grey and has destructive borders with invasive margins. Tumours often show necrotic and haemorrhagic regions, and necrotic yellowish and semi-fluid tissue obtained from intramedullary or subperiosteal lesions may be erroneously interpreted as pus.

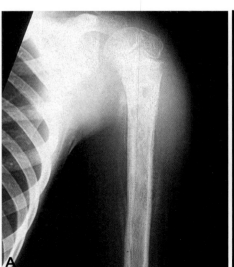
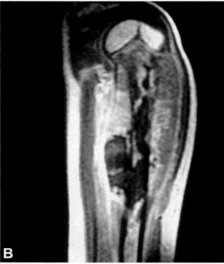

Fig. 19.01 Ewing sarcoma of the left humerus in a 6-year-old boy **A** Periosteal new bone formation showing onion-skin appearance. **B** Coronal T1-weighted MRI of the same lesion. Both intra-osseous and extra-osseous tumours are more clearly demonstrated than on plain film radiographs.

In Ewing sarcoma of bone, the tumour is typically present in the medullary shaft of the involved bones. Soft-tissue extension may be evident. Rare examples of Ewing sarcoma in soft tissue may be associated with a large peripheral nerve.

Histopathology

Although subtle morphological variations can be seen, most cases are composed of uniform small round cells with round nuclei containing fine chromatin, scanty clear or eosinophilic, PAS-positive cytoplasm, and indistinct cytoplasmic membranes (classical Ewing sarcoma) {1644}. In others, the tumour cells are larger, have prominent nucleoli, and irregular contours (atypical Ewing sarcoma) {1688}. Sometimes, a higher degree of neuroectodermal differentiation (ill-defined groups of up to ten cells oriented toward a central space and/or consistent immunophenotype) is present (classically termed as peripheral neuroectodermal tumour) {1644}. The emerging group of "Ewing-like sarcomas" show small to medium-sized cells, with a solid pattern of growth and no stroma; some cells are ovoid, but distinct spindling is only focally seen in occasional cases of this group {1023,1299}.

Immunophenotype

Ewing sarcoma demonstrates a range of neural differentiation. Classic Ewing sarcoma lacks neural differentiation, and typically demonstrates only characteristic diffuse membranous CD99 positivity. Up to 30% show some positivity for keratin. Of note, lymphoblastic leukaemia, lymphoma, and myeloid sarcoma may demonstrate

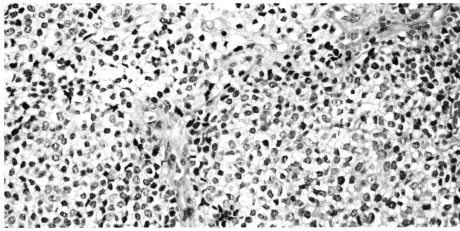

Fig. 19.03 Classical Ewing sarcoma. Notice vaguely lobular pattern and cleared-out cytoplasms, secondary to glycogen deposits.

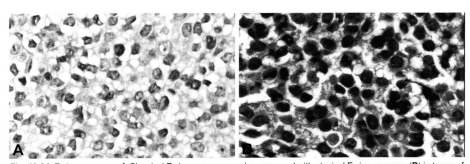

Fig. 19.04 Ewing sarcoma. **A** Classical Ewing sarcoma can be compared with atypical Ewing sarcoma (**B**) in terms of nuclear size, chromatin structure, and cytoplasmic clearing.

membranous CD99 staining identical to that of Ewing sarcoma. Therefore, with leukemic infiltration of soft tissues or extranodal lymphoma, a diagnosis of Ewing sarcoma may be incorrectly made. CD99 can be patchy or negative in "Ewing-like sarcomas" {1023,1299}. Anti-FLI1 and ERG antibodies are available but are not widely used in this context.

Ultrastructure

Ewing sarcoma is composed of primitive cells with round to oval nuclei, and frequent glycogen aggregates in the cytoplasm. No intermediate filaments, neurofilaments, and extracellular matrix are observed. Primitive intercellular junctions are often seen. In addition, PNET can show neurosecretory granules (100–150 nm) and intertwining neurite-like processes.

Genetics

Approximately 85% of Ewing sarcomas harbour a somatic reciprocal chromosomal translocation, t(11;22)(q24;q12), that fuses *EWSR1* to *FLI1* to generate the EWSR1-FLI1 oncoprotein {631,2803}. EWSR1-FLI1 functions as an aberrant transcription factor to dysregulate genes that are required for the oncogenic phenotype of Ewing sarcoma {2270,2588}. In other cases, alternate translocations fuse *EWSR1*

Table 19.01 Chromosomal rearrangements found in Ewing sarcoma and "Ewing-like sarcoma"

Chromosomal rearrangement	Fusion gene	Reference
t(11;22)(q24;q12)	EWSR1-FLI1	2804A
t(21;22)(q22;q12)	EWSR1-ERG	2604
t(7;22)(p22;q12)	EWSR1-ETV1	1330
t(17;22)(q21;q12)	EWSR1-ETV4	1365,2822
t(2;22)(q35;q12)	EWSR1-FEV	2226
t(16;21)(p11;q22)	FUS-ERG	2540
t(2;16)(q35;p11)	FUS-FEV	2028
t(20;22)(q13;q12)[a]	EWSR1-NFATC2	2695
t(6;22)(p21;q12)	EWSR1-POU5F1	3006
t(4;22)(q31;q12)	EWSR1-SMARCA5	2676A
Submicroscopic inv(22) in t(1;22)(p36.1;q12)	EWSR1-PATZ	1754
t(2;22)(q31;q12)	EWSR1-SP3	2894
t(4;19)(q35;q13)	CIC-DUX4	1383

[a] Can occur in ring chromosome and may be amplified.

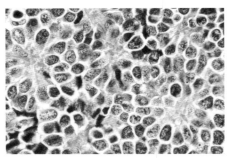

Fig. 19.05 Ewing sarcoma with extensive neural differentiation (PNET) showing well-formed pseudorosettes. Notice the absence of nucleoli and the finely granular quality of chromatin.

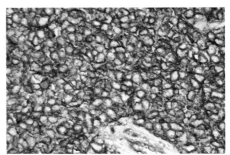

Fig. 19.06 High-power image of Ewing sarcoma showing typical membranous immunohistochemical expression of CD99.

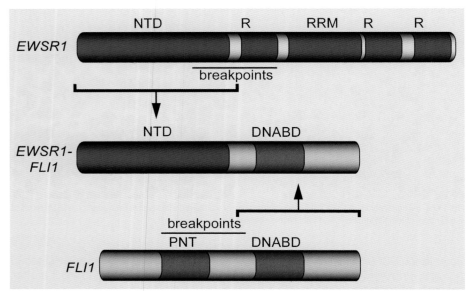

Fig. 19.07 *EWSR1-FLI* translocation in Ewing sarcoma. Schematic diagram of the *EWSR1-FLI1* fusion protein in comparison to wild-type EWSR1 and FLI1 proteins (NTD, amino-terminal domain; R and RRM, RNA-binding domains; PNT, pointed domain; DNABD, DNA-binding domain).

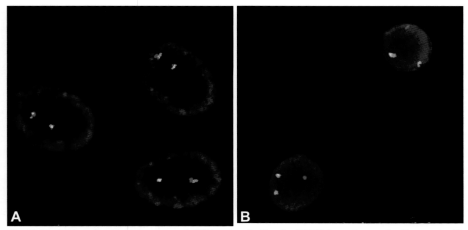

Fig. 19.08 FISH-positive Ewing sarcoma. **A** FISH probes flanking the *EWSR1*locus (orange for 5', green for 3') demonstrate overlap of probes in cells containing two wild-type *EWSR1* alleles. **B** In Ewing sarcoma, in addition to a single wildtype *EWSR1* allele, the second allele is "split" due to the t(11;22)(q24;q12) rearrangement.

to other ETS family members, including t(21;22)(q22;q12), t(7;22)(p22;q12), t(17;22)(q21;q12), or t(2;22)(q35;q12), resulting in *EWSR1-ERG*, *EWSR1-ETV1*, *EWSR1-ETV4*, or *EWSR1-FEV*, respectively {1330,1365,2226,2437,2604,2822}. In additional rare cases, *FUS-ERG* or *FUS-FEV* fusions are present instead {2028,2540}. The FUS protein (TLS) is similar to EWSR1 in amino-acid sequence, and is considered part of the TET family of proteins (including TLS, EWSR1, and TAF15){2711}. In addition to the fusions above, it has recently been appreciated that there are cases of Ewing-like sarcomas that contain fusions between EWSR1 and other, non-ETS, proteins, including NFATc2, SMARCA5, PATZ1, and SP3, and others that lack rearrangement of *EWSR1* or other TET family members, such as t(4;19)(q35;q13) or t(10;19)(q26;q13), encoding a *CIC-DUX4* fusion {1383,1754, 2437,2695,2894,3006}. Whether these cases should be defined as Ewing sarcoma, or represent separate tumour types is unknown {2437}, but currently they are treated in a similar fashion. For the subgroup of "Ewing-like sarcomas" characterized by the *BCOR-CCNB3* fusion, a distinct gene-expression profile and a different pattern of secondary aberrations provide strong arguments for regarding it as a separate entity {2243}. All translocations associated with Ewing sarcoma or "Ewing-like sarcoma" are listed in Table 19.01.

The diagnosis of Ewing sarcoma may be confirmed by the presence of a positive RT-PCR result, or supported by a split *EWSR1* FISH signal (while still considering the diagnoses of other *EWSR1*-rearranged tumours, such as desmoplastic round cell tumour, extraskeletal myxoid chondrosarcoma, myxoid liposarcoma, or clear cell sarcoma, among others). In contrast, while the absence of molecular confirmation should prompt a review of the clinical, histological, and immunohistochemical features, it should not rule out the diagnosis of Ewing sarcoma by itself.

Additional chromosomal abnormalities are often present in Ewing sarcoma {104,217, 690,691,1133,1134,2350,2638,2803}. Trisomies and other gains of chromosome 8 are found in up to 50% of cases, while gains of chromosomes 12 and 1q are found in 25% of cases {104,1132,1134, 1767,1968}, and gains in chromosome 20 are found in 10–20% of cases {2143}. In approximately 20% of cases, an additional unbalanced chromosomal translocation with variable breakpoints, t(1;16), is present in addition to the primary Ewing sarcoma translocations, and results in gains of 1q and losses of 16q {690,1133,1968, 2638,2639}. Losses at 1p36 have also been observed {1134}. The additional Ewing sarcoma chromosomal abnormalities may have prognostic significance, as gains of 1q or 12, and loss of 1p36 or 16q are all associated with an adverse outcome {1132,1134, 1690,2143,2350}. Mutations in *TP53* and alterations in the *CDKN2A* genes have also been identified, and appear to have prognostic significance {586,1242,2915}.

Prognostic factors

The prognosis for patients with Ewing sarcoma has improved considerably with current therapy, and approximately two thirds of patients are cured of their disease {1630}. However, outcome for patients with disseminated disease or early relapse remains dismal {1525}, and the presence of metastatic disease appears to be the major prognostic factor {1674}. Important pathological prognostic features include the stage, anatomical location, and the size of tumour. Histopathological assessment of tumour necrosis after induction chemotherapy has prognostic value. Extent of neural differentiation does not appear to predict outcome {2176}. Several molecular features were reported as having prognostic value, including *TP53* status, *CDKN2A* loss, telomerase expression {586,1132,1242,2104,2915}, and additional chromosomal aberrations such as gains of 1q {1690}, but practical application requires validation in prospective cooperative studies. *EWSR1-ETS* fusion type is no longer thought to be of prognostic significance {1576,2840}.

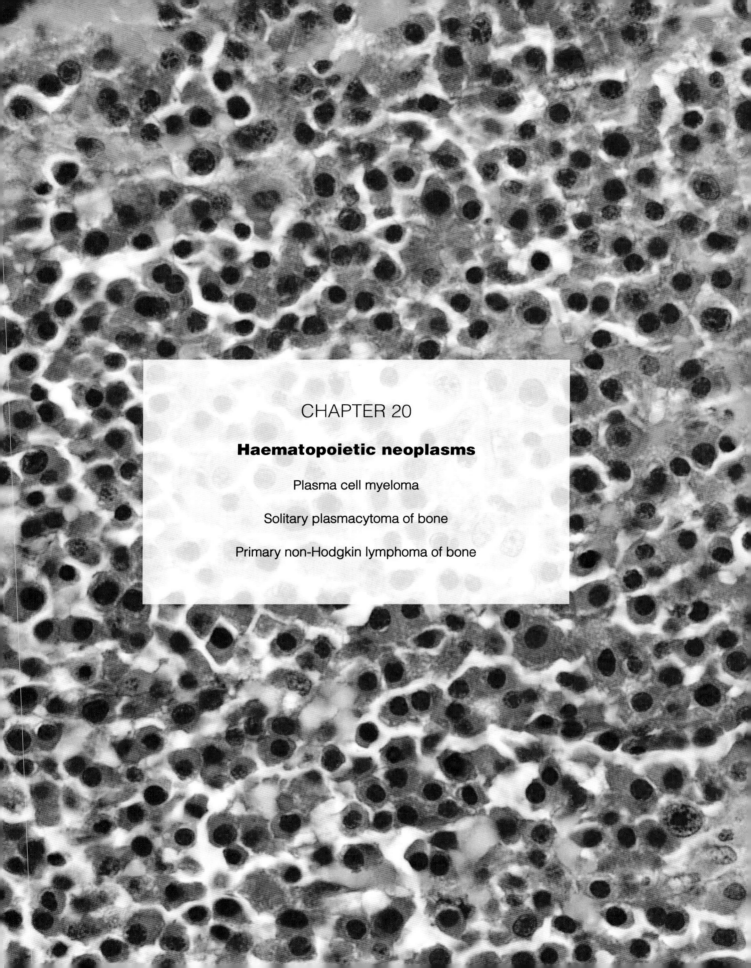

CHAPTER 20

Haematopoietic neoplasms

Plasma cell myeloma

Solitary plasmacytoma of bone

Primary non-Hodgkin lymphoma of bone

Plasma cell myeloma

R. Lorsbach
P.M. Kluin

Definition

A clonal neoplastic proliferation of plasma cells (PCs) of bone-marrow derivation. Plasma cell myeloma (PCM) is usually a multicentric disease that eventually infiltrates various organs and is rarely associated with a leukaemic presentation.

ICD-O code   9732/3

Synonyms

Myeloma; multiple myeloma; Kahler disease

Several variants of PCM have been recognized {1794}: non-secretory myeloma, indolent myeloma, smouldering myeloma, and PC leukaemia. Distinction between these diagnostic entities requires correlation with clinical, laboratory and radiological features. Monoclonal gammopathy of undetermined significance (MGUS) by definition lacks any associated clinical symptoms or end-organ damage, including bone lesions, and is therefore not included in this chapter.

Epidemiology

PCM is the most frequent tumour that occurs primarily in bone and is one of the most common lymphoid neoplasms {673}. Most patients are in the sixth and seven decades of life. The median age at diagnosis is 68 years in males and 70 years in females {1387}. It is rare in individuals younger than 40 years (< 10% of all cases). Both sexes are equally affected.

Sites of involvement

PCM primarily involves bones of the axial skeleton containing haematopoietic marrow. The most frequently involved bones are the vertebrae, ribs, skull, pelvis, femur, clavicle and scapula {1043}.

Clinical and imaging features

Myelomatous osteolytic skeletal lesions cause bone pain, pathological fractures, hypercalcaemia and anaemia. The lumbar or thoracic spinal regions are most often affected by pain. Frequently a pathological fracture is the first symptom and usually affects the spine. Neurological symp-

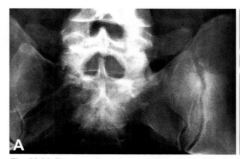
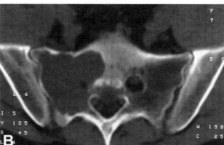

Fig. 20.01 Plasma cell myeloma. **A** Plain X-ray of the lumbosacral region shows subtle radiolucency of the right wing of the sacrum. **B** CT scan of the same patient, at the level of S2, shows loss of the cancellous bone of the right wing of the sacrum, of a large area of the vertebral body, and small scalloping of the endosteal surface of the cortical bone.

toms due to spinal cord or nerve root lesions, secondary to extra-osseous extension of the tumour or pathological fracture, are frequently observed. Peripheral neuropathy is frequently observed with the osteosclerotic variant of multiple myeloma, but it is rare with classic PCM. Anaemia occurs commonly in the setting of PCM; its cause is multifactorial but in many instances reflects anaemia of chronic disease induced, in part, by dysregulated expression of IL-6 {1377}. In other cases it is due to displacement of normal haematopoietic cells. With sensitive techniques such as immunofixation electrophoresis, an M-component can be found in the serum or urine of 99% of patients. In 50% of cases, the monoclonal proteins are of the IgG class, 20–25% are of the IgA class, and rarely, are of the IgM, IgD or IgE classes {1514}. In 15–20%, very little or no heavy chains are detected. Biclonal gammopathies are found in 1% and a monoclonal light chain (Bence-Jones protein) is found in the serum in 75% of the patients. Renal failure is the result of tubular lesions (Bence-Jones proteinuria with formation of tubular casts) due to monoclonal light-chain proteinuria, hypercalcaemia, or more rarely amyloidosis. Patients often have recurrent bacterial infections, in part, because of decreased normal immunoglobulin production due to displacement by the neoplastic clone. Myelomatous bone lesions are lytic, sharply demarcated lesions, a consequence of replacement of bone trabecu-

lae by tumour tissue, and are not usually surrounded by a sclerotic zone. Cortical erosion is commonly observed but prominent periosteal new bone formation is not. Expansion of the affected bone may occur in bones with a small diameter, such as the ribs. The earliest and more severe changes are seen in the skull, vertebrae, ribs and pelvis. About 12–25% of patients have no detectable foci of bone destruction at presentation but may show generalized osteoporosis. Solitary myeloma lesions are also typically lytic and may expand the bone. Infrequently, sclerotic bone lesions are encountered, usually in the context of the rare POEMS syndrome (polyneuropathy, organomegaly, endocrinopathy, monoclonal gammopathy, skin changes) {673}. CT and MRI studies may reveal small, subtle lesions not visible on plain radiographs. The features of MRI are variable, because PCM does not involve the marrow in a homogeneous fashion and because the extent of fatty marrow replacement varies with age. For differential diagnosis, metastatic carcinoma, malignant lymphoma, and hyperparathyroidism have to be considered. The lesions of metastatic carcinoma and lymphoma are usually positive on bone scan, whereas those of myeloma are usually not.

Histopathology

Several patterns of bone-marrow involvement occur in PCM, including interstitial, nodular, focal or obliterative patterns. In occasional cases, prominent fibrosis is present. Cytologically, the neoplastic plasma cells (PCs) manifest a broad spectrum of morphological features depending on the degree of differentiation and, in some cases, on the underlying genetic lesions. Most commonly, myeloma cells closely resemble normal PCs with an eccentrically placed nucleus, condensed chromatin, indistinct nucleolus and abundant basophilic cytoplasm, the so-called Marschalko morphology. In Giemsa-stained preparations, the cytoplasm is basophilic with a perinuclear clear zone that ultrastructurally corresponds to the well-developed RER and prominent Golgi complex, respectively, characteristic of PCs. In a subset of cases, the neoplastic cells have relatively scant cytoplasm and closely resemble lymphocytes, a morphology termed "small lymphocyte-like" or "lymphoplasmacytic". Given their morphology, such cases may be mistaken for a low-grade lymphoma {896,944,1238}. This morphology is typically associated with the t(11;14)(q13;q32) translocation. In less well-differentiated PCM, the neoplastic cells are often significantly larger than normal PCs, and have less condensed chromatin and prominent central nucleoli. In cases with high-grade morphology, the neoplastic cells may have so-called plasmablastic morphology where the neoplastic cells have prominent nucleoli and high nuclear : cytoplasmic ratios. In some poorly differentiated cases, the neoplastic cells closely resemble those seen in large cell lymphoma or acute leukaemia. Occasional cases with anaplastic morphology are seen. In contrast to low-grade cases in which few mitoses are seen, high-grade PCM typically manifests brisk mitotic activity.

Like their benign counterparts, neoplastic PCs may contain a number of different cytoplasmic inclusions, which are gener-

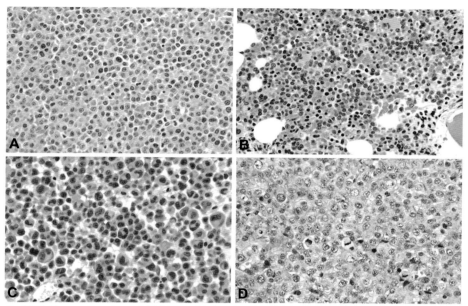

Fig. 20.02 Plasma cell myeloma. **A** Well-differentiated myeloma in which the tumour cells have eccentric round nuclei, no discernible nucleoli and abundant cytoplasm. Mitotic activity is nearly absent. **B** Myeloma with small lymphocyte-like morphology. Interstitial infiltrate of neoplastic plasma cells is present, most of which lack discernible cytoplasm. Such cases closely mimic low-grade lymphoma. **C** Moderately differentiated myeloma. The tumour cells have prominent nucleoli and abundant cytoplasm; frequent multinucleated forms are present. **D** Poorly differentiated myeloma. Most of the tumour cells are large with vesicular nuclei, prominent nucleoli, and lack the abundant cytoplasm typical of low-grade tumours, and the mitotic activity is high. Myeloma with these high-grade features mimics morphologically diffuse large B-cell lymphoma.

ally due to either misfolded or abnormally polymerized immunoglobulin. Cells containing single or multiple cytoplasmic immunoglobulin globules (Russell bodies) or apparently intranuclear globules (Dutcher bodies) are present in some tumours. Crystals resembling Auer rods rarely occur, and may be seen in cases with an associated crystal-storing histiocytosis {1254,1340}. In some PCMs, cytoplasmic inclusions impart a cytological appearance reminiscent of that of the glucocerebroside-containing histiocytes of Gaucher disease {2313}. PCM with signet ring cell morphology, due to the presence of a large immunoglobulin vacuole, are rarely encountered {686,793}. Bone marrow deposition of light-chain amyloid, including localization in the periosteum, occurs in approximately 10–15% of PCM cases {645,1513}.

Immunophenotype

Like their normal counterparts, neoplastic myeloma cells express several pan-plasmacytic markers, including CD138 (syndecan-1) {449,515,2083}, CD38 {1106,2745}, and MUM1 {800}. PCM characteristically expresses monotypic cytoplasmic immunoglobulin (Ig) and

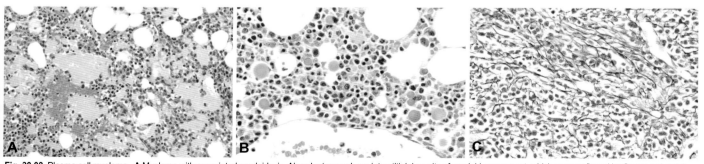

Fig. 20.03 Plasma cell myeloma. **A** Myeloma with associated amyloidosis. Abundant amorphous interstitial deposits of amyloid are present, which was confirmed by Congo red staining. **B** Myeloma in which many tumour cells contain prominent Russell bodies. **C** Reticulin stain on the same case confirming diffuse reticulin fibrosis in association with the myelomatous infiltrate.

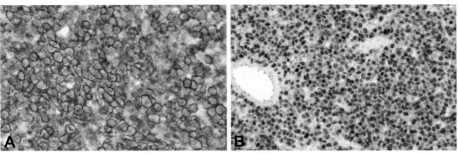

Fig. 20.04 Plasma cell myeloma. **A** Strong, uniform expression of CD138 is present in nearly all myelomas. **B** Strong nuclear expression of the plasma cell transcription factor MUM1.

Table 20.01. Diagnostic criteria for plasma cell myeloma (modified from {68A})

Symptomatic plasma cell myeloma	– M-protein in serum or urine [a]
	– Bone marrow clonal plasma cells or plasmacytoma [b]
	– Related organ or tissue impairment [c]
Asymptomatic (smoldering) myeloma	– M-protein in serum at myeloma levels (> 30 g/dL)
	AND/OR
	– 10% or more clonal plasma cells in bone marrow
	– No related organ or tissue impairment (end-organ damage or bone lesions) or myeloma-related symptoms

[a] No minimal level of serum or urine M-protein is required

[b] No minimal level of myeloma involvement is required; approximately 5% of patients with symptomatic myeloma have <10% plasma cells on routine iliac crest bone-marrow examinations

[c] Typical manifestations of myelomatous tissue impairment include CRAB (hypercalcaemia, renal insufficiency, anaemia, bone lesions). Patients with low-level bone marrow plasmacytosis, amyloidosis, and tissue impairment due solely to amyloid deposition should be classified as primary amyloidosis and not symptomatic myeloma.

lacks surface Ig. In about 85%, both heavy and light chains are produced, but in the remaining cases light chain only is expressed (Bence-Jones myeloma). The monotypic expression of kappa or lambda Ig by the tumour cells establishes the diagnosis of malignancy. CD117 and the natural killer cell antigen, CD56, neither of which is detected in benign PCs, are expressed in 28–58% and 76–88% of cases, respectively {49,376,1106,1629}. Approximately 95% of all PCMs lack expression of the pan-B cell antigen CD19, whereas CD20 is expressed in 20–30% of cases, in particular those harbouring the t(11;14)(q13;q32). In myelomas, the intensity of CD20 expression is usually variable, in contrast to the uniform bright expression typical of most B-cell lymphomas. Cyclin D1 protein is expressed in approximately 35–40% of all myelomas, of which approximately half the cases carry a t(11;14)(q13;q32); other cases with lower or more variable expression may have polysomy of chromosome 11 {2617}. CD138 is highly expressed in virtually all cases, and its expression can be readily assessed by either flow cytometry or immunohistochemistry {449,515, 2083}. However, given that CD138 is expressed by a wide array of carcinomas, CD138 immunohistochemical studies should always be interpreted with caution, particularly in the evaluation of poorly differentiated PCM {461,1359}. Myeloma cells may be positive for EMA {147}. Occasional cases of PCM aberrantly express the myelomonocytic antigen CD33 {2351, 2406}.

Genetics

Cytogenetic and FISH studies genetically define two major groups of PCM. In approximately 40% of cases, a balanced reciprocal translocation targeting the Ig heavy-chain locus (*IGH*) is present. These translocations target several different well-characterized partner genes, mainly in chromosome bands 4p16.3 (*FGFR3/MM-SET*), 6p21 (*CCND3*), 11q13 (*CCND1*), 16q23 (*MAF*), and 20q11 (*MAFB*). At the molecular level, breakpoints are in or near heavy-chain switch regions, which indicates an origin from aberrant class switch events. As a result, the breakpoint in t(11;14)(q13;q32) in PCM is structurally different from that in mantle cell lymphoma. The remaining 60% of cases are characterized by hyper-diploidy with polysomies of several chromosomes, most often chromosomes 3, 5, 7, 9, 11, 15, 19 and 21; this myeloma subgroup infrequently contains an *IGH* trans-location. Secondary translocations in PCM involve other chromosomal partners like 8q24 (*MYC*), which is strongly associated with tumour progression.

Prognostic factors

PCM is generally an incurable disease (median survival, 3 years; 10% survival at 10 years). A shorter survival time is associated with higher clinical stage, renal insufficiency, degree of marrow replacement by tumour cells, increased proliferative activity and certain karyotypic abnormalities. The t(4;14) and the t(14;16) as well as deletions targeting 17p13 (*TP53*) are generally thought to be associated with a poorer prognosis {1978}. Chromosome 1 abnormalities appear to be of prognostic importance; specifically, amplification of genetic material at chromosomal arm 1q and loss at 1p are associated with disease progression and adverse prognosis {422,2525,2996}. Detection of monosomy 13 or del13q by metaphase cytogenetics imparts a negative prognostic impact {121,895}, due in part to its association with known genetic markers of high-risk disease such as t(4;14) {897, 2878}.The prognostic impact of detecting chromosome 13 abnormalities by FISH is less clear. Newer technologies such as array-based gene-expression profiling hold promise in PCM for more precise disease classification and improved prognostication {616,1496,2525, 3056}.

Solitary plasmacytoma of bone

R. Lorsbach
P.M. Kluin

Definition
In contrast to plasma cell myeloma (PCM), solitary plasmacytoma of bone (SPB) is by definition unicentric and characterized by localized bone destruction and an absence of systemic manifestations. Like PCM, SPB is a clonal neoplastic proliferation of plasma cells (PCs) of bone marrow derivation.

ICD-O code
9731/1

Synonym
Solitary osseous plasmacytoma

Epidemiology
SPB occurs in somewhat younger patients than PCM, with a median age at diagnosis of 55 years. It develops more commonly in men than women, with a male to female ratio of approximately 2 : 1 {1282, 2613}.

Sites of involvement
SPB most frequently involves the vertebrae and is the most common primary bone tumour of the spine, comprising approximately 30% of such tumours {668,2534}. Less frequent sites of involvement include ribs, skull, pelvis and femur. SPB must be differentiated from extramedullary (extra-osseous) plasmacytoma, in particular those tumours arising in the upper aerodigestive tract, but also from plasmablastic lymphoma.

Clinical and imaging features
Patients with SPB may manifest skeletal symptoms similar to those seen in PCM, namely bone pain and pathological fractures. Patients with vertebral SPB may manifest neurological symptoms secondary to spinal-cord or nerve-root involvement or compression. Systemic symptomatology (e.g. anaemia) does not occur secondary to SPB.

Histopathology
The diagnosis of SPB is typically straightforward, as most cases manifest overt plasmacytic differentiation. Some SPBs are associated with so-called "break out" lesions in which cortical bone destruction occurs with extension of the tumour into adjacent soft tissue. Such lesions may present as soft-tissue masses. These should not be diagnosed as extramedullary plasmacytoma without correlation with radiological findings. The more refined diagnosis of SPB requires correlation with clinical findings and radiological studies to exclude systemic disease.

Immunophenotype
SPB must be differentiated from primary bone lymphoma that can occasionally have immunoblastic morphology. In this setting, immunohistochemistry for CD20, CD45, CD56, CD138 and EMA, as well as immunoglobulin heavy chain expression

Table 20.02. Clinicopathological diagnostic criteria for solitary plasmacytoma of bone (modified from {68A})

No or little M-protein in serum and/or urine
Single focus of bone destruction due to clonal plasma cells
No other bone marrow involvement
Normal skeletal survey (and MRI of spine and pelvis, if done)
No end-organ damage other than solitary osseous lesions

have diagnostic utility. The latter can be particularly helpful, as in contrast to immunoblastic lymphoma, only rare SPB cases express IgM. Occasional cases may be more poorly differentiated or manifest anaplastic features, making them diagnostically challenging. With such tumours, immunophenotypical studies, including CD138, MUM1 and immunoglobulin light-chain immunohistochemistry, may be essential for confirmation of the diagnosis of SPB. The immunophenotype and genetic features of SPB are similar to those for PCM.

Prognosis
The majority of patients with SPB ultimately progress to PCM, with a 10-year survival of 40–50% {668,2613}. SPB is exquisitely sensitive to radiotherapy. Persistence of a serum paraprotein following radiotherapy is associated with increased risk of progression to PCM {2963}.

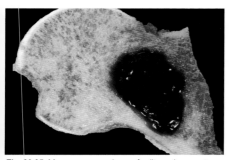

Fig. 20.05 Macroscopy specimen of solitary plasmacytoma of bone.

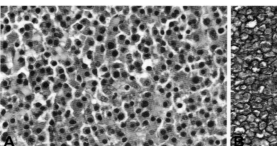
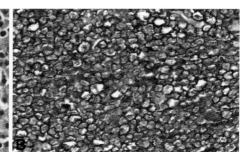

Fig. 20.06 Solitary plasmacytoma of bone. **A** Plasmacytoma composed of sheets of mature-looking plasma cells. **B** The plasma cells in plasmacytomas strongly express CD138.

Primary non-Hodgkin lymphoma of bone

P.C.W. Hogendoorn
P.M. Kluin

Definition
A neoplasm composed of malignant lymphoid cells, producing one or more masses within bone, without any supraregional lymph-node involvement or other extranodal lesions.

ICD-O code   9590/3

Epidemiology
Primary malignant lymphoma of bone is uncommon, accounting for approximately 7% of all bone malignancies. Lymphomas solely involving the bone account for about 5% of all extranodal lymphomas. This lymphoma should not be mistaken for the much more frequent nodal or other extranodal lymphomas with secondary bone involvement. Patients may be of any age group, but there is a tendency to involve adults, especially older adults. There is a male predominance {42,970,1169, 3073}. In "western" countries, more than 95% of primary malignant lymphomas of

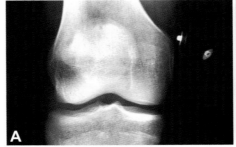 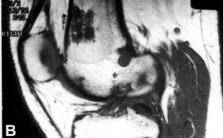

Fig. 20.08 Primary non-Hodgkin lymphoma of bone. **A** Plain X-ray does not reveal the lesion. **B** MRI of the same case shows multifocal involvement of bone with signal changes.

bone consist of B-cell lymphomas; however, in Asian countries this frequency may be slightly lower {1239,2809}. Plasma cell neoplasms are traditionally excluded from this category.

Sites of involvement
The femur is the most commonly involved single site (approximately 25%) {42,970, 1169}. The spine and the pelvic bones are other common sites. The small bones of the hands and feet are rarely involved. When malignant lymphoma presents in the spine or in the maxillary antrum, it is often difficult to assess unambiguously whether the process originates primarily in bone or in the soft tissues. Approximately 15–20% of the patients in "western" countries present with polyostotic disease. This incidence may be higher in Asian populations {1239}.

Clinical and imaging features
The majority of patients with primary bone lymphoma present with bone pain. Some patients present with a palpable mass. In case of spinal involvement, neurological symptoms are common. Patients with primary lymphoma of bone rarely present with systemic or B-cell symptoms, such as fever or night sweats. Serum LDH is infrequently increased. Primary lymphoma of bone can present as a single skeletal lesion with or without regional lymph-node involvement and should be distinguished from secondary bone involvement in systemic lymphoma, since a bone lesion may produce the same presenting symptoms. For instance, some patients with nodal

follicular lymphoma may present with local, intra-osseous transformation to diffuse large B-cell lymphoma (DLBCL) with tumour necrosis causing bone pain, mimicking primary lymphoma of bone. Radiographical studies {304} show that 16% of patients with other lymphomas have evidence of secondary bone involvement. The radiological features are quite variable, somewhat non-specific and at the MRI-level sometimes erroneously suggesting a non-aggressive lesion {1171,1488,1976}. In the long bones, the diaphysis tends to be preferentially involved. The tumour tends to involve a large portion of the bone; it is not unusual to see destruction of up to half of the bone. The process is poorly demarcated with a wide radiological transition area from normal bone. Commonly, there is a mixture of lysis and sclerosis; rarely is the tumour very sclerotic or entirely lytic. The cortex is frequently destroyed and there is often a large soft-tissue mass. In a flat bone such as the pelvis, large areas of destruction with soft tissue extension on either side suggest a diagnosis of lymphoma. If the cortex is not involved and MRI shows signal abnormalities in the marrow, the plain radiographs may even be completely normal. Radionuclide bone scan is almost always positive.

Macroscopy
It is very unusual to see gross specimens of malignant lymphoma involving bone, because the diagnosis is usually made on a needle biopsy and treatment consists

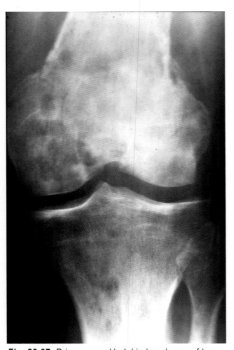

Fig. 20.07 Primary non-Hodgkin lymphoma of bone. Malignant lymphoma of femur and tibia. Note extensive lytic and sclerotic lesions.

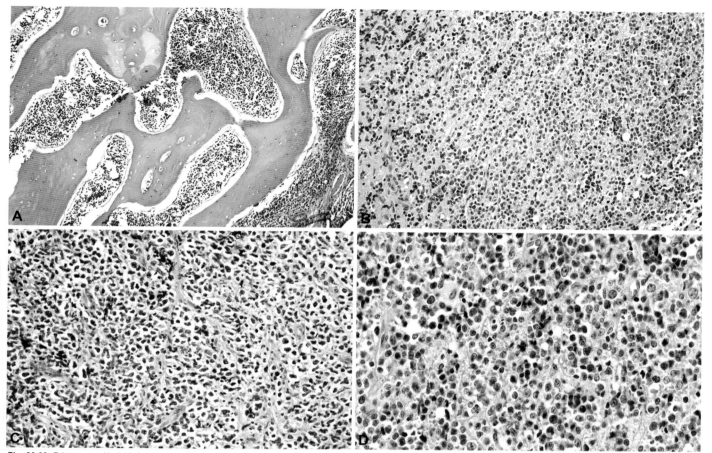

Fig. 20.09 Primary non-Hodgkin lymphoma of bone. **A** In this low-power image, the bony trabeculae are thickened and tumour cells fill up the marrow spaces. **B** Medium-power appearance of the neoplastic infiltrate. **C** In some cases, lymphoma cells may cluster as shown in this photomicrograph. **D** Although nuclei are round and small, there is more variation in their size and shape than is seen in Ewing sarcoma.

of chemotherapy and radiation without any surgery. Grossly, the tumours are tan-white and fleshy with the main mass centred around the metaphyses, and with indistinct bone margins and absence of obvious bone formation.

Histopathology

DLBCL has a characteristic growth pattern and tends to be destructive and obliterative at central sites, but to leave behind normal structures, such as medullary bone and marrow fat cells at the periphery of the lesion. The bony trabeculae may appear normal or may appear thickened or irregular, even Pagetoid. The cytological features show some variation, with a few cases having an immunoblastic appearance that encumbers distinction from solitary plasmacytoma of bone. However, many cases have a more pleomorphic appearance with prominent fibrosis {601, 2236}. The nuclei tend to be large and irregular with a cleaved and/or multilobated

appearance. Nucleoli may be prominent. The cytoplasm is not abundant but may be amphophilic. Fine reticulin fibres are present between individual tumour cells. Occasionally, this gives rise to thick, fibrous bands. Rarely a lymphoma will have so much fibrosis that the tumour cells may spindle, even showing a storiform pattern, leading to an erroneous diagnosis of a sarcoma {1441}. Another common finding is the associated infiltrate of non-neoplastic small lymphocytes. One major diagnostic problem is that the cells tend to be crushed, in particular in trephine biopsies of the long bones. If a biopsy shows such crush artefact, a diagnosis of malignant lymphoma should be suspected and immunohistochemistry should always be performed.

The other more rare variants of primary lymphoma of bone, such as anaplastic large cell lymphoma (either ALK positive or negative) show the characteristic features of their nodal counterparts and

should be diagnosed as such. Extensive staging procedures, including trephine biopsies from the iliac crest should be undertaken to exclude secondary involvement by a systemic/nodal lymphoma.

As a differential diagnosis, Hodgkin lymphoma may involve the skeleton as a manifestation of widespread disease and produce a tumour mass, or, extremely rarely, as a primary (often polyostotic) manifestation of the disease. Classical Reed-Sternberg cells are required for the diagnosis but may be difficult to find. In all cases, a fully convincing immunophenotype should be present to establish a diagnosis of primary Hodgkin lymphoma of bone {2137}. Leukaemic infiltrates may produce a tumour mass centred in the medullary cavity of the bone. Patients with chronic or acute myelogenous leukaemia or granulocytic sarcoma may occasionally present with destructive lesions of bone. Histological features of the infiltrates recapitulate the features of systemic disease.

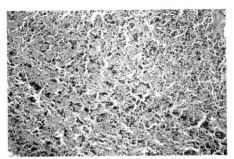

Fig. 20.10 Primary non-Hodgkin lymphoma of bone. Crush artefact is frequently present.

Immunophenotype

Lymphomas involving bone should be worked up by immunohistochemistry in the same way as their lymph node counterparts. Almost all primary lymphomas involving bone are mature B-cell neoplasms, and hence stain with CD20. PAX5 staining may be of help to identify the multilobated nuclear contour of the tumour cells in DLBCL. Most studies show that these lymphomas have a similar distribution with respect to the "cell of origin" as their nodal counterparts, <50% being CD10 positive, and >50% being BCL6 positive. MUM1/IRF4 staining is reported to be variable. BCL2 protein is found in more than half of the cases {10,218,601, 1169,1245,1623}

T-cell lymphomas, including anaplastic large cell lymphomas, should also be immunostained with a panel of antibodies. Anaplastic large cell lymphomas are always strongly CD30 positive and some cases may have expression of ALK protein, indicating chromosomal translocations involving *ALK* at chromosome 2p23.

Genetics

Data from classical cytogenetic analysis are not available. Moreover, very limited studies using interphase FISH have been published for primary DLBCL of bone. *BCL2*/18q21 breakpoints were found in approximately 25% of the cases, *MYC*/8q24 breakpoints in 10%, and *BCL6*/3q27 breakpoints reported variably {218,1623}. Nine DLBCL were analysed by array CGH for numerical and structural abnormalities, suggesting that gain of 1q and amplification of 2p16 may be recurrent events {1170}.

Prognostic factors

In older retrospective series, the prognosis for patients with lymphoma was associated with cell type, and within the DLBCL group with expression of markers such as CD10 or MUM1/IRF4. In many of these series the most important prognostic indicators were the stage of the disease and type of therapy {10,218,1169}. However, with current combined modality treatment protocols, overall survival is excellent and has become independent of these prognostic parameters {42,3073}. One study also suggests that addition of rituximab to CHOP-like chemotherapy may further improve prognosis to an overall survival of >90% {42}.

Table 20.03 Distribution of different types of primary non-Hodgkin lymphoma presenting in bone according to five separate studies

Type of neoplasm	Study				
	Heyning {1169} (n=60)	Gianelli {970} (n=28)	Alencar {42} (n=53)	Zinzani {3073} (n=52)	Hsieh {1239} (n=14)
DLBCL (%)	55 (92)	26 (93)	44 (83)	44 (85)	7 (50)
FL	2	0	3	2	0
SLL/MZL/LPL	1	0	3	2	1
Other B-cell neoplasms	0	0	1	2	0
ALCL	2	1	0	2	5
Other T-cell neoplasms	0	1	2	0	1

DLBCL, diffuse large B-cell lymphoma; FL, follicular lymphoma; SLL, small lymphocytic lymphoma; MZL, marginal zone lymphoma; LPL, lymphoplasmacytic lymphoma; ALCL, anaplastic large-cell lymphoma

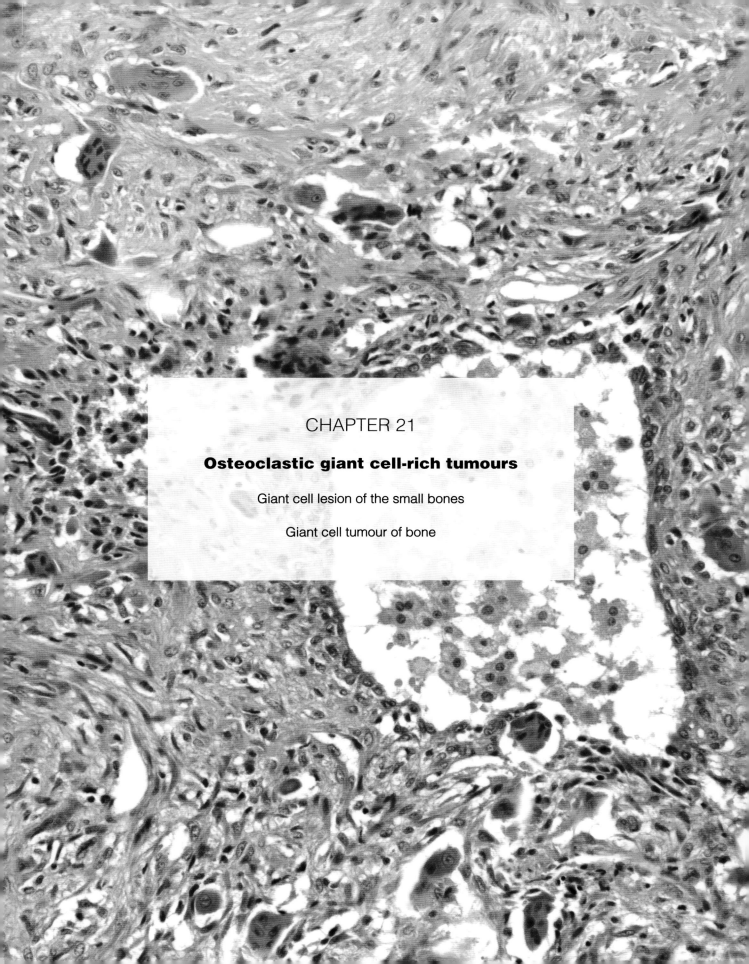

CHAPTER 21

Osteoclastic giant cell-rich tumours

Giant cell lesion of the small bones

Giant cell tumour of bone

Giant cell lesion of the small bones

R. Forsyth
G. Jundt

Definition
Giant cell lesions of the small bones (GCLSB) of the hands and feet are very rare tumour-like lesions consisting of fibrous tissue with haemorrhage, haemosiderin deposits, irregularly distributed giant cells and reactive bone formation.

Synonym
Giant cell reparative granuloma

Epidemiology
GCLSB is most common in the first and second decades of life, although older patients may also be affected. More than 50% of GCLSB are diagnosed in patients aged < 30 years and lesions are distributed equally between the sexes {1982,2981}.

Sites of involvement
Phalangeal, metacarpal and metatarsal bones are more often affected than carpal or tarsal bones. Lesions are rarely seen in long tubular bones or vertebrae {1982}.

Clinical and imaging features
Symptoms at presentation are most commonly pain and swelling. A pathological fracture may complicate GCLSB {2981}. Radiographically, GCLSB appears as a meta(dia)physeal, osteolytic and expansile lesion with distinct circumscription, only rarely extending to the epiphysis, and does not cross the unfused growth plate. The cortex is thinned, but not destroyed. A periosteal reaction is usually absent. Internal trabeculation may be seen. On MRI, cystic areas are uncommon and, if present,

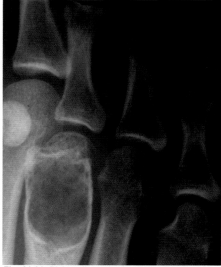

Fig. 21.01 Plain radiograph of a giant cell lesion of the third metatarsal, showing a metaphyseal, osteolytic and slightly expansile lesion with distinct circumscription.

not prominent {1982}. It is also important, as in all giant cell containing lesions of bone, to exclude hyperparathyroid bone disease.

Macroscopy
Typically, GCLSB is a tan-grey/brown, gritty and friable lesion. Haemorrhages are commonly present {1982,2138,3008}.

Histopathology
The lesion consists of fibrous stromal tissue in varying amounts. Spindle-shaped (myo-)fibroblasts without atypia predominate, sometimes arranged in a whorled to fascicular pattern. Osteoclast-like giant cells,

with fewer nuclei than in giant cell tumour of bone, are also present. Key to the histological diagnosis, is the particular distribution and clustering of these giant cells around haemorrhages, separated by bundles of scar-like stromal tissue. Reactive bone formation, comprising immature woven bone, as well as trabeculae with osteoblastic rimming, may be prominent. Mitoses are easily found, atypical mitoses, however, are absent. Focal deposits of haemosiderin are frequently found. Inflammatory cells and occasionally foam cells are also present, as well as small aneurysmal bone cyst (ABC)-like pseudocysts {2981,3008}. Although histologically similar, GCLSB should be separated from giant cell lesions of the jaws and solid variants of ABC according to clinical and preliminary genetic data.

Genetics
Cytogenetic analyses of three tumours have shown unrelated alterations. One tumour showed a t(X;4)(q22;q31.3) {343}, another showed a t(6;13)(q15;q34) and partially deleted 20q {2155}. Various rearrangements of chromosomes 8 and 22, as well as ring chromosomes and telomeric associations similar to those in giant cell tumour of bone, have been described in a third case {1338}.

Prognostic factors
Curettage is the treatment of choice. GCLSBs are associated with a high rate of recurrence (15–50%), but are almost always cured in a second procedure.

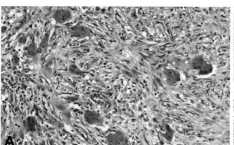
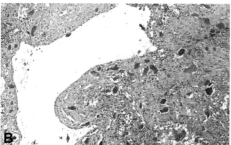
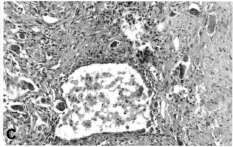

Fig. 21.02 Giant cell lesion of the small bones (GCLSB). A The lesion consists of varying amounts of fibrous stromal tissue. Note the distribution and clustering of the multinucleated giant cells. B Distribution and clustering of giant cells around haemorrhages. C Occasionally, foam cells and small aneurysmal bone cyst-like pseudocysts are present.

Giant cell tumour of bone

N.A. Athanasou
M. Bansal
R. Forsyth
R.P. Reid
Z. Sapi

Definition
A benign but locally aggressive primary bone neoplasm that is composed of a proliferation of mononuclear cells amongst which are scattered numerous macrophages and large osteoclast-like giant cells. A high-grade malignant neoplasm arising in giant cell tumour (GCT) may be identified at the initial diagnosis (primary malignancy in GCT), or subsequent to previous radiation or surgical therapy (secondary malignancy in GCT).

ICD-O code
Giant cell tumour of bone   9250/1
Malignancy in giant cell tumour   9250/3

Synonym
Osteoclastoma

Epidemiology
GCT represents 4–5% of all primary bone tumours {367,683,2454, 2815}. The peak incidence is between the ages of 20 and 45 years, although approximately 10% of cases occur in the second decade of life. GCTs rarely arise in the immature skeleton. There is a slight female predominance in some large series. GCT may rarely complicate Paget disease of bone and can arise in association with focal dermal hypoplasia (Goltz syndrome) {479,1907, 2713}.
Malignant transformation occurs in < 1% of all GCTs, with a slight female predominance. Patients with malignancy in GCT are generally about a decade older than patients with conventional GCT.

Etiology
It is now generally accepted that the numerous large osteoclast-like giant cells in GCT are not neoplastic but reactive in nature. The mononuclear cells are of two types, either macrophage-like osteoclast precursors, or primitive mesenchymal stromal cells that express receptor activator for NF-κβ ligand (RANKL) {3066}; it is the latter that shows mitotic activity and represents the neoplastic component of GCT. Both macrophages and osteoclasts express RANK and, in the presence of

macrophage-colony stimulating factor, the proliferating mononuclear stromal cells induce osteoclast formation by a RANKL-dependent mechanism {1564,3066}. Mononuclear stromal cells also express (pre)osteoblast markers, including alkaline phosphatase, RUNX2 and Sp7 transcription factor (osterix) {1244}.
Most secondary malignancies in GCT follow radiation therapy. Primary malignancies in GCT are the least common type.

Sites of involvement
GCT typically affects the ends of long bones, the distal femur, proximal tibia, distal radius and proximal humerus. In the spine, GCT arises most commonly in the vertebral body of the sacrum, followed by the lumbar, thoracic and cervical vertebrae in decreasing frequency {2436}. Flat bones are uncommonly involved; the ilium is the most frequently involved bone in the pelvis. Fewer than 5% of GCTs affect the tubular bones of the hands and feet. Synchronous or metachronous, multicentric GCTs are rare and commonly involve small bones of the distal extremities {2208} (see Chapter 27). It is important in such cases, as for other GCTs, to exclude hyperparathyroid bone disease.
Malignancy in GCT affects similar bones to those involved in conventional GCT. There have been no cases reported in the small bones of the hands and feet or the skull.

Clinical and imaging features
Patients with GCT typically present with pain and swelling; there may be limitation of joint movement and pathological fracture is seen in 5–10% of patients.
Plain X-rays of lesions in long bones usually show an expansile, eccentric, often lobulated area of osteolysis with a narrow zone of transition. Tumours that have extended into soft tissue are sometimes covered by a sclerotic rim. There is little or no evidence of matrix calcification within the tumour, and relatively little reactive, periosteal new bone formation is seen radiologically. The tumour commonly involves the epiphysis and adjacent metaphysis; it usually extends up to the subchondral bone plate.

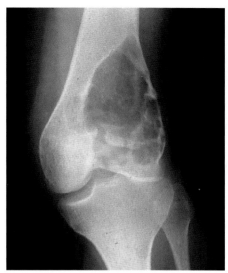

Fig. 21.03 Plain radiography of a giant cell tumour showing a large, expansile area of lysis with a sclerotic border, cortical thinning, and extension to the subchondral plate.

Rarely, the tumour is confined to the metaphysis; this is usually seen in adolescence where the tumour lies in relation to an open growth plate. Diaphyseal lesions are exceptional. GCTs of the sacrum and pelvis are lytic tumours that may involve the sacroiliac or hip joints and surrounding soft tissues. In the spine, GCT is usually located

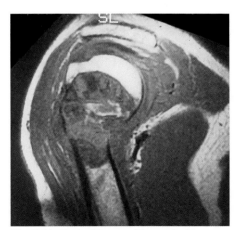

Fig. 21.04 Giant cell tumour of the proximal humerus. MRI shows a well-demarcated lesion with focal destruction of cortex and extension into the epiphysis.

in the vertebral body, but may involve the posterior elements. CT scanning provides a more accurate assessment of cortical integrity than plain radiographs {606}. MRI is useful in assessing the extent of intra-osseous spread and defining soft-tissue and joint involvement {88}. GCT typically shows homogeneous, low to intermediate signal intensity on T1-weighted images and intermediate to high, occasionally heterogeneous, signal intensity on T2-weighted images; large amounts of haemosiderin are often present, giving areas of low signal in both modalities. Dynamic MRI typically shows a fast uptake of contrast and a slow wash-out.

Malignancy in GCT

The recurrence of pain and swelling many years after treatment of a GCT may suggest the possibility of malignant transformation. The symptomatology of primary malignancy in GCT is nonspecific. In primary malignancy in GCT, the tumour presents as a lytic process extending to the end of a long bone. Rarely X-rays show typical features of GCT and a sclerotic destructive tumour juxtaposed to it. In secondary malignancy in GCT, plain radiographs show a destructive process with poor margination situated at the site of a previously diagnosed GCT. Mineralization may be present.

Macroscopy

The tumour is very well defined and often lies eccentrically within the end of a long bone, which is typically expanded and shows thinning of the cortex. Even when the tumour has extended through the cortex, it has a rounded pushing margin. The tumour is often covered by a thin, sometimes incomplete shell of reactive bone. Although the tumour frequently erodes the subchondral bone plate and can focally erode the deep surface of the articular cartilage, it seldom penetrates the articular surfaces. The tumour tissue is usually soft and red-brown and may contain yellow areas, which correspond to xanthomatous change, or firm white areas of abundant fibrous tissue. There are commonly areas of haemorrhage, and blood-filled cystic spaces are sometimes seen. The gross appearance of malignancy in GCT is that of any high-grade sarcoma: a large fleshy tumour often with soft-tissue extension. The underlying GCT is tan-red and haemorrhagic.

Histopathology

GCT is characterized by the presence of very large numbers of osteoclast-like giant cells wthat appear uniformly scattered amongst numerous round or spindle-shaped mononuclear cells. The giant cells morphologically resemble osteoclasts and have plump, eosinophilic cytoplasm and vesicular nuclei which contain prominent nucleoli. Many of the giant cells are larger than normal osteoclasts. They contain a variable number of nuclei but "giant" osteoclasts with > 20 and sometimes > 50 nuclei are not uncommon.

Cells of the mononuclear component are spindle-shaped, round or oval. The nuclei of many of the mononuclear cells have an open chromatin pattern and contain one or two small nucleoli; these macrophage-like nuclear features are similar to those of the osteoclastic giant cells. There is also a population of mononuclear stromal cells with poorly defined cytoplasm and spindle-shaped or ovoid nucleoli; these cells show a variable, occasionally high degree of mitotic activity (up to 20 per 10 HPF). All mitotic figures are typical. The presence of atypical mitotic figures should point to a diagnosis of a sarcoma or other malignancy containing numerous osteoclastic giant cells.

The tumour stroma is often well vascularized and may contain broad bands of cel-

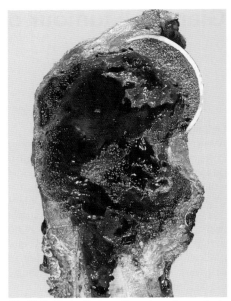

Fig. 21.06 Giant cell tumour of bone. Large haemorrhagic tumour of the proximal humerus with extensive cortical destruction and soft-tissue extension.

lular or collagenous fibrous tissue. Areas of recent haemhorrage, haemosiderin deposition and collections of foamy macrophages may be noted. In some areas of the tumour, giant cells may not be conspicuous and a proliferation of mononuclear cells with round or spindle-shaped nuclei predominates. A fibrous histiocytoma-like storiform pattern may be found in parts of the tumour. Secondary ABC-like change is seen in 10% of cases. Small foci of reactive osteoid or bone formation within the tumour are commonly found, especially after pathological fracture or biopsy. Reactive woven bone formation is also commonly present at the advancing edge of the tumour and focally, some mononuclear cells within the lesion may be associated with osteoid formation. Areas of necrosis and haemorrhage are commonly found in larger lesions. At the metaphyseal (bony) margin of the tumour, a permeative growth pattern may be noted.

When the tumour extends into soft tissue or is present in lung, the histological features are identical to the primary lesion. In one third of cases there may be intravascular invasion, particularly at the periphery of the tumour. Although this does not of itself have prognostic significance, it is commonly seen in cases that metastasize to the lung {36}.

Grading the histological features of GCT has not been shown to have prognostic

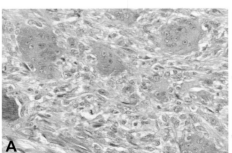
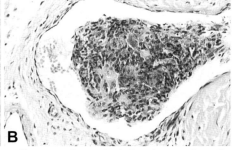

Fig. 21.05 Giant cell tumour of bone. **A** Typical appearance with numerous large osteoclasts and mononuclear cells, some of which show typical mitotic activity. **B** The vascular lumen contains a mixture of spindle and giant cells.

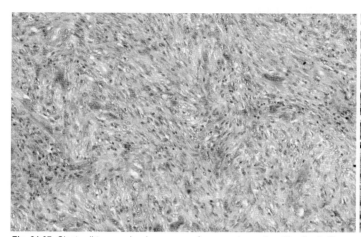

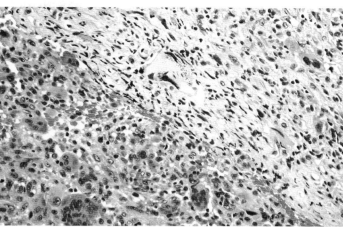

Fig. 21.07 Giant cell tumour showing an area of mononuclear cell proliferation in fibrous tissue. Mononuclear cells lie in a storiform pattern and show focal mitotic activity. There are relatively few giant cells.

Fig. 21.08 Malignancy in giant cell tumour (GCT) of bone. The conventional GCT (lower left), with mononuclear cells uniformly interspersed with multinucleated giant cells, is adjacent to an area of malignant anaplastic tumour cells (upper right).

significance in terms of predicting recurrence or metastasis, although some studies have indicated that assessment of one or more proliferation or cell-cycle markers may provide a guide as to clinical behaviour.

Malignancy in GCT

Primary malignancy in GCT refers to cases where an area or a nodule of highly pleomorphic mononuclear cells is present in an otherwise conventional GCT. The transition between the two components varies. The high-grade sarcoma has no specific morphology; it may or may not produce osteoid. In secondary malignancy in GCT, the pre-existing GCT may or may not be evident.

Immunophenotype

Giant cells have the typical immunophenotype of normal osteoclasts, expressing the vitronectin receptor (CD51) and a restricted range of macrophage markers, including CD45, CD33 and CD68, but not CD14, CD163 or HLA-DR {693,1697}. The giant cells also strongly express tartrate-resistant acid phosphatase and cathepsin K.

Genetics

The most common clonal and non-clonal chromosomal aberration is telomeric association (tas), which is a chromosomal end-to-end fusion without loss of material {2160}. Approximately 50% of GCTs of bone show clonal chromosomal aberrations, including clonal tas and other structural and numerical changes (70, 60, and 30% respectively) {1016}. A moderate reduction in telomere length (average loss of 100–500 base pairs) has been shown in GCT cells {902,2481}. Telomeres most commonly affected are 1q, 11p, 12p, 13p, 14p, 15p, 19q, 20q, 21p and 22p {319, 956,2160,2494}. The frequency of tas, irrespective of clonality, is higher in tumours carrying clonal changes, indicating their precursor role in other types of aberrations {319}; however, the exact mechanism whereby telomere dysfunction leads to tumour formation remains unclear {596,956,2160,2481}. Some GCTs have shown rearrangement of 16q22 and 17p13 {319,2494}, perhaps indicating the presence of an associated ABC.

No clear association between cytogenetic features and adverse clinical outcome has been demonstrated {1016}. Allelic losses of 1p, 9q, and 19q regions are frequent in primary, locally recurrent and metastatic GCTs, whereas LOH of 17p (in proximity to the *TP53* locus) and 9p appear exclusive to pulmonary metastases {2303}. *TP53* and *HRAS* mutations have been identified in secondary malignant GCT of bone (not associated with prior radiation), suggesting a possible role in malignant transformation {2091,2409}. Strong expression of TP53 has been demonstrated in some, but not all secondary malignant GCT {36,1005,2172}. Centrosome amplification is significantly higher in recurrent and malignant GCT {1961}. The lack of an association between centrosome amplification and chromosome-number alteration suggests that alternative causative mechanisms produce genetic instability {1960}.

Prognostic factors

GCT commonly behaves as a benign but locally aggressive tumour; it may be confined to bone or extend through the bone cortex into surrounding soft tissue.

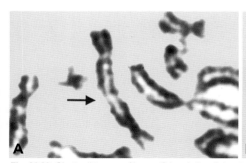

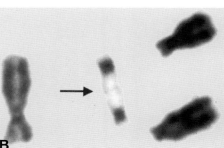

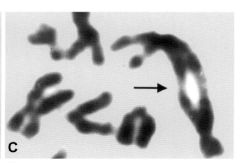

Fig. 21.09 Giant cell tumour of bone. G-banded partial metaphase spreads (**A,B,C**). Telomeric associations are indicated by arrows.

Pulmonary metastases are seen in 2% of GCTs, occurring on average 3–4 years after primary diagnosis {1755,2553}. These metastases are very slow-growing and are thought to represent pulmonary implants that result from embolization of intravascular growths of GCTs {693}. Some of these benign pulmonary implants can regress spontaneously. A small number, however, exhibit progressive enlargement and can lead to the death of the patient. Local recurrence, surgical manipulation and location in the distal radius have been associated with an increased risk of metastasis.

Following curettage, local recurrence occurs in 15–50% of patients, depending on the thoroughness of curettage and the nature of adjuvant therapy employed. Recurrence is usually seen within 2 years. Complete en-bloc excision of the lesion in small bones results in few local recurrences. As osteoclasts form a major component of GCT of bone, therapeutic inhibition of osteoclast formation and activity provides another modality of treatment, particularly in those cases where

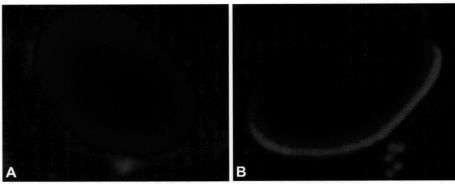

Fig. 21.10 Giant cell tumour of bone. FISH showing expression of γ- tubulin (red staining) in a non-recurring case with a normal centrosome pattern (**A**); and (**B**) a recurrent case showing centrosome amplification.

surgical clearance of a tumour cannot be obtained because it is sited in an inaccessible anatomical location, is very extensive or frequently recurrent. The precise clinical indications for this treatment have not been formalized but treatment with an aminobisphosphonate, such as zoledronate, or more specifically the anti-RANKL antibody denosumab, have been shown to retard or arrest tumour growth {149,2749}. Denosumab-treated tumours

can be devoid of giant cells and mononuclear cells and composed of abundant woven bone and fibrous tissue.

The prognosis for patients with secondary malignant GCTs is similar to that of a high-grade sarcoma, and is reported to be worse than for patients with primary malignant GCT {2007}.

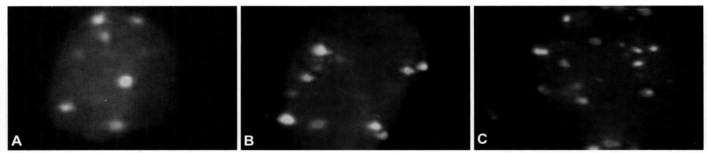

Fig. 21.11 Giant cell tumour of bone (GCTB). Centromeric FISH signals for chromosomes X (blue), 3 (red), 4 (green) and 6 (yellow). **A** Normal disomic cell from a female patient with non-recurring GCTB. **B** Increased random aneusomy is characteristic of recurrent cases (aneusomic cell from a female patient with trisomies of chromosomes 3, 4 and 6). **C** Highly aneusomic cell from a female patient with secondary malignant GCTB. In this case, clonal alteration could also be detected.

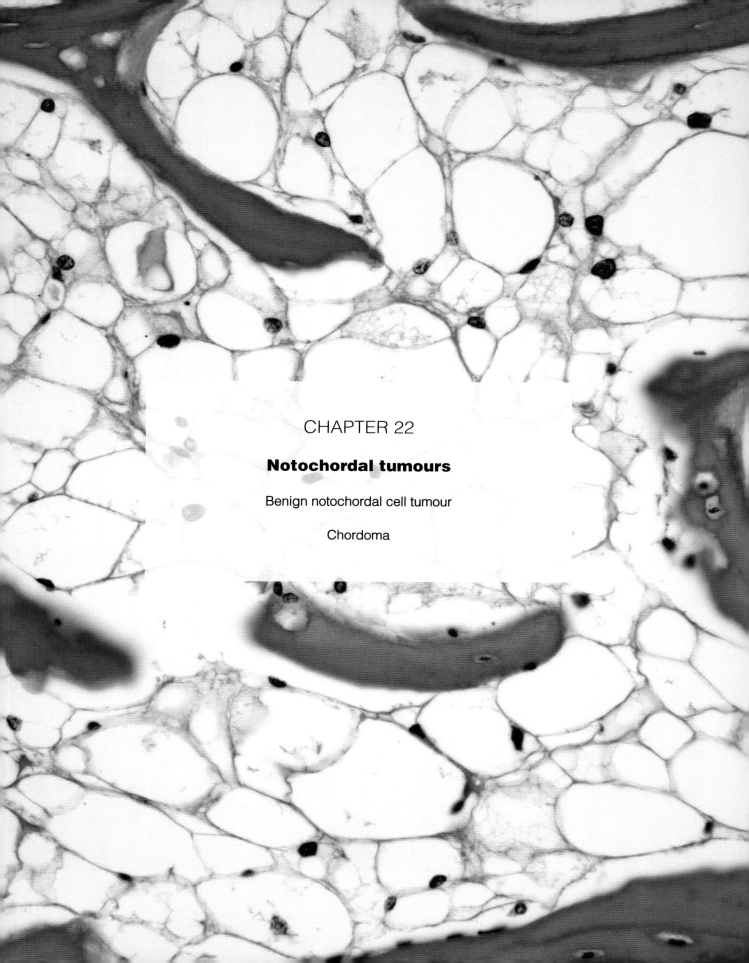

CHAPTER 22

Notochordal tumours

Benign notochordal cell tumour

Chordoma

Benign notochordal cell tumour

A.M. Flanagan
T. Yamaguchi

Definition
A benign tumour showing notochordal differentiation {3010,3011}.

ICD-O code   9370/0

Synonyms
Giant notochordal rest; notochordal hamartoma; ecchordosis physaliphora spheno-occipitalis (EP)

Epidemiology
The incidence of benign notochordal cell tumours (BNCTs) is uncertain, although in a relatively small study they have been reported to occur in at least 20% of cadavers, between the ages of 7 and 82 years {3011}. EP is found in 0.6–2.0% of autopsy cases and 1.7% of patients on MRI {1807}.

Etiology
The origin of BNCT is controversial. Some consider that it derives from persistent no-

tochord, a developmental rod-like structure that is incorporated into the vertebral column during the development of the axial skeleton, and is not normally seen in vertebral bodies after 10 weeks of gestation. Others consider that BNCT may develop after birth {3009}.

Sites of involvement
BNCTs occur in the bones of the base of skull, the vertebral bodies and the sacrococcygeal bones. They can also be sited intradurally in the region of the dorsum of the clivus when the tumour is known as EP. A very small number have been reported in soft tissue {1408}. A unique postmortem study shows that 11.5% of the bones of the clivus, 5% of the cervical vertebrae, none of the thoracic vertebrae, 2% of the lumbar vertebrae, and 12% of the sacrococcygeal vertebrae contain BNCTs. This distribution is similar to that described for the anatomical sites of chordoma previously reported {252}.

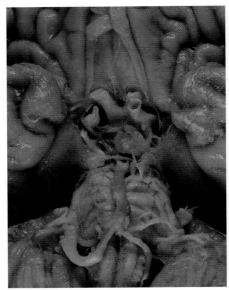

Fig. 22.02 Ecchordosis physaliphora spheno-occipitalis (EP). Jelly-like material representing an EP centred on the Circle of Willis. The histological features are identical to that of a benign notochordal cell tumour.

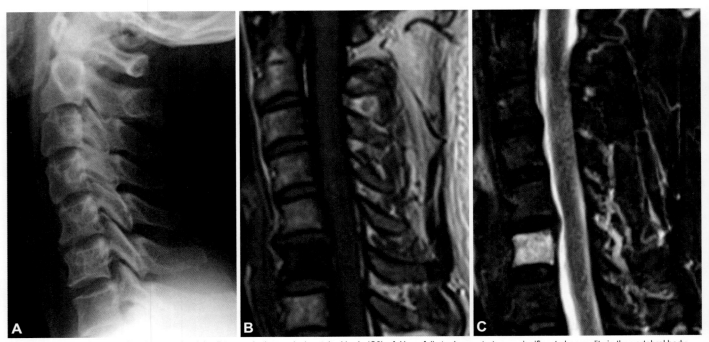

Fig. 22.01 Imaging features of benign notochordal cell tumour in the cervical vertebral body (C6). A X-ray fails to demonstrate any significant abnormality in the vertebral body. B T1-weighted MRI reveals the lesion, which occupies the entire vertebral body, to be of low signal intensity. C Short T1 inversion recovery image reveals the lesion to be of high signal intensity. No extra-osseous tumour mass is evident.

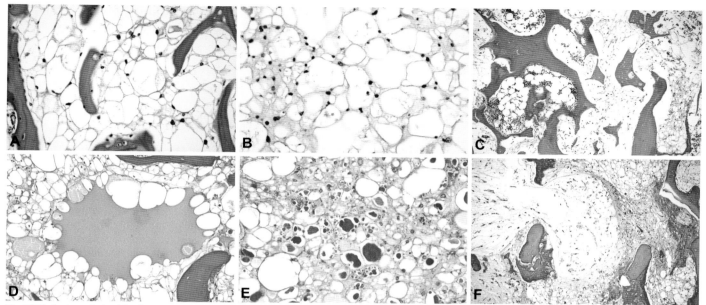

Fig. 22.03 Benign notochordal cell tumour (BNCT). **A** An intra-osseous tumour permeating the trabecular space of the vertebral body. Note the well-defined cell boundaries giving an "adipocyte-like" appearance, the absence of atypia and extracellular matrix. **B** Ecchordosis physaliphora spheno-occipitalis showing similar histological features to an intra-osseous BNCT. **C** The presence of haematopoietic islands set within the BNCT. **D** Cystic-like collection of colloid-type material, and **E** hyaline globules. **F** BNCT on the right with a sharp transition to a chordoma on the left.

Clinical features

Most BNCTs are incidental findings, but lesions that fill the vertebral body, and sufficiently large EPs, may be symptomatic. The risk of transformation to a chordoma is considered to be extremely low {1516}.

Macroscopy features

BNCTs, apart from EPs, which are intradural polypoid notochordal lesions and usually attached to the dorsum of the clivus, are contained within the bone. The average intra-osseous lesion found at autopsy measures approximately 2 × 4 mm {3009,3010}. Larger lesions, also reported as giant notochordal rests, can occupy the entire vertebral body {569,1516}. EPs

are composed of jelly-like material, and usually range from 1 to 2 cm in size {1516, 1807}.

Histopathology

BNCT is a well-defined tumour contained within bone. It lacks lobular architecture, fibrous bands, extracellular myxoid matrix, vasculature and necrosis, all of which are characteristic of its malignant counterpart, the chordoma {3009}. The tumour cells are vacuolated and have centrally or peripherally placed round or oval nuclei, with small nucleoli, without atypia, and can mimic mature adipocytes. Less vacuolated tumour cells can have eosinophilic cytoplasm, which may contain eosinophilic

hyaline globules. No mitotic figures are seen. The affected bone trabeculae are often sclerotic. Bone marrow islands are often entrapped within the tumour. A BNCT may be juxtaposed to a chordoma, raising the possibility that it represents the benign counterpart of the malignant tumour {643,2057,3012}.

EP has similar morphological features to those of BNCT.

Immunophenotype

BNCT, including EP, has the same immunoprofile as chordoma: S100 protein, EMA, AE1/AE3, CAM5.2 and brachyury are expressed {1408,1516,3010}.

Chordoma

A.M. Flanagan
T. Yamaguchi

Definition
A malignant tumour showing notochordal differentiation.

ICD-O code
Chordoma NOS   9370/3
Chondroid chordoma   9371/3
"Dedifferentiated" chordoma   9372/3

Epidemiology
The incidence of chordoma is 0.08 per 100000 people. The male to female ratio is approximately 1.8:1. Chordoma rarely occurs in the black African population but appears to be represented equally in people of other races. The tumour commonly develops in the fifth to seventh decades of life although all age groups are affected.

Etiology
The vast majority of chordomas arise as sporadic disease, and although there is some evidence that chordoma can develop from a benign notochordal cell tumour, this remains unproven {643,2057,

3012}. Very occasionally it occurs in a familial setting, when the inheritance is compatible with an autosomal dominant trait. In some families, the inherited disease is associated with duplication of the brachyury gene (*T* gene) {3025}. Approximately 7% of sporadic chordomas exhibit amplification of the *T* gene, a transcription factor required for notochordal development {2266}. There is also a recognized, although rare association of chordoma, generally in children, with tuberous sclerosis complex {1591,1798}.

Sites of involvement
Chordomas are chiefly located in bones of the base of skull, the vertebral bodies and the sacrococcygeal bone, with only a very small number reported in the extra-axial skeleton, and in soft tissues {2760}. Data from the SEER programme, 1973–1995, reports that in the axial skeleton 32% of cases are cranial-based, and 32.8% and 29.2% occur in the mobile spinal and the sacrococcygeal bones respectively {1797,1973}. This contrasts with other series, which document a cephalic and caudal preponderance {252,1516}. Tumours in children and young adults have a greater propensity to occur in the cranial region {1797,1973}.

Clinical features
Skull-based chordomas most commonly present with headache, neck pain, diplopia, or facial nerve palsy. Retroclival chordoma presents with brain stem symptoms or cranial nerve palsy. Chordoma of the mobile spine and sacrum present with chronic low-back pain, and those in the coccyx may present with coccydynia. Change in bowel and/or bladder function, parasthesia of the limbs, and even a lump, can be presenting symptoms.

Macroscopy
The tumour presents as an expansile, lobulated structure, with the cut surface revealing a blue/slate-grey, gelatinous matrix but other areas may exhibit a more solid chondroid texture. Generally, the tumour extends beyond the cortex.

Histopathology
Chordomas, not otherwise specified (NOS), are classically composed of large cells with clear to eosinophilic cytoplasm separated into lobules by fibrous septa. The tumour cells have copious vacuolated "bubbly" cytoplasm, referred to as "physaliphorous cells". The cells are arranged as small ribbons and cords embedded in abundant extracellular myxoid matrix, or as more densely arranged epithelioid packets. Nuclear atypia and pleomorphism range from low-grade, when it is associated with infrequent mitotic figures, to tumours with high-grade nuclear atypia in which cells may have a more spindled sarcomatoid appearance. The latter is generally associated with greater mitotic activity. However, chordomas often show a significant degree of intratumoral histological heterogeneity. Necrosis is frequently present and may be extensive.
Chondroid chordoma refers to chordoma in which the matrix mimics hyaline cartilaginous tumours. This component can be very focal or extensive. There is no good evidence that tumours behave differently to those without this morphology.
Dedifferentiated chordoma is a biphasic tumour; comprising the features of a chordoma NOS which is juxtaposed to a high-grade undifferentiated spindle cell tumour or osteosarcoma.

Immunophenotype
Chordomas NOS, including those tumours with chondroid foci, express keratins and are usually immunoreactive for EMA, and S100. Brachyury is a highly specific marker for chordoma {2888} and helps distinguish chordoma from morphologically similar neoplasms including carcinoma, chondrosarcoma, and chordoid meningioma. Immunoreactivity for brachyury can be lost following decalcification in formic and nitric acid. Loss of PTEN occurs in a significant number of cases, whereas loss of INI-1 expression is seen in a minority of chordomas {333,1921,2265}. Brachyury, keratins, EMA and S100 are not expressed in the dedifferentiated component of a dedifferentiated chordoma {2888}.

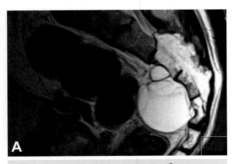

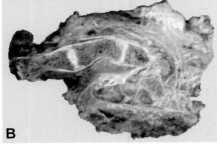

Fig. 22.04 Chordoma. **A** A T2-weighted MR image of a sacral chordoma revealing a high-signal sacral tumour with extra-osseous masses. **B** A sacrectomy specimen showing a coccygeal lobulated tumour composed of myxoid gelatinous material extending from bone into soft tissue.

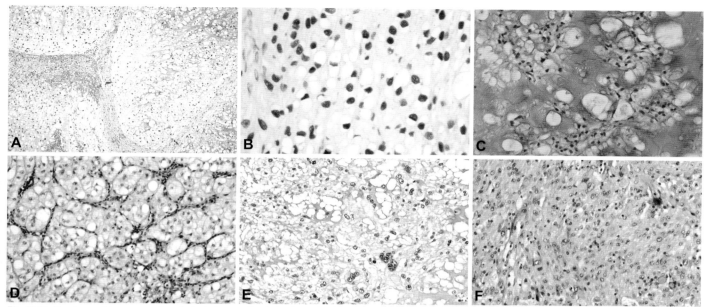

Fig. 22.05 Chordoma. **A** Low-power view of a typical conventional chordoma showing the lobulated architecture and extracellular matrix. **B** The nuclei of chordoma cells showing immunoreactivity for brachyury. **C** Nests and cords of cells with small nuclei set in a rich myxoid matrix. **D** Densely packed epithelioid cells which could be mistaken for renal cell carcinoma. **E** Vacuolated cells in which the nuclei have coarse chromatin. **F** Spindled cells with little intervening matrix.

Ultrastructure

The tumour cells are variably vacuolated and have abundant cytoplasm containing desmosomes, irregular cytoplasmic processes, mitochondria–rough endoplasmic reticulum (ER) complexes, and microtubules within ER in addition to intermediate filaments and glycogen granules {2397,2542}.

Genetics

Most chordomas studied cytogenetically, exhibit near-diploid or moderately hypodiploid karyotypes, with several numerical and structural rearrangements. The most common cytogenetic abnormalities are monosomy of chromosome 1 and gain of chromosome 7 {1022,1396}. An array CGH study revealed that 70% of chordomas harbour either homozygous or heterozygous loss of *CDKN2A* and *CDKN2B* {1086}. Copy-number gain of the brachyury 7q33 locus, and the *EGFR* 7p12 locus are common events {2266,2520}. Silencing of brachyury in a bone-fide chordoma cell line in vitro, results in growth arrest {2266}.

Somatic mutations have not been found in the coding region of brachyury, or in the mutation "hotspots" of other genes, including *EGFR, KRAS, NRAS, HRAS, BRAF, FGFR 1-4* {2265,2520}. *IDH1* and *IDH2* mutations are not detected in chordoma, which helps distinguish them from cartilaginous tumours {54}.

EGFR, PDGFRB, and *IGFR1* and *IGF1* as well as molecules in the mTOR pathway are activated in a significant number of chordomas {2265,2459,2520,2710}.

Prognostic factors

The overall median survival is 7 years, although this varies depending on the site and size of the tumour. Up to 40% of non cranial tumours metastasize. Dedifferentiated tumours appear to have a worse prognosis. The tumours metastasize to lung, bone, lymph nodes and subcutaneous tissue.

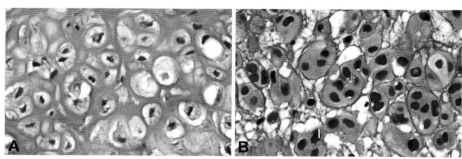

Fig. 22.06 Chondroid chordoma. **A** The cells are embedded in a hyaline matrix and indistinguishable from a cartilaginous tumour except that they express keratin and brachyury. **B** Cells showing a "hepatoid" appearance.

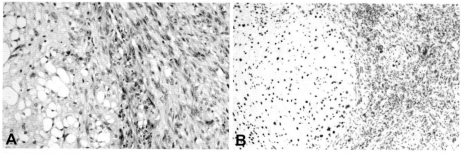

Fig. 22.07 Dedifferentiated chordoma. **A** Typical features of a chordoma with (left) an abrupt change to an undifferentiated spindle cell tumour (right). **B** Immunoreactivity to brachyury is lost in the spindle cell dedifferentiated component.

CHAPTER 23

Vascular tumours

Haemangioma

Epithelioid haemangioma

Epithelioid haemangioendothelioma

Angiosarcoma

Haemangioma

M. Hameed
L.E. Wold

Definition

A benign tumour composed of capillary-like blood vessels of small or large calibre.

ICD-O code   9120/0

Epidemiology

Haemangiomas are common lesions; autopsy studies have identified them in the vertebrae of approximately 10% of the adult population {14}. However, clinically significant, symptomatic tumours are uncommon, and account for < 1% of primary bone tumours {684}. Haemangiomas occur at any age, but most are diagnosed during middle and late middle-age, with the peak incidence in the fifth decade of life {2454}. The male to female ratio is around 2 : 3 {14,684, 2454,2815,2938}.

Sites of involvement

Vertebral bodies are the most commonly affected site, followed by the craniofacial skeleton, and then the long bones where they tend to involve the metaphyses {14, 684, 2938}. Multifocal occurrence is frequent.

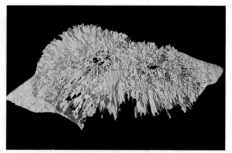

Fig. 23.01 Haemangioma of bone. The radiated spicules are demonstrated on this macerated specimen.

Clinical and imaging features

The majority of haemangiomas, especially those arising in the spine, are incidental radiographical findings. However, large vertebral tumours may cause cord compression, pain and neurological symptoms. Symptomatic tumours occurring elsewhere are painful and may cause a pathological fracture. Radiographically, haemangiomas present as a well-demarcated, lucent mass that frequently contains coarse trabeculations or striations. In flat bones, such as the calvarium, the tumour is expansile and lytic and produces a sunburst pattern of reactive bone formation. Clinically, indolent lesions frequently contain fat and sclerotic trabeculae on CT and MRI. Symptomatic tumours usually show loss of fat and reveal a low signal on T1-weighted images and a high signal on T2-weighted images {684,820, 1655,1758, 2454,2982}.

Macroscopy

Haemangioma manifests as a soft, well-demarcated, dark red mass. It may also have a honeycomb appearance with intralesional, sclerotic, bone trabeculae and scattered blood-filled cavities.

Histopathology

Haemangiomas have variable histological features. Capillary and cavernous haemangiomas are composed of thin-walled, blood-filled vessels lined by a single layer of flat, cytologically banal endothelial cells. The vessels permeate the marrow and surround pre-existing trabeculae. When capillary or cavernous haemangiomas involve a large localized region, or are widespread throughout the skeleton, it is known as angiomatosis.

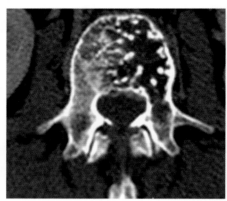

Fig. 23.02 Haemangioma of bone. CT axial image demonstrates a lytic vertebral lesion with the coarse trabeculae known as "polka-dot" pattern .

Immunophenotype

The endothelial cells stain with antibodies to factor VIII, CD31, and CD34. FLI1 and ERG positivity has also been observed.

Prognostic factors

Haemangiomas have an excellent prognosis and low rate of local recurrence.

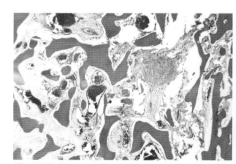

Fig. 23.03 Cavernous haemangioma showing thin-walled blood vessels lined by a single layer of endothelial cells, some filled with blood, within the marrow and between bony trabeculae.

Epithelioid haemangioma

A.E. Rosenberg
J.V.M.G. Bovée

Definition

A locally aggressive neoplasm composed of cells that have an endothelial phenotype and epithelioid morphology.

ICD-O code   9126/0

Synonyms

Histiocytoid haemangioma; angiofollicular hyperplasia with eosinophilia; haemorrhagic epithelioid and spindle cell haemangioma

Epidemiology

Epithelioid haemangioma is uncommon, but the exact incidence is unknown. Patients range in age from the first to ninth decade of life with most being adults; an average age of 35 years has been reported {772,2043}. Male to female ratio is 1.4 : 1 {2043}.

Sites of involvement

Tumours usually involve long tubular bones (40%), distal lower extremities (18%), flat bones, (18%), vertebrae (16%), and small bones of the hands (8%) {2043}. Approximately 18–25% of the tu-

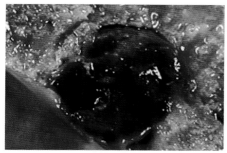

Fig. 23.05 Epithelioid haemangioma. A well-defined, oval, red-brown mass adjacent to cancellous bone.

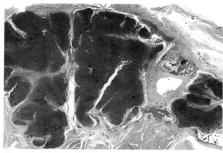

Fig. 23.06 Epithelioid haemangioma. Tumour fills and expands the bone, grows with a lobular architecture, and pushes into the soft tissues.

mours are multifocal with a regional distribution {772,2043}.

Clinical and imaging features

Patients usually present with pain localized to the involved anatomical site; identification as an incidental finding is rare. Imaging studies reveal a well-defined lytic, sometimes expansile, septated mass that may erode the cortex and extend into the soft tissue. On MRI they are hypo- or isointense to muscle on T1-weighted images, and hyperintense on T2-weighted images {772}.

Macroscopy

Tumours range in size from several millimetres to 15 cm; most are < 7 cm and are well defined, nodular, soft, solid, red, and haemorrhagic. They may expand the bone, erode the cortex and extend into the soft tissue.

Histopathology

The tumours have a lobular architecture, replace the marrow cavity, and often infiltrate pre-existing bony trabeculae. The periphery of the lobules may contain

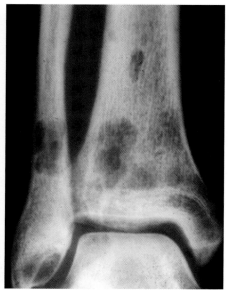

Fig. 23.04 Epithelioid haemangioma. Multiple lytic lesions involving the distal long bones of the leg.

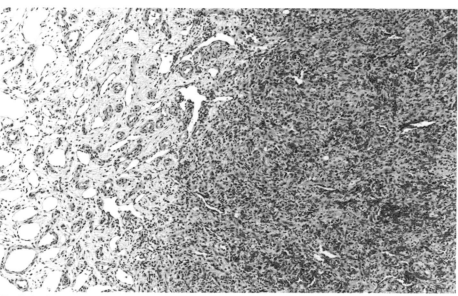

Fig. 23.07 Epithelioid haemangioma. Nodule of tumour surrounded by loose connective tissue containing many small arterioles.

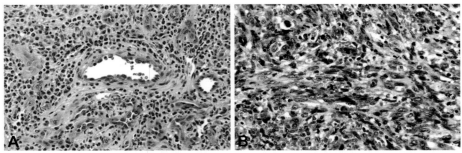

Fig. 23.08 Epithelioid haemangioma. **A** Mixed inflammatory infiltrate with eosinophils that obscures and surrounds a neoplastic vessel. **B** Spindle cells arranged in short fascicles and associated with hemosiderin in the centre of haemorrhagic nodule.

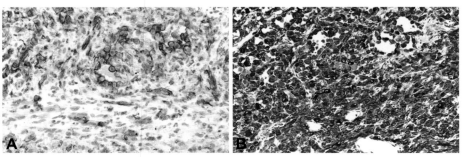

Fig. 23.09 Epithelioid haemangioma. **A** Epithelioid endothelial cells expressing CD31. **B** Epithelioid endothelial cells strongly positive for keratin.

haemorrhage are present in some tumours, especially those involving the short tubular bones of the extremities. These areas also contain proliferating, cytologically banal spindle cells that are arranged in fascicles and may contain haemosiderin deposits {1393}. Infrequent findings include scattered, intratumoral, osteoclast-type giant cells, reactive bone formation, which compartmentalizes the tumour into small nodules, and the presence of a large, dilated vessel lined by epithelioid endothelial cells located within the centre of the tumour.

Immunophenotype

Tumour cells express endothelial markers factor VIII, CD 31, CD34, Fli1, and ERG. Many cases are also positive for keratin and EMA {2084,2869}.

Genetics

In a study of 10 cases of epithelioid haemangioma of bone, none demonstrated the *WWTR1-CAMTA1* fusion, which is seen in epithelioid haemangioendothelioma {772}.

Prognostic factors

Epithelioid haemangioma is a locally aggressive lesion and treatment usually consists of curettage and less frequently, marginal en-bloc excision of the tumour. Radiation has been used for tumours in inaccessible locations. The prognosis is excellent, and in the largest reported series the local recurrence rate is 9%; involvement of regional lymph nodes is rare and it is unclear if this represents multicentric disease or metastatic deposits {772,875,2043,2869}. Clinicopathological features predictive of local recurrence or lymph node involvement have not been reported.

many small arteriolar-like vessels lined by flat endothelial cells. The centres of the lobules are the most cellular and contain epithelioid cells that form vascular lumina or grow in solid sheets {772,2043,2869}. The epithelioid cells are large and polyhedral, and have oval or kidney bean-shaped nuclei, that tend to be hyperlobated or cleaved, and contain finely distributed chromatin. The cytoplasm is abundant, deeply eosinophilic, and occasionally contains one or a few vacuoles that are round, clear, and sometimes contain an intact, or a fragment of an erythrocyte {772,2043,2869}. Cells with vacuoles may aggregate such that neighbouring vacuoles coalesce to form vascular lumens. Most tumours contain many well-formed vessels, lined by the epithelioid cells that sometimes protrude into lumina in a tombstone-like fashion. In some tumours, solid, cellular sheet-like areas predominate, whereas in others, they account for a small portion of the neoplasm. Mitoses are relatively infrequent (< 1 per 10 HPF) and are not atypical. Small foci of necrosis may be present. The stroma consists of loose connective tissue, and may contain a prominent, inflammatory infiltrate, rich in eosinophils. Foci of intralesional

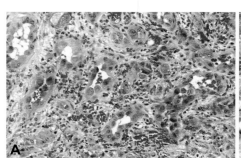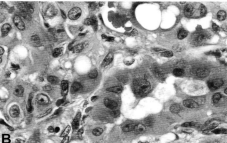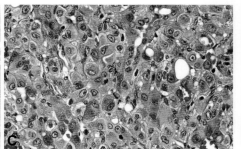

Fig 23.10 Epithelioid haemangioma. **A** Large epithelioid endothelial cells line well-formed vascular spaces. **B** Cord of epithelioid endothelial cells with cytoplasmic vacuoles adjacent to a well-formed neoplastic vessel. **C** Epithelioid endothelial cells growing in sheets.

Epithelioid haemangioendothelioma

A.E. Rosenberg
C.R. Antonescu
J.V.M.G. Bovée

Definition

A malignant neoplasm of low- to intermediate-grade, composed of neoplastic cells that have an endothelial phenotype, epithelioid morphology, and a hyalinized, chondroid, or basophilic stroma.

ICD-O code   9133/3

Epidemiology

Epithelioid haemangioendotheliomas (EHE) are rare, and the true incidence is unknown. The prevalence for all organ sites is < 1 per 10^6 {1560}. The skeleton can be the only organ involved or a component of multiorgan (liver, lung, soft tissue) disease {1560}. The age range is broad (first to eighth decade), with most patients diagnosed during the second and third decades of life. The sexes are equally affected although some studies have reported a male predominance {1432,2085,2869}.

Sites of involvement

Any bone can be affected; 50–60% arise in long tubular bones, especially lower extremity, followed by pelvis, ribs, and spine; 50–64% are multifocal within a single bone or involving separate bones, however, they tend to cluster to an anatomical region {1432,2085,2869}.

Clinical and imaging features

Common symptoms are localized pain and swelling, but sometimes the lesions are asymptomatic. On imaging studies, the tumours manifest as lytic lesions with well- or poorly circumscribed margins, and they may be expansile and erode the cortex.

Macroscopy

The tumours are ovoid, rubbery, and tan, and less frequently, haemorrhagic masses that are < 1–10 cm in size.

Histopathology

The tumours are composed of large epithelioid and spindle endothelial cells with round or elongate nuclei, prominent nucleoli, and abundant eosinophilic cytoplasm. Intracytoplasmic lumina appear as vacuoles that may contain intact or fragmented erythrocytes. Well-formed blood vessels are not prominent in most cases, and instead, the tumour cells are arranged in cords and nests, which are embedded within a myxoid to hyalinized stroma that may resemble cartilaginous matrix. Cytological atypia and mitotic activity is limited, but in some cases, nuclear hyperchromasia and pleomorphism are significant, and mitoses numerous. In these instances the presence of the myxohyaline stroma helps distinguish the neoplasm from high grade angiosarcoma. Composite tumours with areas resembling

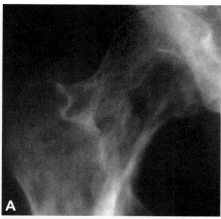

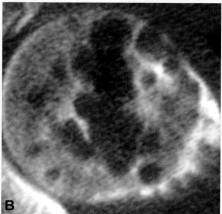

Fig. 23.11 EHE. **A** AP X-ray showing multiple ovoid "moth-eaten" radiolucencies involving the proximal femoral diaphysis, neck, and head. **B** Axial CT through femoral head demonstrating numerous, circular, low-signal regions that have a "punched out" appearance.

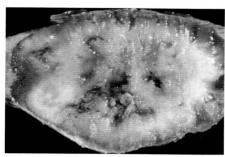

Fig. 23.12 Epithelioid haemangioendothelioma. The tumour is solid, tan-white, focally haemorrhagic, well circumscribed and expands the calvarium.

epithelioid haemangioma, and retiform haemangioendothelioma are very rare.

Immunophenotype

The tumour cells express the endothelial markers CD31, Fli-1, CD34, factor VIII, D2-40, ERG and may be strongly positive for keratin and EMA {977,1432,1491, 2085}.

Genetics

Epithelioid haemangioendothelioma features a t(1;3)(p36;q25) that results in fusion of WWTR1 in 3q25 with CAMTA1 in 1p36 {773,1825,2716}. This fusion event is unique to this neoplasm and is not found in its mimics. Three molecular fusion transcript variants have been described: exon 3 or 4 of WWTR1 fused to either exon 8 or 9 of CAMTA1. The fusion gene encodes a putative transcription factor which places CAMTA1 under control of the WWTR1 promoter and results in overexpression of the C-terminus of CAMTA1, thereby activating a novel transcriptional program. The monoclonal origin of "multifocal" epithelioid haemangioendothelioma has also been established using WWTR1-CAMTA1 breakpoint analysis; indicating that multiple lesions arise from local or metastatic spread from a single primary as opposed to multiple independent primaries {771}.

Prognostic factors

Wide resection is the treatment of choice. The clinical course can be highly variable {2085}. Involvement of two bones is

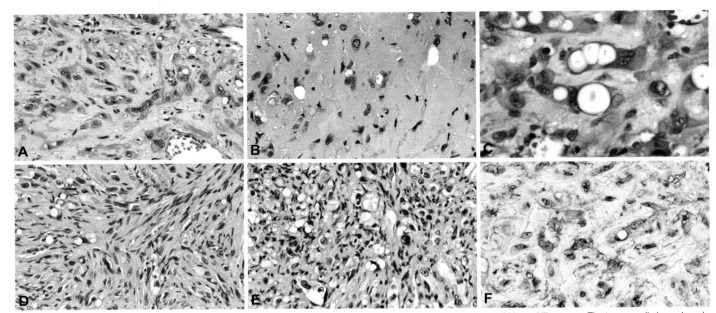

Fig. 23.13 Epithelioid haemangioendothelioma. **A** Cords, clusters and isolated single epithelioid endothelial cells in a solid basophilic stroma. The tumour cells have densely eosinophilic cytoplasm. **B** Chondroid-like matrix surrounds tumour cells that have eosinophilic cytoplasm which also contain round clear vacuoles. **C** Cords of epithelioid endothelial cells in a myxohyaline stroma. Characteristic cytoplasmic vacuoles containing fragments of erythrocytes are prominent. **D** Spindle cells with eosinophilic cytoplasm can be conspicuous in some cases. **E** Infrequently, the tumour cells show significant variation in size and have irregular, large hyperchromatic nuclei. **F** CD34 decorates the cytoplasm of the tumour cells.

associated with a worse prognosis regardless of the number of organs involved {1560}. The mortality rate is approximately 20% {1432,1560}. Histological features do not seem to predict prognosis {1432}.

Angiosarcoma

J.V.M.G. Bovée
A.E. Rosenberg

Definition
A high-grade, malignant neoplasm composed of cells that demonstrate endothelial differentiation.

ICD-O code   9120/3

Epidemiology
Angiosarcoma of bone is rare, accounting for < 1% of malignant bone tumours {1258,1975}. Patients have a broad age range with an almost even distribution between the second and the eighth decades of life. Angiosarcoma is slightly more common in males {644,2868}.

Etiology
The majority of tumours are primary with no known cause, however, a small percentage are associated with either previous radiation {580,1916,1995} or bone infarction {3}.

Sites of involvement
Angiosarcoma shows a wide skeletal distribution with preferential involvement of long and short tubular bones (74%), especially the femur, followed by the pelvis (15%), axial skeleton (7%), and trunk (4%). Approximately one third of cases are multifocal, and affect contiguous (64%) or distant bones (36%) {2868, 2939}.

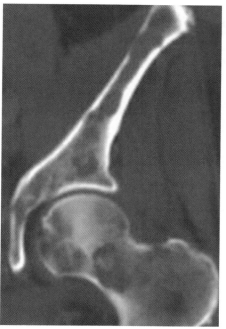

Fig. 23.14 Coronal CT scan of angiosarcoma producing multiple, destructive masses in the bones of the pelvis.

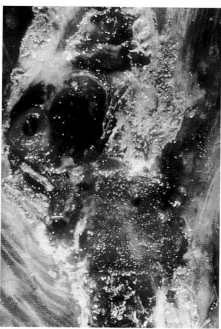

Fig. 23.15 Resected angiosarcoma of a long bone demonstrating a large haemorrhagic tumour that has destroyed the cortex and extended into the soft tissues.

Clinical and imaging features
Angiosarcoma most commonly presents as a painful lesion that may be associated with a palpable mass. Radiographically, it manifests as a single, or regionally multifocal, osteolytic tumour, that may have well- or poorly defined margins. Cortical destruction and extension into the soft tissues are commonplace; however, a periosteal reaction is usually absent {2874}. MRI demonstrates an heterogeneous lesion, with extensive reactive changes (in 58%){2874}.

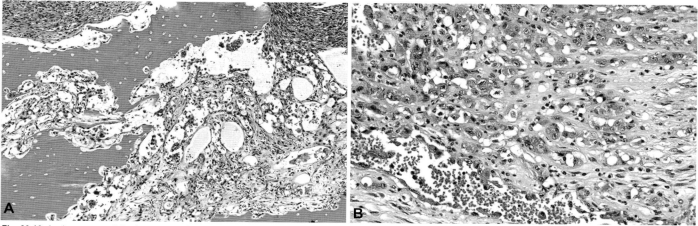

Fig. 23.16 Angiosarcoma. **A** Angiosarcoma infiltrating cancellous bone. Some of the vascular lumina contain tufts of malignant epithelioid cells. **B** Epithelioid angiosarcoma with tumour cells lining vascular lumina and growing in solid nests, the latter mimicking metastatic carcinoma.

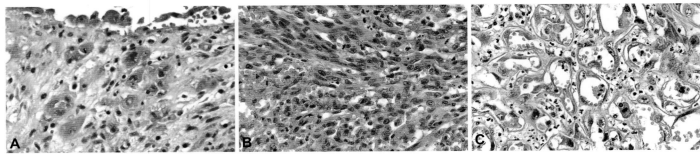

Fig. 23.17 Angiosarcoma. **A** Epithelioid angiosarcoma with tumour cells lining vascular lumina and growing in solid nests, the latter mimicking metastatic carcinoma. **B** Angiosarcoma of bone with spindle cell morphology. **C** Epithelioid angiosarcoma of bone with vasoformative architecture.

Macroscopy

Angiosarcoma is usually > 5 cm in greatest dimension, friable, haemorrhagic and tan-red. The tumour erodes and destroys the cortex and infiltrates into the soft tissues. Areas of necrosis are difficult to identify because of the haemorrhagic appearance of the tumour.

Histopathology

Angiosarcoma is characterized by cytologically malignant cells that are most often epithelioid in appearance (>90% of cases) and less frequently spindled. The nuclei are usually vesicular, and contain one or several small nucleoli or sometimes a prominent macronucleolus. The cytoplasm is deeply eosinophilic and often contains one or more vacuoles, that may be clear and empty, or hold intact or fragmented erythrocytes {790,2085, 2939}. Mitotic figures are often numerous. The tumour cells usually grow in solid sheets; however, in approximately one half of cases they line irregular vascular lumina {2868}. Extravasated erythrocytes can be numerous, and scattered deposits of haemosiderin may also be present. A variable inflammatory infiltrate is seen, generally consisting of lymphocytes and neutrophilic or eosinophilic granulocytes {2868}. Reactive bone formation can sometimes be observed. In the absence of obvious vascular differentiation, abundant intratumoral haemorrhage and intratumoral neutrophils are useful morphological features that may suggest an endothelial phenotype {644}.

Immunophenotype

Expression of various endothelial markers is seen: CD31 (95%), CD34 (39%), vWF (60%) {644,1888,2868}, ERG and FLI1. In addition, individual tumour cells may be positive for SMA (61%) and D2-40 (31%) {2868}. Keratin and EMA are frequently positive, particularly, but not exclusively, in neoplastic cells that have an epithelioid morphology {1880,2106, 2868}. The combination of the multifocality of the tumour, epithelioid morphology and expression of epithelial markers can lead to confusion with metastatic carcinoma {644,2438, 2868,2874}.

Genetics

A t(1;14)(p21;q24) translocation has been described in an angiosarcoma of bone {714}. *MYC* amplification was found in angiosarcoma secondary to irradiation {1728}.

Prognostic factors

The biological behaviour of individual cases is unpredictable, though as a group they are often high grade and clinically extremely aggressive {368,1256, 2983} In a study of 31 patients, the 1-, 2- and 5-year survival rates were 55%, 43% and 33%, respectively {2868}. The presence of a macronucleolus, ≥3 mitoses per 10 HPF and <5 eosinophilic granulocytes per 10 HPF within a tumour has been shown to be associated with an even worse survival {2868}. Lymphangiogenic differentiation as evidenced by the expression of D2-40 also seems to predict a more aggressive course {2868}.

CHAPTER 24

Myogenic, lipogenic and epithelial tumours

Leiomyosarcoma

Lipoma

Liposarcoma

Adamantinoma

Leiomyosarcoma

C.R. Antonescu
E.F. McCarthy

Definition
A primary malignant neoplasm of bone showing smooth-muscle differentiation

ICD-O code   8890/3

Epidemiology
There is a wide age distribution (9–87 years), with a peak incidence in the fifth decade of life and a slight male predominance.

Etiology
A small subset of leiomyosarcoma (LMS) of bone is associated with prior exposure to radiation therapy or with EBV infection {1088,1438}.

Sites of involvement
Most lesions occur in the lower extremity around the knee (distal femoral or proximal tibial metaphysis) {193,1349,1407}, followed by the craniofacial skeleton.

Clinical and imaging features
Patients typically complain of pain and occasionally present with pathological fracture. Metastatic disease from extra-osseous primary lesions (uterus, bowel, soft tissue) should be excluded, as this is much more common than primary LMS of bone. Tumours associated with EBV are found in immunocompromised patients {1438}. Radiographically, they are lytic, aggressive lesions, with a permeative growth pattern and cortical destruction. MRI images show often a hypointense signal on both T1- and T2-weighted studies {2681}.

Macroscopy
The lesions vary widely in size and on cut surface, show a tan, fleshy, creamy appearance, with obvious areas of necrosis.

Histopathology
Lesions resemble LMS from other locations, with cells arranged in long, intersecting fascicles, growing in an infiltrative pattern. The tumour cells have distinctive fibrillary, eosinophilic cytoplasm and elongated, cigar-shaped nuclei with blunted ends. Aggressive behaviour is as-

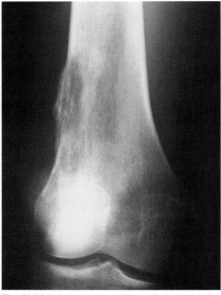

Fig. 24.01 Leiomyosarcoma. X-ray of a tumour in the distal femur showing an aggressive, permeative lytic lesion with cortical destruction.

sociated with necrosis, significant nuclear pleomorphism and mitotic activity.

Immunophenotype
Smooth-muscle differentiation is demonstrated by diffuse staining with desmin, H-caldesmon and SMA. LMP1 immunohistochemistry can be used to document the EBV protein.

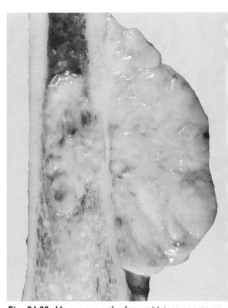

Fig. 24.02 Macroscopy of a femoral leiomyosarcoma. Note both an intra-osseous and an extra-osseous component of the white fleshy tumour.

Genetics
Similar to deep, soft-tissue LMS, intra-osseous lesions show genomic losses and absence of phosphorylated RB {2872}.

Prognostic factors
Histological grade correlates well with clinical outcome {79}. High-grade lesions show a high index of distant spread, often to the lung and eventually 50% of patients succumb to disease {2327}.

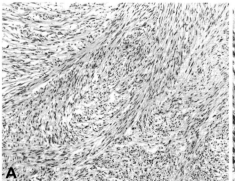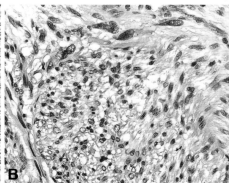

Fig. 24.03 Leiomyosarcoma. **A** Low-power image showing bundles of spindle cells. **B** On high power, cellular pleomorphism of the tumour cells is seen.

Lipoma

A.E. Rosenberg
J.A. Bridge

Definition
A benign neoplasm of adipocytes that arises within the medullary cavity, or on the surface of bone.

ICD-O code   8850/0

Epidemiology
Intra-osseous lipoma is rare, and accounts for < 0.1% of primary bone tumours. They have a wide age range (second to eighth decades); most patients are in their fifth decade of life at the time of diagnosis {1371}. Males are affected more frequently than females (4 : 3) {371}. Parosteal lipoma comprises 15% of bone lipomas and develops during the fifth to sixth decade of life. There is a slight male predominance (9 : 7) {1371}.

Sites of involvement
Tumours commonly affect the calcaneous and metaphysis of long tubular bones, especially the femur, tibia and fibula and infrequently the pelvis, vertebrae, sacrum, skull, mandible, maxilla, and ribs {1371}. Parosteal lipomas develop on the diaphysis of long tubular bones, especially the femur, radius, humerus, and tibia {1371}.

Clinical and imaging features
Intramedullary lipoma may be asymptomatic (30%) or produce aching pain or swelling (70%). Rarely, it presents as a pathological fracture {371,1371}. Radiographically, intramedullary lipoma usually produces a well-defined lytic mass that is surrounded by a thin rim of sclerosis. The lesion may also contain trabeculations or central calcifications. Bony expansion may occur in small calibre bones {371} {2595}. CT shows that the fatty component has a low attenuation value similar to that of subcutaneous fat, and on MRI, the fat has high signal-intensity on both T1- and T2-weighted images {1371}. Parosteal lipoma is frequently asymptomatic and may present as a visible or palpable mass. Radiographs may reveal a radiolucent mass adjacent to the cortex that may show calcification or a periosteal reaction. The CT and MRI findings have the

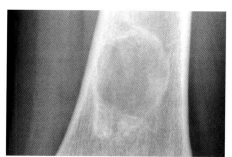
Fig. 24.04 Lipoma. X-ray of distal femur demonstrating an intra-osseous lipoma. The tumour is lytic and contains well-circumscribed, sclerotic margins and scattered calcifications.

same features as subcutaneous fat except when there is calcification, cartilage or ossification within the lesion {247}.

Macroscopy
Intramedullary lipoma is usually 3–5 cm in size, well defined, soft, and yellow. The surrounding bone is often sclerotic. Parosteal lipoma is usually 4–10 cm in greatest dimension, well defined, soft and yellow. Some cases contain gritty spicules of bone or firm nodules of cartilage in the base or scattered throughout the mass.

Histopathology
Intramedullary lipoma consists of lobules of mature-appearing adipocytes that may replace the marrow and encase pre-existing bony trabeculae {371,795,1371,2595}. The adipocytes have a single, large, clear cytoplasmic vacuole that displaces the crescent shaped nucleus to the periphery; rarely is

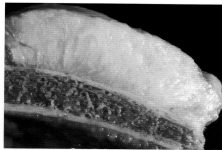
Fig. 24.05 Parosteal lipoma. Parosteal lipoma of rib composed of a juxtacortical, well-defined mass of yellowish fat.

brown fat a component {1495}. Some tumours may demonstrate fat necrosis with foamy macrophages and fibrosis.

In ossifying lipomas, delicate trabeculae of woven and lamellar bone may be present in an irregular fashion throughout the tumour. Parosteal lipoma is a well-defined mass of white fat. At its base, adjacent to the cortex, there may be hyaline cartilage which undergoes endochondral ossification or subperiosteal reactive new bone formation {247}.

Genetics
The translocation t(3;12)(q28;q14) and its associated fusion transcript *HMGA2-LPP* featured in lipoma of soft tissue has also been detected in parosteal lipoma {314, 2231}.

Prognostic factors
Lipoma of bone has an excellent prognosis and rarely recurs.

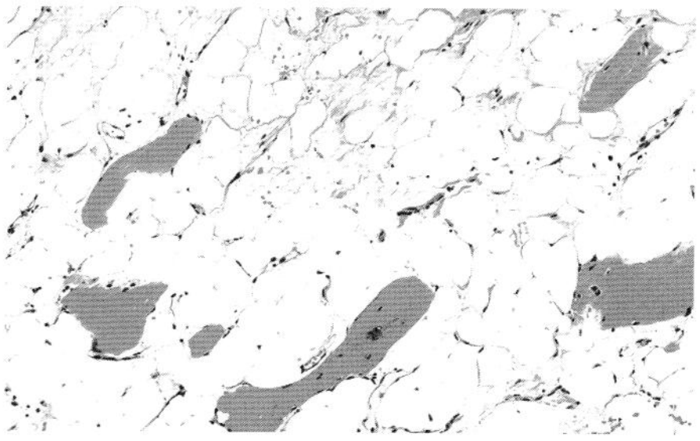

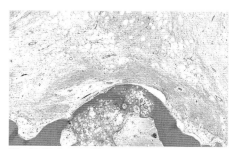

Fig. 24.06 Intra-osseous ossifying lipoma composed of mature white fat and scattered irregular trabeculae of woven bone.

Fig. 24.07 Parosteal lipoma with cartilage undergoing endochondral ossification at its base.

Liposarcoma

A.E. Rosenberg
K.Szuhai

Definition
A malignant neoplasm whose phenotype recapitulates fat and arises within or on the surface of bone.

ICD-O code   8850/3

Epidemiology
Primary liposarcoma of bone is extraordinarily rare; metastases to the bone are more common. It occurs in all age groups although most patients are adults {1398, 1096,1691,2305}. Men are affected slightly more frequently than women.

Sites of involvement
Tumours usually develop in or on the long tubular bones especially the tibia and femur {1096,1398,1691,2305}.

Clinical and imaging features
The tumour presents as a painful mass that is lytic and has well- or poorly defined margins {1096,1398,1691,2305}. The lipid component can be detected on CT and MRI.

Macroscopy
Most liposarcomas are large, lobulated, soft or firm and are yellow to tan-white in colour. Myxoid tumours may be glistening, slimy and mucinous.

Histopathology
The histological variants of liposarcoma in bone are similar to those of soft tissue {1096,1398, 1691,2305,2696}.

Genetics
Supernumerary ring chromosomes, char-

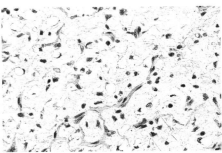

Fig. 24.09 Myxoid liposarcoma consisting of scattered spindle and stellate cells and occasional lipoblasts enmeshed in a frothy myxoid stroma that contains branching small-calibre capillaries.

acteristic of atypical lipomatous tumour/well-differentiated liposarcoma, amplification of 12q14.2–21.2 to include the *HMGA2* and *MDM2* gene regions, and amplification of 1q21.2–31.2 have been detected in a case of parosteal liposarcoma {2696}.

Prognostic factors
The pleomorphic variant of liposarcoma of bone has the worst prognosis {2305}.

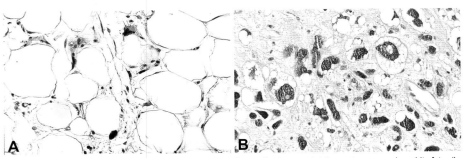

Fig. 24.08 Liposarcoma. **A** Well-differentiated liposarcoma, lipoma-like type, containing mature appearing white fat cells and scattered adipocytes that have enlarged hyperchromatic nuclei. **B** Sheets of pleomorphic cells including lipoblasts characterize pleomorphic liposarcoma.

Adamantinoma

P.C.W. Hogendoorn
M. Kanamori

Definition

A malignant biphasic tumour characterized by a variety of morphological patterns, most commonly clusters of epithelial cells, surrounded by a relatively bland spindle-cell osteofibrous component.

ICD-O code   9261/3

Synonyms

Adamantinoma of long bones; extra-gnathic adamantinoma

Epidemiology

Adamantinoma comprises about 0.4% of all primary bone tumours {1258,1941, 1975}. Patients present with this tumour from age 3 up to 86 years, with a median age of 25–35 years. The youngest age group predominantly includes patients with osteofibrous dysplasia-like adamantinoma, but young children with classic adamantinoma and adults with the osteofibrous dysplasia-like subtype have been reported {1148,1940,2690}. There is a slight predominance in males. Rarely, at middle and advanced age, further progression into dedifferentiated adamantinoma may occur {1147,1303}.

Sites of involvement

The tibia, in particular the anterior metaphysis or diaphysis, is involved in 85–90% of cases. Multifocal involvement of the tibia has been regularly found {2838}. In up to 10% of cases this is combined with one or more lesions in the ipsilateral fibula. Other sites have occasionaly been reported, including the ulna.

Clinical and imaging features

The main complaint is swelling with or without pain. Adamantinoma often displays a protracted clinical behaviour. Clinical symptoms such as swelling or radiographical abnormality may last for >30 years before diagnosis, whereas local recurrences or metastases may develop years after primary, intralesional or marginal surgical treatment. On X-ray, the tumour is typically well circumscribed, cor-

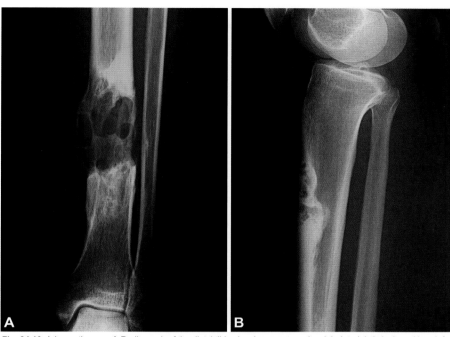

Fig. 24.10 Adamantinoma. **A** Radiograph of the distal tibia showing an expansive, lobulated, lytic lesion with a defect of the outer surface of the cortex. **B** Osteofibrous dysplasia-like adamantinoma. The lateral radiograph of the proximal aspect of the tibia shows a multilocular, lytic lesion with surrounding osteosclerosis of the anterior cortex.

tical, (multi-)lobulated and osteolytic. Intralesional opacities, septation and peripheral sclerosis may also be seen {258,1258}. Multifocality within the same bone is regularly observed. The lesion commonly remains intracortical and extends longitudinally, but may also destroy the cortex and invade the medullary cavity or surrounding periosteum and soft tissue. This is usually accompanied by lamellar or solid periosteal reaction. Aggressive tumours occasionally present as a single, large, lytic lesion. MRI is useful to document multicentricity, the extension of the lesion, and possible soft-tissue involvement {2838}.

Macroscopy

Classic adamantinoma usually presents as a cortical, well-demarcated, yellowish-grey, lobulated tumour of firm to bony consistency with peripheral sclerosis. It may be a single lesion or occasionally multifocal. Small lesions remain intracortical, and are usually white and gritty. Larger tumours

show intramedullary extension and cortical breakthrough, with soft-tissue invasion in a minority of cases. Macroscopically detectable cystic spaces are common, filled with straw-coloured or blood-like fluid.

Histopathology

Classic adamantinomas are characterized by easily recognizable epithelial and osteofibrous components, that may be intermingled in various proportions and differentiation patterns. The four main differentiation patterns of classic adamantinoma are basaloid, tubular, spindle cell, and squamous {2925}. The first two patterns are encountered most commonly, but all patterns may be present in one lesion. The spindle-cell component is more often observed in recurrences, lining cystic spaces, and in metastases. The osteofibrous component is composed of storiform-oriented spindle cells. Woven bone trabeculae are usually present in, or next to the centre of the lesion,

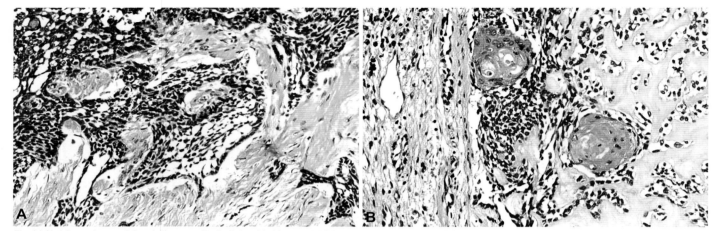

Fig. 24.11 Adamantinoma. **A** Basaloid pattern. Easily distinguishable epithelial fields without clear palisading. **B** Squamoid pattern.

prominently rimmed by osteoblasts, and with varying amounts of transformation to lamellar bone at the periphery of the tumour. Foam cells or myxoid change may be present, and mast cells or multinucleated giant cells are occasionally detected. Mitotic activity is usually low. A fifth histological pattern, the so-called osteofibrous dysplasia-like variant, is characterized by predominance of osteofibrous tissue, in which small groups of epithelial cells are only encountered by careful search or immunohistochemistry.

The majority of classic and osteofibrous dysplasia-like adamantinomas display a "zonal" architecture. In classic adamantinoma, the centre is usually dominated by the epithelial component, and only few, small immature bone trabeculae are present in the fibrous tissue. Towards the periphery, the epithelial islands decrease to inconspicuous elements and the osteofibrous component gradually takes over with increasing amounts of woven bone trabeculae, transforming to lamellar bone. In osteofibrous dysplasia-like adamantinoma, the centre is occupied by fibrous tissue with scanty and thin immature woven bone trabeculae with epithelial elements. Small clusters of epithelial cells are the only features which differentiate osteofibrous dysplasia-like adamantinoma from osteofibrous dysplasia.

Immunophenotype

The fibrous tissue is positive for vimentin. The epithelial cells show coexpression of keratin, EMA, vimentin, p63 and podoplanin {667,1376}. Chain-specific keratin expression {1145,1350} reveals a predominantly basal epithelial-cell differentiation, regardless of subtype, with widespread presence of basal-epithelial-cell keratins 5, 14, and 19. Keratins 1, 13 and 17 are also variably present. Keratins 8 and 18 are virtually absent. E-,P-, and N-cadherins are found in classic, but not in osteofibrous dysplasia-like adamantinoma {1708} In classic adamantinomas, the epithelial component is surrounded by a continuous basement membrane consisting of collagen IV, laminin and galectin-3 {1708}, whereas less distinct epithelial islands show multiple interruptions or no surrounding basement membrane at all {1149}. EGF/EGFR expression is restricted to the epithelial component. FGF2/FGFR1 is present in both components {288}, while in culture the cells express M-CSF and RANKL, which may contribute to the osteolysis observed {2737}.

Ultrastructure

Electron microscopic studies have confirmed the epithelial nature of adamantinoma, showing intracytoplasmic hemidesmosomes, tonofilaments and microfilaments. Irrespective of histological subtype, the epithelial cells are bound by desmosomes and basement membranes have been found to surround the epithelial nests.

Genetics

A recurrent pattern of numerical abnormalities featuring extra copies of chromosomes 7, 8, 12, 19 and/or 21 has been detected in classic as well as osteofibrous dysplasia-like forms of adamantinoma {364,992,1361}. Extra copies of one or more of these chromosomes (except for chromosome 19) have also been identified in osteofibrous dysplasia, supporting a related histopathogenesis {315,992,2174}. In addition to trisomy 19, structural abnormalities including translocations and marker chromosomes have been reported in adamantinoma, but not in osteofibrous dysplasia {364,1150, 1361}. The progressive complexity of the karyotypic aberrations observed in osteofibrous dysplasia, osteofibrous dysplasia-like adamantinoma, and classic adamantinoma may be indicative of a multistep transformation process {992,1146}.

Trisomies 7, 8, and/or 12 have not been observed in osteoblasts or osteoclasts, suggesting that the osseous component is reactive and non-neoplastic, in contrast with the presence of these trisomies in the spindle-cell stroma component of the same lesions {992}. DNA index studies have shown that in aneuploid adamantinomas, the aneuploid population is always restricted to the epithelial component {1144}. TP53 aberrations, as detected immunohistochemically or by LOH analysis, are also restricted to the epithelial component. There have been some cases reported with histological features of adamantinoma as well as Ewing sarcoma, sometimes called "atypical" or "Ewing-like" adamantinoma {258,927, 1289,1429, 1822,2474}, two of which had a t(11;22) {316}; these tumours were hence labelled "adamantinoma-like Ewing sarcoma". The t(11;22)/EWSR1-FLI1 fusion is not present in classic adamantinoma {1136,1721}.

Prognostic factors

Risk factors for recurrence are intralesional or marginal surgery and extracompartmental growth {1148,1350, 1394,2283}. Recurrence after non-radical surgery may rise up to 90% {1148, 1350,1394}. Recurrence is associated

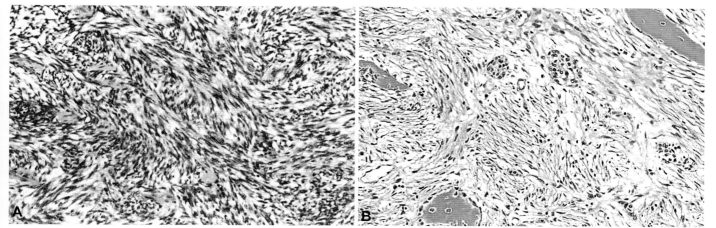

Fig. 24.12 Adamantinoma. **A** Spindle-cell pattern. **B** Osteofibrous dysplasia-like adamantinoma. Small epithelial clusters in a fibro-osseous stroma.

with an increase in epithelium-to-stroma ratio and more aggressive behaviour {1148,1394, 1941}. Additionally, male sex {1350,1394}, females at young age {1941}, pain at presentation {1394}, short duration of symptoms {1148,1394}, young age (< 20 years) {1148} and lack of squa-mous differentiation of the tumour {1148,1394} have been associated with increased rates of recurrence or metasta-sis. Adamantinomas metastasize in 12–29% of patients with comparable mortal-ity rates {1148,1394, 1941,2283}. Metasta-tic tumours are always classic adaman-tinomas, although rarely osteofibrous dys-plasia-like adamantinomas may metasta-size after recurrence and subsequent pro-gression to classic adamantinoma {1148}. The tumour spreads to regional lymph nodes and the lungs, and infrequently to skeleton, liver, and brain.

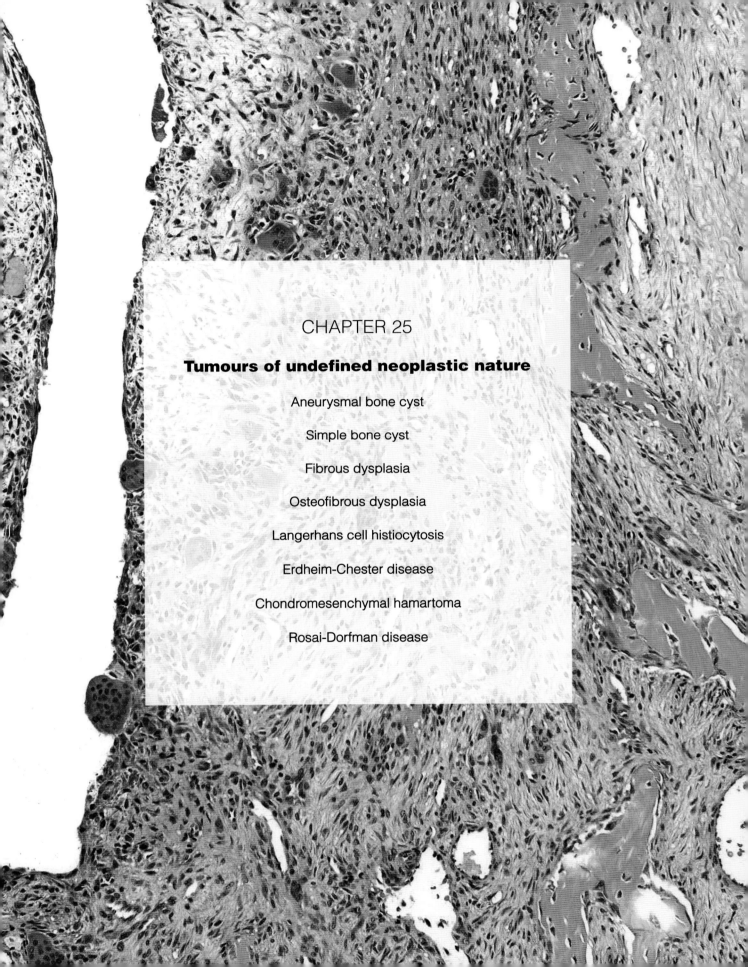

CHAPTER 25

Tumours of undefined neoplastic nature

Aneurysmal bone cyst

Simple bone cyst

Fibrous dysplasia

Osteofibrous dysplasia

Langerhans cell histiocytosis

Erdheim-Chester disease

Chondromesenchymal hamartoma

Rosai-Dorfman disease

Aneurysmal bone cyst

G.P. Nielsen
J.A. Fletcher
A.M. Oliveira

Definition

A destructive, expansile, benign neoplasm of bone composed of multiloculated blood-filled cystic spaces.

ICD-O code   9260/0

Epidemiology

Aneurysmal bone cyst (ABC) affects all age groups, but is most common during the first two decades of life (80%) and both sexes are equally affected {1748, 2873}. The estimated annual incidence is 0.15 per 10^6 {1594}.

Sites of involvement

ABC can affect any bone, but usually arises in the metaphysis of long bones,

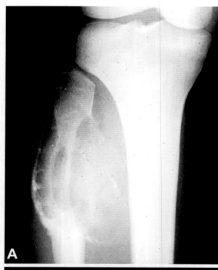

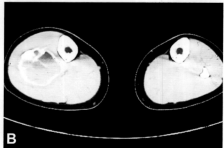

Fig. 25.01 Aneurysmal bone cyst. **A** Plain X-ray of an eccentric lytic mass of the proximal fibula. Note the peripheral shell of reactive bone. **B** CT of the same lesion.

especially the femur, tibia and humerus, and the posterior elements of vertebral bodies. Rare tumours, with morphology identical to primary ABC of bone, have also been described in the soft tissues {59,2035,2244}

Clinical and imaging features

The most common signs and symptoms are pain and swelling, which are rarely secondary to fracture. In the vertebrae, it can compress nerves or the spinal cord and cause neurological symptoms. Radiographically, ABC presents as a lytic, eccentric, expansile mass with well-defined margins. Most tumours contain a thin shell of subperiosteal, reactive bone. CT shows a cystic, expansile and radiolucent tumour. MRI studies show internal septa and the characteristic fluid-fluid levels created by the different densities of the cyst fluid, caused by the settling of erythrocytes {1479,2873}. In secondary ABC, CT and MRI may show evidence of an underlying primary lesion.

Macroscopy

Grossly, ABC is well defined and multiloculated, composed of blood-filled, cystic spaces separated by tan-white, gritty septa. More solid areas can be seen, which may represent either a solid portion of the ABC, or a component of a primary tumour that has undergone secondary ABC-like changes.

Histopathology

ABC is well circumscribed and composed of blood-filled, cystic spaces separated by fibrous septa. The fibrous septa are composed of a moderately dense, cellular proliferation of bland fibroblasts, with scattered, multinucleated, osteoclast-type giant cells and reactive woven bone rimmed by osteoblasts. The woven bone frequently follows the contours of the fibrous septa. In approximately one third of cases, the bone is basophilic and has been termed "blue bone"; however, its presence is not diagnostic, as it can be seen in other entities. Mitoses are commonly present and can be numerous; however, atypical forms

are absent. Necrosis is rare unless there has been a pathological fracture. The solid variant of ABC has the same components and is very similar to giant cell lesion of small bones. Primary ABC accounts for approximately 70% of all cases {203,2433}. ABC-like areas can be seen in other benign and malignant bone tumours that have undergone haemorrhagic cystic change (secondary ABC). The majority of secondary ABC develops in association with benign neoplasms, most commonly giant cell tumour of bone, osteoblastoma, chondroblastoma and fibrous dysplasia {1479,1748,2873}. However, ABC-like changes may also complicate sarcomas, especially osteosarcoma.

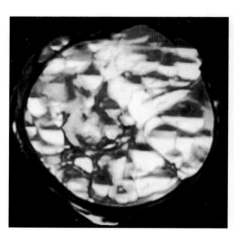

Fig. 25.02 Aneurysmal bone cyst. MRI of a large destructive lesion of the distal femur. Note numerous fluid-fluid levels.

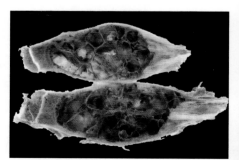

Fig. 25.03 Aneurysmal bone cyst. Macroscopy of a resected specimen of the fibula with characteristic sponge-like appearance and numerous septations.

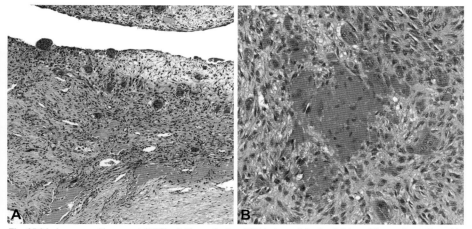

Fig. 25.04 Aneurysmal bone cyst (ABC). **A** The wall of an ABC lacks a distinct cell-lining of the cystic cavity and is composed of bland spindle-shaped cells with scattered osteoclast-type giant cells and reactive, woven bone with osteoblastic rimming. **B** Solid ABC. The tumour is composed of bland looking spindle-shaped cells and clusters of osteoclast-type giant cells that tend to aggregate around areas of haemorrhage. This tumour is identical to the so-called "giant cell lesion of small bones".

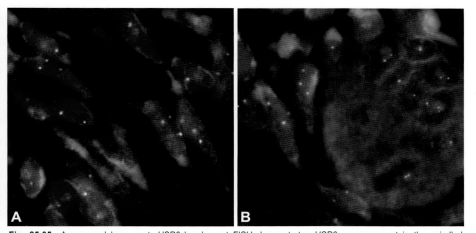

Fig. 25.05 Aneurysmal bone cyst. *USP6* break-apart FISH demonstrates *USP6* rearrangement in the spindled myofibroblastic-like cells (**A**), but not in the multinucleated giant cells (**B**).

Genetics

ABC contains cytogenetic rearrangements of the *USP6* (ubiquitin specific peptidase 6/Tre-2) gene at chromosome band 17p13. The most common translocation t(16;17)(q22;p13) {554,2117,2163,2237, 2494} leads to fusion of the cadherin 11 gene (*CDH11*) with *USP6,* with resultant upregulation of *USP6* transcription {2117, 2120}. *USP6* rearrangements are found in approximately 70% of primary ABC but not in secondary ABC {2121}. *USP6* rearrangements do not seem to be associated with distinct biological behaviour {2121}. While the most frequent *USP6* fusion partner is *CDH11* (30% of *USP6* fusion genes), others include *TRAP150, ZNF9, OMD,* and *COL1A1* {2120}. The ABC neoplastic component, containing the *USP6* rearrangements, is a spindle-cell population, indistinguishable from normal fibroblasts and myofibroblasts {2121}. Other cells commonly seen in ABC, including inflammatory cells, endothelial cells, metaplastic bone-associated osteoblasts, and multinucleated osteoclast-like giant cells, do not contain a *USP6* rearrangement and are presumably reactive {2121}.

Prognostic factors

ABC is a potentially locally recurrent neoplasm. The recurrence rate following curettage is variable (20–70%). Spontaneous regression following incomplete removal is very unusual.

Simple bone cyst

R.K. Kalil
E. Santini Araujo

Definition
An intramedullary, usually unilocular, cystic bone cavity lined by a fibrous membrane and filled with serous or sero-sanguineous fluid.

Synonyms
Solitary bone cyst; unicameral bone cyst

Epidemiology
Males predominate in a ratio of 3 : 1. About 80% of patients are in the first two decades of life.

Sites of involvement
Any bone can be affected. The most common sites are the proximal humerus (50%), proximal femur (25%) and proximal tibia. The ilium and calcaneus are less commonly affected in older patients. Metaphyseal areas, close to growth plates, are most commonly affected.

Clinical and imaging features
Most patients are asymptomatic. Simple bone cysts are generally discovered after a pathological fracture or incidentally, after roentgenological examination for other reasons. Some patients may experience mild pain, swelling or limitation of motion. Roentgenograms show a well-outlined, centrally located, metaphyseal–diaphyseal lucency, expanding and thinning the cortices, not wider than the epiphyseal plate. It usually abuts but rarely transgresses the growth plate. Cysts located near the plate are called "active", and those separated from the plate by normal cancellous bone are termed "inactive" or "latent".

A multilocular appearance may be seen due to prominent bony ridges in the inner cortical wall. True septation is unusual. Periosteal reaction is absent except at sites of fracture. MRI usually confirms its fluid content, which can be bloody in fractured lesions {1731}. Solid areas in intact lesions may suggest that the cyst is not primary.

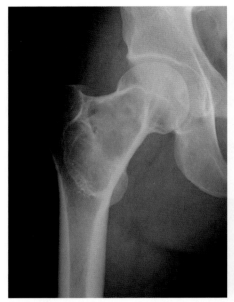

Fig. 25.07 Simple bone cyst. A lesion in the neck of the femur, a common location

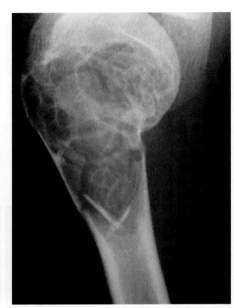

Fig. 25.08 Simple bone cyst. X-ray demonstrating the "fallen leaf" signal of a fractured lesion which, when present, is highly suggestive of a hollow lesion.

Macroscopy
A simple bone cyst consists of a unicameral cavity filled with serous or serosanguineous fluid. Its inner surface shows bony ridges separating depressed zones, lined by a thin, smooth, greyish-white to reddish-brown membrane. Partial septae may be seen.

Histopathology
The inner lining and septae of the cyst consist of connective tissue, containing

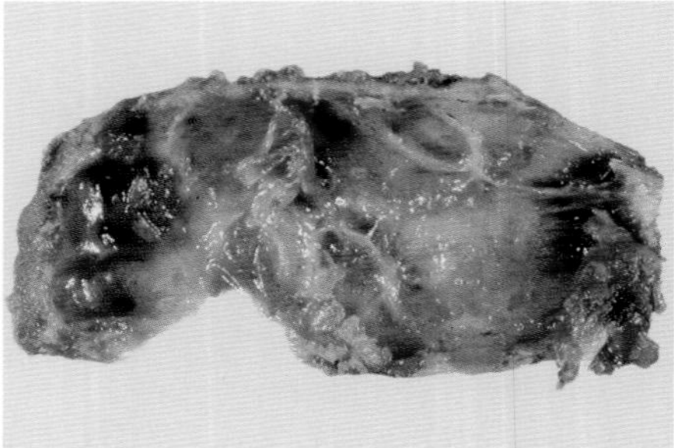

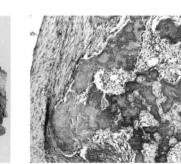

Fig. 25.06 Simple bone cyst. Unicameral cavity filled with serous or serosanguineous fluid. Its inner surface shows membrane-lined bony ridges.

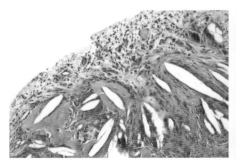

Fig. 25.09 Simple bone cyst. Fibrinous deposits are sometimes mineralized, resembling cementum.

Fig. 25.10 Simple bone cyst. Haemosiderin pigment, scattered giant cells, cholesterol clefts and occasional foamy histiocytes are seen.

foci of reactive new bone, haemosiderin pigment and scattered giant cells. Cholesterol clefts and foamy histiocytes may be present. Collagen deposition, sometimes resembling fibrin is often seen. Some of these are mineralized, resembling cementum. Occasionally, histological features of fracture callus may be prominent. Rare "solidified" cases of simple bone cyst have been described in older subjects.

Genetics

The translocation t(16;20)(p11.2;q13) has been reported as the sole anomaly in one case {2334} and complex karyotypic abnormalities have been described in a second case which, in a later recurrence, demonstrated a *TP53* mutation {2863, 2864}.

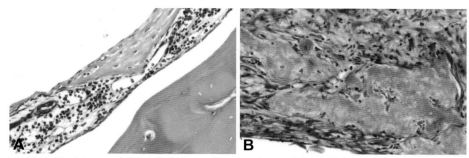

Fig. 25.11 Simple bone cyst **A** Variable thickness of inner membranous lining. **B** Fibrinous deposits are often seen.

Prognostic factors

Recurrence is reported in 10–20% of cases, especially in younger subjects and in large cysts {377,994}. Large cysts are also related to limb shortening {995}. Growth arrest of the affected bone, and avascular necrosis of the head of the femur after pathological fracture can occur {2637}. Spontaneous healing after fracture has been described {57}.

Fibrous dysplasia

G.P. Siegal
P. Bianco
P. Dal Cin

Definition

A benign, medullary, fibro-osseous lesion, which may involve one or more bones.

ICD-O code   8818/0

Epidemiology

Fibrous dysplasia occurs in children and adults worldwide, and affects all racial groups with an equal sex distribution. The monostotic form is six to ten times more common than the polyostotic form.

Sites of involvement

Craniofacial bones and the femur are the two most common sites, both in monostotic and polyostotic forms, but every bone can be affected {223,1285,2101}. In the monostotic form, a substantial number of cases involve the femur, skull, and tibia, and an additional 20% in the ribs. In the polyostotic form, the femur, pelvis, and tibia are involved in the majority of cases {1116}.

Clinical and imaging features

Fibrous dysplasia can be monostotic or polyostotic, and in the latter case, can be confined to one extremity or one side of the body or be diffuse. Fibrous dysplasia presents in childhood or adolescence, but the monostotic form may remain hidden until adulthood. The polyostotic form often manifests earlier in life than the monostotic form {1116}. The lesion is often asymptomatic, but pain and fractures are common presenting features {427}. Fibrous dysplasia infrequently produces excess FGF-23 causing osteomalacia similar to tumour-induced osteomalacia {2187, 2339}. Fibrous dysplasia combines with endocrinopathies and skin pigmentation abnormalities in McCune-Albright syndrome, and with intramuscular myxomas in Mazabraud syndrome {798,1333}. Roentgenographic studies often show a non-aggressive geographical lesion with a ground-glass matrix, and this can be sig-nificantly modified by lesion age and secondary changes (e.g., cyst formation and fracture). A cartilaginous component can sometimes be identified. "Shepherd-crook" deformity of the proximal femur is highly diagnostic when present. Generally, there is neither soft-tissue extension nor periosteal reaction unless there is a complicating fracture. Bone scintigraphy, CT and MRI best delineate the features and the extent of disease {540,1324, 2766}.

Macroscopy

The bone is often expanded and the lesional tissue has a tan-grey colour with a firm to gritty consistency. There may be cysts, which may contain some yellow-tinged fluid {2554}. When cartilage is present (a rare event), it often stands out as sharply circumscribed, blue-tinged, translucent material {2815}.

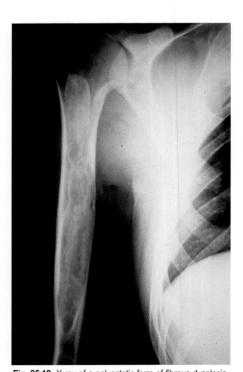

Fig. 25.12 X-ray of a polyostotic form of fibrous dysplasia. There is a well-defined lucency with sclerotic margins.

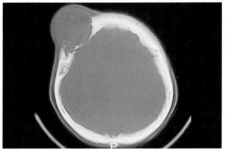

Fig. 25.13 CT of skull with fibrous dysplasia. In flat bones the process is often expansile.

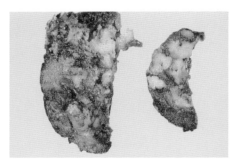

Fig. 25.14 Fibrous dysplasia with gross cartilaginous components.

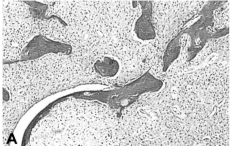

Fig. 25.15 Fibrous dysplasia. **A** Characteristic C-shaped bony spicules with hypocellular spindle cell stroma. **B** Typical appearance of bone, which seems to be dissected by spindle cell proliferation. Note that there is no osteoblastic rimming.

Histopathology

Fibrous and osseous tissue are present in varying proportions. The fibrous tissue is composed principally of bland fibroblastic cells. Mitoses are uncommon but are more often seen in the setting of a fracture. The osseous component is comprised of irregular, curvilinear, trabeculae of woven (or rarely lamellar) bone {1435}. Nodules of benign hyaline cartilage, which undergo endochondral ossification can be seen. Osteoblasts are present but inconspicuous and spindle-shaped {2341}. Occasionally, rounded psammomatous or cementum-like bone may be seen {2571}. Secondary changes including ABC-like changes, foam cells, multinucleated osteoclastic giant cells, or extensive myxoid change may occur {682}.

Genetics

Fibrous dysplasia is caused by post zygotic, activating missense mutations in the *GNAS* gene (20q13) that encodes the α-subunit of the stimulatory G-protein-α (GSα) {222,491,2530,2921}. These activating mutations have been detected in up to 93% of cases and include R201H (57%), R201C (38%), and Q227L (5%) {223,1277}. *GNAS* mutations have been also associated with McCune-Albright syndrome and non-skeletal isolated endocrine lesions, suggesting a spectrum of phenotypic expressions of the same basic disorder

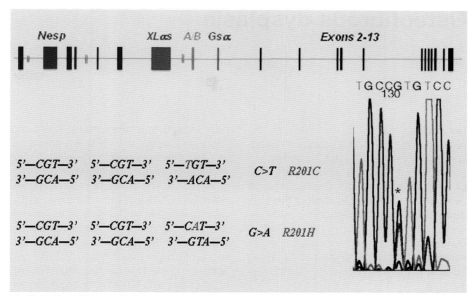

Fig. 25.16 The *GNAS* gene. Multiple promoters and first exons are spliced onto a common downstream coding sequence (exons 2–13) to generate different transcripts (Nesp, Xlas, A/B, Gsα). Mutations causing fibrous dysplasia are point mutations that replace arginine 201 of the Gsα protein with either a cysteine or a histidine. Sequencing analysis of genomic DNA from a fibrous dysplasia patient shows the G>A (R201H) mutation (*) .

{222}. With regard to clonal chromosome aberrations, the only recurrent changes described to date have been trisomy 2 and structural aberrations of 12p13 {557}.

Prognostic factors

The prognosis for many patients with fibrous dysplasia is excellent. However, monostotic fibrous dysplasia can cause skeletal deformities, leg-length discrepancies or impinge on cranial nerves, while extensive polyostotic disease may be crippling. Malignant transformation very rarely occurs {1657}.

Osteofibrous dysplasia

V. J. Vigorita
P.C.W. Hogendoorn
J.R. Sawyer

Definition

A benign fibro-osseous lesion of bone. Usually self-limited, but reported to progress into adamantinoma in some cases, it characteristically involves cortical bone of the anterior mid-shaft of the tibia during infancy and childhood.

Synonyms

Kempson-Campanacci lesion; ossifying fibroma of long bones

Epidemiology

The lesion is most commonly detected during the first two decades of life. Considered a rare condition, osteofibrous dysplasia (OFD) may be under-reported as most cases are asymptomatic. OFD has been reported in neonates where extensive involvement of the cortical and medullary compartments of the tibia may be seen. It is extremely rare after skeletal maturation.

Etiology

The etiology is obscure. Familial cases have recently been reported {1374A} and there is evidence that OFD is a precursor to adamantinoma on the basis of genetic and immunohistochemical as well as clinical studies. The occurrence of so-called osteofibrous-like adamantinoma, to be distinguished from classic epithelium-rich adamantinoma but different from classic OFD, raises the possibility of an association (i.e. progression) between OFD and adamantinoma {144A, 1148,1405,1504A}. Most cases of OFD arise de novo and are not originally related to adamantinoma.

Sites of involvement

The proximal or middle third of the tibial cortex is the most frequent site of involvement {369}. Lesions can be bilateral with ipsilateral or contralateral involvement of the fibula. Ipsilateral involvement of the fibula is seen in about 20% of cases. Very rare sites include other long bones such as the ulna, radius and humerus {2925}. Multifocal or large confluent lesions oriented longitudinally along the cortical axis are not unusual.

Clinical and imaging features

The lesion is rare after the age of 15 years, when the clinical differential diagnosis of osteofibrous dysplasia-like adamantinoma should be seriously considered. The most common presenting symptoms are swelling or a painless deforming anterior bowing of the tibia. Pain, if present, is usually associated with a pathological fracture. Pseudo-arthrosis may occur. OFD is typically epicentred in the cortical bone, but may modestly involve the medullary cavity by extension. Although slow growth is characteristic of OFD, some lesions are periodically aggressive and may involve the entire bone with a significant bowing deformity. Often well demarcated, it is associated with a thinning, expanding or even missing cortex. The expanding cortex is often sclerotically rimmed near the medullary bone. Separate or confluent oval, scalloped, saw-toothed or bubbly multiloculated, lytic lesions are often noted, oriented parallel to the shaft of the bone. Perilesional sclerosis may be considerable. The radiodensity of the

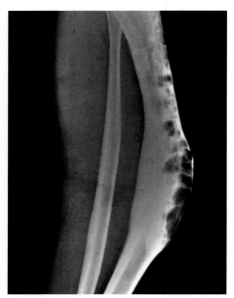

Fig. 25.17 Osteofibrous dysplasia. Expansile lucent, longitudinally oriented tibial lesion, surrounded by sclerosis and thinning of the anterior cortex of the diaphysis of the tibia. Note the anterior bowing of the tibia.

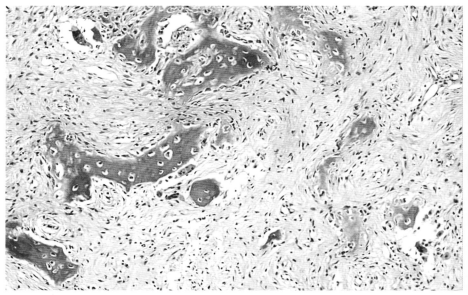

Fig. 25.18 Osteofibrous dysplasia. Hypocellular spindle-cell proliferation and spicules of bone. The bony spicules display prominent osteoblastic rimming.

interior of the lytic foci are typically more radiodense than soft tissue. Periosteal reactions and soft tissue extensions are unusual. Bone scans are typically hot. CT scans classically delineate a cortical epicentre to the lesion not breaking through into the soft tissue and demarcated from medullary bone by sclerosis. MRI findings show high-intensity lesions on T2-weighted images and mixed signals on T1- and fat-suppressed images. Adamantinoma can be distinguished from OFD by its imaging features which show an extensive lesion with "moth-eaten" margins and complete involvement of the medullary cavity on axial MRI {1405}.

Macroscopy

OFD is solid with a whitish-yellow and soft or gritty texture, blending into the surrounding cortical bone. The periosteum often appears intact, but the cortex is thin or absent. Medullary extension is usually demarcated by a sclerotic rim.

Histopathology

The histopathological findings in OFD are irregular fragments of woven bone often rimmed by lamellar layers of bone laid down by well-defined osteoblasts. Osteoclasts may be present. The fibrous component consists of bland spindle cells with collagen production and a matrix that varies from a myxoid component to one that is moderately fibrous. Mitoses are extremely rare. Zonal architecture is delineated with thin spicules and woven bone

or even fibrous tissue predominating in the centre of the lesion with more abundant anastomosing and lamellar bone peripherally, the latter often blending into the surrounding host bone {369}. Secondary changes of hyalinization, haemorrhage, xanthomatous change, cyst formation and foci of giant cells are rare. Cartilage or clusters of epithelial cells are absent.

The differential diagnosis of OFD is essentially that of fibrous dysplasia, with which it shares some histological features, and adamantinoma, which also commonly occurrs in the tibia. Fibrous dysplasia can be distinguished by the presence of mutations in the GNAS gene and the absence of keratin-positive epithelial cells and the fact that it is epicentred in the medullary compartment of the bone. Adamantinoma can be distinguished by the presence of clusters of epithelial cells.

Immunophenotype

OFD is positive for vimentin and occasionally for S100 and Leu7. Isolated keratin-positive cells, not identifiable on routine H&E staining, have been reported in as many as 90% of cases if there is adequate sampling and careful examination. A tumour should be considered OFD-like adamantinoma when abundant keratin-positive cells are found {1148,1997}, and classic adamantinoma, if easily identifiable clusters of epithelial tissue are present. Podoplanin has been found to be expressed both in OFD and adamantinoma {1376}.

Genetics

Recurrent cytogenetic and FISH findings in OFD include trisomies of chromosomes 7, 8, and 12 {315,322,992}, supporting a relationship to adamantinoma {315,992, 1146}. Causative molecular genetic aberrations have not been identified, but proto-oncogenes FOS and JUN are expressed {1708,2418}. Additionally, GNAS mutations appear to be absent in OFD {1609}.

Prognostic factors

The natural history of OFD in most cases is that of gradual growth during the first decade of life with stabilization at about 15 years of age, followed by healing or spontaneous resolution. Bowing of the tibia may persist for years. The progression of OFD-like adamantinoma (or "OFD with small clusters of keratin-positive cells") to classic adamantinoma has been shown in a few patients {716,1148, 1335,2619, 2623}. Dogmatic recommendations regarding the role of surgery are suspect due to the rareness of the entity, lack of randomized studies, variation in progression that is probably age-related, and lack of long-term follow-up. Some would agree that the risk of significant deformity or pseudoarthrosis, impending or existing pathological fracture, the desire for definitive diagnosis and possibly the severity of symptoms warrant surgical intervention.

Langerhans cell histiocytosis

B. De Young
R.M. Egeler
B.J. Rollins

Definition
A clonal and likely neoplastic proliferation of pathological Langerhans cells.

ICD-O code
Monostotic	9752/1
Polystotic	9753/1

Synonym
Eosinophilic granuloma

Epidemiology
Langerhans cell histiocytosis (LCH) accounts for < 1% of all osseous lesions, with a wide age distribution ranging from birth to the eighth decade of life, although 80% of cases are seen in patients under the age of 30 years. The disease affects males more frequently than females (2 : 1 sex ratio) {1311,1612,2943}.

Sites of involvement
Although any bone may be involved, LCH most commonly involves bones of the

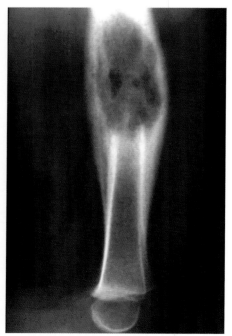

Fig. 25.19 Langerhans cell histiocytosis. Plain X-ray showing lucency in the shaft of the femur associated with thick periosteal new-bone formation.

skull, notably the calvarium. Other frequently involved sites include the femur, the pelvis, and the mandible {1612,2943}. In adults, the rib is the most frequently involved site. Monostotic disease is three to four times more common than polyostotic disease.

Clinical and imaging features
The most common presenting symptoms are pain and swelling of the affected area, with rare pathological fracture. Other findings vary with the bone involved. In temporal bone involvement, the presentation can show significant clinical overlap with otitis media or mastoiditis. With mandibular involvement, loosening or loss of teeth can be encountered. Vertebral body disease may result in compression fracture and possible neurological impairment. Early lesions may appear aggressive on radiographs. Roentgenograms generally show a purely lytic, well-demarcated lesion, usually associated with thick periosteal new-bone formation. Skull lesions are sometimes described as a "hole in a hole" due to uneven involvement of the two osseous tables. Clinical presentation can be restricted to the skeletal system, or affect other organ systems {1155}.

Histopathology
The diagnosis depends on the recognition of lesional Langerhans cells, which are of intermediate size and have indistinct cytoplasmic borders, eosinophilic to clear cytoplasm and oval nuclei, which are frequently indented, irregular in outline and typically possess nuclear grooves. Chromatin is either diffusely dispersed or condensed along the nuclear membrane. In osseous LCH, the Langerhans cells are found in nests or clusters. Diffuse sheet-like architecture is rare, and, if present, should raise the suspicion of haemato-lymphoid malignancy. The Langerhans cells are frequently admixed with inflammatory cells, including large numbers of eosinophils, as well as lymphocytes, neutrophils and plasma cells. Necrosis is common and does not portend an aggressive clinical course. Multinucleated

osteoclast-like giant cells and lipid-laden histiocytes may occasionally be present. The cells of LCH can exhibit a relatively brisk mitotic rate, with up to 5–6 mitoses per 10 HPF.

Immunophenotype
Langerhans cells have a characteristic immunophenotype: CD1a and CD 207/ Langerin membrane positivity {743,958}; nuclear and cytoplasmic expression of S100 and CD45 negative immunostaining.

Ultrastructure
Langerhans cells contain unique intracytoplasmic "tennis racket" shaped inclusions known as Birbeck granules which are thought to arise from the cell membrane.

Genetics
Despite evidence from small series that LCH may have a heritable component, no germline risk-alleles have been identified. Studies of X-chromosome inactivation demonstrated that non-pulmonary LCH is clonal {2973,3043}. Pathological Langerhans cells are diploid and show no recurrent cytogenetic abnormalities {1604}. The oncogenic *BRAF* mutation encoding

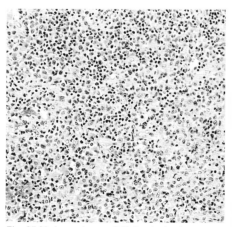

Fig. 25.20 Langerhans cell histiocytosis. Low-power magnification shows loose aggregates of histiocytic-appearing cells in a mixed inflammatory background with prominent eosinophilia and evidence of recent haemorrhage.

BRAF V600E is present as a somatic mutation in over half of LCH cases {135}. To date, there appears to be no correlation between the presence of BRAF V600E and LCH clinical behaviour, however, larger studies are needed before such associations can be definitively excluded {136}. TP53 is frequently overexpressed but only one *TP53* mutation has been reported (TP53 R175H) {135}.

Prognostic factors

The prognosis for patients with either monostotic or limited polyostotic diseases is good. Spontaneous healing is not uncommon; however reactivations may occur in approximately 10% of monostotic cases and up to 25% of polyostotic LCH.

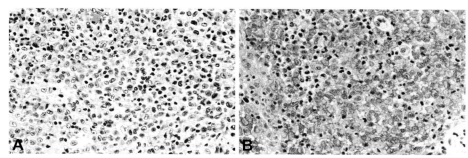

Fig. 25.21 Langerhans cell histiocytosis. **A** High-power image depicting Langerhans cells with ovoid to reniform nuclei with irregular notches and grooves. **B** Langerhans cells show distinct membrane-based immunoreactivity for CD1a.

LCH-related mortality is associated with disseminated disease involving viscera, and usually occurs in individuals aged < 2 years at diagnosis.

Erdheim-Chester disease

R. Jaffe

Definition
A xanthogranulomatous histiocytosis involving bone, soft tissues, viscera and CNS, leading to osteosclerosis, fibrosis and critical organ failure {2879}.

ICD-O code   9750/1

Epidemiology
There is a slight male predominance (sex ratio is 5:4) and the age range is 18–84 years with a mean of 50 years. Childhood cases are very rare and overlap with systemic juvenile xanthogranuloma.

Sites of involvement
Long bones of the distal extremities are most commonly affected, and frequent bilateral symmetrical involvement is characteristic. Orbital and facial bones, pelvis, lung, CNS, posterior pituitary, meninges, heart, peri-aortic and retroperitoneal tissues, skin, breast and testis can be involved. The spleen, lymph nodes and liver are generally spared.

Clinical and imaging features
The variable clinical effects are determined by the extent of disease and sites of involvement. Systemic symptoms include fever, weakness and weight loss. Bone pain is common in the lower limbs; exophthalmos arises from orbital involvement; skin lesions include eyelid xanthelasmas and skin papules; abdominal pain and hydronephrosis result from retroperitoneal disease and dyspnea from infiltrating lung lesions. Cardiovascular involvement includes aortic and coronary artery coating, precordial and myocardial infiltration. Diabetes insipidus and focal CNS lesions create a wide range of effects. {671,700,1114}. The serum lipid profile is usually normal. X-rays of Erdheim-Chester disease show bilateral, symmetrical lower limb osteosclerosis of diaphyseal and metaphyseal medullary cavities, partially sparing the epiphyses. Periostitis and endostitis are seen in half of cases, lytic lesions in one third. Bone scans highlight increased tracer uptake in involved bones. CT scans reveal orbital, dural, peri-aortic, mediastinal and retroperitoneal lesions extending through perirenal fat producing a "hairy kidney" pattern. Chest CT shows diffuse pulmonary infiltrates, with pleural, septal, intralobular and peribronchial thickening. MRI reveals marrow replacement on T1-weighted images that enhance with gadolinium, and mixed signal intensity on T2-weighted images {106,335,2875}.

Macroscopy
Bone lesions are irregularly sclerotic. Soft tissue lesions are firm and golden-yellow.

Histopathology
Histologically, the lesion is composed of foamy histiocytes and scattered Touton-type giant cells enmeshed in reactive fibrous tissue also containing lymphocytes, plasma cells, and occasional eosinophils. The involved bone is usually sclerotic {2246,2786}.

Immunophenotype
The histiocytes express CD14, CD68, CD163, factor X111a and fascin. Late xanthomatous lesions may lose factor

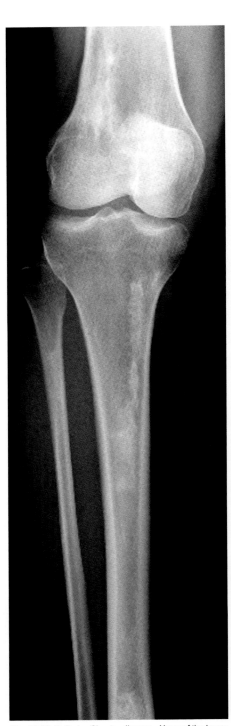

Fig. 25.23 Erdheim-Chester disease. X-ray of the lower limb reveals patchy sclerosis involving the medullary cavity of the tibia, fibula and femoral bones.

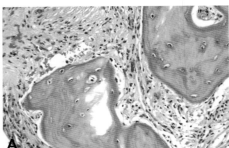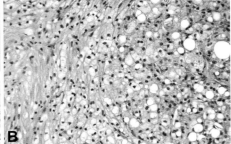

Fig. 25.22 Erdheim-Chester disease. A Low-power image. B High-power image.

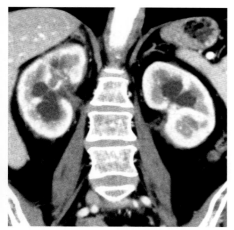

Fig. 25.24 Erdheim-Chester disease. Coronal reformatted image of contrast-enhanced abdominal CT highlights the coating of the thoracic aorta and the characteristic "hairy-kidney" appearance.

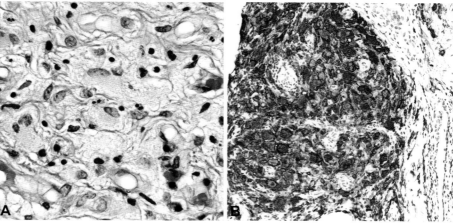

Fig. 25.25 Erdheim-Chester disease. **A** High-power view reveals early foamy transformation at the periphery of the histiocytes. Totally xanthomatous cells may lack the full phenotype and are of less diagnostic specificity. **B** The phenotype reveals immunostaining for CD163.

X111a/fascin, widening the differential diagnosis. S100 immunoexpression is weak or absent and Langerhans cell histiocytosis markers, CD1a and Langerin are absent {242, 2934}.

Ultrastructure

Histiocytes contain intracytoplasmic lipid vacuoles and sparse organelles, Birbeck granules are absent.

Genetics

Half the lesions examined have been shown to be clonal {441}.The same *BRAF* V600E mutation that is seen in Langerhans cell histiocytosis has recently been reported in 13 of 24 patients with Erdheim-Chester disease {1114A}.

Prognostic factors

Widespread systemic involvement, especially with CNS and/or cardiovascular lesions has a worse prognosis than lesions solely involving bone alone {106}.

Chondromesenchymal hamartoma

E.M.I. Amstalden

Definition
A rare, benign lesion of early infancy. It typically arises in the rib cage, producing a mass composed of a varying admixture of spindle cells, cartilage and haemorrhagic cysts.

Synonym
Chest wall hamartoma

Epidemiology
A little more than 100 cases have been identified {1070}. The reported incidence is 1 per 3000 among primary bone tumours {2302}. Most occur in infants but may be congenital {536,1351}. Rare cases have been discovered in adults, the eldest being 26 years old {677}. The male to female ratio is 2 : 1 {2514}.

Sites of involvement
Lesions commonly arise within the medullary cavity or on the surface of a rib. Bilaterality or multicentricity is well recognized {1209,

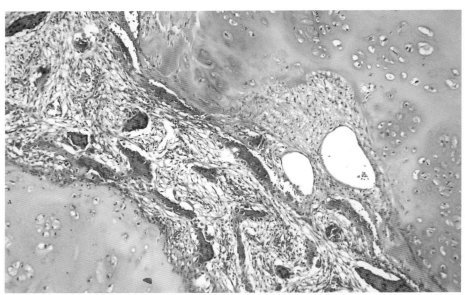

Fig. 25.26 Chondromesenchymal hamartoma. Lobules of mature cartilage intervening with connective septae associated with trabecular new bone formation and ectatic blood vessels.

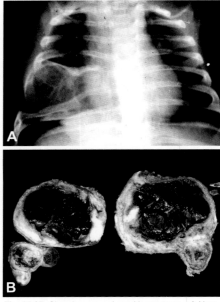

Fig. 25.27 Chondromesenchymal hamartoma. **A** X-ray of a 4-month-old infant. Expansile, lytic, trabeculated lesion involving the lateral portion of the fifth right rib with thinning of the lower rib. **B** Cut surface of the lobulated mass contains cavernous blood-filled cystic spaces with small glistening nodules of cartilage at the periphery.

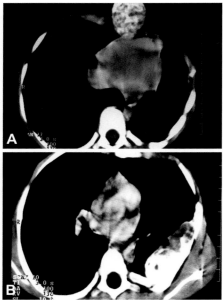

Fig. 25.28 Chondromesenchymal hamartoma. CT scans in a 7-year-old boy. **A** Nodular calcified lesion arising from the anterior aspect of the sternum. **B** Expansile, well-circumscribed mass with significant calcification, arising from the posterior lateral portion of the rib with bone destruction and intrathoracic extension.

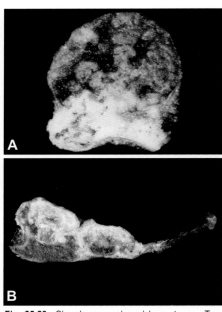

Fig. 25.29 Chondromesenchymal hamartoma. Two lesions in a 7-year-old boy. Both ressected tumours have a prominent solid cartilaginous appearance. **A** Scattered haemorrhagic spaces are seen in the sternum mass. **B** The rib lesion arises in the medullary cavity with destruction and erosion of the bone, forming an exophytic mass.

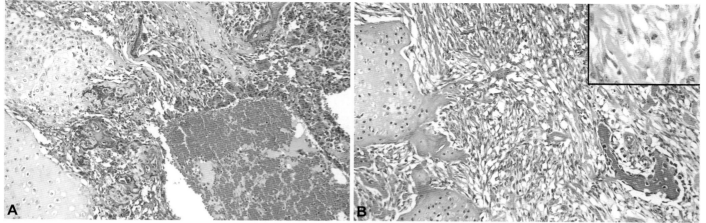

Fig. 25.30 Chondromesenchymal hamartoma. **A** Nodules of cartilage surrounding the aneurysmal bone cyst-like area. The cystic spaces are filled with blood. Walls and septae are composed of connective tissue stroma with collagenized areas, scattered osteoid trabeculae and multinucleated, osteoclastic giant cells. **B** Fascicles of mesenchymal spindle cells are permeated by collagen fibres and merge on the left with nodules of immature cartilage and on the right with a focus of active woven bone. Inset: spindle-cell component similar to fibroblasts in tissue culture, with a typical mitotic figure.

2782}. Other uncommon sites include the spine, sternum, and nasal sinuses {60, 1412, 2404A}.

Clinical and imaging features

Patients can be asymptomatic or may have respiratory distress {123,490}. Frequently, the tumour presents as a palpable chest wall mass, or may be detected incidentally {1414}. X-ray films and CT-scans usually demonstrate an expansile tumour with well-defined sclerotic margins, containing matrix calcification and ossification. MRI shows masses with solid and cystic components, giving heterogeneous signal intensities on T1- and T2-weighted images {1051}.

Macroscopy

Lesions can be of considerable size. The cut surface shows solid and cystic haemorrhagic areas in variable proportions. Solid areas consist mainly of cartilage {60}.

Histopathology

Solid areas are composed of fibroblast-like cells containing variable amounts of collagen, woven bone and cartilage, frequently with enchondral ossification. The haemorrhagic spaces are similar to aneurysmal bone cysts. Walls and septae are composed of fibrous tissue, reactive bone and scattered osteoclast-like giant cells.

Genetics

A chondromesenchymal hamartoma arising in the nasal septum showed a t(12;17)(q24.1;q21) as the sole anomaly {180A}.

Prognostic factors

Surgical excision is usually curative and secondary scoliosis can occur {692}. Sporadic fatal cases due to severe respiratory insufficiency have been reported {1160, 1796}. Asymptomatic patients can be managed conservatively {294,363}. Spontaneous regression has been described {911}.

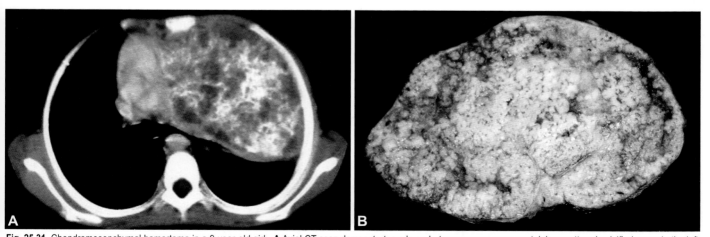

Fig. 25.31 Chondromesenchymal hamartoma in a 9-year-old girl. **A** Axial CT scan demonstrates a large heterogeneous mass containing scattered calcified areas in the left hemithorax that dislocates the heart and mediastinum. **B** The large well-circumscribed tumour (largest diameter, 16 cm; weight, 1062 g) is composed mainly of cartilage with occasional haemorrhagic foci.

Rosai-Dorfman disease

A.E. Rosenberg

Definition
A disease characterized by the proliferation of histiocytes.

Synonym
Sinus histiocytosis with massive lymphadenopathy

Epidemiology
Rosai-Dorfman disease is a rare disorder that usually presents as nodal disease. Approximately 2–10% of patients have bone involvement; primary bone disease is rare {635}. There is equal gender distribution and patients range in age from 3 to 56 years (mean, 27 years) {635, 1066}.

Sites of involvement
The metaphyseal region of long bones and the craniofacial skeleton are most commonly affected {635}. Most cases are solitary, but 20% may have involvement of two or more separate bones {635}.

Clinical and imaging features
Patients usually present with pain, localized to the involved anatomical site. Imaging studies reveal a well-defined, lytic, sometimes expansile, septated mass. Cortical thickening and periosteal reaction present in minority of cases {635,1066, 2890}.

Macroscopy
The size of tumours is 1–7 cm; most <5 cm and are well defined, tan-grey, soft or gritty.

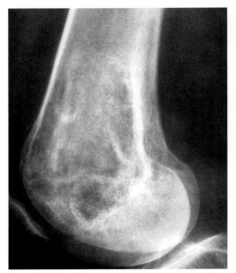

Fig. 25.32 Rosai-Dorfman disease. Lateral X-ray of the distal femur showing an irregular lytic lesion that has a sclerotic margin.

Histopathology
The lesions consist of numerous, characteristic, large histiocytes, enmeshed in a variably cellular, mixed inflammatory infiltrate composed of plasma cells, often containing Russell bodies, lymphocytes, neutrophils, foamy macrophages, and rare eosinophils. The large histiocytes contain abundant eosinophilic cytoplasm and demonstrate conspicuous emperipolesis (lymphocytophagocytosis) with intracytoplasmic lymphocytes, plasma cells, or neutrophils {903}. The histiocyte

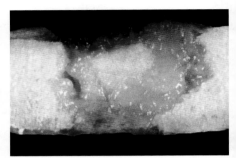

Fig. 25.33 Rosai-Dorfman disease. Resected segment of calvarium containing a tan-grey, pink lesion.

nuclei range from round or oval to kidney-bean shaped, with fine or vesicular chromatin and prominent nucleoli, which can be large. The histiocytes are variable in number and distribution; they may be absent in large regions, which is a potential problem in relation to sampling. Microabscesses may be present.

Immunophenotype
The large histiocytes express S100, CD68, and CD163 and are negative for CD1a {938}.

Prognostic factors
The disease has a good prognosis; approximately 40% of patients develop extraosseous foci of disease. The bone lesions are effectively treated by curettage {635}.

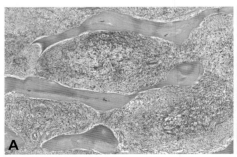
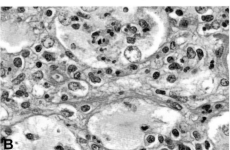
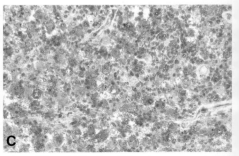

Fig. 25.34 Rosai-Dorfman disease. **A** Dense inflammatory infiltrate replacing the marrow and encompassing the cancellous bone. **B** Large histiocytes with lymphocyes present within the abundant cytoplasm. **C** Large histiocytes strongly express S100 protein.

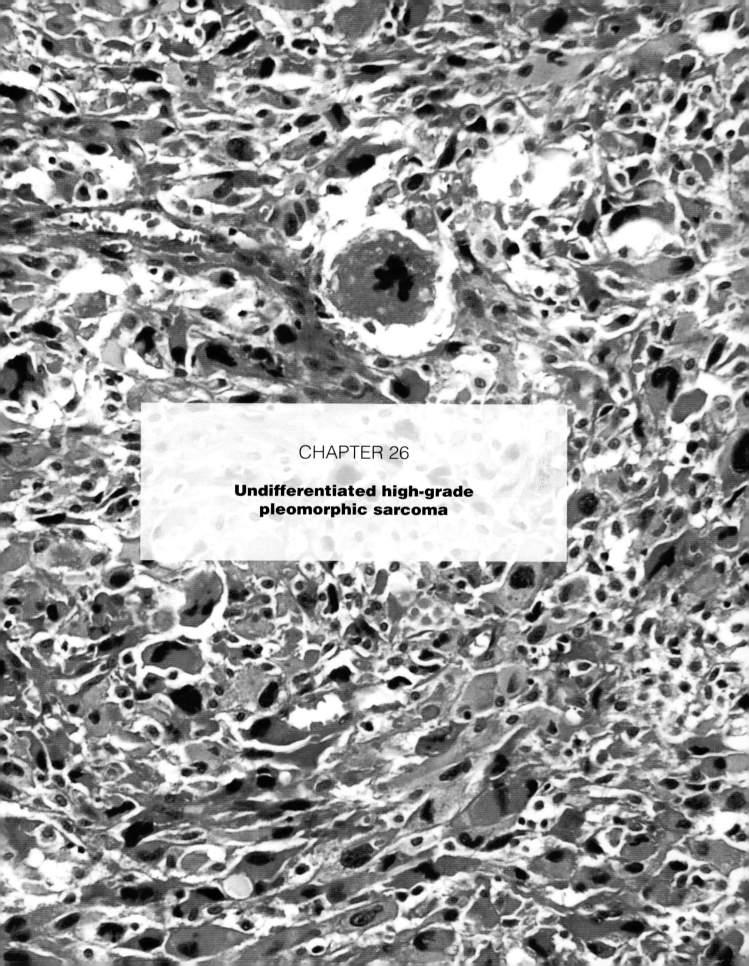

CHAPTER 26

Undifferentiated high-grade pleomorphic sarcoma

Undifferentiated high-grade pleomorphic sarcoma

S. Romeo
J.V.M.G. Bovée
G. Jundt

Definition
A high-grade malignant neoplasm characterized by tumour cells with diffuse pleomorphism in the absence of a specific line of differentiation.

ICD-O code   8830/3

Synonym
Malignant fibrous histiocytoma (MFH) of bone

Epidemiology
Undifferentiated high-grade pleomorphic sarcoma (UPS) of bone is a rare tumour that represents < 2% of all primary malignant bone lesions. Males are more frequently affected than females. The age of patients at the time of diagnosis varies from the second to eighth decade of life, with a higher incidence in adults aged > 40 years and only 10–15% of cases occurring in patients aged < 20 years.

Etiology
The etiology of UPS of bone is unclear; however some predisposing conditions are known. UPS may arise as a primary bone tumour or may develop secondary to pre-existing bone conditions, such as Paget disease or bone infarct, or at the site of an irradiated bone {642,1265,778}. Secondary UPS accounts for approximately 28% of all UPS {1260,1265, 2055, 2171}.

An autosomal dominant predisposing condition has been identified: diaphyseal medullary stenosis with UPS {109,1109, 1738,1980,2075}. UPS has occurred in 13 out of 40 patients affected by this rare bone dysplasia, characterized by diffuse diaphyseal medullary stenosis with overlying endosteal cortical thickening, metaphyseal striations, scattered infarctions and sclerotic areas throughout the long bones {109,1109,1738,1980,2075}.

Sites of involvement
Primary UPS predominantly affects the long bones of the lower extremities, particularly the femur (30–45%), followed by tibia and humerus. The knee is a common location, with concurrent involvement of the distal femur and proximal tibia {230}. Among the bones of the trunk, the pelvis is most frequently involved. Almost all UPS are solitary lesions.

Clinical and imaging features
Most patients present with pain and less frequently, swelling, varying from 1 week to 3 years (average, 7–9 months). Rarely, a pathological fracture may be the initial presenting symptom. The tumours are essentially lytic, aggressive, and poorly limited with cortex destruction and soft-tissue involvement. In secondary UPS arising in Paget disease and bone infarct, radiographs indicate the presence of an underlying bone process in most cases.

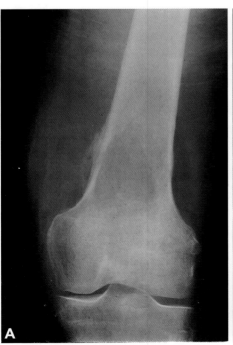
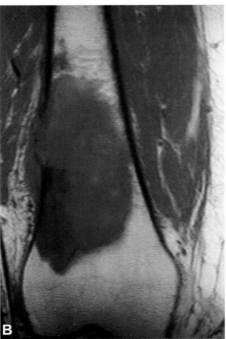

Fig. 26.01 Undifferentiated high-grade pleomorphic sarcoma. **A** Radiograph showing a large, lytic lesion of the distal femur, with ill-defined margins and focal periosteal reaction. **B** Coronal T1-weighted MRI showing a large medullary lesion with focal soft-tissue extension.

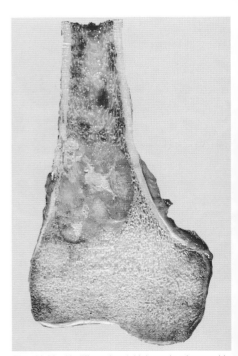

Fig. 26.02 Undifferentiated high-grade pleomorphic sarcoma. A greyish-white, circumscribed tumour with yellowish necrotic area, focally destroying the cortex.

Macroscopy

The gross appearance of this tumour is not characteristic. It varies in colour from tan to greyish-white and soft to firm in consistency. Areas of yellowish discoloration, necrosis and haemorrhage are frequently seen. Irregular margins, cortical destruction and soft-tissue infiltration are often present.

Histopathology

Since UPS of bone is a diagnosis of exclusion, extensive sampling is mandatory to rule out the focal deposition of osteoid, indicative of osteosarcoma. Microscopically, the appearance of UPS is quite heterogeneous, with mainly spindle-shaped cells and less often polygonal or epithelioid cells with more abundant cytoplasm. Varying numbers of multinucleated giant cells, often frankly atypical, are also present. An inflammatory infiltrate consisting of lymphocytes and histiocytes is frequently found. The nuclei of the tumour cells are often quite pleomorphic with numerous typical and atypical mitoses. A spindle cell storiform pattern commonly involves fibroblastic areas. Some would regard these tumours as pleomorphic fibrosarcomas {2358A}.
UPS may have foci of osteoid or primitive bone formation at the periphery in the areas of soft-tissue involvement representing periosteal reactive bone {1260, 1993}.

Immunophenotype

Immunohistochemistry must be applied to rule out other malignant neoplasms that may resemble UPS, such as leiomyosarcoma, metastatic carcinoma and melanoma {858}. Focal positivity for SMA can be found in almost half of the cases {2358,2358A, 2810}. Keratin can be positive, which can confound the differential diagnosis with metastatic sarcomatoid carcinoma.

Genetics

UPS have complex karyotypes {1854, 2725}. A low frequency of TP53 mutations (11–22%) {1381,2732}, MDM2 amplification (17%) {1381} and CDKN1A expression (33%) {1381} has been reported. Although loss of 9p21–22 can be found in both sporadic and diaphyseal medullary stenosis-related UPS {1739,2561}, mutational studies suggest that CDKN2A is not the critical gene {2732}. Copy-number increase of 8q24 and overexpression of MYC have been shown in a subset of tumours {2725}.

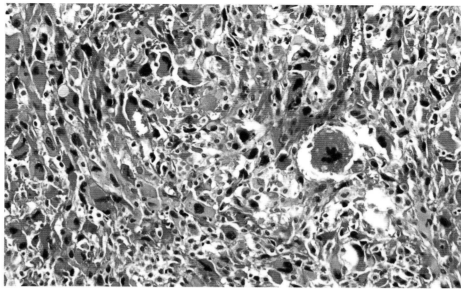

Fig. 26.03 Giant cells in an undifferentiated high-grade pleomorphic sarcoma of bone. Both reactive and neoplastic multinucleated giant cells may be present.

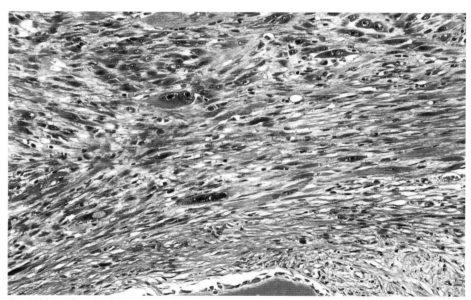

Fig. 26.04 Undifferentiated high-grade pleomorphic sarcoma of bone.

Prognostic factors

UPS is a highly malignant neoplasm with frequent metastases, particularly to the lungs (45–50%). Generally, treatment is wide surgical excision preceded by chemotherapy in those patients with resectable lesions {3034}. The degree of tumour necrosis in the resected specimen after chemotherapy is an important prognostic factor, as in the management of osteosarcoma {230,1329,2171}. In patients with localized disease, 5-year disease-free survival has been reported to be > 50% {298,2171}. Favourable prognostic factors are younger age at manifestation (< 40 years) and adequate surgical margins. Incomplete expression of myogenic markers is not thought to affect the prognosis {2358}.

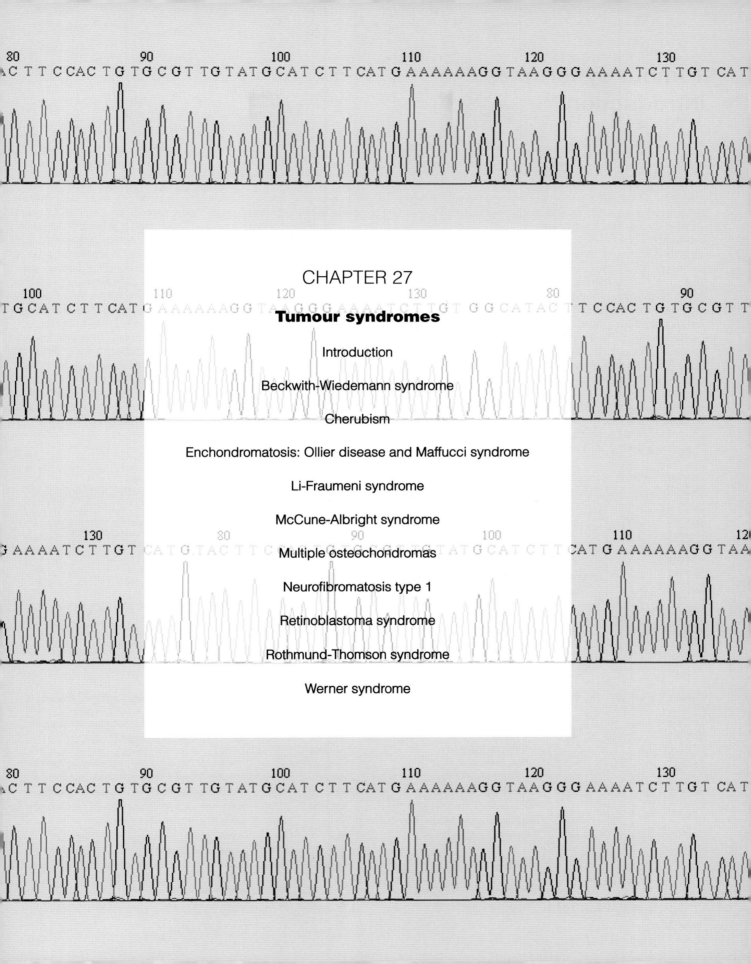

CHAPTER 27

Tumour syndromes

Tumour syndromes: Introduction

J.A. Bridge
F. Mertens

Hereditary etiologies complying with Mendelian inheritance principles, in addition to congenital malformation syndromes lacking a clear inheritance pattern, have increasingly been recognized as responsible for a subset of tumours of bone and soft tissue in children and adults. A continuing rise in the identification of cancer-causing germline mutations for which molecular testing is available, coupled with a heightened awareness of the importance of a detailed family history for patients with sarcoma, has improved diagnosis, prevention, surveillance, and therapy for affected families. Moreover, for some disorders such as Cowden disease, which have variable expression and subtle clinical features, incidence rates were underestimated before the identification of the responsible gene; a fact further underscoring the significance of these gene-mutation discoveries. Importantly, the genetic breakthroughs that have resulted from the investigation of inherited cancer syndromes have not only benefited patients with heritable tumour predisposition, but have also shed light on the regulatory molecular pathways involved in in the development of sporadic tumours, thus also advancing the care of sarcoma patients without known risk factors. And yet, although the genetic causes of many hereditary cancer syndromes have been established, it can be presumed that there remain other, still undiscovered, causative genes.

For some sarcomas, such as osteosarcoma, affiliations with multiple, distinct, hereditary tumour syndromes exist. In contrast, for others such as Ewing sarcoma, no significant connection with a classic syndrome of tumour susceptibility has been identified. On the following pages, we provide a schematic depicting recognized relationships between individual subtypes of bone and soft tissue tumours with corresponding predisposition syndromes. The data are also presented in Table 27.01, which lists the underlying genetic causes of congenital and hereditary syndromes associated with tumours of soft tissue and bone. This chapter also presents more detailed descriptions of the clinical, histopathological, and genetic data for select syndromes that are well characterized at the DNA level, or for which the associated neoplasms display features that are distinct from those of their sporadic counterparts.

Table 27.01 Hereditary disorders associated with tumours of soft tissue and bone, ordered by genes known to be involved (continued on facing page)

Gene	Locus	Inherited syndrome	Inheritance	MIM No.	Associated tumours
ACP5	19p13	Spondyloenchondrodysplasia	AR	271550	Enchondromas
ACVR1	2q24	Fibrodysplasia ossificans progressiva	Sporadic/AD	135100	Progressive heterotopic ossification (myositis ossificans progressiva), proximal tibial osteochondromas
AKT1	14q32	Proteus syndrome	Sporadic	176920	Lipomas
ANTXR1	2p13	Haemangioma, capillary infantile	AD	602089	Haemangiomas
ANTXR2	4q21	Fibromatosis, juvenile hyaline	AR	228600	Fibromatosis
APC	5q21	Desmoid disease, hereditary	AD	135290	Desmoid tumours
		Familial adenomatous polyposis 1 (Gardner syndrome included)	AD	175100	Craniofacial osteomas, desmoid tumours, Gardner fibromas
BLM	15q26	Bloom syndrome	AR	210900	Osteosarcomas
BRAF	7q34	Cardiofaciocutaneous syndrome	AD	115150	Giant cell lesions of small bones (central)
BUB1B	15q15	Mosaic variegated aneuploidy syndrome 1	AR	257300	Embryonal rhabdomyosarcomas
CHEK2	22q12	Li-Fraumeni syndrome 2	AD	151623	Osteosarcomas, rhabdomyosarcomas and other soft tissue sarcomas
Complex, incl. CDKN1C, KCNQ1OT1, IGF2 and H19	11p15	Beckwith-Wiedemann syndrome	Sporadic/AD	130650	Embryonal rhabdomyosarcomas, myxomas, fibromas, hamartomas
CREBBP	16p13	Rubinstein-Taybi syndrome 1	AD	180849	Rhabdomyosarcomas, leiomyosarcomas, haemangiomas
DICER1	14q32	PPB familial tumour and dysplasia syndrome (DICER1 syndrome)	AD	601200	Embryonal rhabdomyosarcomas
EXT1	8q24	Multiple osteochondromas	AD	133700	Osteochondromas, secondary peripheral chondrosarcomas
		Tricho-rhino-phalangeal syndrome type 2	Sporadic	150230	Osteochondromas, secondary peripheral chondrosarcomas
EXT2	11p11	Multiple osteochondromas	AD	133701	Osteochondromas, secondary peripheral chondrosarcomas
		Potocki-Shaffer syndrome	Sporadic	601224	Osteochondromas, secondary peripheral chondrosarcomas
FH	1q42	Hereditary leiomyomatosis and renal cell cancer	AD	150800	Leiomyomas of the skin and uterus
GLMN	1p22	Glomovenous malformations	AD	138000	Glomus tumours
GNAS	20q13	Pseudohypoparathyroidism, type 1A	AD	103580	Cutaneous osteomas
		McCune-Albright syndrome, incl. Mazabraud syndrome	Sporadic	174800	Polyostotic fibrous dysplasia, osteosarcomas, (Mazabraud syndrome: intramuscular myxomas)
		Osseous heteroplasia, progressive	AD	166350	Cutaneous osteomas
		Pseudopseudohypoparathyroidism	AD	612463	Cutaneous osteomas

Gene	Locus	Inherited syndrome	Inheritance	MIM No.	Associated tumours
HRAS	11p15	Costello syndrome	AD	218040	Embryonal rhabdomyosarcomas
IDH1	2q34	Enchondromatosis (Ollier disease and Maffucci syndrome)	Sporadic	166000	Enchondromas, chondrosarcomas (Maffucci syndrome: haemangiomas, angiosarcomas)
IDH2	15q26	Enchondromatosis (Ollier disease and Maffucci syndrome)	Sporadic	166000	Enchondromas, chondrosarcomas (Maffuci syndrome: haemangiomas, angiosarcomas)
KDR	4q12	Haemangioma, capillary infantile	AD	602089	Haemangiomas
KIT	4q12	GIST, familial	AD	606764	GISTs
LEMD3	12q14	Buschke-Ollendorff (osteopoikilosis isolated incl.)	AD	166700	Enostoses
MAP2K1	15q22	Cardiofaciocutaneous syndrome	AD	115150	Giant cell lesions of small bones (central)
MEN1	11q13	Multiple endocrine neoplasia, type 1	AD	131100	Lipomas
MID1	Xp22	Opitz GBBB syndrome, X-linked	XR	300000	Cranial osteomas
MTAP	9p21	Diaphyseal medullary stenosis	AD	112250	Undifferentiated pleomorphic sarcomas of bone
NBN	8q21	Nijmegen breakage syndrome	AR	251260	Rhabdomyosarcomas
NF1	17q11	Neurofibromatosis, type 1	AD	162200	Neurofibromas, malignant peripheral nerve sheath tumours, GISTs, giant cell lesions of small bones (central), rhabdomyosarcomas, glomus tumours
NF2	22q12	Neurofibromatosis, type 2	AD	101000	Schwannomas
PDGFRA	4q12	GIST, familial	AD	606764	GISTs
PMS2	7p22	Mismatch repair cancer syndrome	AR	276300	Rhabdomyosarcomas
PORCN	Xp11	Focal dermal hypoplasia	XD	305600	Giant cell tumours of bone
PRKAR1A	17q24	Carney complex, type 1	AD	160980	Osteochondromyxomas, cardiac and other myxomas, melanocytic schwannomas
PTCH1	9q22	Basal cell naevus syndrome	AD	109400	Cardiac fibromas, rhabdomyosarcomas, fetal rhabdomyomas
PTEN	10q23	Bannayan-Riley-Ruvalcaba syndrome	AD	153480	Lipomas, haemangiomas
		Cowden disease	AD	158350	Lipomas, haemangiomas
		Proteus syndrome	Sporadic	176920	Lipomas
PTH1R	3p21	Enchondromatosis (Ollier disease and Maffucci syndrome)	Sporadic	166000	Enchondromas, chondrosarcomas (Maffucci syndrome: haemangiomas, angiosarcomas)
PTPN11	12q24	LEOPARD syndrome 1	AD	151100	Granular cell tumours
		Metachondromatosis	AD	156250	Enchondromas, osteochondroma-like lesions
		Noonan syndrome 1	AD	163950	Granular cell tumours, giant cell lesions of small bones (central)
RB1	13q14	Retinoblastoma	AD	180200	Osteosarcomas, soft tissue sarcomas
RECQL4	8q24	Baller-Gerold syndrome	AR	218600	Osteosarcomas
		RAPADILINO syndrome	AR	266280	Osteosarcomas
		Rothmund-Thomson syndrome	AR	268400	Osteosarcomas
SDHB	1p36	Paraganglioma and GIST (Carney-Stratakis syndrome)	AD	606864	Paragangliomas, GISTs
SDHC	1q21	Paraganglioma and GIST (Carney-Stratakis syndrome)	AD	606864	Paragangliomas, GISTs
SDHD	11q23	Paraganglioma and GIST (Carney-Stratakis syndrome)	AD	606864	Paragangliomas, GISTs
SH3BP2	4p16	Cherubism	AD	118400	Giant cell lesions of small bones
SMARCA4	19p13	Rhabdoid tumour predisposition syndrome 2	AD	613325	Malignant rhabdoid tumours
SMARCB1	22q11	Rhabdoid tumour predisposition syndrome 1	AD	609322	Malignant rhabdoid tumours
SOS1	2p22	Noonan syndrome 4	AD	610733	Embryonal rhabdomyosarcomas, granular cell tumours, giant cell lesions including giant cell lesions of small bones (central) and pigmented villonodular synovitis
SQSTM1	5q35	Paget disease of bone	AD	602080	Osteosarcomas
T	6q27	Chordoma, familial	AD	215400	Chordomas
TEK	9p21	Venous malformations, multiple cutaneous and mucosal	AD	600195	Haemangiomas
TNFRSF11A	18q22	Paget disease of bone	AD	602080	Osteosarcomas
		Polyostotic osteolytic dysplasia, hereditary expansile	AD	174810	Osteosarcomas
TP53	17p13	Li-Fraumeni syndrome 1	AD	151623	Osteosarcomas, rhabdomyosarcomas and other soft tissue sarcomas
TSC1	9q34	Tuberous sclerosis 1	AD	191100	Fibromas, cardiac rhabdomyomas, angiomyolipomas, chordomas
TSC2	16p13	Tuberous sclerosis 2	AD	613254	Fibromas, cardiac rhabdomyomas, angiomyolipomas, chordomas, PEComas
VHL	3p25–26	Von Hippel-Lindau syndrome	AD	193300	Haemangioblastomas
WRN	8p12	Werner syndrome	AR	277700	Bone and soft tissue sarcomas

AD, autosomal dominant; AR, autosomal recessive; GIST, gastrointestinal stromal tumour; XD, X-linked dominant; XR, X-linked recessive

Angiosarcoma — Maffucci syndrome

Chondrosarcoma
- Enchondromatosis (Maffucci syndrome, Ollier disease)
- Osteochondromas, multiple, nonsyndromic
- Tricho-rhino-phalangeal syndrome type 2

Chordoma
- Chordoma, familial
- Tuberous sclerosis

Enchondroma
- Enchondromatosis (Maffucci syndrome, Ollier disease)
- Metachondromatosis
- Spondyloenchondrodysplasia

Fibroma
- Basal cell nevus syndrome (cardiac fibromas)
- Beckwith-Wiedemann syndrome
- Familial adenomatous polyposis 1 (Gardner fibromas)
- Jaffe-Campanacci syndrome (non-ossifying fibromas)
- Tuberous sclerosis 1 and 2

Fibromatosis (desmoid and non-desmoid types)
- Desmoid disease, hereditary
- Familial adenomatous polyposis 1 (Gardner syndrome)
- Fibromatosis, congenital generalized (myofibromatosis) and Fibromatosis, juvenile hyaline

Fibrous dysplasia
- McCune-Albright syndrome (polyostotic)
- Mazabraud syndrome (polyostotic)

Gastrointestinal stromal tumour
- Carney triad
- Gastrointestinal stromal tumour, familial
- Neurofibromatosis, type 1
- Paraganglioma and gastrointestinal stromal tumour (Carney-Stratakis syndrome)

Giant cell lesions
- Cardiofaciocutaneous syndrome (giant cell reparative granulomas, central)
- Cherubism (giant cell reparative granulomas, central)
- Noonan syndrome 1 and 4 (giant cell reparative granulomas, central and PVNS)

Glomus tumour
- Venous malformations with glomus cells
- Glomuvenous malformations
- Neurofibromatosis, type 1

Granular cell tumour
- LEOPARD syndrome 1
- Noonan syndrome 1 and 4

Haemangioma
- Bannayan-Riley-Ruvalcaba syndrome
- Cowden disease
- Maffucci syndrome
- Haemangioma, capillary infantile
- Klippel-Trenauny-Weber syndrome (cutaneous)
- Rubinstein-Taybi syndrome 1
- Venous malformations, multiple cutaneous and mucosal

Leiomyoma — Hereditary leiomyomatosis and renal cell cancer

Leiomyosarcoma
- Hereditary leiomyomatosis and renal cell cancer
- Rubinstein-Taybi syndrome 1

Lipoma
- Bannayan-Riley-Ruvalcaba syndrome
- Cowden disease
- Lipomatosis, familial multiple and Lipomatosis, multiple symmetric
- Multiple endocrine neoplasia, type 1
- Proteus syndrome

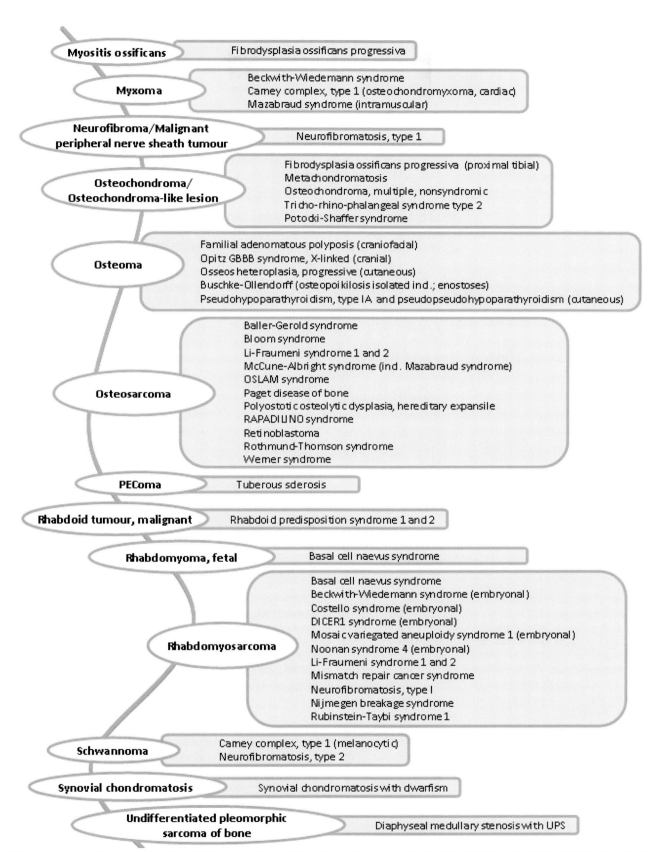

Myositis ossificans — Fibrodysplasia ossificans progressiva

Myxoma
- Beckwith-Wiedemann syndrome
- Carney complex, type 1 (osteochondromyxoma, cardiac)
- Mazabraud syndrome (intramuscular)

Neurofibroma/Malignant peripheral nerve sheath tumour — Neurofibromatosis, type 1

Osteochondroma/Osteochondroma-like lesion
- Fibrodysplasia ossificans progressiva (proximal tibial)
- Metachondromatosis
- Osteochondroma, multiple, nonsyndromic
- Tricho-rhino-phalangeal syndrome type 2
- Potocki-Shaffer syndrome

Osteoma
- Familial adenomatous polyposis (craniofacial)
- Opitz GBBB syndrome, X-linked (cranial)
- Osseous heteroplasia, progressive (cutaneous)
- Buschke-Ollendorff (osteopoikilosis isolated ind.; enostoses)
- Pseudohypoparathyroidism, type IA and pseudopseudohypoparathyroidism (cutaneous)

Osteosarcoma
- Baller-Gerold syndrome
- Bloom syndrome
- Li-Fraumeni syndrome 1 and 2
- McCune-Albright syndrome (incl. Mazabraud syndrome)
- OSLAM syndrome
- Paget disease of bone
- Polyostotic osteolytic dysplasia, hereditary expansile
- RAPADILINO syndrome
- Retinoblastoma
- Rothmund-Thomson syndrome
- Werner syndrome

PEComa — Tuberous sclerosis

Rhabdoid tumour, malignant — Rhabdoid predisposition syndrome 1 and 2

Rhabdomyoma, fetal — Basal cell naevus syndrome

Rhabdomyosarcoma
- Basal cell naevus syndrome
- Beckwith-Wiedemann syndrome (embryonal)
- Costello syndrome (embryonal)
- DICER1 syndrome (embryonal)
- Mosaic variegated aneuploidy syndrome 1 (embryonal)
- Noonan syndrome 4 (embryonal)
- Li-Fraumeni syndrome 1 and 2
- Mismatch repair cancer syndrome
- Neurofibromatosis, type I
- Nijmegen breakage syndrome
- Rubinstein-Taybi syndrome 1

Schwannoma
- Carney complex, type 1 (melanocytic)
- Neurofibromatosis, type 2

Synovial chondromatosis — Synovial chondromatosis with dwarfism

Undifferentiated pleomorphic sarcoma of bone — Diaphyseal medullary stenosis with UPS

Fig. 27.01 A schematic depicting recognized relationships between subtypes of bone and soft tissue tumours (listed in alphabetical order) with corresponding predisposition syndromes. PVNS, pigmented villonodular synovitis

Beckwith-Wiedemann syndrome

M. Mannens

Definition
The Beckwith-Wiedemann syndrome (BWS) is a complex overgrowth disorder caused by a number of genes that are subject to genomic imprinting.

MIM No.
130650

Synonyms
Exomphalos-macroglossia-gigantism (EMG) syndrome; Wiedemann-Beckwith syndrome (WBS)

Epidemiology
The syndrome occurs with an estimated incidence of 1 per 13700 and most cases (85%) are sporadic.

Diagnostic criteria
Patients can be classified as having BWS according to the clinical criteria proposed by Elliot or DeBaun {612,741,2550,2935}, although cases of BWS are known that do not comply with either set of criteria. Elliot classifies patients as having BWS when they present with three major features or two major features plus three or more minor features. Most important major features are: anterior abdominal wall defects, macroglossia and pre- and/or postnatal growth > 90th percentile. Some examples of minor features include ear creases or pits, naevus flammeus, hypoglycaemia, nephromegaly and hemihypertrophy. DeBaun is less strict in his classification, i.e. two or more of the five most common features are needed for the diagnosis (macroglossia, birth weight > 90th percentile, hypoglycaemia in the first month of life, ear creases/pits and abdominal wall defects).
BWS can be diagnosed in the laboratory by chromosome banding analysis (< 5%) or DNA diagnostics. The current major DNA tests involve methylation assays at two loci, scanning for microdeletions at these loci and finally mutation analysis. Most cases (50–80%) demonstrate aberrant methylation of KCNQ1OT1, with or without aberrant methylation of IGF2/H19. These cases often show uniparental disomy (UPD) for 11p15, in a mosaic form, which explains this aberrant methylation of both genes. However, the majority of cases with KCNQ1OT1 defects and some cases with IGF2/H19 defects have no UPD 11p15. Therefore, an imprinting switch can be assumed, involving an imprinting centre, analogous to the Prader-Willi and Angelman syndromes. The current data are most compatible with two distinct imprinting centres for either KCNQ1OT1/ CDKN1C (IC2) or IGF2/H19 (IC1). CDKN1C mutation analyses might be considered, especially in familial cases of BWS. The increased risk of tumours (especially Wilms tumour) for BWS patients seems to be associated with UPD in general and H19 methylation defects in particular. Methylation defects limited to KCNQ1OT1 seem to be a favourable prognostic factor since tumours are only very rarely associated with this group of patients. Recurrence risks for a second pregnancy can be assessed with UPD studies. In case of a UPD in a mosaic form, there is no increased risk of recurrence of BWS in a second pregnancy since the genetic defect occurred post-fertilization.

Clinical features
The BWS is a disorder first described by Beckwith in 1963. Later, Wiedemann described the syndrome in more detail {175,2958}. BWS is characterized by a great variety of clinical features, among which are abdominal wall defects, macroglossia, pre- and postnatal gigantism, earlobe pits or creases, facial naevus flammeus, hypoglycaemia, renal abnormalities and hemihypertrophy {2550,2935}.

Clinical management
Screening for hypoglycaemia is of particular importance during the first days of life. Surgical intervention can be necessary (e.g. repair of omphalocele, tongue reduction in case of macroglossia or corrections of hemihypertrophic growth). Tumour surveillance, especially in high-risk children, is indicated. Protocols vary throughout the world {2935}, but include α-fetoprotein (AFP) screening every 2–3 months to the age of 4 years for early detection of hepatoblastoma, and ultrasound imaging to the age of 8 years to discover abdominal tumours. Positive findings should be examined in detail with other imaging techniques such as CT or MRI.

Neoplastic disease spectrum
BWS patients have an increased risk of 7.5% for the development of (mostly intra-abdominal) childhood tumours. Tumours most frequently found are Wilms tumour, adrenocortical carcinoma, embryonal rhabdomyosarcoma, and hepatoblastoma. Myxomas, fibromas, and hamartomas have also been reported to occur at increased frequencies.

Genetics
BWS is caused by genetic changes in chromosome band 11p15, as shown by linkage studies, and the detection of chromosome abnormalities, loss of imprinting (LOI), and gene mutations. The syndrome is subject to genomic imprinting since maternal transmission seems to be predominant. In addition, chromosomal translocations are of maternal origin, duplications and UPD of paternal origin. All hitherto-known causative genes are imprinted {2642,2935}.
The 11p15 region consists of a number of imprinted genes. There are two distinct imprinting centres (IC1 and IC2). BWS translocation breakpoints disrupt KCNQ1OT1, which shows aberrant methylation in 50–80% of BWS cases. It does not code for a protein and may function through its RNA. CDKN1C is an inhibitor of cyclin dependent kinases and heterozygous mutations have been identified in about 20% of BWS patients in two studies. Others, however, have not been able to confirm this mutation frequency. In addition, it has been reported that this gene is more frequently involved in familial cases of BWS. Mouse models with mutated Cdkn1c revealed some of the clinical BWS features such as omphalocele and renal adrenal cortex anomalies. In humans, CDKN1C and IC2 anomalies also seem to be more frequently associated with abdominal wall defects.

Another gene involved in the etiology of BWS is the insulin growth factor type 2 gene (*IGF2*) located at IC1. Mouse models overexpressing Igf2 display a phenotype overlapping with that of BWS. *IGF2* LOI is often seen in BWS patients. Downstream from *IGF2* lies *H19*, also a noncoding gene. The roles of *IGF2* and *H19* seem to be linked. *H19* is important for the maintenance of the imprinting status of *IGF2*. Mouse studies have underlined the link between *IGF2* and *H19* expression and overgrowth phenotypes. *H19* LOI is frequently seen in BWS cases, although not always in combination with *IGF2* LOI.

Other genetic events reported in BWS
Rare *NLRP2* and *ZFP57* mutations have been reported in cases with LOI at IC2. Translocation breakpoints that disrupted the *ZNF215/ZNF214* region at 11p15 were seen in one case. Methylation alterations at multiple imprinted loci throughout the genome have been described in BWS cases recently, but the clinical significance of these findings is under investigation.

Genotype/phenotype correlations
As mentioned, risk of developing a tumour is particularly associated with UPD and IC1 defects. Omphalocele seems to be associated with IC2 defects or

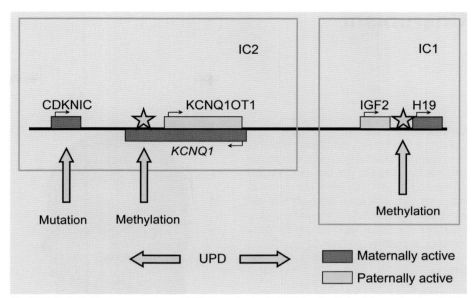

Fig. 27.02 Beckwith-Wiedemann syndrome (BWS). Genes involved in BWS localized to imprinting centres 1 and 2 (IC1, IC2), their imprinting status and the DNA tests used for diagnostics. UPD, uniparental disomy; the stars indicate differentially methylated sites.

CDKN1C mutations. Familial cases are more often seen in carriers of *CDKN1C* mutations or IC1 microdeletions, but rarely present in patients with IC2 defects. Developmental delay is associated with large paternal duplications.

Cherubism

E.J. Reichenberger
A.M. Flanagan

Definition

Cherubism is a benign, symmetric, bilateral, fibro-osseous tumour, limited to mandibular and maxillary bones. The bone lesions are composed of spindled mononuclear stromal cells and osteoclast-like cells that expand during childhood, resulting in the characteristic facial features that typically stabilize at puberty.

MIM No.   118400

Synonyms

Familial fibrous dysplasia of the jaws {1345}; familial multilocular cystic disease of the jaws {1344}

Epidemiology

Cherubism is a very rare disorder. An estimated 300 cases have been reported in patients with various ethnic and racial backgrounds. Males and females are affected with equal frequency.

Diagnostic criteria

Clinical diagnosis is based on the age of onset, family history, radiographical and histological findings and can be confirmed by the identification of a germline mutation in *SH3BP2* {2167}. Histologically, cherubism is indistinguishable from other giant cell lesions of bone {1345}.

Clinical features

Classically, cherubism presents between the ages of 2 and 6 years, as painless, symmetrical, bilateral swellings of the jaw, but in its milder form, or during the earlier phase of the disease, the bone defect may only be detected by imaging. The disease solely involves the maxillary and mandibular bones. A high V-shaped mandibular arch is often observed. In the severe form of the disease the lesional tissue can extend into the floor or the walls of the orbits, displacing the globes and result in retraction of the eyelids {898}. This may not only lead to the cherubic appearance, which gave name to the disorder, but can displace the optic nerves and cause proptosis {2758}. Occasionally, upper airway obstruction or obliteration of

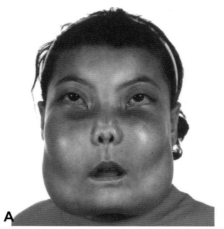

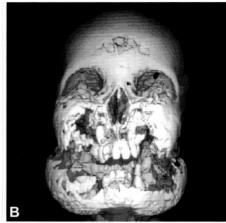

Fig. 27.03 Cherubism. **A** Patient with severe cherubism. **B** 3D CT scan shows extensive bone resorption in maxilla and mandible in this patient {2812}.

the nasal airway may lead to mouth breathing, chronic nasal infection and sleep apnoea {166,1526}. More significant is the impact on secondary dentition as teeth may be absent, displaced, or roots may be "free floating" in a lesion, or partially resorbed {797,1373}.

Lymphadenopathy in children, especially at the early stages, has been reported but not systematically followed, through disease progression.

If a cherubism phenotype is associated with extragnathic skeletal osteoclast-rich lesions, scoliosis, *café-au-lait* spots and short stature, a diagnosis of Noonan syndrome and neurofibromatosis type 1 (NF1) should be considered {854}.

Cherubism lesions usually stabilize at puberty and can regress in some affected individuals, but this appears to be related to the severity of the disease and those who are severely affected may display cherubism features in adulthood {390}.

Serum markers for calcium, parathyroid hormone (PTH), parathyroid-like hormone (PTHLH) and calcitonin are typically within normal range {2614}.

Imaging

Radiographical examination reveals bilateral multicystic radiolucencies, with irregular bony septa involving the mandible and maxilla. Early signs of cherubism are

often seen at the mandibular angle. In most instances, the radiolucency resolves as a result of infilling of the lesions with bone. However, in severe cases the radiological abnormality persists.

Microscopic features

Cherubism lesions contain osteoclast-like cells intermingled with spindled mononuclear stromal cells. The number and size of the osteoclast-like cells appear to depend on the phase of the disease, with the lesion becoming more fibroblastic and collagen-rich, and less osteoclast-rich with time. In the osteolytic, early phase of the disease, the osteoclasts can have as many as 100 nuclei, but in the later phase the osteoclasts can be significantly smaller. The tumour contains little bone

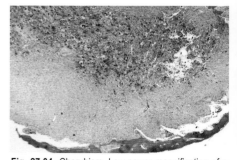

Fig. 27.04 Cherubism. Low-power magnification of a lesion showing a peripheral rim of bone.

formation other than an interrupted eggshell-like rim of woven bone surrounding the lesion. The osteoclast-like cells express tartrate-resistant acid phosphatase (TRAP) and macrophage markers, including CD68. Osteolytic, reparative and bone forming stages have been suggested {452}.

Neoplastic disease spectrum

For the management of cherubism it is important to exclude brown tumour of hyperparathyroidism, giant cell lesions, Noonan/multiple giant cell lesion syndrome, fibrous dysplasia, ossifying fibroma, aneurysmal bone cyst, NF1, and the hyper-parathyroidism-jaw tumour syndrome (HPT-JT) {72}.

Previously, some patients were treated with radiotherapy, but this can be associated with malignant transformation.

Genetics

Cherubism is inherited as an autosomal dominant trait, involving mutations in the SH3-domain binding protein 2 (*SH3BP2*) {2812} located in 4p16.3, with variable penetrance and expression levels {1725, 2762}. Approximately 50% of cases are without family history and are presumed to be de novo mutations {854}. Genetic heterogeneity exists, and recessive inheritance cannot be excluded {1471}. The cherubism phenotype has also been found in patients with Noonan syndrome {492,2729} and NF1 {1071,2832}. In a study of 49 families presenting with a cherubism phenotype, 75% harboured a *SH3BP2* germline mutation, 4% a *PTPN11* mutation that characterizes Noonan syndrome, and a *NF1* mutation in a patient with NF1. In addition, isolated cases with *SOS1* mutations have been identified {187,1101}. Mutations in these genes were not identified in the remaining families/individuals, some of whom had extragnathic skeletal giant cell tumours {854}.

SH3BP2 is a 561 amino-acid adaptor protein encoded by 13 exons. It directs signal transduction pathways by forming complexes with other signalling proteins (reviewed in {617,2315A}). The protein consists of an N-terminal pleckstrin homology (PH) domain, a proline-rich (PR) domain and a C-terminal Src-homology 2 domain (SH2). Canonical cherubism mutations are located in exon 9, within a 6-amino-acid interval (RSPPDG) in the pro-

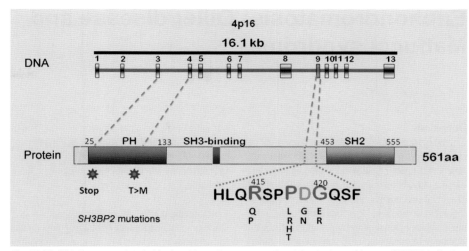

Fig. 27.05 Mutations associated with cherubism. Gene map and protein structure of human *SH3BP2* indicating mutations in the canonical cherubism mutation interval (amino acids 415–420) and mutations reported in the pleckstrin homology (PH) domain. Modified from {2812}.

Table 27.02 Documented mutations in *SH3BP2*[a] associated with cherubism (modified from {2315A})

Nucleotide change	Amino acid change	Exon	Reference
c.1244G>C	p.Arg415Pro	9	{2812}
c.1244G>A	p.Arg415Gln	9	{2812}
c.1253C>T	p.Pro418Leu	9	{2812}
c.1253C>G	p.Pro418Arg	9	{2812}
c.1253C>A	p.Pro418His	9	{2812}
c.1252C>A	p.Pro418Thr	9	{600}
c.1256A>G	p.Gln419Gly	9	{1605}
c.1255G>A	p.Asp419Asn	9	{1620}
c.1258G>C	p.Gly420Arg	9	{2812}
c.1258G>A	p. Gly420Arg	9	{1645}
c.1259G>A	p.Gly420Glu	9	{2812}
c.147delC translation stop at nt 325 (TGA)	p.Arg49ArgfsX26	3	{392}
c.320C>T	p.Thr107Met	4	{391}
[a]See also http://INFEVERS.org			

line-rich domain proximal to the SH2 domain of *SH3BP2* (Table 26.02) {600, 1605,1620,1645,2812}. Mutations have also been reported in exons 3 and 4 for one patient each {391,392}. A genotype–phenotype correlation has not been possible due to variable expressivity {854}, however, the exon 3 mutation is associated with an aggressive form of the disease.

A knock-in mouse model for *SH3BP2* {2811} demonstrated that a mutation for cherubism (Pro416Arg) stimulates bone resorption and causes inflammatory lesions by increasing TNF-α levels in blood.

This mutation inhibits the tankyrase-mediated destruction of *SH3BP2* and therefore stabilizes the protein, which in turn leads to hyperactivation of certain signalling pathways {1598}. How *SH3BP2* mutations lead to temporal and spacial specificity of expression remains unknown.

Enchondromatosis: Ollier disease and Maffucci syndrome

J.V.M.G. Bovée
B.A. Alman

Definition

Enchondromatosis refers to a group of rare, skeletal disorders in which patients have multiple enchondromas. Ollier disease and Maffucci syndrome are the most common subtypes, while the others (metachondromatosis, genochondromatosis, spondyloenchondrodysplasia, dysspondyloenchondromatosis and cheirospondyloenchondromatosis) are much less frequent. Ollier disease is a non-hereditary developmental disorder characterized by the occurrence of multiple cartilaginous masses, particularly affecting the short and long tubular bones of the limbs. When cutaneous, soft tissue or visceral haemangiomas are also present, the disorder is referred to as Maffucci syndrome.

MIM No.   16600

Synonyms

Ollier disease: dyschondroplasia; multiple cartilaginous enchondromatosis; enchondromatosis Spranger type I; multiple enchondromas; dyschondroplasia
Maffucci syndrome: dyschondrodysplasia with haemangiomas; enchondromatosis with multiple cavernous haemangiomas; Kast syndrome; haemangiomatosis chondrodystrophica; enchondromatosis Spranger type II

Epidemiology

Enchondromatosis is rare, but the exact incidence is unknown. Enchondromatosis has been described in many different ethnic groups, and there is no significant gender bias.

Diagnostic criteria

The diagnosis is based on radiographical appearance and clinical features.

Clinical features

The different enchondromatosis subtypes can be distinguished based on the distribution of the enchondromas, other accompanying symptoms and the mode of inheritance.
Ollier disease is non-hereditary and usually manifests in early childhood; 75% of the patients are diagnosed before the age of 20 years {2870}. The enchondromas primarily affect the short and long tubular bones of the extremities, but flat bones, such as the pelvis and ribs, may also be involved. There is a tendency for one side of the body, or one extremity, to be more severely affected. The craniofacial bones and vertebrae are usually spared. Enchondromas in the metaphyseal regions of long bones result in deformity and limb asymmetry, and occasional pathological fractures. The extent of orthopaedic complications is dependent on the number and skeletal distribution of enchondromas. There is wide clinical variability with respect to size, number, location, age of onset and requirement of surgery.
Maffucci syndrome is non-hereditary and presents at birth or in early childhood with cavernous haemangiomas of the dermis, subcutis or internal organs. In addition, spindle cell haemangioma, a vascular lesion with a high propensity for local recurrence, is overrepresented among patients with Maffucci syndrome {803,2209}. The skeletal features in Maffucci syndrome are indistinguishable from those in Ollier disease.
Orthopaedic surgical intervention may be needed to treat the deformities. Excision of a lesion, osteotomy to correct malalignment, or bone lengthening is performed on symptomatic patients {1584}.

Imaging

Roentgenographic features of Ollier disease and Maffucci syndrome are similar, except for the presence of haemangioma-associated phleboliths in Maffucci syndrome. Enchondromas present as multiple, oval, linear and/or pyramidal osteolytic lesions, with well-defined margins in the metaphysis and/or diaphysis of bone. When cortical destruction and soft-tissue extension with indistinct borders and lack of mineralization are seen, this is suspicious of malignant transformation towards chondrosarcoma.

Microscopic features

Enchondromas present as well-circumscribed nodules. The cartilage is hypercellular and the nuclei are enlarged and irregular. Within the context of Ollier disease and Maffucci syndrome, increased cellularity and some nuclear atypia are not sufficient to diagnose low-grade chondrosarcoma; the distinction should be made using a multidisciplinary team approach with consideration of radiological features, such as cortical destruction and soft-tissue extension.

Neoplastic disease spectrum

In addition to enchondromas and chondrosarcomas, patients with Ollier disease have an increased incidence of gliomas and juvenile granulosa cell tumours {2164}. In Maffucci syndrome, angiosarcomas, astrocytomas, pituitary adenomas, juvenile granulosa cell tumours, pancreatic adenocarcinomas and isolated cases of other tumours have been reported {2164,2299}.

Tumours of soft tissue and bone

Patients with Ollier disease have an approximately 40% risk (ranging from 5 to

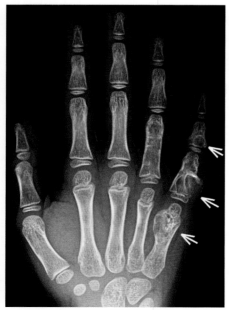

Fig. 27.06 Ollier disease. Multiple enchondromas in the fifth ray of the hand of a young patient.

50%) of developing secondary conventional chondrosarcoma {1638, 2453, 2484, 2870}. When patients have enchondromas restricted to hands and feet, the risk is less (15%) as compared with patients in which long bones are also affected (43–46%) {2870}. Approximately 25% of patients develop multiple chondrosarcomas {2870}. Continued or renewed growth in adults should raise the suspicion of malignant transformation. The risk of developing chondrosarcoma is possibly even higher among patients with Maffucci syndrome, with incidence of up to 53% reported {2870}.

Genetics

Ollier disease and Maffucci syndrome are not inherited. These patients harbour mutations in the isocitrate dehydrogenase genes *IDH1* and *IDH2* within their enchondromas (87%), chondrosarcomas and spindle cell haemangiomas (70%) {56,2165}. In total, 65 of 75 (87%) patients with Ollier disease and 17 of 21 (81%) patients with Maffucci syndrome were shown to carry mutations in their tumours {56,2165}. Mutations mostly affect the Arg132 position in exon 4 of *IDH1* and include R132C (65%), R132H (15%), R132G (5%) or other very rare variants affecting the R132 position. Mutations in *IDH2* (R172S) are described for only two patients with Ollier disease {56,2165}. In Maffucci syndrome only the R132C substitution is found. Multiple tumours within the same patient were shown to carry identical mutations. Also, mutations are found at a very low frequency in normal tissue in these patients {56,2165}. Thus, *IDH1* and *IDH2* mutations probably occur in the mesoderm early after gastrulation causing a somatic mosaic distribution of mutations leading to multiple enchondromas and haemangiomas.

IDH1 and IDH2 are metabolic enzymes involved in the tricarboxylic acid cycle. *IDH* mutations were previously found in other tumours, mainly gliomas and acute myeloid leukaemia. *IDH1* mutations lead to gain of function and the increased production of the metabolite D-2-hydroxyglutarate (2HG) {56} as well as DNA hypermethylation and downregulation of several genes in enchondromas {2165}.

In addition, < 5% of patients with Ollier disease carry mutations in the *PTHLH* gene {56,1210,1751,2165,2382}, encoding a receptor for parathyroid hormone and parathyroid hormone-like hormone

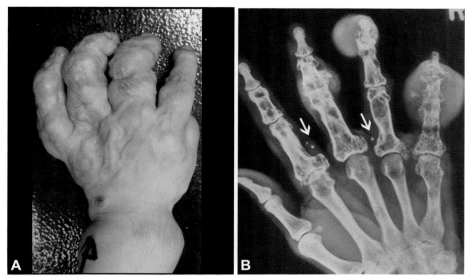

Fig. 27.07 Maffucci syndrome. **A** Deformed hand due to multiple enchondromas in a patient with Maffucci syndrome; note the superficial haemangioma. **B** Multiple enchondromas with and without soft tissue extension in the second to fifth digit and the fifth metacarpal bone of another patient. In addition phleboliths can be seen in the soft tissue at the bases of the second and fourth finger (arrows) indicating haemangiomas.

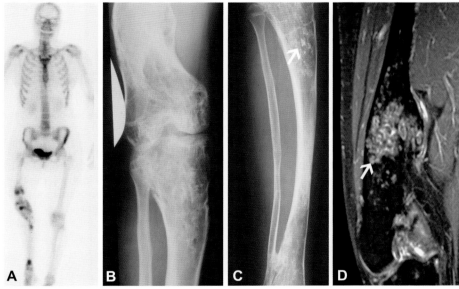

Fig. 27.08 Ollier disease. **A** Technetium-99m bone scintigraphy demonstrates unilateral occurrence with deformity of the right lower limb showing multiple areas of focally increased uptake of the tracer in the femur and tibia. **B** Anteroposterior radiograph of the right knee and lower leg of same patient shows structural changes in the marrow cavity and cortical bone of the femur and tibia consisting of osteolysis and osteosclerosis. **C** In the proximal tibia, areas with mineralization (calcifications) can be appreciated (arrow). **D** Coronal fat-suppressed T1-weighted MRI of the femur after intravenous administration of contrast shows multiple, partially lobulated, areas with increased signal intensity due to enhancement of the chondromatous lesions. There is a large lesion in the distal diaphysis of the femur suggestive of chondrosarcoma (arrow). The enhancement demonstrates rings and arcs (also known as septal or nodular enhancement) consistent with the chondromatous nature of the lesion.

(PTHLH), which is associated with constitutively active IHH signalling {1210}. Mutations include R150C, G121E, A122T and R255H {1210,1751}.

For some other enchondromatosis sub-

types, the genetic background has also been elucidated. *PTPN11*, a protein tyrosine phosphatase involved in Ras/MAPK signalling, was found to be mutated in patients with metachondromatosis {292, 2592}.

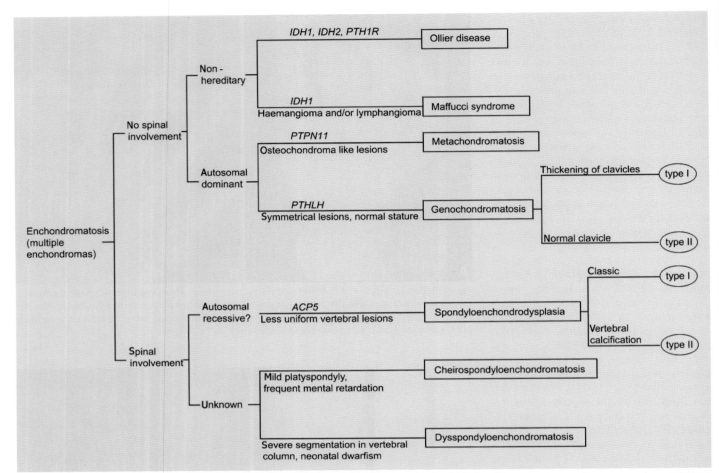

Fig. 27.09 Chart for the classification of different types of enchondromatosis. Distinction is made based on the distribution of the enchondromas, other accompanying symptoms as well as the mode of inheritance. Known responsible genes are shown in italics.

Duplication of 12p11.23 to 12p11.22 containing *PTHLH*, normally involved in growth plate signalling, was found in one patient with symmetrical enchondromato-sis (genochondromatosis features) {504}. Mutations in *ACP5* were found in patients with spondyloenchondrodysplasia {324, 1568}. *ACP5* encodes for tartrate-resis-tant phosphatase (TRAP) which is re-quired for maintenance of osteopontin, a bone matrix protein.

Li-Fraumeni syndrome

D. Malkin

Definition
Classical Li-Fraumeni syndrome is an autosomal dominant disorder in which the proband is diagnosed with a sarcoma at age < 45 years, has a first-degree relative with any cancer diagnosed at age < 45 years, and another first- or second-degree relative with any cancer at age < 45 years or a sarcoma at any age.

MIM No. 151623

Synonym
SBLA (sarcoma, breast cancer, leukaemia/lymphoma/lung carcinoma, adrenocortical carcinoma) syndrome

Epidemiology
Over 600 families have been reported worldwide with complete or partial (Li-Fraumeni syndrome-like [LFL]) phenotypes, and many more families have been identified but not reported. The *TP53* carrier rate is between 1 per 5000 to 1 per 20000 births {1008,1531}. The cumulative risks in kindred, ascertained on the basis of childhood soft tissue sarcomas are estimated by ages 20, 30, 40 and 50 years to be 18%, 49%, 77% and 93% respectively in female carriers, and 10%, 21%, 33% and 68% respectively, in male carriers {2993}. On average, females exhibit an earlier age of onset (29 years versus 40 years in men) {2531}. The differences in risk remain, after exclusion of breast, ovary and prostate cancer {453, 1268}. Gene carriers harbour an overall relative risk of additional malignancies of 5.3 (95% CI, 2.8–7.8), with a cumulative probability of a second cancer occurrence of 57% {1184}. However, it is not clear whether risk of second cancers is increased in the radiation field of treated primary tumours.

A unique population of *TP53* mutation carriers is found in the south-east states of Brazil where a 10-fold incidence of adrenocortical carcinoma (ACC) had been observed. Most of these individuals share a distinct germline mutation (p.R337H) within the oligomerization domain of *TP53* {1558,2331}. The carrier rate

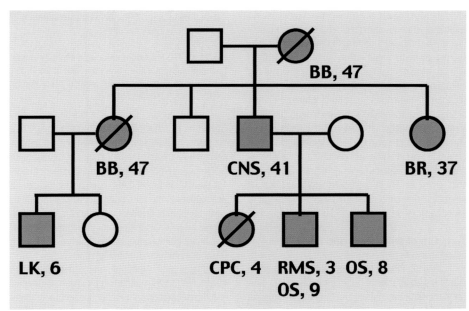

Fig. 27.10 Pedigree of a family with Li-Fraumeni syndrome. Filled circles/squares represent affected members; slashes represent deceased family members. Numbers represent age at diagnosis. BB, bilateral breast cancer; CNS, brain tumour; BR, unilateral breast cancer; LK, leukaemia; CPC, choroid plexus carcinoma; RMS, rhabdomyosarcoma; OS, osteosarcoma.

of this mutation in this region is approximately 1 in 300 {950,2248}. Analysis of tumour patterns in R337H carriers and their families reveals common features of LFS/LFL, clearly establishing that this mutant predisposes to a wide spectrum of multiple cancers.

Diagnostic criteria
The diagnostic criteria for LFS and LFL are summarized in Table 27.03.

Imaging
There are no unique radiological features of the tumours in LFS patients as compared with their sporadic counterparts. However, evidence suggests that tumours detected "early" using a comprehensive clinical surveillance protocol {2881}, are smaller, less invasive and of lower stage.

Microscopic features
There are no histopathological features of the tumours in LFS patients that are unique from their sporadic counterparts.

Where TP53 immunostaining is performed, the presence of heterozygous missense mutant TP53 expression in tumour cells typically confers intense staining.

Neoplastic disease spectrum
Breast cancer (usually invasive carcinoma of no special type) is the most common tumour in *TP53* mutation carriers (24–31.2%), followed by soft tissue sarcomas (11.6–17.8%), brain tumours (3.5–14%), osteosarcomas (12.6–13.4%), and adrenocortical tumours (6.5–9.9%) {1433,2123}. Most (69%) LFS-associated brain tumours are astrocytic (astrocytoma or glioblastoma), followed by medulloblastoma/primitive neuroectodermal tumours (17%) {1433}. Other tumours including haematological malignancies, gastric, colorectal, bronchoalveolar, cervical and ovarian cancers occur less frequently, but as with the common LFS tumours, do so at ages strikingly younger than in the general population {2030,2123}.

The age at diagnosis of tumours associated with *TP53* germline mutations show marked organ-specific differences. ACC occurs primarily in children; bone sarcomas occur mainly in adolescents, with a tendency shifted to the latter part of the first decade of life; brain tumours and soft tissue sarcomas exhibit a biphasic age distribution, with a first peak in very early childhood (< 5 years) and a second peak between 20–40 years; 10% of LFS patients develop gliomas, typically before the age of 45 years. Up to 5% of patients develop supratentorial primary neuroectodermal tumours, choroid plexus carcinomas and medulloblastomas {2735}; breast carcinomas are most prevalent in the third and fourth decades of life. Sex distribution shows an excess of brain tumours, haematopoietic cancers and gastric cancer in men, and an excess of breast cancer, ACC and non-melanoma skin cancer in women {2151}.

Tumours of soft tissue and bone

Sarcomas represent 17.4% of all cancers in the IARC TP53 database and 36.8% of all cancers in patients aged < 20 years. The most common types are osteosarcoma (40.4%), sarcoma NOS (17%), rhabdomyosarcoma (RMS) (16.5%), leiomyosarcoma (9.1%), and liposarcoma (4.9%) {2098}. The incidence of osteosarcoma among female *TP53* mutation carriers is slightly increased compared with a SEER

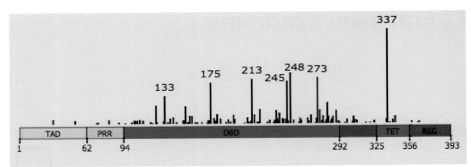

Fig. 27.11 *TP53* mutations associated with Li-Fraumeni syndrome. Relative frequency of germline mutations in *TP53* by codon adjacent to the primary structure of the TP53 protein. TAD, transactivation domain; PRR, proline rich region; DBD, DNA-binding domain; TET, tetramerization domain; REG, regulatory domain.

dataset, but for other sarcomas there are no substantive sex ratio differences. Sixty-seven percent of sarcomas in carriers of germline *TP53* mutation occur before age 19 years. While RMS and osteosarcoma are almost exclusively observed before age 19 years, liposarcoma and leiomyosarcoma arise predominantly in adults. With respect to genotype:phenotype correlations, RMS and osteosarcoma show a higher than expected proportion of missense mutations in the TP53 DNA-binding domain, whereas the liposarcomas and leiomyosarcomas are more frequently associated with frameshift, splice and nonsense mutations.

Genetics

Germline *TP53* mutations are found in approximately 80% of all individuals or fam-

ilies that meet the classic criteria for LFS, and in fewer than 20% where a broader LFS-like definition is applied. TP53 is a transcriptional activator that mediates cellular stress responses, and initiates DNA repair, cell-cycle arrest, senescence and apoptosis. Almost 4000 different *TP53* mutations have been reported, most localized to the DNA-binding domain (http://www-p53.iarc.fr/index.html) {2232}. TP53 loss-of-function, dominant-negative and gain-of-function properties all contribute to tumorigenesis {816,2347}. Disruption of function results primarily from *TP53* missense mutations that lead to the synthesis of a stable full length protein {2612} with a mutant DNA-binding core domain. The most common *TP53* germline mutations occur at codons 175, 248, 249,

Table 27.03 Clinical criteria for classic Li-Fraumeni syndrome (LFS) and LFS-like (LFL)

Definition	Clinical criteria
Classic LFS {1607}	Proband diagnosed with a sarcoma before age 45 years **AND**
	A first-degree[a] relative with cancer diagnosed before age 45 years **AND**
	Another first- or second-degree[b] relative on the same side of the family with cancer diagnosed before age 45 years or a sarcoma at any age.
LFS, Chompret criteria {2759}	Proband diagnosed with a tumour belonging to the LFS tumour spectrum (sarcoma, brain tumour, premenopausal breast cancer, adrenocortical carcinoma, leukaemia, lung bronchoalveolar cancer) before age 46 years, and at least one first- or second-degree relative affected with a LFS tumour (other than breast cancer if the proband is affected by breast cancer) before age 56 years, or a relative with multiple primary tumours at any age; **OR**
	A proband with multiple primary tumours (except multiple breast tumours), two of which belong to the LFS tumour spectrum and the first of which occurred before age 46 years, regardless of family history; **OR**
	A proband with adrenocortical carcinoma or choroid plexus tumour, regardless of family history.
LFL, from Birch {240}	Proband with any childhood cancer or sarcoma, brain tumour, or adrenocortical carcinoma diagnosed before age 45 years; **AND**
	First- or second-degree relative with a typical LFS cancer (sarcoma, breast cancer, brain tumour, leukaemia, or adrenocortical carcinoma) diagnosed at any age; **AND**
	A first- or second-degree relative on the same side of the family with any cancer diagnosed before the age of 60 years
LFL, Eeles definition {726}	Two first- or second degree relatives with LFS related malignancies (sarcoma, breast cancer, brain tumour, leukaemia, adrenocortical tumour, melanoma, prostate cancer, pancreatic cancer) at any age.

[a] First-degree relative is defined as a parent, sibling, or child.

[b] Second-degree relative is defined as a grandparent, aunt, uncle, niece, nephew, or grandchild.

Table 27.04 Clinical surveillance protocol for carriers of germline mutations in *TP53* {2881}

Tumour type	Surveillance strategy
Children	
Adrenocortical carcinoma	Ultrasound of abdomen/pelvis every 3–4 months Complete urine analysis every 3–4 months Bloodwork every 4 months: ESR, LDH, βHCG, α-fetoprotein, 17-OH-progesterone, testosterone, DHEAS, androstenedione
Brain tumour	Annual MRI of the brain
Soft tissue and bone sarcoma	Annual rapid total-body MRI
Leukaemia/lymphoma	Bloodwork every 4 months: CBC profile
In general	Regular evaluation by family physician with close attention to any medical concerns/ complaints
Adults	
Breast cancer	Monthly breast self examination starting at age 18 years Biennial clinical breast examination starting at age 20–25 years, or 5–10 years before the earliest known breast cancer in the family Annual (mammogram) and breast MRI screening starting at age 20–25 years, or individualized based on earliest age of onset in family Consider risk-reducing bilateral mastectomy
Brain tumour	Annual MRI of the brain
Soft tissue and bone sarcoma	Total-body MRI to be used as a baseline
Colon cancer	Biennial colonoscopies beginning at age 40 years, or 10 years before the earliest known colon cancer in the family
Melanoma	Annual dermatology examination
Leukaemia/lymphoma	CBC profile every 6 months for indications of leukaemia/lymphoma Annual abdominal ultrasound
In general	Regular evaluation by family physician with close attention to any medical concerns/complaints

βHCG, human chorionic gonadotropin; CBC, complete blood count; DHEAS, dehydroepiandrosterone sulfate; ESR, erythrocyte sedimentation rate; LDH, lactate dehydrogenase

273 and 281 (http://www-p53.iarc.fr/index.html) {2232}. While these are similar to the somatic mutation "hot spots", splice-acceptor mutations are found more frequently in the germline {2860}. Germline *TP53* deletions are rare. A recent report suggests that when the deletion breakpoint is within the open reading frame (ORF), an LFS cancer phenotype is observed; however, if the deletion breakpoints fall outside the ORF, the ensuing phenotype is restricted to a spectrum of congenital anomalies including developmental delay, hypotonia and hand/foot abnormalities with no associated cancer occurrence {2543}. These observations suggest that qualitative defects in TP53 structure are more conducive to aberrant DNA binding and dysfunctional transcriptional activation leading to malignant transformation of cells. *TP53* and *MDM2* SNPs may affect the natural course {266,1041, 2700,2947}.

The observation of genetic anticipation (earlier age of onset of cancer in successive generations) suggests a role of higher mutator phenotypes with each generation. This observation may be explained by accelerated telomere attrition from generation to generation {2700,2778}. In both adults and children, telomere length is shorter in *TP53* mutation carriers affected by cancer than in non-affected carriers and wild-type controls. Further evidence that profound genomic instability is associated with accelerated phenotypes in LFS, are found in the observation of increased frequency and complexity of DNA copy number variable regions in *TP53* mutation carriers {2544}. Evidence that early *TP53* mutation (germline or early somatic event) induces catastrophic, irreversible DNA damage is found in the high frequency of chromothripsis ("shattered chromosomes") in *TP53* mutation carriers who develop medulloblastoma {2307}. The inheritance of a *TP53* mutation coupled with a somatic defect in another developmental pathway (in this case, SHH signalling) leads to a sudden catastrophic shattering and rearrangement of chromosomes leading to dramatic telomere dysfunction, and rapid cellular proliferation. In summary, while germline *TP53* mutations establish a baseline risk of tumour development in LFS, a complex relationship of modifying genetic cofactors, likely defines the specific phenotypes of individual patients.

McCune-Albright syndrome

S.A. Lietman
M.A. Levine
G.P. Siegal

Definition

A sporadic syndrome characterized by polyostotic fibrous dysplasia, café-au-lait skin lesions, precocious puberty, and additional hyperfunctional endocrinopathies.

MIM No.   174800

Epidemiology

McCune-Albright syndrome (MAS) is rare, and the prevalence has been estimated to be 1:100000 to 1:1000000 people {712,2344}. All racial and ethnic groups are affected equally. Females are affected two to three times more than males {2344}.

Diagnostic criteria

MAS is diagnosed on the basis of the clinical triad of fibrous dysplasia, café-au-lait skin lesions and autonomous endocrine hyperfunction. Molecular tests may have a role in confirming the diagnosis. Affected patients carry a somatic mutation in the *GNAS* gene that leads to ligand-independent activation of the encoded protein, the α subunit of the heterotrimeric GTP-binding protein Gs that stimulates adenylyl cyclase {2487,2488,2920,2921}. Detection of the *GNAS* mutation in genomic DNA from involved cells, present either in the circulation or in lesional tissue, can aid in the diagnosis of MAS in selected patients, but as identical mutations are pres-

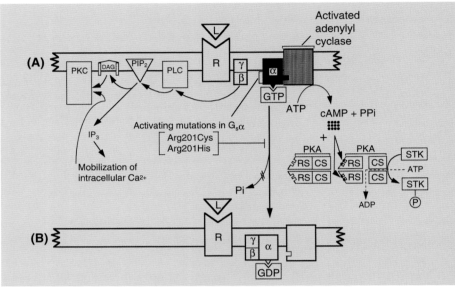

Fig. 27.12 A Activating mutations (Arg201Cys or Arg201His) in the gene encoding the α subunit of stimulatory G protein abrogating the endogenous GTPase of the α subunit, and hence leading to ligand-independent stimulation of adenylyl cyclase. The protein kinase A or cAMP-dependent protein kinase pathway (PKA) is shown on the right. The protein kinase C pathway (PKC) is shown on the left. The inability to hydrolyse GTP leads to persistent binding of Gsα to adenylyl cyclase and continuous synthesis of cAMP, which, in turn, overactivates the PKA pathway. PKA is composed of two regulatory subunits (RS) that have binding sites for cAMP, and two catalytic subunits (CS) that, when dissociated, phosphorylate serine/threonine kinases (STK). The dissociated βγ Gs subunits overactivates the PKC pathway. PLC (phospholipase C) cleaves PIP2 (phosphatidylinositol bisphosphate) into two intracellular messengers: DAG (diacylglycerol) and IP3 (inositol trisphosphate). The latter triggers the release of sequestered calcium ions (Ca^{2+}) which together with DAG activate PKC. **B** Normally, hydrolysis of GTP associated with Gsα leads to dissociation of Gsα-GDP from adenylyl cyclase and reassociation with the βγ dimer to form the inactive heterotrimer. Ligand binding causes repetition of the cycle {492A}.

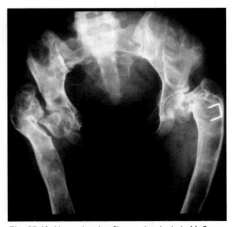

Fig. 27.13 X-ray showing fibrous dysplasia in McCune-Albright syndrome.

ent in patients with isolated fibrous dysplasia, this test lacks specificity {1619}. In addition, it can be difficult to detect the mutation if a sufficient number of involved cells are not available for analysis, thus most assays have only modest sensitivity {1619}.

Clinical features

The clinical features of MAS are variable in each individual and are dependent on the particular distribution of affected cells that carry the somatic mutation in *GNAS* and the specific role of adenylyl cyclase, and the second messenger, cyclic AMP in affected tissues {2344}. Fibrous dysplasia can be monostotic or polyostotic {662, 2680}. Typical endocrinopathies are precocious puberty, more common in females

than males, and hyperthyroidism, growth hormone excess, hyperprolactaemia, and hypercortisolism. The onset of these manifestations is usually during infancy and childhood {330}.

Nonendocrine manifestations can include renal phosphate wasting due to excess production of FGF23 from fibrous dysplasia {2187,2339}. Testicular abnormalities can also be detected by ultrasound in approximately 80% of boys with MAS, with both hyperechoic (49%) and hypoechoic (30%) lesions {293A}. Microlithiasis, which is normally uncommon, is present in 30–80% of males with MAS {293A,2906A}. Although large foci of Leydig cell hyperplasia that cannot be definitively distinguished from Leydig cell tumours are commonly found in the testes, malignancy is very uncommon. Additional nonendocrine features of MAS include hepatic involvement with cirrhosis and cardiac disturbances in function and rhythm {2344}.

Imaging
Imaging shows typical non-aggressive geographical lesions, except they are present in more than one bone (polyostotic). Radiographically the lesions often have a hazy mineralization producing a "ground-glass" appearance. They can occur in any bone, but the lesions are generally metaphyseal or diaphyseal, and their radiographical appearance has been described as a "long lesion in a long bone" {662,2680}. Many MAS patients have craniofacial lesions.

Microscopic features
The lesions are composed of proliferating fibroblasts that produce a collagenous matrix. Osteoid trabeculae are present throughout the lesions and these trabeculae are haphazard and nonfunctional in their orientation {662}. The haphazard osteoid pattern within a fibrous stroma is that of curvilinear trabeculae of woven bone {662}. Cystic degeneration and/or fat may also be seen within the lesions {2680}

Neoplastic disease spectrum
This is a benign condition with very rare conversion to malignancy. When malignant transformation occurs, the tumour type is usually either osteosarcoma, chondrosarcoma, fibrosarcoma or undifferentiated pleomorphic sarcoma. Patients with MAS appear to have a greater risk for sarcomatous change than individuals with fibrous dysplasia alone, while patients with both Mazabraud syndrome and MAS have a still greater risk {1657}.

Tumours of soft tissue and bone
Fibrous dysplasia is a bone disorder that can also be associated with intramuscular myxomas (Mazabraud syndrome).

Genetics
The molecular basis for MAS is a post-zygotic somatic mutation in exon 8 of GNAS that replaces the residue arginine at position 201 with histidine or cysteine {2487, 2920}. Infrequently, the arginine is replaced by serine, glycine, or leucine {372,373,689,1675,1710,2340}. Although missense mutations that replace the nearby glutamine at position 227 (exon 9) have been identified in solitary endocrine tumours and fibrous dysplasia, they have not been described in patients with MAS {1277}. GNAS encodes several proteins, but most relevant to MAS is the α subunit of the stimulatory G protein called Gs, that couples heptahelical receptors for hormone and neurotransmitters to activation of adenylyl cyclase. These somatic mutations activate Gsα which leads to constitutive (i.e. ligand-independent) activation of adenylyl cyclase and production of cyclic AMP {1621,2487, 2488,2920,2921}.

Multiple osteochondromas

W. Wuyts
J.V.M.G. Bovée
P.C.W. Hogendoorn

Definition
Multiple osteochondromas (MO) is an autosomal dominant condition. It is caused by mutations in one of the *EXT* genes; *EXT1* or *EXT2*. MO can be present as an isolated condition or as part of the clinical spectrum in the contiguous gene syndromes Tricho-rhino-phalangeal syndrome type II (Langer-Giedion syndrome) or Potocki-Shaffer syndrome.

MIM Nos
According to the gene involved, the following MIM Nos have been assigned:

EXT1	133700
EXT2	133701
TRPS2/Langer Giedion syndrome	150230
Potocki-Shaffer syndrome	601224

Synonym
Hereditary multiple exostoses

Epidemiology
The incidence of MO is approximately 1 per 50 000 persons within the general population {2466}, although this may be an underestimation. The solitary (sporadic) form of osteochondroma is approximately six times more common. The prevalence seems to be higher in males (sex ratio, 1.5 : 1), which is probably due to the fact that females tend to have a milder phenotype and are therefore more easily overlooked {1592,2955}. Approximately 80% of the patients with multiple osteochondromas have a positive family history {1326}. There are no recorded racial differences.

Diagnostic criteria
MO can be diagnosed when at least two osteochondromas of the juxta-epiphyseal region of long bones are observed radiographically or in the presence of a positive family history or germline mutation in one of the *EXT* genes.

Clinical features
Osteochondromas develop and increase in size in the first two decades of life, ceasing to grow when the growth plates close at the end of puberty. They are pedunculated or sessile (broad base) and can vary widely in size. The majority are asymptomatic and located in bones that develop by enchondral ossification, especially the long bones of the extremities, predominantly around the knee. The number of osteochondromas may vary significantly within and between families. In addition, a variety of orthopaedic deformities can be found, such as deformities of the forearm (shortening of the ulna with secondary bowing of radius) (39–60%) {2466}, inequality in limb length (10–50%) varus or valgus angulation of the knee (8–33%), deformity of the ankle (2–54%) {2466, 2523}, and disproportionate short stature (37–44%) {1592,2955}. The most important complication of MO is malignant transformation of an osteochondroma towards secondary peripheral chondrosarcoma, which is estimated to occur in 0.5–5% of MO patients {1592,2466, 2955}.

The suspicion of secondary chondrosarcoma is indicated by tumour growth after puberty, increase in pain, or a thickness over 1.5–2 cm of the cartilaginous cap in adults. Although there are no universally accepted guidelines for surveillance of individuals with MO to date, it is evident that patients should be well instructed to seek earlier medical attention if their clinical condition changes, and should have a regular follow-up (every year or every 2 years) to discover potential malignant transformation at an early stage for optimal treatment {1093}.

Other complications of osteochondromas include bursa formation, arthritis (14%) and impingement on adjacent tendons, nerves (23%), vessels (11%) or spinal cord (0.6%) {2955} and 84% of MO patients report frequent pain {571}. MO patients may also show abnormal scar formation {1228}, malformed and/or displaced teeth with abnormal enamel {478,2636} and bear the risk of fracture of the bony stalk of the osteochondromas during physical exercise {385}.

Imaging
The clinical diagnosis of MO can be confirmed by conventional radiographs. To evaluate possible malignant transforma-

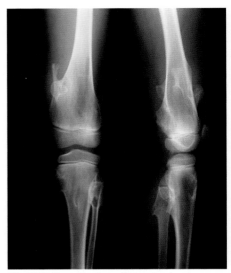

Fig. 27.14 X-ray showing multiple osteochondromas.

tion, the size of the cartilaginous cap can be accurately established with T2-weighted MRI and CT imaging {198,957}. A cartilage cap > 1.5–2 cm should be regarded as a cause for concern. The role of 18FDG-PET in the evaluation of osteochondroma needs to be further established {823}.

For screening purposes, a baseline bone scan should be considered after skeletal maturation. Furthermore, baseline plain radiographs of areas that cannot be manually examined, like the chest, pelvis and scapula can be performed. If lesions change over time, further examination, using MRI including contrast-enhanced sequences, is indicated {1093}.

Tumours of soft tissue and bone
Hereditary osteochondromas and secondary peripheral chondrosarcomas developing within the cartilaginous cap of hereditary osteochondromas are histopathologically similar to their sporadic counterparts. Morphologically, two types of osteochondroma can be recognized: broad-based sessile lesions with irregular cartilaginous linings and those with a well-defined cartilaginous cap. Both may occur within and outside the context of MO. When malignant transformation of

an osteochondroma occurs, it most commonly leads to a secondary peripheral chondrosarcoma (94%). Occasionally, osteo-sarcomas and spindle cell sarcomas develop in the stalk of the osteochondroma {285,1535}. These osteosarcomas and undifferentiated spindle cell sarcomas display an indistinguishable phenotype from their non-osteochondroma-related counterparts. No soft-tissue neoplasms are described within the context of MO.

Genetics

MO is a genetically heterogeneous disorder for which two genes, *EXT1* at 8q24 {20} and *EXT2* {2655,3001} at 11p11–12, have been isolated. With currently employed technical approaches, *EXT* point mutations or gross deletions are detected in > 90% of MO patients. In the remaining MO cases, other alterations such as deep intronic or promoter mutations, inversions, translocations or somatic mosaicism may be the underlying cause {1326,2697}.
Both *EXT* genes are also involved in a contiguous gene-deletion syndrome. Patients carrying an 8q24 deletion to include the *EXT1* {20} and *TRPS1* genes {1928}, demonstrate the tricho-rhino-phalangeal syndrome type II (TRPS2 or Langer-Giedion syndrome), which is characterized by craniofacial dysmorphism and mental retardation in addition to multiple osteochondromas {1539}. Patients carrying an 11p11–12 deletion to include the *EXT2* and *ALX4* genes {2999} demonstrate Potocki-Shaffer syndrome (proximal 11p deletion syndrome, DEFECT11, 11p11.2 contiguous gene-deletion syndrome) with enlarged parietal foramina, multiple osteochondromas, and sometimes craniofacial dysostosis and mental retardation {158}.
Three additional genes, *EXTL1* {2978}, *EXTL2* {3000} and *EXTL3* {2847} have been identified based on their homology with the *EXT1* and *EXT2* genes, but no association with disease has been documented for these genes.

Gene structure

The *EXT1* gene is composed of 11 exons, and spans approximately 350 kb of genomic DNA {1673}. The cDNA has a coding region of 2238 bp {20}. The *EXT2* gene spans 108 kb and contains 16 exons, two of which (1a and 1b) are alternatively spliced {481}. It encodes a 718 amino acid protein with significant simi-

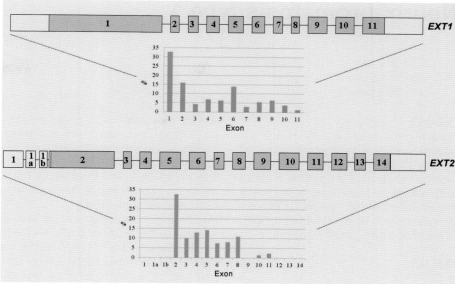

Fig. 27.15 Genomic structure of the *EXT1* (top) and *EXT2* (bottom) genes. Grey boxes represent coding regions. The mutation spectrum for each gene is illustrated below the genomic structure to include the frequency of exon involvement.

larity to the *EXT1* gene product, especially in the carboxy terminal region {2655, 3001}.

Gene function

Both *EXT1* and *EXT2* mRNA are ubiquitously expressed {20,2655,3001}. The gene products, exostosin-1 (EXT1) and exostosin-2 (EXT2), are endoplasmic reticulum localized type II transmembrane glycoproteins which form a Golgi-localized heterooligomeric complex that catalyses heparan sulfate (HS) polymerization {1631,1786,2559}.
Osteochondromas result from the presence of EXT-deficient (EXT-/-) and therefore HS-lacking chondrocytes that overproliferate due to a disturbed fibroblast growth factor and IHH signalling.

Mutations

Heterozygous *EXT* mutations are detected in 70–95% of the patients. Of these, *EXT1* mutations are detected in approximately 65% of cases, versus approximately 35% *EXT2* mutations. Inactivating mutations (nonsense, frameshift, and splice-site mutations) represent the majority of MO causing mutations (75–80%). In *EXT1*, mutations are more or less randomly distributed taking into account the exon size, while in *EXT2* most mutations are found in exons 2–8 {1326}. An overview of the reported variants is provided by the online Multiple Osteochondromas Mutation Database (http://medgen.ua.ac.be/LOVDv.2.0)

{1326}. In osteochondroma tissue, loss of the remaining wildtype allele has been demonstrated {283,2317}.
Mutations in *EXT1* seem to be associated with a more severe phenotype compared to *EXT2* mutations {51,52,1315,2257} but additional (genetic) factors also contribute to the final clinical presentation {1327}.

Neurofibromatosis type 1

E. Legius
H. Brems

Definition

Neurofibromatosis type 1 (NF1) is an autosomal dominant disorder characterized by café-au-lait spots (CALs), axillary and inguinal freckling, Lisch nodules of the iris and multiple neurofibromas. Malignant tumours can arise in all ages, with malignant peripheral nerve sheath tumours (MPNSTs) in adulthood being most common.

MIM No.   162200

Synonyms

Von Recklinghausen disease; peripheral neurofibromatosis

Epidemiology

NF1 is a common autosomal dominant disorder with an annual incidence of 1 per 3000 births and a prevalence of 1 per 4000 {1252}.

Diagnostic criteria

Diagnostic criteria for NF1 were established during a consensus conference of the NIH. Seven main criteria were defined {2048} and patients must exhibit two or more of the following features: (i) six or more CALs (> 5 mm diameter in children, > 15 mm in adults); (ii) two or more cutaneous or subcutaneous neurofibromas or one plexiform neurofibroma; (iii) axillary/inguinal freckling; (iv) optic pathway glioma (OPG); (v) two or more Lisch nodules in the iris; (vi) bone dysplasia; and (vii) first-degree relative with NF1 (by the above criteria).

Adults with NF1 easily fulfil these diagnostic criteria, but in young children the clinical diagnosis is more difficult since CALs are often the only manifestation. Patients with Legius syndrome, caused by SPRED1 mutations, also present with similar CALs and freckling, clinically indistinguishable from NF1 patients (especially at young age). Molecular genetic testing may be helpful {310,1859}.

Clinical features

Multiple cutaneous neurofibromas are benign peripheral nerve sheath tumours which typically develop during puberty

and are present in > 90% of NF1 individuals {827}. In contrast, clinical and mouse studies suggest that plexiform neurofibromas are of congenital origin {1579} and occur in 30–50% of NF1 individuals {827}. Plexiform neurofibromas have a risk of malignant transformation.

Additional typical manifestations include multiple CALs, axillary/inguinal freckling, Lisch nodules and OPGs {827}. CALs, the hallmark of NF1, may be present at birth and develop further during the first few years. Lisch nodules are asymptomatic iris hamartomas easily detected by slit-lamp examination in most NF1 individuals. Eighty-five percent of NF1 individuals will show axillary/inguinal freckling, usually after the age of 3 years. OPGs arise in 15–20% of NF1 children with a mean age at diagnosis of 4.5 years {254,2694}. Only one third of children with OPGs develop symptoms such as visual impairment.

Bone abnormalities can cause serious complications in NF1 individuals. Dystrophic scoliosis, sphenoid wing dysplasia, non-ossifying fibromas of long bones and similar lesions in the facial bones, and congenital tibial bowing are skeletal abnormalities typically associated with NF1. Congenital tibial bowing is present at birth in 5% of NF1 children. Progressive tibial bowing usually results in pathological fracture with development of a pseudarthrosis {738}.

Other clinical signs are short stature, macrocephaly, deficits in attention and cognitive function. Six to seven percent of NF1 individuals are intellectually disabled. Less common complications include epilepsy and cardiovascular problems.

Imaging

Plain film studies are commonly used to diagnose and follow skeletal abnormalities (scoliosis, non-ossifying fibromas, tibial bowing), but CT and MRI detect potentially associated tumours (OPGs, other brain and spinal tumours, internal plexiform neurofibromas, MPNSTs, pheochromocytomas). Even digital glomus tumours can be detected by MRI {2654}.

Whole-body MRIs of young adults with

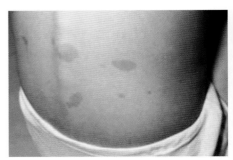

Fig. 27.16 Typical multiple café-au-lait spots in a child with neurofibromatosis type 1.

NF1 have been studied to detect individuals with a large (internal) tumour burden and who might be at increased risk of developing malignancies {1768}.

The use of FDG-PET is a helpful diagnostic tool in differentiating benign neurofibromas from atypical neurofibromas and MPNSTs {826}.

Unidentified bright objects (UBOs) are focal areas of T2 hyperintensities on brain MRI. UBOs are identified in the majority of NF1 children. An association between UBOs and cognitive dysfunction has been suggested, but not all studies confirm a relationship {824,1269}.

Neoplastic disease spectrum

NF1 children (aged < 5 years) have a higher risk of developing juvenile myelomonocytic leukaemia (JMML) than children without NF1, although the annual incidence is low (1 per 2000 to 1 per 5000) {2046}. NF1 individuals are at increased risk of developing benign and malignant solid tumours from both nervous and non-nervous system {309}.

Somatostatinomas (duodenal carcinoids) are rarely detected in NF1 individuals but are often metastatic when diagnosed {309}. About 1% of NF1 patients are diagnosed with pheochromocytomas, commonly with metastases at initial presentation {309,2332}.

Tumours of the optic pathway occur in 15–20% of children with NF1 {1636}. Most NF1-associated brain tumours in children are classified as pilocytic astrocytoma WHO grade I. Brain tumours in adults with

NF1 are less common. Grade IV astrocytomas (glioblastoma multiforme) are aggressive invasive tumours which infiltrate the brain and have a poor prognosis.

Tumours of soft tissue and bone
Non-nervous-system tumours
An association between digital glomus tumours and NF1 has been described {311}. NF1 children may develop non-ossifying fibromas of the long bones, sometimes reported as Jaffe-Campanacci syndrome {501}. Individuals with NF1 have a lifetime risk as high as 6% of developing gastrointestinal stromal tumours (GISTs) {309,1881}. NF1-associated GISTs mostly affect the small intestine and are multifocal {309}. Rhabdomyosarcomas have a prevalence of 0.5% in NF1 children {309}, typically affecting bladder, prostate, head and neck, trunk and extremities.

Peripheral nervous system tumours
Neurofibromas are the most frequent tumour identified in NF1 individuals, manifesting as focal cutaneous, subcutaneous or diffuse lesions. Cutaneous neurofibromas are typically benign, whereas plexiform neurofibromas have a risk of becoming malignant. NF1 individuals have an 8–13% lifetime risk of MPNST development {777}. Individuals with a germline NF1 microdeletion have a 16–26% risk {603}. MPNSTs are difficult to diagnose in the early phase and they often metastasize and have a poor prognosis. Atypical neurofibromas are thought to be premalignant lesions {178}.
Rarely, an association between neuro-blastoma and NF1 has been reported {1507}.

Genetics
Gene structure and expression
NF1 is caused by inactivating mutations in the NF1 gene that encodes neurofibromin {405,2882,2891}. NF1 (located in 17q11.2) is large (285 kb genomic region) and composed of 57 constitutive- and four alternatively-spliced exons (9a, 10a-2, 23a, 48a). Three genes are embedded in intron 27b

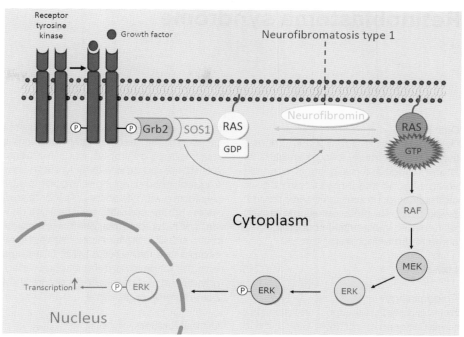

Fig. 27.17 The function of neurofibromin in the RAS-MAPK pathway. ERK, extracellular-signal-regulated kinase; MEK, MAP kinase kinase.

and transcribed in the opposite direction, EVI2A, EVI2B and OMGP. Neurofibromin is widely expressed during embryonic development, but most abundantly in the central nervous system. Neurofibromin is expressed in Schwann cells, neurons and oligodendrocytes {575}, leukocytes, adrenal medulla and many other cell types.

Gene function
Neurofibromin acts as a tumour suppressor. Different interaction partners of neurofibromin have been described, but two unequivocal functional domains are identified in neurofibromin, the Sec14-plextrin homology module and the RAS-GAP (GTPase-activating protein) related domain. Neurofibromin is a negative regulator of the RAS-MAPK pathway and stimulates intrinsic GTPase activity of RAS, resulting in the conversion of RAS-GTP into inactive RAS-GDP {1742}.

Mutations
Although no mutational hotspot has been identified, a pathogenic NF1 mutation is detected in 95% of NF1 individuals {1860}. Nonsense, frameshift, and splice-site mutations, small insertions, small deletions or small duplications all result in NF1 inactivation. In 5% of cases a NF1 microdeletion has been identified {1442}. Three types of microdeletions are known {188,1658,2225}. The NF1-associated tumours show somatic mutations; a second hit in NF1 has been reported in MPNSTs {1593}, neurofibromas {2513}, neuroblastomas {1749}, astrocytomas {1561}, GISTs {1694}, pheochromocytomas {3005}, glomus tumours {311} and JMML {2551}. A second hit has also been reported in CALs {1693} and pseudarthrosis tissue {2652}.

Retinoblastoma syndrome

W.K. Cavenee
O. Bogler
T. Hadjistilianou
I.F. Newsham

Definition

Retinoblastoma is a malignant tumour of the embryonic neural retina. Familial or bilateral retinoblastoma patients often develop second-site primary tumours including osteosarcoma, chondrosarcoma, Ewing sarcoma, pinealoblastoma, epithelial tumours, leukaemia, lymphoma, melanoma and brain tumours.

MIM No.   180200

Epidemiology

Retinoblastoma is the most common intraocular tumour of children, with a worldwide incidence between 1 per 3500 and 1 per 25 000 with no significant differences between the sexes or races {37,172,650, 2432}.

Diagnostic criteria

Presentation is "leukocoria", a white, pink-white, or yellow-white pupillary reflex that results from replacement of the vitreous humour by tumour, or by a large tumour growing in the macula {907}. Strabismus (exotropia or esotropia), can also occur alone or associated with leukocoria. Less frequent presenting signs include a red, painful eye with secondary glaucoma, low-vision orbital cellulitis, unilateral mydriasis, and heterochromia {3072}. Retinoblastoma occurs as a mass between the choroid and retina (exophytic) or a bulge from the retina toward the vitreous (endophytic) and most advanced tumours show both patterns of growth.

Clinical features

Retinoblastoma can be unifocal or multifocal. In bilateral cases, one eye is usually in a more advanced stage, with the contralateral eye having one or more tumour foci. The average age at diagnosis is 12 months for bilateral and 18 months for unilateral cases, with 90% of cases being diagnosed before the age of 3 years {38, 1464,2435,2772}. Retinoblastoma can be a part of the chromosome 13q14 deletion syndrome, in association with moderate growth and mental retardation, broad, prominent nasal bridge, short nose, ear and dental abnormalities, and muscular hypotonia {44,906}.

Trilateral retinoblastoma describes the association between bilateral retinoblastoma and midline brain tumours, usually in the pineal region {708}. Pineal tumours, resembling well-differentiated retinoblastomas, are also called ectopic retinoblastomas. CT scanning and MRI have reduced the misinterpretation of pineal tumours as intracranial spread of retinoblastoma {3072}. This is clinically important since ectopic intracranial retinoblastoma requires therapy to the whole neuraxis as well as high-dose equivalent radiotherapy to the primary tumour.

Imaging

Differentiation from a variety of simulating lesions, such as persistent hyperplastic primary vitreous, retrolental fibroplasia, Coats disease, toxocara canis infection, retinal dysplasia, or chronic retinal detachment can be difficult {1232,1233, 1628}, but can be accomplished using CT, MRI, ultrasonography or fine-needle aspiration biopsy (FNAB) and a careful history of the family and affected child {1628}.

Microscopic features

The tumour is histologically characterized by rosettes and fleurettes, likely representing matured or differentiated neoplastic cells. Rosettes are spherical structures (circular in section) of uniform cuboidal or short columnar cells, arranged about a small, round lumen (Flexner-Wintersteiner rosette) or without any lumen (Homer-Wright rosette). The latter also appears in other neuroectodermal tumours such as medulloblastoma. Fleurettes are arranged with short, thin stromal axes surrounded by differentiated neoplastic cells with their apical part facing the externum. Tumours can be necrotic, with surviving cells around blood vessels creating "pseudorosettes". Calcified foci and debris from nucleic acids can also be found in

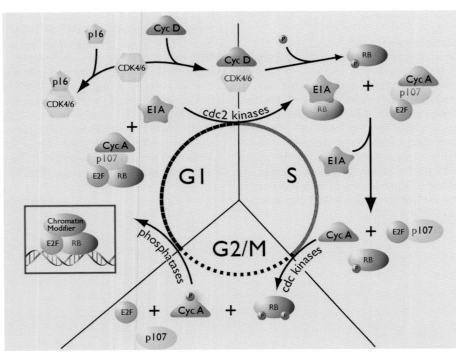

Fig. 27.18 Regulation of cell growth by the retinoblastoma protein (RB). Regulation of the cell cycle through oscillating phosphorylation of p105RB. Regulation of chromatin structure by RB is shown in G1.

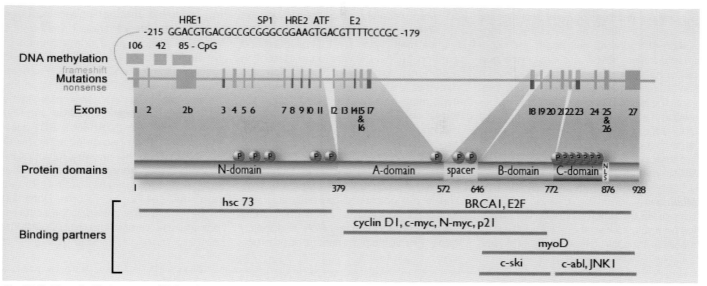

Fig. 27.19 The retinoblastoma gene (*RB1*) and mutations that are associated with the retinoblastoma syndrome. Genomic and protein domain organization of the 105 kD retinoblastoma protein. Mutational hotspots for frameshift and nonsense mutations are identified above individual exons. Orange rectangles represent regions of identified CpG methylation. The upstream DNA region between -215 and -175, representing the RB1 promoter, contains binding sites for a variety of transcription factors. Examples of some of the known cellular binding proteins and their region of interaction are depicted below the protein domains. Sites of phosphorylation are also indicated (P).

necrotic areas, giving rise to basophilic vessel walls {38,2435,2772}.

Growth patterns, degree of differentiation, number of mitoses and other histological parameters are not very useful for determining prognosis. Stronger relationships exist with invasion of the choroid, optic nerve and sclera. Progressive invasion of the eye coats, even in the horizontal plane, is highly informative for determining prognosis {1464,2772}.

Neoplastic disease spectrum

Retinoblastoma is the prototypic example of a genetic predisposition to cancer. About 60% of cases are nonhereditary and unilateral, 15% are hereditary and unilateral, and 25% are hereditary and bilateral. The latter two types occur with autosomal dominant inheritance and nearly complete penetrance. Epidemiological/cytogenetic {905,1167,1448,2616,2625,2668}, molecular genetic {402,403} and molecular biological {715,1225} analyses suggest that two stochastic mutational events are required in the *RB1* locus for tumour formation. The first mutation can be inherited through the germline or somatically acquired, whereas the second occurs somatically in either case. *RB1* locus inactivation is also found in non hereditary retinoblastoma {704}, osteosarcoma and other sarcomas occurring as second primary tumours in retinoblastoma patients, as well as some primary sarcomas in the absence of retinoblastoma involvement {915,1102}. Heterozygous *Rb1* knock-out mice, or mice harbouring a heterozygous germline *Rb1* defect, have a significant increase in the incidence of osteosarcomas after radiation exposure {1010}. The RB1 protein appears to function as a direct transcriptional coactivator of osteoblast differentiation that may explain why osteosarcomas are the most frequent secondary malignancy seen in patients with bilateral retinoblastoma following radiotherapy {2750}.

Tumours of soft tissue and bone

Second-site, primary malignant tumours (nonmetastatic tumours arising in "disease-free" patients treated for initial disease) associated with retinoblastoma include osteosarcoma, fibrosarcoma, chondrosarcoma, epithelial tumours, Ewing sarcoma, leukaemia, lymphoma, melanoma, brain tumours, and pinealoblastoma {8,639,697,2349,2405}. These second-site tumours are classified as: (i) tumours in the irradiated area; (ii) tumours outside and remote from the irradiated area; (iii) tumours in patients not receiving radiotherapy; (iv) tumours unable to be determined as primary or metastases; and (v) tumours in members of retinoblastoma families who were free of retinal tumours. The great majority of children in whom second neoplasms develop have bilateral retinoblastoma, and their incidence of second neoplasms is similar whether they received radiation or not. Osteosarcomas are the most frequent second-site neoplasms in all published series {8,639,697,2349,2405}.

Genetics

Gene structure and protein expression

The *RB1* locus in 13q14.1 {402,905,2616, 2668} encompasses 200 kb of genomic DNA organized into 27 exons {270, 928,1588} and encodes the 105 kD RB1 protein, which is ubiquitously expressed in normal human tissues. The RB1 protein is differentially phosphorylated {1589}, with the unphosphorylated form predominantly found in the G1 stage of the cell cycle, and an initial phosphorylation occurring at the G1/S boundary {338,615}. Viral proteins bind the p105RB protein {614,718,2952} using regions necessary for their transforming function. Over 100 intracellular pRB-binding proteins have also been identified, including the E2F family of transcription factors, lineage-specific transcription factors, the tumour suppressor BRCA1, DNA-modifying enzymes, members of chromatin remodelling complexes and RB-like proteins p107 and p130 {1953}. Complexing with the two latter factors also oscillates in a cell-cycle-dependent manner, linking the tumour-suppressing function of RB1 with transcriptional regulation. These protein interactions translate into many, somewhat paradoxical, biological roles for RB1, such as

G1 checkpoint control, control of cellular differentiation during embryogenesis, regulation of apoptotic cell death and autophagy, maintenance of senescence and quiescence, and preservation of chromosomal stability. Although RB1 clearly prevents the initiation of retinoblastoma, osteosarcoma and small cell lung cancer, most other tumour types display *RB1* alterations later in their progression, supporting a broader, tissue-specific contextual role for *RB1* in cancer {349,450,2880}.

Mutations

Loss of RB1 function has been described for retinoblastoma patients and their tumours at the DNA, RNA, and protein levels. More recently, epigenetic events at the *RB1* locus have been discovered. Differential methylation in a 1.2 kb CpG island in intron 2 (CpG 85) was found to result in preferential expression of *RB1* from the maternal allele {342,1362}. Furthermore, hypermethylation in the 5' *RB1* promoter region can also affect expression by reducing promoter activity. Such epigenetic alterations are significantly correlated with the incidence of unilateral, sporadic tumours {2107}. The observed differential penetrance and age at diagnosis variations in retinoblastoma patients may therefore result from altered methylation states and/or imprinted expression of the *RB1* gene. Exonic point mutations not disrupting the gene product have also been shown to create variance in penetrance and expression, as a consequence of residual function of these alleles in retinoblastoma precursor cells. Promoter haplotypes associated with *RB1* can further contribute to penetrance diversity by influencing transcriptional activity and *RB1* expression levels {518,1650}. *RB1* alterations have also been detected in a variety of second-site primary tumours including osteosarcoma, as well as other non-secondary tumours, such as breast and small-cell lung carcinoma. Detection of *RB1* mutations provides for accurate prenatal risk assessment {404,1226,2961, 3018}.

Rothmund-Thomson syndrome

N.M. Lindor
M.J. Hicks

Definition

Rothmund-Thomson syndrome (RTS) is an autosomal recessive genodermatosis with a diagnostic hallmark of a facial rash presenting in infancy (poikiloderma), and variable clinical findings, including skeletal abnormalities, sparse scalp hair, juvenile cataracts, premature ageing, skeletal abnormalities, and early onset of osteosarcoma, skin cancers and other tumours {1542,1543,2897,2899}. *RECQL4* (8q24.3) mutations have been identified in about two thirds of patients. This syndrome has been divided into two types {1543,2896}. The above description is for RTS type II with truncating *RECQL4* mutations. RTS type I, with poikiloderma and juvenile cataracts, lacks truncating *RECQL4* mutations.

MIM No.   268400

Synonym
Poikiloderma congenitale

Epidemiology
RTS is a rare disorder with 300 reported cases affecting all ethnic and racial groups {1543,2896,2897,2899}.

Diagnostic criteria
The hallmark of RTS is poikiloderma, presenting in infancy with skin erythema, swelling and blistering of the cheeks and face {1543,2899}. The rash spreads to the extremities and buttocks, with truncal and abdominal sparing. The rash enters a chronic lifelong phase with reticulated hypopigmentation or hyperpigmentation, telangiectasia and atrophy. Probable RTS is suggested with an atypical rash and two of the following features: (i) sparse scalp hair, eyelashes, or eyebrows; (ii)

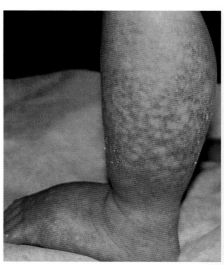

Fig. 27.20 Poikiloderma in Rothmund-Thomson syndrome. Extensor surface of the lower leg demonstrating the chronic phase with skin atrophy, marbleized mixed hypo- and hyperpigmentation with telangiectasia.

short stature; (iii) gastrointestinal disturbance; (iv) radial ray defects; (v) radiological bone abnormalities; (vi) dental abnormalities; (vii) nail abnormalities; (viii) hyperkeratosis; (ix) cataracts; and (x) cancer {1543,2899}.

Clinical features

The dermatological hallmark of RTS is an erythematous, oedematous and blistering rash followed by a chronic lifelong phase, as described previously {1543,2896,2897, 2899}. Additional findings include skeletal dysplasia (75%), sparse to absent eyelashes/eyebrows (73%), short stature with normal growth hormone (66%), low birth weight (66%), sparse scalp hair with premature greying (50–75%), cataracts (7–50%), photosensitivity (35%), dental abnormalities (27–59%), radial ray defects (20%), and dystrophic nails {1543,2897, 2899}. Gastrointestinal abnormalities reported include oesophageal/pyloric stenosis, anal atresia, annular pancreas, rectovaginal fistula, feeding problems, emesis and diarrhoea. RTS ocular lesions include exophthalmos, corneal atrophy/-scleralization, congenital bilateral glaucoma, retinal atrophy/coloboma, strabismus, photophobia/photosensitivity, iris dysgenesis and blue sclerae. Haematological abnormalities include leukopoenia, chronic microcytic hypochromic anaemia, myelodysplasia and aplastic anaemia. Normal neurological milestones and intelligence are the rule. Hypogonadism and infertility may occur. There is an increased malignancy risk, most commonly osteosarcoma and skin cancer {1175,1543, 2897,2899}.

Potential guidelines in suspected RTS cases include: a baseline radiographical skeletal survey by age 5 years for dysplasias; examination for cataracts; and parental counselling regarding protection from excess sun exposure and awareness of RTS medical risks {1175,2896,2897, 2899}. Ongoing care may include: (i) annual evaluation by physician familiar with RTS; (ii) annual eye examination; (iii) skin cancer screening; and (iv) skeletal radiographs if osteosarcoma is suspected {1175,2896, 2897,2899}.

Imaging

Radiological skeletal abnormalities occur in 75% of cases {1808,2897,2899}. Most common are metaphyseal trabeculation (64%), brachymesophalangy (64%), thumb agenesis/hypoplasia (43%), osteopenia (43%), patellar hypoplasia, aplasia or multicentric ossification (25%), radial head dislocation (21%), radial agenesis/hypoplasia (21%), radioulnar synostosis (18%), ulnar hypoplasia/bowing (18%), butterfly vertebrae (4%) and 13 rib pairs (4%) {1808}.

Neoplastic disease spectrum

Osteosarcoma (32%; mean age, 11 years) and basal and squamous cell carcinomas (5%; mean age, 34 years) occur at an earlier age than in the general population {1175,1543,2896,2897,2899}. Other primary and secondary malignancies include myelodysplastic syndrome, acute myeloid leukaemia, Hodgkin/non-Hodgkin

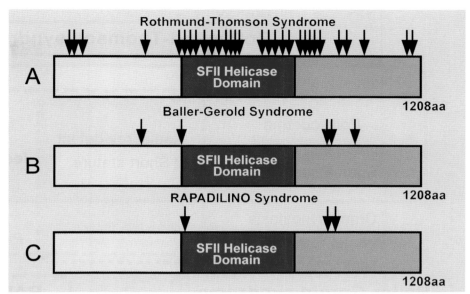

Fig. 27.21 Mutations in RECQL4 protein. In Rothmund-Thomson syndrome (A), most mutations occur in the helicase region of the RECQL4 protein, whereas in the Baller-Gerold (B) and RAPADILINO syndromes (C), most mutations occur in the flanking regions outside of the helicase region.

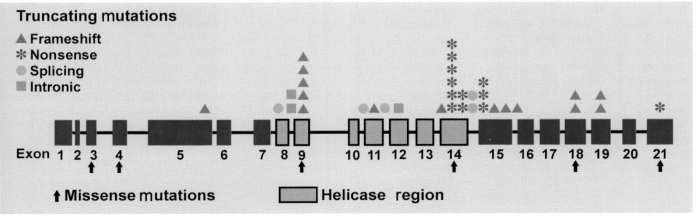

Fig. 27.22 Schematic of the *RECQL4* gene, indicating location and type of mutations occurring in Rothmund-Thomson syndrome.

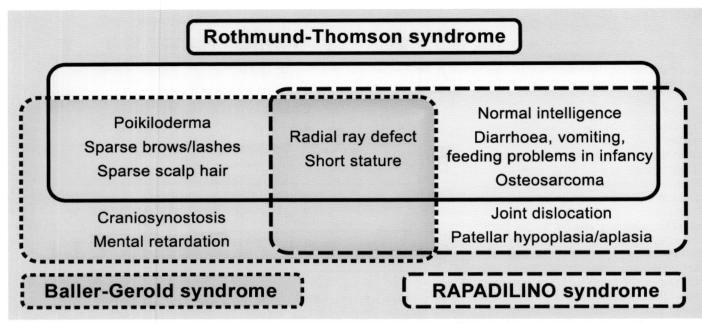

Fig. 27.23 The diagram ilustrates how the clinical features of Rothmund-Thomson syndrome overlap with those of Baller-Gerold and RAPADILINO syndromes; these autosomal recessive syndromes are all associated with mutations in the *RECQL4* gene.

lymphoma, gastric carcinoma, malignant eccrine poroma, fibrosarcoma and undifferentiated pleomorphic sarcoma {1542, 1543, 2897,2899}.

Tumours of soft tissue and bone
Reported sites of RTS osteosarcoma are distal femur (50%), proximal tibia (25%), proximal humerus (25%), distal fibula (7%), distal ulna (7%), distal radius (7%) and patella (7%). Around 30% may be multicentric. Histological subtypes included osteoblastic (72%), fibroblastic (14%), chondroblastic (7%) and telangiectatic/giant cell rich (7%). Following chemotherapy, the histological response is similar to that for sporadic osteosarcoma. Second malignancies develop in 16% of cases, with non-Hodgkin lymphoma, Hodgkin lymphoma and squamous cell carcinoma being reported {1175,2897,2899}. Conventional chemotherapy is recommended, with close observation for doxorubicin sensitivity.

Genetics
The *RECQL4* helicase gene (8q24.3) spans 21 exons, including binding sites for AP1, AP2CRE and PAE3 transcription factors {967,1542,1543,1640}. It encodes a 133 kDa protein (RECQ protein-Like 4) comprised of an ATP-dependent, superfamily II helicase. *RECQL4* mutations may result in RTS, Baller-Gerold syndrome or RAPADILINO syndrome, with overlapping features among these autosomal recessive syndromes {1542,1543,2899}. Baller-Gerold syndrome is associated with radial ray defects, skeletal dysplasia, short stature and craniosynostosis. RAPADILINO includes radial hypoplasia/-aplasia, patellar hypoplasia/aplasia, cleft/-high-arched palate, diarrhoea, dislocated joints, small size, limb malformations, slender nose and normal intelligence.

Most RTS mutations occur within the superfamily II helicase domain, and less frequently within the N-terminus and C-terminus. RECQL4 functions include: single-stranded DNA annealing; stabilizing complex for chromosome segregation and apoptosis; DNA replication; DNA repair and homologous recombination; oxidative-stress reduction; UV-induced DNA-damage repair; and telomere maintenance with shelterin (TRF1, TRF2, POT1) and WRN interaction {967,1542, 1543, 1640}. *RECQL4* mutations include: nonsense mutations; insertions/deletions with frameshifts; splicing alterations with exon skipping, frameshift and intron deletions; and missense mutations. Most RTS mutations are nonsense or frameshift mutations, resulting in mRNA destabilization. Truncating *RECQL4* mutations occur in RTS patients with osteosarcoma, and nontruncating mutations in RTS patients without osteosarcoma {1542,1543,2896}. Truncating mutations are clustered in the helicase region. Chromosomal instability with mosaic aneuploidy and isochromosomes is present. Acquired cytogenetic abnormalities include chromosome 8 (trisomy, partial 8q duplication, tetrasomy, isochromosome 8q), trisomy 7 and trisomy 2 {1542,1543,2896,2899}. In a young child with only poikiloderma, the differential diagnosis includes: acrogeria, hereditary sclerosing poikiloderma, dyskeratosis congenita, Kindler syndrome, xeroderma pigmentosum, poikiloderma with neutropenia, exocrine pancreatic hypofunction and atrophy, Bloom syndrome, Werner syndrome, Fanconi anaemia, ataxia telangiectasia, and Cockayne syndrome {1542,1543,2897}. *RECQL4* molecular analyses are helpful in providing an accurate diagnosis.

Werner syndrome

R.J. Monnat Jr

Definition

Werner syndrome (WS) is a rare, autosomal recessive, genetic instability syndrome with a phenotype that mimics premature aging and is caused by inactivation of the *WRN* gene.

MIM No.   277700

Synonyms

Werner syndrome; progeria of the adult

Epidemiology

Patients with WS have been identified worldwide, with the largest number in Japan {1017}. Estimates of the frequency or prevalence of WS, obtained from case-counting and consanguinity data, range from 1 per 22000 to 1 per 10^6 {2464}. The frequency of WS is strongly influenced by the presence of local founder mutations and consanguinity. WS is likely to be under-diagnosed by virtue of its variable, slowly developing and incompletely penetrant clinical phenotype {762,1017, 1967,2464}.

Clinical features and diagnostic criteria

Patients develop a prematurely aged appearance in the second and third decades of life, and are at increased risk of developing age-associated neoplastic and non-neoplastic diseases. The elevated risk of neoplasia in WS is selective, and divided almost equally between epithelial and non-epithelial neoplasms. The most common causes of death are cancer and atherosclerotic cardiovascular disease.

The most consistent clinical findings, seen after age 10 years, include bilateral cataracts; scleroderma-like skin changes; short stature; and premature greying and loss of scalp hair. There may be affected siblings, as well as parental consanguinity (third cousin or closer). Additional, less consistent findings include diabetes mellitus; hypogonadism; osteoporosis; soft tissue calcification, most notably of the Achilles tendon; premature atherosclerotic cardiovascular disease; a high pitched, "squeaky" or hoarse voice; and flat feet {762,1017,1967,2134,2464}. Clinical find-

ings and family history, if scored consistently, allow the reliable identification of definite, probable or possible WS patients {71,2134,2464}. A definitive diagnosis can be established by *WRN* mutation typing in conjunction with demonstration of loss of expression of the WRN protein (see below).

Neoplastic disease spectrum

WS patients are at increased risk of developing both sarcomas and epithelial neoplasms {1018,1932}. The elevated risk of neoplasia in WS is selective. Table 26.05 summarizes a recent, quantitatively rigorous analysis of tumour spectrum and risk in a cohort of 189 WS patients with

Table 27.05 Histopathological spectrum of neoplasia in Werner syndrome

Frequent neoplasms (67% of total)[a]	Less common neoplasms (33% of total)
Thyroid neoplasms (15.8%) Follicular carcinoma Papillary thyroid carcinoma Anaplastic thyroid carcinoma Thyroid adenoma	**Non-melanoma skin cancer (4.9%)** Squamous cell carcinoma Basal cell carcinoma
Malignant melanoma (13.0%) Acral lentiginous melanoma (ALM) Malignant mucosal melanoma Malignant melanoma non-ALM	**Gastrointestinal (4.9%)** Oesophageal carcinoma Gastric adenocarcinoma Pancreatic adenocarcinoma
Meningioma (11.3%)	**Uterus/ovary (4.0%)** Ovarian cystadenocarcinoma Uterine carcinoma Uterine leiomyoma
Soft tissue sarcomas (9.7%) Undifferentiated pleomorphic sarcoma Leiomyosarcoma Fibrosarcoma Malignant peripheral nerve sheath tumour Rhabdomyosarcoma Synovial sarcoma	**Hepatobiliary (4.0%)** Cholangiocarcinoma Hepatocellular carcinoma
Haematologic/lymphoid (9.3%) Acute myeloid leukaemia (M1–M5, M6, M7) Pre-leukaemic marrow disorders 　Myelofibrosis 　Myelodysplasia 　Refractory anaemia with excess blasts T-cell leukaemia Plasmacytoma	**Genito-urinary (3.6%)** Ureteral transitional cell carcinoma Bladder transitional cell carcinoma Vulvar carcinoma Prostrate carcinoma
Osteosarcoma/bone (7.7%) Conventional osteosarcoma Extraskeletal osteosarcoma	**Head and neck neoplasms (3.2%)** Nasal carcinoma NOS Hard/soft palate squamous cell carcinoma Tongue squamous cell carcinoma Laryngeal carcinoma NOS
Osteochondroma	**Breast carcinoma (2.8%)**
	Lung (2.0%) Squamous cell carcinoma Adenocarcinoma Bronchioloalveolar carcinoma Carcinoid
	CNS (2.0%) Astrocytoma Spinal cord haemangiolipoma
	Adrenal (1.6%) Cortical carcinoma Pheochromocytoma

[a] Table data are from a recent, quantitatively rigorous analysis of tumour spectrum and risk that included 189 WS patients with 247 neoplasms reported between 1939 and 2011, where 139 patients were resident in Japan and the remaining 50 were from a diversity of locations outside of Japan {1565A}. WS patients are at a substantially elevated risk of developing all of the frequent neoplasms listed in the left column of the table.

NOS, not otherwise specified.

247 neoplasms reported between 1939 and 2011 {1565A}. This cohort included 139 resident in Japan WS patients and 50 patients from a diversity of locations outside Japan. The most frequent neoplasms in WS patients, representing two thirds of all reports, were, in order of decreasing frequency: thyroid neoplasms, malignant melanoma, meningioma, soft tissue sarcomas, leukaemia and pre-leukaemic conditions, and osteosarcoma. These frequent neoplasms occur at significantly elevated risk in Japanese WS patients compared with population controls {1565A}. Thyroid neoplasms and melanoma are significantly under-represented in WS patients outside Japan for unknown reasons. Many other neoplasms, including common adult epithelial malignancies, have been observed in WS patients (Table 27.05). However, it is not clear whether these neoplasms are significantly more frequent in WS patients compared with population controls. Multiple neoplasia is common: 21.7% of patients (41 of 189) had one to four additional, concurrent or sequential neoplasms, and these were often at different sites {1018, 1565A}.

Several features of neoplasia in WS are of diagnostic or pathogenetic interest. The risk of malignant melanoma is confined almost exclusively to relatively rare variants that arise on the palms and soles (acral lentigenous melanoma, ALM), or in mucosa (e.g. the nasal cavity or oesophagus). Thyroid neoplasms include frequent follicular and less frequent papillary and anaplastic neoplasms. Leukaemias cover the full spectrum of acute myelogenous leukaemia. Atypical leukaemias have been reported, as have many cases of preleukaemic marrow disorders such as myelodysplasia, myelofibrosis and refractory anaemia with an excess of blasts (RAEB). Rare lymphoid neoplasms (T-cell leukaemia, plasmacytoma) have also been reported. The elevated risk of developing marrow-associated premalignant or malignant disease in WS, may be related to the progressive accumulation of genetic damage in bone marrow {1956}. The histopathological spectrum of neoplasia in WS overlaps with, although distinct from, two other RecQ helicase deficiency syndromes, Bloom syndrome and Rothmund-Thomson syndrome {1932}.

Tumours of soft tissue and bone

Soft tissue sarcomas in WS include, in order of decreasing frequency: undifferentiated pleomorphic sarcoma, leiomyosarcoma, fibrosarcoma, malignant and benign nerve sheath tumours, pleomorphic rhabdomyosarcoma and synovial sarcoma. Osteosarcomas, the only well-documented malignant bone tumour in WS, display osteoblastic or fibroblastic differentiation and may be extraskeletal.

Genetics

The WRN (RECQL2) gene consists of 35 exons in a 165 kb region at 8p11–12 {3041}. The WRN protein has DNA helicase and exonuclease activities that play important physiological roles in DNA metabolism {1933}. Werner syndrome patients have pathogenic null mutations in both WRN alleles, which result in loss of the WRN protein {914,1019,1957,1967, 2813}. Molecular confirmation can be especially helpful in the diagnosis of WS in young patients, or where the diagnosis is suspected but inconclusive on clinical grounds alone. Pathogenic WRN mutations and polymorphisms have been summarized in the WRN Mutational Database {69}. Additional information on WS diagnosis and molecular testing can be obtained from the International Registry of Werner Syndrome {71} and from GeneTests {70}.

Contributors

Dr Thomas AIGNER
Medical Center Coburg
Klinikum Coburg GmbH
Coburg D-96450
GERMANY
Tel. +49 9561 226213
Fax +49 9651 227590
thomas.aigner@klinikum-coburg.de

Dr Benjamin A. ALMAN
Dept of Surgery, Division of Orthopaedics
Hospital for Sick Children
University of Toronto
Toronto, ON MSG1X8
CANADA
Tel. +1 416 813 7980
Fax +1 416 813 6414
benjamin.alman@sickkids.ca

Dr Eliane M. I. AMSTALDEN
Dept of Pathology, School of Medical Sciences
State University of Campinas (UNICAMP)
Rua Tessália Vieira de Camargo, 126
Campinas, CEP 13083-887, SP
BRAZIL
Tel. +55 19 32893897
Fax +55 19 32893897
ingrid@fcm.unicamp.br

Dr Cristina R. ANTONESCU*
Dept of Pathology
Memorial Sloan-Kettering Cancer Center
New York, NY 10065
USA
Tel. +1 212 639 5905
Fax +1 212 717 3203
antonesc@mskcc.org

Dr Nicholas A. ATHANASOU*
Dept of Histopathology
Nuffield Dept of Orthopaedics, Rheumatology
and Musculoskeletal Sciences
Oxford OX3 7LD
UK
Tel. +44 1 865 738 136
Fax +44 1 865 738140
Nick.Athanasou@ndorms.ox.ac.uk

Dr Manjula BANSAL
Dept of Pathology / Laboratory Medicine
Hospital for Special Surgery
535 E 70th Street
New York, NY 10021
USA
Tel. +1 212 606 1105
Fax +1 212 606 1910
bansalm@hss.edu

Dr Frederic G. BARR
Laboratory of Pathology
National Cancer Institute
Bethesda, MD 20892
USA
Tel. +1 301 594 3780
Fax +1 301 480 0853
barrfg@mail.nih.gov

Dr Daniel BAUMHOER
Bone Tumor Reference Center
Institute of Pathology
University Hospital Basel
Basel, CH-4031
SWITZERLAND
Tel. +41 61 328 6892
Fax +41 61 265 3194
dbaumhoer@mac.com

Dr Alfred BEHAM
Institute of Pathology
University of Graz Medical School
Graz, A-8036
AUSTRIA
Tel. +43 316 380 4410
Fax +43 316 373 890
alfred.beham@medunigraz.at

Dr Paolo BIANCO
Anatomic Pathology, Stem Cell Laboratory
Dept of Molecular Medicine
Viale Regina Elena 324
Rome, 00161 Rome
ITALY
Tel. +39 06 444 1049
Fax +39 06 494 0896
paolo.bianco@uniroma1.it

Dr Jaclyn A. BIEGEL
The Children's Hospital of Philadelphia
Abramson Research Building, Room 1002
Philadelphia, PA 19104
USA
Tel. +1 215 590 3856
Fax +1 215 590 3764
biegel@mail.med.upenn.edu

Dr Beata BODE-LESNIEWSKA
Institute of Surgical Pathology
University Hospital Zurich
Zurich, CH-8091
SWITZERLAND
Tel. +41 44 255 4051
Fax +41 44 255 4416
beata.bode@usz.ch

Dr Oliver BOGLER
Academic Affairs
MD Anderson Cancer Center
1515 Holcombe Boulevard
Houston, TX 77030-4009
USA
Tel. +1 713 792 0873
Fax +1 713 745 4277
obogler@mdanderson.org

Dr Fred BOSMAN*
University Institute of Pathology
Rue du Bugnon 25
1011 Lausanne
SWITZERLAND
Tel. +41 21 314 7202
Fax. +41 21 314 7205
fred.bosman@chuv.ch

Dr Judith V. M. G. BOVEE*
Dept of Pathology
Leiden University Medical Center
PO Box 9600, L1-Q
Leiden, 2300 RC
THE NETHERLANDS
Tel. +31 71 526 6617
Fax +31 71 526 6952
j.v.m.g.bovee@lumc.nl

*The asterisk indicates participation in the Working Group Meeting on the Classification of Tumours of the Soft Tissue and Bone that was held in Zurich, Switzerland, April 18–20, 2012

Dr Johannes BRAS
Academisch Medisch Centrum
Amsterdam, 1105 AZ
THE NETHERLANDS
Tel. +31 20 566 2827
Fax +31 20 566 9523
j.bras@amc.uva.nl

Dr Hilde BREMS
Dept of Human Genetics
Catholic University of Leuven
Leuven, 3000
BELGIUM
Tel. "+32 16 34 13 20
Fax +32 16 346051
Hilde.Brems@med.kuleuven.be

Dr Thomas BRENN
Dept of Pathology, NHS Lothian University Hos-
pitals Trust and the University of Edinburgh
Alexander Donald Building
Western General Hospital
Edinburgh EH4 2XU
SCOTLAND
Tel. +44 131 537 1957
Fax +44 131 537 3618
t_brenn@yahoo.com

Dr Julia A. BRIDGE*
Depts of Pathology/Microbiology,
Pediatrics and Orthopaedic Surgery
University of Nebraska Medical Center
Omaha, NE 68198-3135
USA
Tel. +1 402 559 7212
Fax +1 402 559 6018
jbridge@unmc.edu

Dr J. Eduardo CALONJE*
St John's Institute of Dermatology
St Thomas' Hospital
Lambeth Palace Road
London SE1 7EH
UK
Tel. +44 207 1886408
Fax +44 207 1886382
jaime.calonje@kcl.ac.uk

Dr J. Aidan CARNEY
Dept of Laboratory Medicine and Pathology
Mayo Clinic
Plummer North 10
Rochester, MN 55905
USA
Tel. +1 507 284 2691
Fax +1 507 284 5036
carney.aidan@mayo.edu

Dr Webster K. CAVENEE
Ludwig Institute for Cancer Research
University of California, San Diego
Cellular and Molecular Medicine East
La Jolla, CA 92093-0660
USA
Tel. +1 858 534 7805
Fax +1 858 534 7750
wcavenee@ucsd.edu

Dr John K.C. CHAN
Dept of Pathology
Queen Elizabeth Hospital
Kowloon
HONG KONG SAR CHINA
Tel. +852 2958 6830
Fax +852 2385 2455
jkcchan@ha.org.hk

Dr Frederic CHIBON
Dept of Pathology
Institut Bergonié
Bordeaux Cedex, 33076
FRANCE
Tel. +33 3 56 330439
Fax +33 5 56 330438
chibon@bergonie.org

Dr Anne-Marie CLETON-JANSEN
Dept of Pathology
Leiden University Medical Center
PO Box 9600, L1-Q
Leiden, 2300 RC
THE NETHERLANDS
Tel. +31 71 5266515
Fax +31 71 5266952
a.m.cleton-jansen@lumc.nl

Dr Cheryl M. COFFIN*
Dept of Pathology, Microbiology, & Immunobiology
Vanderbilt University Medical Center North
C3324
Nashville, TN 37232-2561
USA
Tel. +1 615 322 2302
Fax +1 615 322 5551
cheryl.coffin@vanderbilt.edu

Dr Jean-Michel COINDRE*
Dept of Pathology
Institut Bergonié
Bordeaux Cedex, 33076
FRANCE
Tel. +33 556 333 333
Fax +33 556 333 389
coindre@bergonie.org

Dr Christopher L. CORLESS
Dept of Pathology
Oregon Health and Science University
Portland, OR 97239-3098
USA
Tel. +1 503 494 6776
Fax +1 503 494 6787
corlessc@ohsu.edu

Dr Bogdan A. CZERNIAK
Dept of Pathology
The University of Texas
M.D. Anderson Cancer Center
Houston, TX 77030
USA
Tel. +1 713 794 1025
Fax +1 713 792 4094
bczernia@mdanderson.org

Dr Paola DAL CIN
Dept of Pathology
Brigham and Women's Hospital
Boston, MA 02115-6195
USA
Tel. +1 857 307 5124
Fax +1 857 307 1522
pdalcin@partners.org

Dr Enrique DE ALAVA*
Dept of Pathology
Centro de Investigacion del Cancer and
Salamanca University Hospital
Salamanca, E-37007
SPAIN
Tel. +34 923 294 820
Fax +34 923 294 795
edealava@usal.es

Dr Carlos E. DE ANDREA
Dept of Histology and Pathology
University of Navarra
c/Irunlarrea 1
Pamplona, 31008
SPAIN
Tel. +34 948 42 6215 (ext. 6231)
Fax +34 948 425 649
ceandrea@unav.es

Dr Diederik DE BRUIJN
Dept of Human Genetics
Radboud University
Nijmegen Medical Center
Nijmegen, 6500 HB
THE NETHERLANDS
Tel. +31 24 361 9635
Fax +31 24 366 8752
d.debruijn@antrg.umcn.nl

Dr Gonzague DE PINIEUX
Dept of Pathology
Hôpital Trousseau - CHU de Tours
Tours Cedex 9, 37044
FRANCE
Tel. + 33 247 478 111
Fax + 33 247 474 622
depinieux@med.univ-tours.fr

Dr Nicolas DE SAINT AUBAIN SOMERHAUSEN
Service d'Anatomie Pathologique, Cytologie,
et Cytogénétique
Institut Jules Bordet
Brussels, 1000
BELGIUM
Tel. +32 484 942 668
Fax +32 541 32 81
nicolas.desaintaubain@bordet.be

Dr Barry DE YOUNG
Dept of Pathology
University of Iowa Hospitals and Clinics
200 Hawkins Drive
Iowa City, IA 52242
USA
Tel. +1 319 356 4433
Fax +1 319 384 9613
barry-deyoung@uiowa.edu

Dr Maria DEBIEC-RYCHTER
Dept of Human Genetics
Catholic University of Leuven
Leuven, 3000
BELGIUM
Tel. +32 16 347218
Fax +32 16 346210
maria.debiec-rychter@med.kuleuven.be

Dr Angelo Paolo DEI TOS*
Depts of Oncology and Anatomic Pathology
General Hospital of Treviso
Treviso, 31100
ITALY
Tel. +39 0422 322 707
Fax +39 0422 322 705
apdeitos@ulss.tv.it

Dr Andrea T. DEYRUP
Pathology Consultants
Greenville, SC 29605
USA
Tel. +1 864 455 3455
Fax +1 864 455 8926
atdeyrup@yahoo.com

Dr Sarah M. DRY
Dept of Pathology and Laboratory Medicine
David Geffen School of Medicine
University of California Los Angeles
Los Angeles, CA 90095-1732
USA
Tel. +1 310 794 9311
Fax +1 310 267 2058
sdry@mednet.ucla.edu

Dr R. Maarten EGELER
Division of Haematology/Oncology
Hospital for Sick Children
555 University Avenue
Toronto ON M5G 1X8
CANADA
Tel. +1 416 813 7654
Fax +1 416 813 5327
maarten.egeler@sickkids.ca

Dr Harry L. EVANS
Division of Anatomic Pathology
University of Texas MD Anderson Cancer
Center
Houston, TX 77030
USA
Tel. +1 713 792 2143
Fax +1 713 792 5531
hevans@mdanderson.org

Dr Julie C. FANBURG-SMITH
Dept of Pathology/
Surgical Pathology Consultation Services
Sibley Memorial Hospital ofJohns Hopkins Medicine
Washington, DC 20016
USA
Tel. +1 703 623 7013
Fax +1 202 537 4466
jcfsmd@gmail.com

Dr John F. FETSCH
Dept of Soft Tissue Pathology
Joint Pathology Center
Silver Spring, MD 20910
USA
Tel. +1 301 295 7275
Fax +1 301 295 5675
john.fetsch@us.army.mil

Dr Adrienne M. FLANAGAN*
University College London Cancer Institute
London WC1E 6BT
UK
Tel. +44 20 8909 5354
Fax +44 20 7679 6470
a.flanagan@ucl.ac.uk

Dr Christopher D. M. FLETCHER*
Dept of Pathology
Brigham and Women's Hospital
Boston, MA 02115
USA
Tel. +1 617 732 8558
Fax +1 617 566 3897
cfletcher@partners.org

Dr Jonathan A. FLETCHER*
Dept of Pathology
Brigham and Women's Hospital
Harvard Medical School
Boston, MA 02115
USA
Tel. +1 617 732 7883
Fax +1 617 278 6921
jfletcher@partners.org

Dr Uta FLUCKE
Dept of Pathology
Radboud University Nijmegen Medical Center
Nijmegen, 6500HB
THE NETHERLANDS
Tel. +31 24 361 4387
Fax +31 24 366 8750
U.Flucke@pathol.umcn.nl

Dr Andrew L. FOLPE*
Department of Laboratory Medicine and
Pathology
Mayo Clinic
Rochester, MN 55901
USA
Tel. +1 507 284 8730
Fax +1 507 284 1599
folpe.andrew@mayo.edu

Dr Ramses FORSYTH
Pathlicon, Histopathological and Molecular
Laboratories
Reibroekstraat 13
Evergem (Ghent) OVL, BE-9940
BELGIUM
Tel. +32 925 360 30
Fax +32 925 355 37
ramses.forsyth@pathlicon.be

Dr Ad GEURTS VAN KESSEL
Dept of Human Genetics
University Hospital Nijmegen
Nijmegen, 6500 HB
THE NETHERLANDS
Tel. +31 24 361 4107
Fax +31 24 366 8752
A.GeurtsVanKessel@antrg.umcn.nl

Dr Briana C. GLEASON
Diagnostic Pathology Medical Group, Inc.
Sacramento, CA 95816
USA
Tel. +1 916 446 0424
Fax +1 916 446 9330
bgleason@dpmginc.com

Dr John R. GOLDBLUM
Dept of Anatomic Pathology
The Cleveland Clinic Foundation
Cleveland, OH 44195
USA
Tel. +1 219 444 8238
Fax +1 216 445 6967
goldblj@ccf.org

Dr Robert J. GRIMER
The Royal Orthopaedic Hospital
NHS Foundation Trust, Northfield
Birmingham, B31 2AP
UK
Tel. +44 121 685 4019
Fax +44 121 685 4146
Robert.Grimer@nhs.net,
rob.grimer@btopenworld.com

Dr Alessandro GRONCHI
Dept of Surgery
Istituto Nazionale dei Tumori
Milan, 20133
ITALY
Tel. +39 022 3993 234
Fax +39 022 3902 404
alessandro.gronchi@istitutotumori.mi.it

Dr Theodora HADJISTILIANOU
Dept of Ophthalmology, Ocular Oncology Unit
School of Medicine
University of Siena, Siena
ITALY
Tel. +39 0577 585 784
Fax +39 0577 233 358
hadjistilian@unisi.it

Dr Meera HAMEED
Memorial Sloan-Kettering Cancer Center
1275 York Avenue
New York, 10065
USA
Tel. +1 212 639 5905
Fax +1 646 422 2070
hameedm@mskcc.org

Dr Esther HAUBEN
Dept of Pathology
University Hospitals Leuven
Leuven, 3000
BELGIUM
Tel. +32 16 341658
Fax +32 16 336640
esther.hauben@uzleuven.be

Dr Sverre HEIM
Oslo University Hospital
The Norwegian Radium Hospital Institute for
Medical Informatics
Section for Cancer Cytogenetics
Oslo, N-0310
NORWAY
Tel. +47 2 293 4468
Fax +47 2 293 5477
sverre.heim@medisin.uio.no

Dr Dominique HEYMANN
Pathophysiology of Bone Resorption and
Therapy of Primary Bone Tumors
University of Nantes
Faculty of Medicine
Nantes Cedex 1, 44035
FRANCE
Tel.+33(0)240 412 845
Fax +33(0)240 412 860
Dominique.heymann@univ-nantes.fr

Dr M. John HICKS
Dept of Pathology, Baylor College of Medicine
Texas Children's Hospital
Abercrombie Building, MC 1-2261
Houston, TX 77030
USA
Tel. +1 832 824 1869
Fax +1 832 825 1032
mjhicks@texaschildrenshospital.org

Dr Masanori HISAOKA
Dept of Pathology & Oncology
University of Occupational & Environmental Health
Fukuoka, 807-8555
JAPAN
Tel. +81 93 691 7425
Fax +81 93 692 0189
hisaoka@med.uoeh-u.ac.jp

Dr Pancras C. W. HOGENDOORN*
Dept of Pathology
Leiden University Medical Center
Building 1, Room H-01-34
Postzone L1Q
Leiden, 2300 RC
THE NETHERLANDS
Tel. +31 71 526 2559
Fax +31 71 524 8126
p.c.w.hogendoorn@lumc.nl

Dr Jason L. HORNICK*
Dept of Pathology
Brigham and Women's Hospital
Boston, MA 02115
USA
Tel. +1 617 525 7257
Fax +1 617 566 3897
jhornick@partners.org

Dr Andrew HORVAI
University of California, San Francisco
San Francisco, CA 94115
USA
Tel. +1 415-885-7313
Fax +1 415-673-9726
Andrew.horvai@ucsf.edu

Dr Hsuan-Ying HUANG
Dept of Anatomical Pathology
Kaohsiung Chang Gung Memorial Hospital
and Chang Gung University College of Medicine
Kaohsiung City, 833
TAIWAN, CHINA
Tel. +88 6 7 731 7123 ext. 2537
Fax +88 6 7 733 3198
a120600310@yahoo.com

Dr Carrie INWARDS*
Dept of Pathology
Mayo Clinic
Rochester, MN 55905
USA
Tel. +1 507 284 8730
Fax +1 507 284 1599
Inwards.carrie@mayo.edu

Dr Yoko IWASA
Dept of Pathology
Osaka City University
Graduate School of Medicine
Osaka, 545-8585
JAPAN
Tel. +81 6 6645 3741
Fax +81 6 6645 3742
yiwasa@med.osaka-cu.ac.jp

Dr Ronald JAFFE
Dept of Pediatric Pathology
Children's Hospital of Pittsburgh
Pittsburgh, PA 15224
USA
Tel. +1 412 692 5650
Fax +1 412 692 6550
ronald.jaffe@chp.edu

Dr Gernot JUNDT*
Bone Tumor Reference Center
Institute of Pathology
University Hospital Basel
Basel, CH-4031
SWITZERLAND
Tel. +41 61 328 7867
Fax +41 61 265 3194
gernt.jundt@unibas.ch

Dr Ricardo K. KALIL
Area de Patologia Cirurgica
Rede Sarah de Hospitals do Aparelho Locomotor
Brasilia DF, 70.335-901
BRAZIL
Tel. +55 61 33191183
Fax +55 61 33192902
rkkalil@gmail.com, 201199@sarah.br

Dr Masahiko KANAMORI
Dept of Orthopaedic Surgery and Human Science
University of Toyama
Toyama, 930-0194
JAPAN
Tel. +81 76 434 7405
Fax +81 76 434 5186
kanamori@med.u-toyama.ac.jp

Dr Hiroyuki KAWASHIMA
Division of Orthopedic Surgery
Dept of Regenerative and Transplant Medicine
Niigata University Graduate School of
Medical and Dental Science
Chuo-ku, Niigata, 951-8510
JAPAN
Tel. +81 25 227 2272
Fax +81 25 227 0782
inskawa@med.niigata-u.ac.jp

Dr Scott E. KILPATRICK
Pathologists Diagnostic Services
Winston-Salem, NC 27103-3013
USA
Tel. +1 336 718 5856
Fax +1 336 718 9259
sekilpatrick@novanthealth.org

Dr Lars-Gunnar KINDBLOM
Dept of Musculoskeletal Pathology
Robert Aitken Institute of Clinical Research
The Medical School
University of Birmingham
Birmingham, B15 2TT
ENGLAND
Tel. +44 (0)121 414 7643
Fax +44 (0)121 414 7640
lars.kindblom@nhs.net

Dr Michael KLEIN*
Dept of Pathology and Laboratory Medicine
Hospital for Special Surgery
New York, NY 10021
USA
Tel. +1 212 606 1807
Fax +1 212 606 1910
KleinM@HSS.EDU

Dr Philip M. KLUIN
Dept of Pathology and Medical Biology
Groningen University Hospital
Groningen, 9700 RB
THE NETHERLANDS
Tel. +31 50 3616161
Fax +31 50 3619107
p.m.kluin@umcg.nl

Dr Sakari KNUUTILA
Dept of Pathology
Haartman Institute and HUSLAB
University of Helsinki and
Helsinki University Central Hospital
Helsinki, FI-00290
FINLAND
Tel. +358 9 191 26527
Fax +358 9 191 26675
sakari.knuutila@helsinki.fi

Dr Paul KOMMINOTH
Dept of Pathology
Stadtspital Triemli
Zurich, 8063
SWITZERLAND
Tel. +41 44 466 21 20
Fax +41 44 466 21 38
paul.komminoth@zuerich.ch

Dr Heinz KUTZNER
Dermatopathologie Friedrichshafen
Siemensstrasse 6/1
Friedrichshafen, 88048
GERMANY
Tel. +49 7541 6044 0
Fax +49 7541 6044 23
kutzner@dermpath.de

Dr Michael KYRIAKOS
Dept of Pathology
Washington University
School of Medicine
St Louis, MD 63110
USA
Tel. +1 314 362 0119
Fax +1 314 747 2040
mkyriakos@path.wustl.edu

Dr Marc LADANYI*
Dept of Pathology
Memorial Sloan-Kettering Cancer Center
New York, NY 10065
USA
Tel. +1 212 639 6369
Fax +1 212 717 3515
ladanyim@mskcc.org

Dr Janez LAMOVEC
Dept of Pathology
Institute of Oncology
Ljubljana, 1105
SLOVENIA
Tel. +386 1 5879 719 (or 726)
Fax +386 1 5879 802
jlamovec@onko-i.si

Dr William B. LASKIN
Dept of Pathology
Northwestern Memorial Hospital
Feinberg Pavilion 7th Floor-325
Chicago, IL 60611-2908
USA
Tel. +1 312 926 1367
Fax +1 312 926 3127
wbl769@northwestern.edu

Dr Jerzy LASOTA
Laboratory of Pathology
National Cancer Institute
Building 10, Room B1B47
Bethesda, MD 20892-1500
USA
Tel. +1 301 402 8411
Fax +1 301 402 7575
jerzy.lasota@nih.gov,

Dr Alexander LAZAR
Dept of Pathology, Sections of Sarcoma
Pathology and Dermatopathology
Sarcoma Research Center
The University of Texas M.D. Anderson
Cancer Center
Houston, TX 77030-4009
USA
Tel. +1 713 563 1843
Fax +1 713 563 1849
alazar@mdanderson.org

Dr Jen-Chieh LEE
Dept of Pathology
National Taiwan University Hospital
Taipei, 10001
TAIWAN, CHINA
Tel. +886 2 23123456
Fax +886 2 23934172
leejenchieh@ntuh.gov.tw

Dr Eric LEGIUS
Dept of Human Genetics
Catholic University of Leuven
Leuven, 3000
BELGIUM
Tel. +32 163 459 03
Fax +32 163 460 51
Eric.Legius@uzleuven.be

Dr Stephen L. LESSNICK
Center for Children's Cancer Research
Huntsman Cancer Institute
2000 Circle of Hope, Room 4242
Salt Lake City, UT 84112
USA
Tel. +1 (801) 585-9268
Fax +1 (801) 585-5357
stephen.lessnick@hci.utah.edu

Dr Michael A. LEVINE
Division of Endocrinology and Diabetes
The Children's Hospital of Philadelphia
34th and Civic Center Boulevard
Philadelphia, Pennsylvania 19104
USA
Tel. +1 215 590 3618
Fax +1 215 590 3053
levinem@chop.edu

Dr Bernadette LIEGL-ATZWANGER
Institut für Pathologie
Medizinische Universität Graz
Graz, A-8036
AUSTRIA
Tel. +43 316 385 80459
Fax +43 316 385 13432
bernadette.liegl-atzwanger@medunigraz.at

Dr Steven A. LIETMAN
Dept of Orthopedic Surgery
Cleveland Clinic Foundation
Crile Building A41
Cleveland, OH 44195
USA
Tel. 216 444 2600
Fax 216 445-6255
lietmas@ccf.org

Dr Noralane M. LINDOR
Dept of Health Science Research
Mayo Clinic Arizona
Scottsdale, AZ 85259
USA
Tel. +1 480 301 6817
Fax +1 480 301 8387
nlindor@mayo.edu

Dr Robert LORSBACH
Dept of Pathology
University of Arkansas for Medical Sciences
Little Rock, AR 72205
USA
Tel. +1 501 603 1963
Fax +1 501 603 1479
RLorsbach@uams.edu

Dr Ragnhild A. LOTHE
Dept of Cancer Prevention
Institute for Cancer Research
Radium Hospitalet
Oslo University Hospital
Oslo, 0310
NORWAY
Tel. +47 2278 1728
Fax +47 2278 1745
Ragnhild.A.Lothe@rr-research.no

Dr David R. LUCAS
Dept of Pathology
University of Michigan Hospital
2G332 UH
Ann Arbor, MI 48109-0054
USA
Tel. +1 734 232 0022
Fax +1 734 763 4095
drlucas@umich.edu

Dr David MALKIN
Genetics & Genome Biology Program
The Hospital for Sick Children
555 University Avenue
Toronto, ON M5G1X8
CANADA
Tel. +1 416 813 5348
Fax +1 416 813 5327
david.malkin@sickkids.ca

Dr Nils MANDAHL*
Dept of Clinical Genetics
University and Regional Laboratories
Lund, S-221 85
SWEDEN
Tel. +46 46 172889
Fax +46 46 131061
Nils.Mandahl@med.lu.se

Dr Marcel MANNENS
Dept of Clinical Genetics
Academic Medical Center
University of Amsterdam
P.O. Box 22700
Amsterdam, 1100 DE
THE NETHERLANDS
Tel. +31 20 5667899
Fax +31 20 5669389
kg_dna@amc.uva.nl

Dr Adrian MARINO-ENRIQUEZ
Dept of Pathology
Brigham and Women's Hospital
Boston, MA 02115
USA
Tel. +1 617 732 7883
Fax +1 617 278 6921
amarinoenriquez@partners.org

Dr Edward F. MCCARTHY
Division of Surgical Pathology, Bone and Joint
Pathology
Dept of Pathology
Johns Hopkins Hospital
Baltimore, MD 21231-2410
USA
Tel. +1 410 614 3653
Fax +1 614 3766
mccarthy@jhmi.edu

Dr Mairin MCMENAMIN
Dept of Histopathology
St James's Hospital
Dublin, 8
IRELAND
Tel. +353 141 62994
Fax +353 141 03514
MMcMenamin@stjames.ie

Dr Jeanne M. MEIS
Dept of Pathology
University of Texas MD Anderson Cancer
Center
Houston, TX 77030
USA
Tel. +1 713 792 2575
Fax +1 713 745 8228
jmmeis@mdanderson.org

Dr Thomas MENTZEL
Dermatohistopathologische
Gemeinschaftspraxis
Postfach 16 46
Friedrichshafen, D-88006
GERMANY
Tel. +49 7541 604431
Fax +49 7541 604410
mentzel@dermpath.de

Dr Fredrik MERTENS*
Dept of Clinical Genetics
University and Regional Laboratories
Lund, S-221 85
SWEDEN
Tel. +46 46 173387
Fax +46 46 131061
Fredrik.Mertens@med.lu.se

Dr Michal MICHAL
Sikl's Dept of Pathology
Medical Faculty Hospital
Charles University
Pilsen, 304 60
CZECH REPUBLIC
Tel. +420 6038 86633
Fax +420 3771 04650
michal@medima.cz

Dr Markku M. MIETTINEN*
Laboratory of Pathology
General Surgical Pathology Section
National Cancer Institute
Building 10, Magnuson CC, Room 2B50
Bethesda, MD 20892
USA
Tel. +1 301 594 3930
Fax +1 301 480 9488
miettinenmm@mail.nih.gov

Dr Raymond J. MONNAT Jr
Dept of Pathology
University of Washington
Box 357705
Seattle, WA 98195
USA
Tel. +1 206 616 7392
Fax +1 206 543 3967
monnat@u.washington.edu

Dr Anthony G. MONTAG
The University of Chicago Medical Center
Chicago, IL 60637
USA
Tel. +1 773 702 9318
Fax +1 773 834 7644
amontag@bsd.uchicago.edu

Dr Elizabeth A. MONTGOMERY
Dept of Pathology
The Johns Hopkins School of Medicine
Baltimore, MD 21231
USA
Tel. +1 410 614 2308
Fax +1 443 287 3818
emontgom@jhmi.edu

Dr Yasuaki NAKASHIMA
Laboratory of Anatomic Pathology
Kyoto University Hospital
Sakyo-Ku Kyoto, 606-8507
JAPAN
Tel. +81 75 751 3488
Fax +81 75 751 3499
nakashim@kuhp.kyoto-u.ac.jp

Dr Alessandra F. NASCIMENTO
Dept of Pathology
Brigham and Women's Hospital
Boston, MA 02115
USA
Tel. +1 617 525 7813
Fax +1 617 566 3897
anascimento1@me.com

Dr Irene F. NEWSHAM
Genitourinary Medical Oncology Dept
UT-MD Anderson Cancer Center
Houston, TX 77030
USA
Tel. +1 713 792 6941
Fax +1 713 563 2067
Inewsham@mdanderson.org

Dr G. Petur NIELSEN
Dept of Pathology
Massachusetts General Hospital
Boston, MA 02114-2696
USA
Tel. +617 724 1469
Fax +617 726 9312
gnielsen@partners.org

Dr Jun NISHIO
Dept of Orthopaedic Surgery
School of Medicine
Fukuoka University
Fukuoka, 814-0180
JAPAN
Tel. +81 92 801 1011
Fax +81 92 864 9055
nishio@minf.med.fukuoka-u.ac.jp

Dr John X. O'CONNELL
Dept of Pathology
Surrey Memorial Hospital
Surrey, BC V3V 1Z2
CANADA
john.Oconnell@fraserhealth.ca

Dr Yoshinao ODA*
Dept of Anatomic Pathology
Kyushu University
3-1-1 Maidashi
Fukuoka, 812-8582
JAPAN
Tel. +81 92 642 6061
Fax +81 92 642 5968
oda@surgpath.med.kyushu-u.ac.jp

Dr Hiroko OHGAKI*
Section of Molecular Pathology
International Agency for Research on Cancer
150 cours Albert Thomas
69372 Lyon
FRANCE
Tel. +33 4 72 73 85 34
Fax +33 4 72 73 86 98
ohgaki@iarc.fr

Dr Kyoji OKADA
Department of Physical Therapy
Akita University Graduate
School of Health Sciences
Akita, 010-8543
JAPAN
Tel. +81 18 884 6532
Fax +81 18 884 6532
cshokada@med.akita-u.ac.jp

Dr Andre M. OLIVEIRA
Dept of Laboratory Medicine and Pathology
Mayo Clinic
Hilton Building, 11th Floor
Rochester, MN 55905
USA
Tel. +1 507 538 4908
Fax +1 507 284 1599
oliveira.andre@mayo.edu

Dr Nelson G. ORDONEZ
Dept of Pathology
The University of Texas
MD Anderson Cancer Center
Houston, TX 77030
USA
Tel. +1 713 792 3167
Fax +1 713 792 3696
nordonez@mdanderson.org

Dr Chin-Chen PAN
Dept of Pathology
Taipei Veterans General Hospital
Taipei, 11217
TAIWAN, CHINA
Tel. +886 228757055
Fax +886 228757056
ccpan@vghtpe.gov.tw

Dr David M. PARHAM*
Pediatric Pathology
OUHSC College of Medicine
940 SL Young Blvd, BMSB 451
Oklahoma City, OK 73104
USA
Tel. +1 405 271 2753
Fax +1 405 271 1804
david-parham@ouhsc.edu

Dr Florence PEDEUTOUR*
Laboratoire de Génétique des Tumeurs Solides
Nice University Hospital and Institute for
Research on Cancer and Aging (IRCAN)
Faculty of Medicine
28 avenue de Valombrose
Nice Cedex 2, 06107
FRANCE
Tel. +33 493 37 70 12
Fax +33 493 37 70 07
florence.pedeutour@unice.fr

Dr Arie PERRY
Dept of Pathology, Division of Neuropathology
University of California, San Francisco (UCSF)
Box 0102
San Francisco, CA 94143
USA
Tel. +1 415 476 5236
Fax +1 415 476 7963
Arie.Perry@ucsf.edu

Dr Brad QUADE
Dept of Pathology
Brigham and Women's Hospital
Boston, MA 02115-6195
USA
Tel. +1 617 732 7980
Fax +1 617 738 6996
bquade@partners.org

Dr Ernst J. REICHENBERGER
University of Connecticut Health Center
Center for Regenerative Medicine
and Skeletal Development
Dept of Reconstructive Sciences
Farmington, CT 06030-3705
USA
Tel. +1 860 679 2062
Fax +1 860 679 2910
reichenberger@uchc.edu

Dr Robin P. REID
0/1 13 Kirklee Terrace
Glasgow, G12 0TH
UK
Tel. +44 141 339 7755
Robinpreid@btinternet.com

Dr Barrett J. ROLLINS
Dept of Medical Oncology
Dana-Farber Cancer Institute
Dept of Medicine
Boston, MA 02115
USA
Tel. +1 617 632 3896
Fax +1 617 632 5998
barrett_rollins@dfci.harvard.edu

Dr Salvatore ROMEO
Dept of Pathology
Treviso General Hospital
Piazza Ospedale 1
Treviso, 31100
ITALY
Tel. +39 04 223 22707
Fax +39 04 223 22705
sromeo@ulss.tv.it

Dr Andrew E. ROSENBERG*
Miller School of Medicine
University of Miami Hospital
1400 NW 12th Avenue
Miami, FL 33136
USA
Tel. +1 305 243 8730
Fax +1 305 689 1326.
arosenberg@med.miami.edu

Dr Sabrina ROSSI
Dept of Pathology
Treviso General Hospital
Piazza Ospedale 1
Treviso, 31100
ITALY
Tel. +39 04 233 22707/8105
Fax +39 04 223 22705
sr920@yahoo.it

Dr Brian ROUS*
Eastern Cancer Registry and Information Centre
Unit C - Magog Court
Shelford Bottom, Hinton Way
CB22 3AD Cambridge
UK
Tel. +1 223 213 625
Fax +1 223 213 571
brian.rous@ecric.nhs.uk

Dr Brian P. RUBIN*
Dept of Anatomic Pathology
Cleveland Clinic Main Campus
Mail Code L25
Cleveland, OH 44195
USA
Tel. +1 216 445 5551
Fax +1 216 445 3707
rubinb2@ccf.org

Dr Eduardo SANTINI ARAUJO
School of Medicine and Dentistry, University of
Buenos Aires
Department of Pathology, Central Army Hospital
Laboratory of Orthopedic Pathology
Paraguay 2302. 11th floor. Of. 1.
Buenos Aires, C1121 ABL
ARGENTINA
Tel. +54 11 4966 1224
Fax +54 11 4964 0379
santiniaraujo@laborpat.com.ar

Dr Zoltan SAPI
First Dept of Pathology and Experimental
Cancer Research
Semmelweis University
Budapest, 1085
HUNGARY
Tel. +36 1 459 1500/4457
Fax +36 1 317 1074
sapi.zoltan.dr@gmail.com

Dr Jeffrey R. SAWYER
Dept of Pathology
Myeloma Institute for Research and Therapy
University of Arkansas for Medical Sciences
Freeway Medical Tower, Suite 200
Little Rock, AR 72204
USA
Tel. +1 501 526 8000 (ext 1)
Fax +1 501 526 7468
SawyerJeffreyR@uams.edu

Dr Alan SCHILLER
Dept of Pathology
Mount Sinai School of Medicine
One Gustave L Levy Place
New York, NY 10029
USA
Tel. +1 212 241 8014
Fax: +1 212 426 5129
Alan.schiller@mssm.edu

Dr Raf SCIOT*
Dienst Pathologische Ontleedkunde
UZ St Rafael
Leuven, B-3000
BELGIUM
Tel. +32 16 3365 93
Fax +32 16 3365 48
Raf.Sciot@uzleuven.be

Dr Janet SHIPLEY
Sarcoma Molecular Pathology
Divisions of Molecular Pathology and Cancer
Therapeutics
The Institute of Cancer Research
15 Cotswold Road
Sutton, SM2 5NG
UK
Tel. +44 20 8722 4273
Fax +44 20 8722 4084
janet.shipley@icr.ac.uk

Dr Gene P. SIEGAL
Dept of Anatomic Pathology
University of Alabama at Birmingham
Birmingham, AL 35233
USA
Tel. +1 205 934 6608
Fax +1 205 975 7284
gsiegal@uab.edu

Dr Samuel SINGER
Dept of Surgery
Memorial Sloan-Kettering Cancer Center
New York, NY 10021
USA
Tel. +1 212 639 2940
Fax +1 212 717 3053
singers@mskcc.org

Dr Poul SORENSEN
Dept of Molecular Oncology
British Columbia Cancer Research Center
Vancouver, BC V5Z 1L3
CANADA
Tel. +1 604 675 8202
Fax +1 604 675 8218
phbsorensen@gmail.com

Dr Jeremy SQUIRE
Queen's University
Dept of Pathology and Molecular Medicine
Kingston
Ontario, K7L3N6
CANADA
Tel. +1 613 533 2345
Fax +1 613 533 2907
squirej@queensu.ca

Dr Goran STENMAN
Lundberg Laboratory for Cancer Research
Dept of Pathology
Goteborg University
Sahlgrenska University Hospital
Goteborg, SE-413 45
SWEDEN
Tel. +46 31 342 2922
Fax +46 31 820 525
goran.stenman@llcr.med.gu.se

Dr Constantine A. STRATAKIS
SEGEN/PDEGEN
National Institute of Child Health
and Human Development
NIH, Building 10 CRC, Room 1-3330
Bethesda, MD MSC1103
USA
Tel. +1 301 496 4686
Fax +1 301 402 0574
stratakc@mail.nih.gov

Dr Albert J.H. SUURMEIJER
Dept of Pathology
University Medical Center Groningen
PO Box 30.001
Groningen, 9700 RB
THE NETHERLANDS
Tel. +31 50 3612827
Fax +31 50 3619107
a.j.h.suurmeijer@umcg.nl

Dr Karoly SZUHAI
Dept of Molecular Cell Biology
Leiden University Medical Center
Leiden, 2333ZC
THE NETHERLANDS
Tel. +31 71 5269211
Fax +31 71 5268270
K.Szuhai@lumc.nl

Dr Lester D. R. THOMPSON
Dept of Pathology
Woodland Hills Medical Center
Woodland Hills, CA 91367
USA
Tel. +1 818 719 2613
Fax +1 818 719 2309
lester.d.thompson@kp.org

Dr William Y. W. TSANG
Institute of Pathology
Queen Elizabeth Hospital
Kowloon
HONG KONG SAR CHINA
Tel. +852 2958 6830
Fax +852 2385 2455
tsangyw@ha.org.hk

Dr Matt VAN DE RIJN
Dept of Pathology
Stanford University Medical Center
Stanford, CA 94305
USA
Tel. +1 650 498 7154
Fax +1 650 725 6902
mrijn@stanford.edu

Dr Daniel VANEL*
Rizzoli Orthopedic Institute
Bologna 40136
ITALY
Tel. +39 051 6366931
daniel.vanel@ior.it

Dr Vincent J. VIGORITA
Dept of Pathology
Maimonides Medical Center
Brooklyn, New York 11219
USA
Tel. +1 631 267 8726
Fax +1 631 267 2296
vvigorita1@aol.com

Dr Sharon W. WEISS
Dept of Pathology and Lab Medicine
Emory University Hospital, H-180
Atlanta, GA 30322
USA
Tel. +1 404 712 0708/0707
Fax +1 404 712 4454
swweiss@emory.edu

Dr Lester E. WOLD
Dept of Pathology
Mayo Clinic Health System - Austin
1000 First Drive NW
Austin, MN 55912
USA
Tel. +1 507 434 1247
Fax +1 507 434 1494
lwold@mayo.edu

Dr James M. WOODRUFF
6500 Flotilla Drive, Unit 205
Holmes Beach, Florida, 34217
USA
Tel. +1 413 977 1082
woodrufj@earthlink.net

Dr Wim WUYTS
Dept of Medical Genetics
University of Antwerp
Edegem, 2650
BELGIUM
Tel. +32 3 275 9706
Fax +32 3 275 9722
wim.wuyts@ua.ac.be

Dr Takehiko YAMAGUCHI
Dept of Pathology
Jichi Medical University
Tochigi, 329-0498
JAPAN
Tel. +81 285 58 7327
Fax +81 285 44 8467
takehiko@jichi.ac.jp

Dr Eduardo ZAMBRANO
Dept of Pathology
Medical College of Wisconsin
Milwaukee, WI 53226
USA
Tel. +1 414 805 8786
Fax +1 414 805 8444
ezambrano@mcw.edu

IARC/WHO Committee for the International Classification of Diseases for Oncology (ICD-O)

Dr Christopher D. M. FLETCHER
Deptartment of Pathology
Brigham and Women's Hospital
Boston, MA 02115
USA
Tel. +1 617 732 8558
Fax +1 617 566 3897
cfletcher@partners.org

Dr David FORMAN
Section of Cancer Information
International Agency for Research on Cancer
150 cours Albert Thomas
69372 Lyon Cedex 08
FRANCE
Tel. +33 4 72 73 80 56
Fax +33 4 72 73 86 96
formand@iarc.fr

Mrs April FRITZ
A. Fritz and Associates, LLC
21361 Crestview Road
Reno, NV 89521
USA
Tel. +1 775 636 7243
Fax +1 888 891 3012
april@afritz.org

Dr Pancreas C. W. HOGENDOORN
Deptartment of Pathology
Leiden University Medical Center
Building 1, Room P-01-34
Postzone L1Q
Leiden, 2300 RC
THE NETHERLANDS
Tel. +31 71 526 6625
Fax +31 71 526 6952
p.c.w.hogendoorn@lumc.nl

Dr Robert JAKOB
Classifications and Terminologies
Evidence and Information for Policy
World Health Organization (WHO)
20 Avenue Appia
1211 Geneva 27
SWITZERLAND
Tel. +41 22 791 58 77
Fax +41 22 791 48 94
jakobr@who.int

Dr Paul KLEIHUES
Department of Pathology
University Hospital
Schmelzbergstrasse 12
8091 Zurich
SWITZERLAND
Tel. +41 44 362 2110
Fax +41 44 251 0665
kleihues@pathol.uzh.ch

Dr Hiroko OHGAKI
Section of Molecular Pathology
International Agency for Research on Cancer
150 cours Albert Thomas
69372 Lyon Cedex 08
FRANCE
Tel. +33 4 72 73 85 34
Fax +33 4 72 73 86 98
ohgaki@iarc.fr

Dr D. Maxwell PARKIN
Clinical Trials Service & Epidemiology Studies Unit
University of Oxford
Richard Doll Building, Old Road Campus
Roosevelt Drive, Headington
Oxford OX3 7LF
UK
Tel. +44 1865 743663
Fax +44 1865 743985
ctsu0138@herald.ox.ac.uk

Dr Brian ROUS
Eastern Cancer Registry and Information Centre
Unit C - Magog Court
Shelford Bottom, Hinton Way
CB22 3AD Cambridge
UK
Tel. +1 223 213 625
Fax +1 223 213 571
brian.rous@ecric.nhs.uk

Dr K. SHANMUGARATNAM
Department of Pathology
National University Hospital
5 Lower Kent Ridge Road
Singapore 119074
SINGAPORE
Tel. +65 6772 4312
Fax +65 6773 6021
k_shanmugaratnam@nuhs.edu.sg

Dr Leslie H. SOBIN
Frederick National Laboratory for Cancer Research
The Cancer Human Biobank
National Cancer Institute
11400 Rockville Pike, Suite 700
Rockville, MD 20852
USA
Tel. +1 301 827 4361
Fax +1 301 480 1069
leslie.sobin@nih.gov

Source of figures and tables

Sources of figures

2.01A,B	Nielsen G.P.
2.02A,B	Nielsen G.P.
2.03A,B	Nielsen G.P.
2.04	Mertens F.
2.05	Fanburg-Smith J.
2.06	Fanburg-Smith J.
2.07A,B	Nielsen G.P.
2.08A,B	Nielsen G.P.
2.09A,B	Coffin C.M.
2.10A,B	Coffin C.M.
2.11A,B	Sciot R.
2.12A,B	Meis J.M.
2.13A	Dei Tos A.P.
2.13B	Kindblom L.G.
2.14A,B	Huang D, Sumegi J, Dal Cin P et al. (2010). C11orf95-MKL2 is the resulting fusion oncogene of t(11;16)(q13;p13) in chondroid lipoma. Genes Chromosomes Cancer 49: 810–818. Copyright (2010), with permission from Wiley.
2.15A,B	Fletcher C.D.M
2.16	Miettinen M.M.
2.17A	Fletcher C.D.M
2.17B	Fanburg-Smith J.
2.17C,D	Fletcher C.D.M
2.18A-C	Miettinen M.M.
2.19	Mertens F.
2.20A,B	Miettinen M.M.
2.21A-C	Dei Tos A.P.
2.22	Dei Tos A.P.
2.23A,B	Dei Tos A.P.
2.23C	Fletcher C.D.M
2.24A	Coindre J.M.
2.24B	Dei Tos A.P.
2.25A,B	Pedeutour F.
2.26	Pedeutour F.
2.27	Pedeutour F.
2.28A,B	Dei Tos A.P.
2.29	Nascimento A.G.
2.30A-C	Dei Tos A.P.
2.31	Dei Tos A.P.
2.32	Dei Tos A.P.
2.33A,B	Antonescu C.R.
2.34A-C	Antonescu C.R.
2.35A,B	Antonescu C.R.
2.36	Antonescu C.R
2.37A	Antonescu C.R.
2.37B	Mertens F.
2.38A-C	Coindre J.M.
2.39	Coindre J.M.
2.40	Coindre J.M.
2.41	Coindre J.M.
2.42A,B	Coindre J.M
2.43	Pedeutour F.
2.44	Pedeutour F.
3.001A,B	Lazar A.
3.002A,B	Lazar A.
3.002C,D	Kempson
3.003	Oliveira A.
3.004A	Fletcher C.D.M
3.004B	Lazar A.
3.005A	Wei-Lien Wang, Houston, Texas
3.005B	Lazar A.
3.006	Rosenberg A.E.
3.007A	Lamovec J.
3.007B	Fletcher C.D.M
3.008A,B	Rosenberg A.E.
3.009A-C	Rosenberg A.E.
3.010A,B	Rosenberg A.E.
3.011	Liegl-Atzwanger B.
3.012A-C	Liegl-Atzwanger B.
3.013	Hisaoka M.
3.014A-C	Nielsen G.P.
3.015A-D	Coffin C.M.
3.016	Coffin C.M.
3.017	Coffin C.M.
3.018A,B	Fletcher C.D.M
3.019	Ojeda V.J.
3.020A,B	O'Connell J.X.
3.021	Fletcher C.D.M
3.022	Laskin WB, Miettinen M, Fetsch J. Infantile digital fibroma/fibromatosis. A clinicopathologic and immunohistochemical study of 69 tumors from 57 patients with long-term follow-up. Am J Surg Pathol 2009;33(1):1–13. Copyright © (2009), with permission from Wolters Kluwer Health.
3.023	Laskin WB, Miettinen M, Fetsch J. Infantile digital fibroma/fibromatosis. A clinicopathologic and immunohistochemical study of 69 tumors from 57 patients with long-term follow-up. Am J Surg Pathol 2009;33(1):1–13. Copyright © (2009), with permission from Wolters Kluwer Health.
3.024	Laskin W.B.
3.025A	Laskin WB, Miettinen M, Fetsch J. Infantile digital fibroma/fibromatosis. A clinicopathologic and immunohistochemical study of 69 tumors from 57 patients with long-term follow-up. Am J Surg Pathol 2009;33(1):1–13. Copyright © (2009), with permission from Wolters Kluwer Health.
3.025B	Laskin W.B.
3.026	Laskin W.B.
3.027	De Smet L.

3.028A,B	Sciot R.
3.029	Fetsch J
3.030A,B	Miettinen M.M.
3.031	Miettinen M.M.
3.032	Bridge JA
3.033A,B	Mc Menamin M.E.
3.034A-C	Mc Menamin M.E.
3.035A,B	Kilpatrick S.E.
3.036	Kilpatrick S.E.
3.037A,B	Fletcher C.D.M
3.038A-D	Fletcher C.D.M
3.039	Laskin W.B.
3.040A,B	Laskin W.B.
3.041A,B	Fletcher C.D.M
3.042	Michal M.
3.043A,B	Coffin C.M.
3.044	Nascimento A.G.
3.045A,B	Nascimento A.G.
3.046A,B	Fletcher C.D.M
3.047A,B	Fletcher C.D.M
3.047C	Goldblum J.R.
3.047D	Fletcher C.D.M
3.048	Nascimento A.G.
3.049A-C	Goldblum J.R.
3.050	Fanburg-Smith J.
3.051A,B	Goldblum J.R.
3.052A,B	Fletcher C.D.M
3.053A	Fletcher C.D.M
3.053B	Miettinen M.M.
3.053C	Fletcher C.D.M
3.054	Coindre J.M.
3.055	Coindre J.M.
3.056A,B	Coindre J.M.
3.057	Coindre J.M.
3.058A,B	Coindre J.M.
3.059	Coindre J.M.
3.060	Coindre J.M.
3.061A,B	Bridge J.A.
3.062A	Mentzel T.
3.062B	Gianotti R.
3.063A,B	Mentzel T.
3.064	Mentzel T.
3.065	Mentzel T.
3.066	Mentzel T.
3.067	Calonje E.
3.068	Mentzel T.
3.069	Pedeutour F.
3.070	Pedeutour F.
3.071	Guillou L.
3.072A,B	Guillou L.
3.073A-D	Guillou L.
3.074A-C	Guillou L.
3.075A-C	Guillou L.
3.076A-C	Fletcher C.D.M
3.077A,B	Guillou L.
3.078	Coffin C.M.
3.079A-C	Coffin C.M.
3.080A,B	Coffin C.M.
3.081	Mentzel T.
3.082A,B	Mentzel T.

3.083A,B	Mentzel T.
3.084A,B	Mentzel T
3.085	Meis J.M.
3.086A-D	Meis J.M.
3.087A,B	Meis J.M.
3.088	Reprinted with permission from John Wiley & Sons, from Hallor KH, et al. Two genetic path ways, t(1;10) and amplification of 3p11-12, in myxoinflammatory fibroblastic sarcoma, haemosiderotic fibrolipomatous tumour, and morphologically similar lesions. J Pathol (2009);217:716–727.
3.089	Coffin C.M.
3.090A,B	Coffin C.M.
3.091A,B	Coffin C.M.
3.092A,B	Coffin C.M.
3.093A,B	Coffin C.M.
3.094	Folpe A.L.
3.095A,B	Folpe A.L.
3.096	Mentzel T.
3.097A-F	Mentzel T.
3.098A	Antonescu C.R.
3.098B-D	Mentzel T.
3.099	Hsuan-Ying Huang
3.100A,B	Folpe A.L.
3.101A,B	Folpe A.L.
3.102A	Folpe A.L.
3.102B	Fanburg-Smith J.
3.103A,B	Hornick J.L.
3.104	Mertens F.
3.105	Kindblom L.G.
3.106	Hornick J.L.
3.107A-C	Kindblom L.G.
4.01A,B	de Saint Aubain N.
4.02A	Fletcher C.D.M
4.02B	de Saint Aubain N.
4.03A	de Saint Aubain N.
4.03B	Folpe A.L.
4.04A,B	de Saint Aubain N.
4.05A-C	de Saint Aubain N.
4.06A,B	Fanburg-Smith J.
4.07	Mertens F.
4.08	Fletcher C.D.M
4.09	Coindre J.M.
4.10A,B	Coindre J.M.
4.11	Moosavi C, Jha P, Fanburg-Smith JC, An update on plexiform fibrohistiocytic tumor and addition of 66 new cases from the Armed Forces Instiute of Pathology, in honor of Franz M. Enzinger, MD, Reprinted from Annals of Diagnostic Pathology.11:313-319. Copyright (2007), with permission from Elsevier
4.12	Moosavi C, Jha P, Fanburg-Smith JC, An update on plexiform fibrohistiocytic tumor and addition of 66 new cases from the Armed Forces Instiute of Pathology, in honor of Franz M. Enzinger, MD, Reprinted from Annals of Diagnostic Pathology.11:313-319. Copyright (2007), with permission from Elsevier

4.13	Moosavi C, Jha P, Fanburg-Smith JC, An update on plexiform fibrohistiocytic tumor and addition of 66 new cases from the Armed Forces Instiute of Pathology, in honor of Franz M. Enzinger, MD, Reprinted from Annals of Diagnostic Pathology.11:313-319. Copyright (2007), with permission from Elsevier.
4.14	Fanburg-Smith J.C
4.15	Nascimento A.G.
4.16	Nascimento A.G.
4.17A	Fletcher C.D.M
4.17B	Nascimento A.G.
4.18A	Oliveira A.
4.18B,C	Nascimento A.G.
5.01A,B	Miettinen M.
5.02A-C	Miettinen M.
5.03	Fletcher C.D.M
5.04A,B	Lazar A.
5.05	Fletcher C.D.M
5.06A	Fletcher C.D.M
5.06B	Demicco E.
5.07	Lazar A.
5.08	Wang R.
6.01A,B	Folpe A.L.
6.02	Folpe A.L.
6.03	Folpe A.L.
6.04	Fletcher C.D.M
6.05A,B	Folpe A.L.
6.06	Mentzel T.
6.07A,B	Mentzel T.
6.08	Mentzel T.
6.09	Fletcher C.D.M
6.10A,B	Mentzel T.
6.11	Mentzel T.
6.12A	Coffin C.M.
6.12B	Rubin B.P.
6.13	Coffin C.M.
6.14	Hisaoka M.
6.15A-D	Hisaoka M.
7.01A,B	Kapadia S.B.
7.02A,B	Kapadia S.B.
7.03A-C	Kapadia S.B.
7.04	Kapadia S.B.
7.05A-D	Kapadia S.B.
7.06A-C	Kapadia S.B.
7.07A,B	Parham D.M.
7.08	Parham D.M.
7.09A,B	Parham D.M.
7.10A,B	Parham D.M.
7.11A	Fletcher C.D.M
7.11B	Parham D.M.
7.12	Parham D.M.
7.13	Antonescu C.R.
7.14	Parham D.M.
7.15	Parham D.M.
7.16	Parham D.M.
7.17A,B	Parham D.M.

7.18A,B	Parham D.M.
7.19	Bridge J.A.
7.20	Barr F.G.
7.21A,B	E. Montgomery E.
7.22A,B	E. Montgomery E.
7.23A,B	E. Montgomery E.
7.24A,B	E. Montgomery E.
7.25	Fisher C.
7.26	Nascimento A.G.
7.27A,B	Nascimento A.G.
7.29	Nascimento A.G.
8.01	Calonje E.
8.02A	Fletcher C.D.M
8.02B	Calonje E.
8.03A-C	Calonje E.
8.04	Calonje E.
8.05A-C	Calonje E.
8.06	Fetsch J.
8.07A-C	Fetsch J.
8.08A,B	Fetsch J.
8.09A,B	Weiss S.W.
8.10A-C	Beham A.
8.11A,B	Beham A.
8.12A-C	Beham A.
8.13A-D	Weiss S.W.
8.14	Calonje E.
8.15A-D	Calonje E.
8.16	Fanburg-Smith J.C
8.17A-C	Fanburg-Smith J.C
8.18	Dr. B. Azadeh, Dept. of Pathology, Hamad General Hospital, Doha, Qatar.
8.19	Rubin B.P.
8.20A,B	Rubin B.P.
8.21A,B	Rubin B.P.
8.22A-C	Lamovec J.
8.23A,B	Mentzel T.
8.24	Mentzel T.
8.25A	Kutzner H.
8.25B-D	Mentzel T.
8.26	Kutzner H.
8.27	Hornick J.L.
8.28A-C	Hornick J.L.
8.29A,B	Hornick J.L.
8.30A,B	Weiss S.W.
8.31	Fletcher C.D.M
8.32A,B	Weiss S.W.
8.33A,B	Antonescu C.R.
8.34A,B	Weiss S.W.
8.35A,B	Weiss S.W.
8.36A,B	Weiss S.W.
8.37	Antonescu C.R.
9.01	Rosenberg A.E.
9.02	Rosenberg A.E.
9.03	Rosenberg A.E.
9.04	Rosenberg A.E.
9.05	Rosenberg A.E.
9.06	Rosenberg A.E.
9.07A,B	Rosenberg A.E.

12.60A-C	Antonescu C.R.
12.61A,B	Antonescu C.R.
12.62	Antonescu C.R.
12.63	Bridge J.A.
12.64	Lucas D.
12.65	Lucas D.
12.66A,B	Lucas D.
12.67	Stenman G.
12.68A-F	Lucas D.
12.69	Antonescu C.R.
12.70	Antonescu C.R.
12.71A,B	Antonescu C.R.
12.72A-F	Antonescu C.R.
12.73A-C	Antonescu C.R.
12.74A,B	Antonescu C.R.
12.75	Antonescu C.R.
12.76	Antonescu C.R.
12.77	Antonescu C.R.
12.78	Oda Y.
12.79A,B	Oda Y.
12.80	Oda Y.
12.81A-C	Oda Y.
12.82	Biegel J. A.
12.83	Hornick J.L.
12.84	Fletcher C.D.M
12.85A,B	Hornick J.L.
12.86	Hornick J.L.
12.87A,B	Hornick J.L.
12.88	Chin-Chen Pan
12.89A-D	Hornick J.L.
12.90	Bode-Lesniewska B.
12.91	Bode-Lesniewska B.
12.92A-D	Bode-Lesniewska B.
12.93A,B	Bode-Lesniewska B.
12.94	Debiec-Rychter M.
13.01A,B	Fletcher C.D.M
13.02	Chibon F.
13.03A,B	Fletcher C.D.M
14.01	Modified from Mukherjee D, Chaichana KL, Gokaslan ZL et al. (2011). Survival of patients with malignant primary osseous spinal neoplasms: results from the Surveillance, Epidemiology, and End Results (SEER) database from 1973 to 2003. J Neurosurg Spine 14: 143–150.
14.02	Lazar A.
15.01	Rosenberg A.E.
15.02	Heymann D.
15.03A,B	Heymann D.
15.04	Bovee J.V.M.G
15.05A,B	Heymann D.
15.06	Bovee JV. (2010). EXTra hit for mouse osteochondroma. Proc Natl Acad Sci U S A. 107:1813–1814. Reprinted with permission from PNAS.
15.07	Lucas D.
15.08A,B	Lucas D.

15.09A,B	Lucas D.
15.09C	Lucas D.
15.09D	Lucas D.
15.10A,B	Lucas D.
15.11	Lucas D.
15.12	Ostrowski M.L.
15.13	Ostrowski M.L.
15.14A-C	Ostrowski M.L.
15.15A-D	Bridge J.A.
15.16	Romeo S, Duim RA, Bridge JA et al. Heterogeneous and complex rearrangements of chromosome arm 6q in chondromyxoid fibroma: delineation of breakpoints and analysis of candidate target genes. Am J Pathol 177:1365–1376. Copyright (2010), with permission from Elsevier.
15.17	Carney J.A.
15.18A,B	Carney J.A.
15.19A,B	Carney J.A.
15.20A-C	Carney J.A.
15.21	Sciot R.
15.22	Sciot R.
15.23	Brys P.
15.24A,B	Sciot R.
15.25	Brys P.
15.26	Sciot R.
15.27	Kilpatrick S.E.
15.28	Kilpatrick S.E.
15.29A,B	Kilpatrick S.E.
15.30	Kilpatrick S.E.
15.31	Bridge J.A.
15.32	Bertoni F.
15.33	Bovee J.V.M.G
15.34	Bertoni F.
15.35A-C	Bertoni F.
15.36	Bovee J.V.M.G
15.37	Bovee J.V.M.G
15.38A,B	Bertoni F.
15.39A,B	Bertoni F.
15.40A,B	Bertoni F.
15.41A,B	Bertoni F.
15.42	Bovee J.V.M.G
15.43A-C	Inwards C.
15.44	Inwards C.
15.45A-C	Inwards C.
15.46A-D	Nakashima Y.
15.47	Nakashima Y.
15.48A-C	Nakashima Y.
15.49	Unni K.K.
15.50A,B	Unni K.K.
15.51A,B	Unni K.K.
16.01A,B	Bras J.
16.02	Bras J.
16.03	Bras J.
16.04	Horvai A.
16.05	Horvai A.
16.06	Klein M.J.
16.07A	Klein M.J.
16.07B,C	Horvai A.
16.08A,B	Schiller A.

23.17A	Rosenberg A.E.
23.17B,C	Bovee J.V.M.G
24.01	McCarthy E.F.
24.02	McCarthy E.F.
24.03A,B	McCarthy E.F.
24.04	Rosenberg A.E.
24.05	Rosenberg A.E.
24.06	Rosenberg A.E.
24.07	Rosenberg A.E.
24.08A,B	Rosenberg A.E.
24.09	Rosenberg A.E.
24.10A,B	Hogendoorn P.C.W.
24.11A,B	Hogendoorn P.C.W.
24.12A,B	Hogendoorn P.C.W.
25.01A,B	Rosenberg A.E.
25.02	Rosenberg A.E.
25.03	Hogendoorn PCW
25.04A,B	Nielsen G.P.
25.05A,B	Fletcher J.
25.06	Araujo E.S.
25.07	Kalil R.K.
25.08	Kalil R.K.
25.09	Araujo E.S.
25.10	Kalil R.K.
25.11A,B	Kalil R.K.
25.12	Siegal G.
25.13	Siegal G.
25.14	Siegal G.
25.15A,B	Unni K.K.
25.16	Siegal G.
25.17	Vigorita V.
25.18	Unni K.K.
25.19	Unni K.K.
25.20	De Young B.R.
25.21A,B	De Young B.R.
25.22A,B	Klein M.J.
25.23	Jaffe R.
25.24	Jaffe R.
25.25A,B	Jaffe R.
25.26	Amstalden E.M.I.
25.27A,B	Amstalden E.M.I.
25.28A,B	Amstalden EMI, Carvalho RB, Pacheco BEM, Oliveira-Filho A, Stragea-Neto L, Rosenberg AE, Int J Surg Pathol 14, pp 119-126, copyright © 2006 by SAGE Publications. Reprinted by Permission of SAGE Publications.
25.29A,B	Amstalden EMI, Carvalho RB, Pacheco BEM, Oliveira-Filho A, Stragea-Neto L, Rosenberg AE, Int J Surg Pathol 14, pp 119-126, copyright © 2006 by SAGE Publications. Reprinted by Permission of SAGE Publications.
25.30A,B	Amstalden E.M.I.
25.31A	Amstalden EMI, Carvalho RB, Pacheco BEM, Oliveira-Filho A, Stragea-Neto L, Rosenberg AE, Int J Surg Pathol 14, pp 119-126, copyright © 2006 by SAGE Publications. Reprinted by Permission of SAGE Publications.
25.31B	Amstalden E.M.I.
25.32	Rosenberg A.E.
25.33	Rosenberg A.E.
25.34A-C	Rosenberg A.E.
26.01A,B	Steiner G.C.
26.02	Steiner G.C.
26.03	Romeo S.
26.04	Romeo S.
27.01	Bridge J.A.
27.02	Mannens M.
27.03A,B	Modified from Ueki et al. Mutations in the gene encoding c-Abl-binding protein SH3BP2 cause cherubism. Nature Genetics, copyright (2001), with permission from Macmillan Publishers Ltd, Nature Publishing Group.
27.04	Flanagan A.
27.05	Modified from Ueki et al. Mutations in the gene encoding c-Abl-binding protein SH3BP2 cause cherubism. Nature Genetics, copyright (2001), with permission from Macmillan Publishers Ltd, Nature Publishing Group.
27.06	Alman B.
27.07A,B	Pansuriya TC, Kroon HM, Bovee JV. Enchondromatosis: insights on the different subtypes. Int J Clin Exp Pathol 3:557–569.Copyright (2010), with permission from IJCEP.
27.08A-D	Pansuriya TC, Kroon HM, Bovee JV. Enchondromatosis: insights on the different subtypes. Int J Clin Exp Pathol 3:557–569. Copyright (2010), with permission from IJCEP.
27.09	Pansuriya TC, Kroon HM, Bovee JV. Enchondromatosis: insights on the different subtypes. Int J Clin Exp Pathol 3:557–569. Copyright (2010), with permission from IJCEP.
27.10	Malkin D. Li-Fraumeni syndrome. Genes Cancer. 2:475–484. Copyright © Malkin D (2011), reprinted with permission from SAGE publications.
27.11	Malkin D. Li-Fraumeni syndrome. Genes Cancer. 2:475–484. Copyright © Malkin D (2011), reprinted with permission from SAGE publications.
27.12	Cohen M.M. Jr.
27.13	Siegal G.
27.14	Wuyts W.
27.15	Wyuts W.
27.16	Legius E.
27.17	Brems H.
27.18	Bogler O.
27.19	Bogler O.
27.20	Wang L.L.
27.21	Modified from Liu Y. Rothmund-Thomson syndrome helicase, RECQ4: on the crossroad between DNA replication and repair. DNA Repair. 9:325-30. Copyright (2010), with permission from Elsevier.
27.22	Wang LL, Gannavarapu A, Kozinetz CA et al.

(2003). Association between osteosarcoma and deleterious mutations in the RECQL4 gene in Rothmund-Thomson syndrome. J Natl Cancer Inst 95: 669–674. Copyright (2003), with permission of Oxford University Press.

27.23   Modified from Larizza L, Magnani I, Roversi G. Rothmund-Thomson syndrome and RECQL4 defect: splitting and lumping. Cancer Letters 232:107-120, Copyright (2006), with permission from Elsevier.

Sources of tables

1.01   Coindre JM . Grading of soft tissue sarcomas: review and update. Arch Pathol Lab Med 130:1448–1453. Copyright © 2010 College of American Pathologists.

1.02   Coindre JM . Grading of soft tissue sarcomas: review and update. Arch Pathol Lab Med 130:1448–1453. Copyright © 2010 College of American Pathologists.

10.01   Miettinen M, Lasota J . Gastrointestinal stromal tumors: review on morphology, molecular pathology, prognosis, and differential diagnosis. Arch Pathol Lab Med 130: 1466–1478. Copyright © 2010 College of American Pathologists.

14.01   Czerniak B.A.

14.02   Grimer R.J.

14.03   Rubin BP, Antonescu CR, Gannon FH et al. (2010). Protocol for the examination of specimens from patients with tumors of bone. Arch Pathol Lab Med 134: e1–e7. Copyright © 2010 College of American Pathologists.

15.01   Carney JA, Boccon-Gibod L, Jarka DE et al. (2001). Osteochondromyxoma of bone: a congenital tumor associated with lentigines and other unusual disorders. Am J Surg Pathol 25: 164–176. Copyright © (1999), with permission from Wolters Kluwer Health

16.01   Rosenberg A.E.

19.01   de Alava E., Lessnick S.L. and Sorenson P.

20.01   Criteria for the classification of monoclonal gammopathies, multiple myeloma and related disorders: a report of the International Myeloma Working Group.Br J Haematol. (2003).121:749-757. With permission from John Wiley & Sons.

20.02   Criteria for the classification of monoclonal gammopathies, multiple myeloma and related disorders: a report of the International Myeloma Working Group. Br J Haematol (2003)121:749-757. Reprinted with permission from John Wiley & Sons.

20.03   Hogendoorn P.C.W.

27.01   Bridge J.A.

27.02   Reichenberger E.J.

27.03   Malkin D.

27.04   Reprinted from Villani A, Tabori U, Schiffman J et al. (2011). Biochemical and imaging surveillance in germline TP53 mutation carriers with Li-

Fraumeni syndrome: a prospective observational study. Lancet Oncol 12: 559–567. Copyright 2011, with permission from Elsevier.

27.05   Monnat R.J.

Sources of figures for front cover

Top left   Matsuno T.

Top centre   Kalil R.K.

Top right   Mentzel T.

Middle left   Fletcher C.

Middle centre   Coffin C.

Middle right   Thompson L.D.R.

Bottom left   Romeo S, Duim RA, Bridge JA et al. Heterogeneous and complex rearrangements of chromosome arm 6q in chondromyxoid fibroma: delineation of breakpoints and analysis of candidate target genes. Am J Pathol177:1365–1376. Copyright (2010), with permission from Elsevier.

Bottom centre   Debiec-Rychter M.

Bottom right   Lessnick S.

References

1. Abbas M, Ajrawi T, Tungekar MF (2004). Mesenchymal chondrosarcoma of the thyroid — a rare tumour at an unusual site. APMIS 112: 384–389.

2. Abbasi NR, Brownell I, Fangman W (2007). Familial multiple angiolipomatosis. Dermatol Online J 13: 3

3. Abdelwahab IF, Klein MJ, Hermann G et al. (1998). Angiosarcomas associated with bone infarcts. Skeletal Radiol 27: 546–551.

4. Abdul-Karim FW, el-Naggar AK, Joyce MJ et al. (1992). Diffuse and localized tenosynovial giant cell tumor and pigmented villonodular synovitis: a clinicopathologic and flow cytometric DNA analysis. Hum Pathol 23: 729–735.

5. Abe S, Yamamoto A, Tamayama M et al. (2011). Synovial hemangioma of the hip joint with pathological femoral neck fracture and extra-articular extension. J Orthop Sci. In press.

6. Abraham SC, Krasinskas AM, Hofstetter WL et al. (2007). "Seedling" mesenchymal tumors (gastrointestinal stromal tumors and leiomyomas) are common incidental tumors of the esophagogastric junction. Am J Surg Pathol 31: 1629–1635.

7. Abraham Z, Rozenbaum M, Rosner I et al. (1997). Nuchal fibroma. J Dermatol 24: 262–265.

8. Abramson DH, Ellsworth RM, Kitchin FD et al. (1984). Second nonocular tumors in retinoblastoma survivors. Are they radiation-induced? Ophthalmology 91: 1351–1355.

9. Adamicova K, Fetisovova Z, Mellova Y et al. (1998). [Microstructure of subcutaneous lesions in juvenile hyaline fibromatosis]. Cesk Patol 34: 99–104.

10. Adams H, Tzankov A, d'Hondt S et al. (2008). Primary diffuse large B-cell lymphomas of the bone: prognostic relevance of protein expression and clinical factors. Hum Pathol 39: 1323–1330.

11. Adams SC, Potter BK, Mahmood Z et al. (2009). Consequences and prevention of inadvertent internal fixation of primary osseous sarcomas. Clin Orthop Relat Res 467: 519–525.

12. Adem C, Gisselsson D, Dal Cin P et al. (2001). ETV6 rearrangements in patients with infantile fibrosarcomas and congenital mesoblastic nephromas by fluorescence in situ hybridization. Mod Pathol 14: 1246–1251.

13. Adeniran A, Al-Ahmadie H, Mahoney MC et al. (2004). Granular cell tumor of the breast: a series of 17 cases and review of the literature. Breast J 10: 528–531.

14. Adler CP (2000). Hemangioma of the bone. In: Bone DiseasesSpringer: Berlin: pp 370–374.

15. Agaimy A, Bihl MP, Tornillo L et al. (2010). Calcifying fibrous tumor of the stomach: clinicopathologic and molecular study of seven cases with literature review and reappraisal of histogenesis. Am J Surg Pathol 34: 271–278.

16. Agaimy A, Michal M (2011). Hybrid schwannoma-perineurioma of the gastrointestinal tract: a clinicopathologic study of 2 cases and reappraisal of perineurial cells in gastrointestinal schwannomas. Appl Immunohistochem Mol Morphol 19: 454–459.

17. Agaimy A, Wunsch PH, Hofstaedter F et al. (2007). Minute gastric sclerosing stromal tumors (GIST tumorlets) are common in adults and frequently show c-KIT mutations. Am J Surg Pathol 31: 113–120.

18. Agaimy A, Wunsch PH, Schroeder J et al. (2008). Low-grade abdominopelvic sarcoma with myofibroblastic features (low-grade myofibroblastic sarcoma): clinicopathological, immunohistochemical, molecular genetic and ultrastructural study of two cases with literature review. J Clin Pathol 61: 301–306.

19. Agesen TH, Florenes VA, Molenaar WM et al. (2005). Expression patterns of cell cycle components in sporadic and neurofibromatosis type 1-related malignant peripheral nerve sheath tumors. J Neuropathol Exp Neurol 64: 74–81.

20. Ahn J, Ludecke HJ, Lindow S et al. (1995). Cloning of the putative tumour suppressor gene for hereditary multiple exostoses (EXT1). Nat Genet 11: 137–143.

21. Aideyan UO, Kao SC (1998). Case report: Urinary bladder rhabdomyosarcoma associated with Beckwith-Wiedemann syndrome. Clin Radiol 53: 457–459.

22. Aigner T, Dertinger S, Belke J et al. (1996). Chondrocytic cell differentiation in clear cell chondrosarcoma. Hum Pathol 27: 1301–1305.

23. Akbarnia BA, Wirth CR, Colman N (1976). Fibrosarcoma arising from chronic osteomyelitis. Case report and review of the literature. J Bone Joint Surg Am 58: 123–125.

24. Akhlaghpoor S, Aziz Ahari A, Ahmadi SA et al. (2010). Histological evaluation of drill fragments obtained during osteoid osteoma radiofrequency ablation. Skeletal Radiol 39: 451–455.

25. Al Dhabi R, Powell J, McCuaig C et al. (2010). Differentiation of vascular tumors from vascular malformations by expression of Wilms tumor 1 gene: evaluation of 126 cases. J Am Acad Dermatol 63: 1052–1057.

26. Al-Abbadi MA, Almasri NM, Al-Quran S et al. (2007). Cytokeratin and epithelial membrane antigen expression in angiosarcomas: an immunohistochemical study of 33 cases. Arch Pathol Lab Med 131: 288–292.

27. Al-Daraji WI, Miettinen M (2008). Superficial acral fibromyxoma: a clinicopathological analysis of 32 tumors including 4 in the heel. J Cutan Pathol 35: 1020–1026.

28. Al-Saleh S, Mei-Zahav M, Faughnan ME et al. (2009). Screening for pulmonary and cerebral arteriovenous malformations in children with hereditary haemorrhagic telangiectasia. Eur Respir J 34: 875–881.

29. Alaggio R, Barisani D, Ninfo V et al. (2008). Morphologic overlap between infantile myofibromatosis and infantile fibrosarcoma: a pitfall in diagnosis. Pediatr Dev Pathol 11: 355–362.

30. Alaggio R, Bisogno G, Rosato A et al. (2009). Undifferentiated sarcoma: does it exist? A clinicopathologic study of 7 pediatric cases and review of literature. Hum Pathol 40: 1600–1610.

31. Alaggio R, Cecchetto G, Bisogno G et al. (2010). Inflammatory myofibroblastic tumors in childhood: a report from the Italian Cooperative Group studies. Cancer 116: 216–226.

32. Alaggio R, Coffin CM, Weiss SW et al. (2009). Liposarcomas in young patients: a study of 82 cases occurring in patients younger than 22 years of age. Am J Surg Pathol 33: 645–658.

33. Alaggio R, Collini P, Randall RL et al. (2010). Undifferentiated high-grade pleomorphic sarcomas in children: a clinicopathologic study of 10 cases and review of literature. Pediatr Dev Pathol 13: 209–217.

34. Alaggio R, Ninfo V, Rosolen A et al. (2006). Primitive myxoid mesenchymal tumor of infancy: a clinicopathologic report of 6 cases. Am J Surg Pathol 30: 388–394.

35. Albagha OM, Wani SE, Visconti MR et al. (2011). Genome-wide association identifies three new susceptibility loci for Paget's disease of bone. Nat Genet 43: 685–689.

36. Alberghini M, Kliskey K, Krenacs T et al. (2010). Morphological and immunophenotypic features of primary and metastatic giant cell tumour of bone. Virchows Arch 456: 97–103.

37. Albert DM, Lahav M, Lesser R et al. (1974). Recent observations regarding retinoblastoma. I. Ultrastructure, tissue culture growth, incidence, and animal models. Trans Ophthalmol Soc U K 94: 909–928.

38. Albert DM, McGhee CN, Seddon JM et al. (1984). Development of additional primary tumors after 62 years in the first patient with retinoblastoma cured by radiation therapy. Am J Ophthalmol 97: 189–196.

39. Albertini AF, Brousse N, Bodemer C et al. (2011). Retiform hemangioendothelioma developed on the site of an earlier cystic lymphangioma in a six-year-old girl. Am J Dermatopathol 33: e84–e87.

40. Albores-Saavedra J, Manivel JC, Essenfeld H et al. (1990). Pseudosarcomatous myofibroblastic proliferations in the urinary bladder of children. Cancer 66: 1234–1241.

41. Aleixo PB, Hartmann AA, Menezes IC et al. (2009). Can MDM2 and CDK4 make the diagnosis of well differentiated/dedifferentiated liposarcoma? An immunohistochemical study on 129 soft tissue tumours. J Clin Pathol 62: 1127–1135.

42. Alencar A, Pitcher D, Byrne G et al. (2010). Primary bone lymphoma—the University of Miami experience. Leuk Lymphoma 51: 39–49.

43. Alguacil-Garcia A, Unni KK, Goellner JR (1978). Giant cell tumor of tendon sheath and pigmented villonodular synovitis: an ultrastructural study. Am J Clin Pathol 69: 6–17.

44. Allderdice PW, Davis JG, Miller OJ et al. (1969). The 13q-deletion syndrome. Am J Hum Genet 21: 499–512.

45. Allen PW (1972). Nodular fasciitis. Pathology 4: 9–26.

46. Allen PW (1972). Recurring digital fibrous tumours of childhood. Pathology 4: 215–223.

47. Allen PW, Enzinger FM (1970). Juvenile aponeurotic fibroma. Cancer 26: 857–867.

48. Allen PW, Enzinger FM (1972). Hemangioma of skeletal muscle. An analysis of 89 cases. Cancer 29: 8–22.

49. Almeida J, Orfao A, Ocqueteau M et al. (1999). High-sensitive immunophenotyping and DNA ploidy studies for the investigation of minimal residual disease in multiple myeloma. Br J Haematol 107: 121–131.

50. Alqahtani A, Nguyen LT, Flageole H et al. (1999). 25 years' experience with lymphangiomas in children. J Pediatr Surg 34: 1164–1168.

51. Alvarez C, Tredwell S, De Vera M et al. (2006). The genotype-phenotype correlation of hereditary multiple exostoses. Clin Genet 70: 122–130.

52. Alvarez CM, De Vera MA, Heslip TR et al. (2007). Evaluation of the anatomic burden of patients with hereditary multiple exostoses. Clin Orthop Relat Res 462: 73–79.

53. Alvegard TA, Sigurdsson H, Mouridsen H et al. (1989). Adjuvant chemotherapy with doxorubicin in high-grade soft tissue sarcoma: a randomized trial of the Scandinavian Sarcoma Group. J Clin Oncol 7: 1504–1513.

54. Amary MF, Bacsi K, Maggiani F et al. (2011). IDH1 and IDH2 mutations are frequent events in central chondrosarcoma and central and periosteal chondromas but not in other mesenchymal tumours. J Pathol 224: 334–343.

55. Amary MF, Berisha F, Del Carlo Bernardi F et al. (2007). Detection of SS18-SSX fusion transcripts in formalin-fixed paraffin-embedded neoplasms: analysis of conventional RT-PCR, qRT-PCR and dual color FISH as diagnostic tools for synovial sarcoma. Mod Pathol 20: 482–496.

56. Amary MF, Damato S, Halai D et al. (2011). Ollier disease and Maffucci syndrome are caused by somatic mosaic mutations of IDH1 and IDH2. Nat Genet 43: 1262–1265.

57. Ambacher T, Maurer F, Weise K (1999). [Spontaneous healing of a juvenile bone cyst of the tibia after pathological fracture]. Unfallchirurg 102: 972–974.

58. Amin MB, Patel RM, Oliveira P et al. (2006). Alveolar soft-part sarcoma of the urinary bladder with urethral recurrence: a unique case with emphasis on differential diagnoses and diagnostic utility of an immunohistochemical panel including TFE3. Am J Surg Pathol 30: 1322–1325.

59. Amir G, Mogle P, Sucher E (1992). Case report 729. Myositis ossificans and aneurysmal bone cyst. Skeletal Radiol 21: 257–259.

60. Amstalden EM, Carvalho RB, Pacheco EM et al. (2006). Chondromatous hamartoma of the chest wall: description of 3 new cases and literature review. Int J Surg Pathol 14: 119–126.

61. Andaluz N, Balko G, Bui H et al. (2000). Angiolipomas of the central nervous system. J Neurooncol 49: 219–230.

62. Anderson MW, Temple HT, Dussault RG et al. (1999). Compartmental anatomy: relevance to staging and biopsy of musculoskeletal tumors. AJR Am J Roentgenol 173:

1663–1671.

63. Andresen KJ, Sundaram M, Unni KK et al. (2004). Imaging features of low-grade central osteosarcoma of the long bones and pelvis. Skeletal Radiol 33: 373–379.

64. Andronesi OC, Kim GS, Gerstner E et al. (2012). Detection of 2-hydroxyglutarate in IDH-mutated glioma patients by in vivo spectral-editing and 2D correlation magnetic resonance spectroscopy. Sci Transl Med 4: 116ra4

65. Angervall L, Dahl I, Kindblom LG et al. (1976). Spindle cell lipoma. Acta Pathol Microbiol Scand A 84: 477–487.

66. Angervall L, Kindblom LG, Haglid K (1984). Dermal nerve sheath myxoma. A light and electron microscopic, histochemical and immunohistochemical study. Cancer 53: 1752–1759.

67. Angervall L, Nielsen JM, Stener B et al. (1979). Concomitant arteriovenous vascular malformation in skeletal muscle: a clinical, angiographic and histologic study. Cancer 44: 232–238.

68. Anninga JK, Gelderblom H, Fiocco M et al. (2011). Chemotherapeutic adjuvant treatment for osteosarcoma: where do we stand? Eur J Cancer 47: 2431–2445.

68A. Anon. (2003). Criteria for the classification of monoclonal gammopathies, multiple myeloma and related disorders: a report of the International Myeloma Working Group. Br J Haematol 121:749–757.

69. Anon. (2007). Werner syndrome mutational database. Department of Pathology, University of Washington, Seattle (http://www.pathology.washington.edu/research/werner/database/).

70. Anon. (2011). GeneTests: medical genetics information resource [database online]. University of Washington, Seattle (http://www.genetests.org).

71. Anon. (2011). The International Registry of Werner Syndrome. Department of Pathology at the University of Washington, Seattle (http://www.wernersyndrome.org/registry/registry.html).

72. Anon. (2012). OMIM - Online Mendelian Inheritance in Man [online database]. McKusick-Nathans Institute of Genetic Medicine, Johns Hopkins University School of Medicine (http://omim.org/).

73. Antaya RJ, Cajaiba MM, Madri J et al. (2007). Juvenile hyaline fibromatosis and infantile systemic hyalinosis overlap associated with a novel mutation in capillary morphogenesis protein-2 gene. Am J Dermatopathol 29: 99–103.

74. Antman K, Ryan L, Borden E (1990). Pooled results from three randomized adjuvant studies of doxorubicin versus observation in soft tissue sarcoma: 10-year results and review of the literature. In: Adjuvant Therapy of Cancer VI. Salmon SE. WB Saunders Co: Philadelphia: pp 529–544.

75. Antonescu CR, Argani P, Erlandson RA et al. (1998). Skeletal and extraskeletal myxoid chondrosarcoma: a comparative clinicopathologic, ultrastructural, and molecular study. Cancer 83: 1504–1521.

76. Antonescu CR, Dal Cin P, Nafa K et al. (2007). EWSR1-CREB1 is the predominant gene fusion in angiomatoid fibrous histiocytoma. Genes Chromosomes Cancer 46: 1051–1060.

77. Antonescu CR, Elahi A, Healey JH et al. (2000). Monoclonality of multifocal myxoid liposarcoma: confirmation by analysis of TLS-CHOP or EWS-CHOP rearrangements. Clin

Cancer Res 6: 2788–2793.

78. Antonescu CR, Elahi A, Humphrey M et al. (2000). Specificity of TLS-CHOP rearrangement for classic myxoid/round cell liposarcoma: absence in predominantly myxoid well-differentiated liposarcomas. J Mol Diagn 2: 132–138.

79. Antonescu CR, Erlandson RA, Huvos AG (1997). Primary leiomyosarcoma of bone: a clinicopathologic, immunohistochemical, and ultrastructural study of 33 patients and a literature review. Am J Surg Pathol 21: 1281–1294.

80. Antonescu CR, Gerald WL, Magid MS et al. (1998). Molecular variants of the EWS-WT1 gene fusion in desmoplastic small round cell tumor. Diagn Mol Pathol 7: 24–28.

81. Antonescu CR, Nafa K, Segal NH et al. (2006). EWS-CREB1: a recurrent variant fusion in clear cell sarcoma—association with gastrointestinal location and absence of melanocytic differentiation. Clin Cancer Res 12: 5356–5362.

82. Antonescu CR, Rosenblum MK, Pereira P et al. (2001). Sclerosing epithelioid fibrosarcoma: a study of 16 cases and confirmation of a clinicopathologically distinct tumor. Am J Surg Pathol 25: 699–709.

83. Antonescu CR, Tschernyavsky SJ, Decuseara R et al. (2001). Prognostic impact of P53 status, TLS-CHOP fusion transcript structure, and histological grade in myxoid liposarcoma: a molecular and clinicopathologic study of 82 cases. Clin Cancer Res 7: 3977–3987.

84. Antonescu CR, Tschernyavsky SJ, Woodruff JM et al. (2002). Molecular diagnosis of clear cell sarcoma: detection of EWS-ATF1 and MITF-M transcripts and histopathological and ultrastructural analysis of 12 cases. J Mol Diagn 4: 44–52.

85. Antonescu CR, Yoshida A, Guo T et al. (2009). KDR activating mutations in human angiosarcomas are sensitive to specific kinase inhibitors. Cancer Res 69: 7175–7179.

86. Antonescu CR, Zhang L, Chang NE et al. (2010). EWSR1-POU5F1 fusion in soft tissue myoepithelial tumors. A molecular analysis of sixty-six cases, including soft tissue, bone, and visceral lesions, showing common involvement of the EWSR1 gene. Genes Chromosomes Cancer 49: 1114–1124.

87. Antonescu CR, Zhang L, Nielsen GP et al. (2011). Consistent t(1;10) with rearrangements of TGFBR3 and MGEA5 in both myxoinflammatory fibroblastic sarcoma and hemosiderotic fibrolipomatous tumor. Genes Chromosomes Cancer 50: 757–764.

88. Aoki J, Tanikawa H, Ishii K et al. (1996). MR findings indicative of hemosiderin in giant-cell tumor of bone: frequency, cause, and diagnostic significance. AJR Am J Roentgenol 166: 145–148.

89. Aoki T, Hisaoka M, Kouho H et al. (1997). Interphase cytogenetic analysis of myxoid soft tissue tumors by fluorescence in situ hybridization and DNA flow cytometry using paraffin-embedded tissue. Cancer 79: 284–293.

90. Aoki Y, Niihori T, Kawame H et al. (2005). Germline mutations in HRAS proto-oncogene cause Costello syndrome. Nat Genet 37: 1038–1040.

91. Araki N, Uchida A, Kimura T et al. (1991). Involvement of the retinoblastoma gene in primary osteosarcomas and other bone and soft-tissue tumors. Clin Orthop Relat Res 271–277.

92. Arata MA, Peterson HA, Dahlin DC (1981). Pathological fractures through non-ossifying fibromas. Review of the Mayo Clinic

experience. J Bone Joint Surg Am 63: 980–988.

93. Argani P, Antonescu CR, Illei PB et al. (2001). Primary renal neoplasms with the ASPL-TFE3 gene fusion of alveolar soft part sarcoma: a distinctive tumor entity previously included among renal cell carcinomas of children and adolescents. Am J Pathol 159: 179–192.

94. Argani P, Aulmann S, Illei PB et al. (2010). A distinctive subset of PEComas harbors TFE3 gene fusions. Am J Surg Pathol 34: 1395–1406.

95. Argani P, Facchetti F, Inghirami G et al. (1997). Lymphocyte-rich well-differentiated liposarcoma: report of nine cases. Am J Surg Pathol 21: 884–895.

96. Argani P, Fritsch M, Kadkol SS et al. (2000). Detection of the ETV6-NTRK3 chimeric RNA of infantile fibrosarcoma/cellular congenital mesoblastic nephroma in paraffin-embedded tissue: application to challenging pediatric renal stromal tumors. Mod Pathol 13: 29–36.

97. Argani P, Fritsch MK, Shuster AE et al. (2001). Reduced sensitivity of paraffin-based RT-PCR assays for ETV6-NTRK3 fusion transcripts in morphologically defined infantile fibrosarcoma. Am J Surg Pathol 25: 1461–1464.

98. Argani P, Lal P, Hutchinson B et al. (2003). Aberrant nuclear immunoreactivity for TFE3 in neoplasms with TFE3 gene fusions: a sensitive and specific immunohistochemical assay. Am J Surg Pathol 27: 750–761.

99. Argenyi ZB (1990). Immunohistochemical characterization of palisaded, encapsulated neuroma. J Cutan Pathol 17: 329–335.

100. Argenyi ZB, Cooper PH, Santa Cruz D (1993). Plexiform and other unusual variants of palisaded encapsulated neuroma. J Cutan Pathol 20: 34–39.

101. Argenyi ZB, Penick GD (1993). Vascular variant of palisaded encapsulated neuroma. J Cutan Pathol 20: 92–93.

102. Argenyi ZB, Santa Cruz D, Bromley C (1992). Comparative light-microscopic and immunohistochemical study of traumatic and palisaded encapsulated neuromas of the skin. Am J Dermatopathol 14: 504–510.

103. Argenyi ZB, Van Rybroek JJ, Kemp JD et al. (1988). Congenital angiomatoid malignant fibrous histiocytoma. A light-microscopic, immunopathologic, and electron-microscopic study. Am J Dermatopathol 10: 59–67.

104. Armengol G, Tarkkanen M, Virolainen M et al. (1997). Recurrent gains of 1q, 8 and 12 in the Ewing family of tumours by comparative genomic hybridization. Br J Cancer 75: 1403–1409.

105. Armour A, Williamson JM (1993). Ectopic cervical hamartomatous thymoma showing extensive myoid differentiation. J Laryngol Otol 107: 155–158.

106. Arnaud L, Hervier B, Neel A et al. (2011). CNS involvement and treatment with interferon-alpha are independent prognostic factors in Erdheim-Chester disease: a multicenter survival analysis of 53 patients. Blood 117: 2778–2782.

107. Arndt CA, Hammond S, Rodeberg D et al. (2006). Significance of persistent mature rhabdomyoblasts in bladder/prostate rhabdomyosarcoma: Results from IRS IV. J Pediatr Hematol Oncol 28: 563–567.

108. Arndt CA, Stoner JA, Hawkins DS et al. (2009). Vincristine, actinomycin, and cyclophosphamide compared with vincristine, actinomycin, and cyclophosphamide alternating

with vincristine, topotecan, and cyclophosphamide for intermediate-risk rhabdomyosarcoma: children's oncology group study D9803. J Clin Oncol 27: 5182–5188.

109. Arnold WH (1973). Hereditary bone dysplasia with sarcomatous degeneration. Study of a family. Ann Intern Med 78: 902–906.

110. Arsenovic N, Abdulla KE, Shamim KS (2011). Mammary-type myofibroblastoma of soft tissue. Indian J Pathol Microbiol 54: 391–393.

111. Arsenovic N, Ramaiya A, Moreira R (2011). Symplastic glomangioma: information review and addition of a new case. Int J Surg Pathol 19: 499–501.

112. Arthaud JB (1972). Pigmented nodular synovitis: report of 11 lesions in non-articular locations. Am J Clin Pathol 58: 511–517.

113. Arya M, Garcia-Montes F, Patel HR et al. (2001). A rare tumour in the pelvis presenting with lower urinary symptoms: 'sclerosing epithelioid fibrosarcoma'. Eur J Surg Oncol 27: 121–122.

114. Ashar HR, Fejzo MS, Tkachenko A et al. (1995). Disruption of the architectural factor HMGI-C: DNA-binding AT hook motifs fused in lipomas to distinct transcriptional regulatory domains. Cell 82: 57–65.

115. Asp J, Sangiorgi L, Inerot SE et al. (2000). Changes of the p16 gene but not the p53 gene in human chondrosarcoma tissues. Int J Cancer 85: 782–786.

116. Assoun J, Richardi G, Railhac JJ et al. (1994). Osteoid osteoma: MR imaging versus CT. Radiology 191: 217–223.

117. Atiye J, Wolf M, Kaur S et al. (2005). Gene amplifications in osteosarcoma-CGH microarray analysis. Genes Chromosomes Cancer 42: 158–163.

118. Attwooll C, Tariq M, Harris M et al. (1999). Identification of a novel fusion gene involving hTAFII68 and CHN from a t(9;17)(q22;q11.2) translocation in an extraskeletal myxoid chondrosarcoma. Oncogene 18: 7599–7601.

119. Ausmus GG, Piliang MP, Bergfeld WF et al. (2007). Soft-tissue perineurioma in a 20-year-old patient with neurofibromatosis type 1 (NF1): report of a case and review of the literature. J Cutan Pathol 34: 726–730.

120. Austin RM, Mack GR, Townsend CM et al. (1980). Infiltrating (intramuscular) lipomas and angiolipomas. A clinicopathologic study of six cases. Arch Surg 115: 281–284.

121. Avet-Loiseau H, Attal M, Moreau P et al. (2007). Genetic abnormalities and survival in multiple myeloma: the experience of the Intergroupe Francophone du Myelome. Blood 109: 3489–3495.

122. Ayadi L, Charfi S, Ben Hamed Y et al. (2008). Pigmented lipofibromatosis in unusual location: case report and review of the literature. Virchows Arch 452: 115–117.

123. Ayala AG, Ro JY, Bolio-Solis A et al. (1993). Mesenchymal hamartoma of the chest wall in infants and children: a clinicopathological study of five patients. Skeletal Radiol 22: 569–576.

124. Ayala AG, Ro JY, Raymond AK et al. (1989). Small cell osteosarcoma. A clinicopathologic study of 27 cases. Cancer 64: 2162–2173.

125. Aydingoz IE, Demirkesen C, Serdar ZA et al. (2009). Composite haemangioendothelioma with lymph-node metastasis: an unusual presentation at an uncommon site. Clin Exp Dermatol 34: e802–e806.

126. Aymard B, Boman-Ferrand F, Vernhes L

et al. (1987). [Fibrolipomatous hamartoma of the peripheral nerves. Anatomico-clinical study of 5 cases, including 2 with ultrastructural study]. Ann Pathol 7: 320–324.
127. Azouz EM (1995). Benign fibrous histiocytoma of the proximal tibial epiphysis in a 12-year-old girl. Skeletal Radiol 24: 375–378.
128. Azumi N, Curtis J, Kempson RL et al. (1987). Atypical and malignant neoplasms showing lipomatous differentiation. A study of 111 cases. Am J Surg Pathol 11: 161–183.
129. Bacchini P, Inwards C, Biscaglia R et al. (1999). Chondroblastoma-like osteosarcoma. Orthopedics 22: 337–339.
130. Bacci G, Ferrari S, Bertoni F et al. (2000). Prognostic factors in nonmetastatic Ewing's sarcoma of bone treated with adjuvant chemotherapy: analysis of 359 patients at the Istituto Ortopedico Rizzoli. J Clin Oncol 18: 4–11.
131. Bacci G, Ferrari S, Ruggieri P et al. (2001). Telangiectatic osteosarcoma of the extremity: neoadjuvant chemotherapy in 24 cases. Acta Orthop Scand 72: 167–172.
132. Bacci G, Longhi A, Ferrari S et al. (2002). Prognostic significance of serum alkaline phosphatase in osteosarcoma of the extremity treated with neoadjuvant chemotherapy: recent experience at Rizzoli Institute. Oncol Rep 9: 171–175.
133. Bacci G, Longhi A, Forni C et al. (2007). Neoadjuvant chemotherapy for radioinduced osteosarcoma of the extremity: The Rizzoli experience in 20 cases. Int J Radiat Oncol Biol Phys 67: 505–511.
134. Bacci G, Longhi A, Versari M et al. (2006). Prognostic factors for osteosarcoma of the extremity treated with neoadjuvant chemotherapy: 15-year experience in 789 patients treated at a single institution. Cancer 106: 1154–1161.
135. Badalian-Very G, Vergilio JA, Degar BA et al. (2010). Recurrent BRAF mutations in Langerhans cell histiocytosis. Blood 116: 1919–1923.
136. Badalian-Very G, Vergilio JA, Degar BA et al. (2012). Recent advances in the understanding of Langerhans cell histiocytosis. Br J Haematol 156: 163–172.
137. Bague S, Folpe AL (2008). Dermatofibrosarcoma protuberans presenting as a subcutaneous mass: a clinicopathological study of 15 cases with exclusive or near-exclusive subcutaneous involvement. Am J Dermatopathol 30: 327–332.
138. Bahrami A, Dalton JD, Krane JF et al. (2012). A subset of cutaneous and soft tissue mixed tumors are genetically linked to their salivary gland counterpart. Genes Chromosomes Cancer 51: 140–148.
139. Bahrami A, Folpe AL (2010). Adult-type fibrosarcoma: A reevaluation of 163 putative cases diagnosed at a single institution over a 48-year period. Am J Surg Pathol 34: 1504–1513.
140. Bahrami A, Weiss SW, Montgomery E et al. (2009). RT-PCR analysis for FGF23 using paraffin sections in the diagnosis of phosphaturic mesenchymal tumors with and without known tumor induced osteomalacia. Am J Surg Pathol 33: 1348–1354.
141. Bai H, Aswad BI, Gaissert H et al. (2001). Malignant solitary fibrous tumor of the pleura with liposarcomatous differentiation. Arch Pathol Lab Med 125: 406–409.
142. Baird PA, Worth AJ (1976). Congenital generalized fibromatosis: an autosomal recessive condition? Clin Genet 9: 488–494.
143. Bajaj MS, Kashyap S, Wagh VB et al. (2005). Glial heterotopia of the orbit and extranasal region: an unusual entity. Clin Experiment Ophthalmol 33: 513–515.
144. Baker AC, Rezeanu L, O'Laughlin S et al. (2007). Juxtacortical chondromyxoid fibroma of bone: a unique variant: a case study of 20 patients. Am J Surg Pathol 31: 1662–1668.
144A. Baker PL, Dockerty MB, Coventry MB (1954). Adamantinoma (so-called) of the long bones; review of the literature and report of three new cases. J Bone Joint Surg Am. 36:704–20.
145. Balachandran K, Allen PW, MacCormac LB (1995). Nuchal fibroma. A clinicopathological study of nine cases. Am J Surg Pathol 19: 313–317.
146. Baldini EH, Goldberg J, Jenner C et al. (1999). Long-term outcomes after function-sparing surgery without radiotherapy for soft tissue sarcoma of the extremities and trunk. J Clin Oncol 17: 3252–3259.
147. Baldus SE, Palmen C, Thiele J (2007). MUC1 (EMA) expressing plasma cells in bone marrow infiltrated by plasma cell myeloma. Histol Histopathol 22: 889–893.
148. Bale PM, Hughes L, de Silva M (1990). Sequestrated meningoceles of scalp: extracranial meningeal heterotopia. Hum Pathol 21: 1156–1163.
149. Balke M, Campanacci L, Gebert C et al. (2010). Bisphosphonate treatment of aggressive primary, recurrent and metastatic Giant Cell Tumour of Bone. BMC Cancer 10: 462
150. Balsaver AM, Butler JJ, Martin RG (1967). Congenital fibrosarcoma. Cancer 20: 1607–1616.
151. Baratti D, Pennacchioli E, Casali PG et al. (2007). Epithelioid sarcoma: prognostic factors and survival in a series of patients treated at a single institution. Ann Surg Oncol 14: 3542–3551.
152. Barnoud R, Sabourin JC, Pasquier D et al. (2000). Immunohistochemical expression of WT1 by desmoplastic small round cell tumor: a comparative study with other small round cell tumors. Am J Surg Pathol 24: 830–836.
153. Barr FG (2001). Gene fusions involving PAX and FOX family members in alveolar rhabdomyosarcoma. Oncogene 20: 5736–5746.
154. Barr FG, Duan F, Smith LM et al. (2009). Genomic and clinical analyses of 2p24 and 12q13-q14 amplification in alveolar rhabdomyosarcoma: a report from the Children's Oncology Group. Genes Chromosomes Cancer 48: 661–672.
155. Barr FG, Qualman SJ, Macris MH et al. (2002). Genetic heterogeneity in the alveolar rhabdomyosarcoma subset without typical gene fusions. Cancer Res 62: 4704–4710.
156. Barretina J, Taylor BS, Banerji S et al. (2010). Subtype-specific genomic alterations define new targets for soft-tissue sarcoma therapy. Nat Genet 42: 715–721.
157. Barry HC (1969). Paget's disease of bone. E & S Livingstone Ltd: Edinburgh.
158. Bartsch O, Wuyts W, Van Hul W et al. (1996). Delineation of a contiguous gene syndrome with multiple exostoses, enlarged parietal foramina, craniofacial dysostosis, and mental retardation, caused by deletions in the short arm of chromosome 11. Am J Hum Genet 58: 734–742.
159. Bartuma H, Domanski HA, Von Steyern FV et al. (2008). Cytogenetic and molecular cytogenetic findings in lipoblastoma. Cancer Genet Cytogenet 183: 60–63.
160. Bartuma H, Hallor KH, Panagopoulos I et al. (2007). Assessment of the clinical and molecular impact of different cytogenetic subgroups in a series of 272 lipomas with abnormal karyotype. Genes Chromosomes Cancer 46: 594–606.
161. Bartuma H, Nord KH, Macchia G et al. (2011). Gene expression and single nucleotide polymorphism array analyses of spindle cell lipomas and conventional lipomas with 13q14 deletion. Genes Chromosomes Cancer 50: 619–632.
162. Bartuma H, Panagopoulos I, Collin A et al. (2009). Expression levels of HMGA2 in adipocytic tumors correlate with morphologic and cytogenetic subgroups. Mol Cancer 8: 36
163. Baruffi MR, Volpon JB, Neto JB et al. (2001). Osteoid osteomas with chromosome alterations involving 22q. Cancer Genet Cytogenet 124: 127–131.
164. Baser ME, Friedman JM, Evans DG (2006). Increasing the specificity of diagnostic criteria for schwannomatosis. Neurology 66: 730–732.
165. Batstone P, Forsyth L, Goodlad J (2001). Clonal chromosome aberrations secondary to chromosome instability in an elastofibroma. Cancer Genet Cytogenet 128: 46–47.
166. Battaglia A, Merati A, Magit A (2000). Cherubism and upper airway obstruction. Otolaryngol Head Neck Surg 122: 573–574.
167. Bauer TW, Dorfman HD, Latham JT, Jr. (1982). Periosteal chondroma. A clinicopathologic study of 23 cases. Am J Surg Pathol 6: 631–637.
168. Bayani J, Zielenska M, Pandita A et al. (2003). Spectral karyotyping identifies recurrent complex rearrangements of chromosomes 8, 17, and 20 in osteosarcomas. Genes Chromosomes Cancer 36: 7–16.
169. Bayat A, Cunliffe EJ, McGrouther DA (2007). Assessment of clinical severity in Dupuytren's disease. Br J Hosp Med (Lond) 68: 604–609.
170. Bayat A, McGrouther DA (2006). Management of Dupuytren's disease—clear advice for an elusive condition. Ann R Coll Surg Engl 88: 3–8.
171. Beall DP, Ly J, Bell JP et al. (2008). Pediatric extraskeletal osteosarcoma. Pediatr Radiol 38: 579–582.
172. Bech K, Jensen OA (1961). Bilateral retinoblastoma in Denmark, 1928-1957. Acta Ophthalmol (Copenh) 39: 561–568.
173. Beck AH, Lee CH, Witten DM et al. (2010). Discovery of molecular subtypes in leiomyosarcoma through integrative molecular profiling. Oncogene 29: 845–854.
174. Beckett JH, Jacobs AH (1977). Recurring digital fibrous tumors of childhood: a review. Pediatrics 59: 401–406.
175. Beckwith JB (1963). Extreme cytomegaly of the adrenal cortex, omphalocele, hyperplasia of kidneys and pancreas, and Leydig-cell hyperplasia: Another syndrome? West Soc Ped Res. Los Angeles November 11
176. Beer TW (2005). Cutaneous angiomyolipomas are HMB45 negative, not associated with tuberous sclerosis, and should be considered as angioleiomyomas with fat. Am J Dermatopathol 27: 418–421.
177. Beer TW, Drury P, Heenan PJ (2010). Atypical fibroxanthoma: a histological and immunohistochemical review of 171 cases. Am J Dermatopathol 32: 533–540.
178. Beert E, Brems H, Daniels B et al. (2011). Atypical neurofibromas in neurofibromatosis type 1 are premalignant tumors. Genes Chromosomes Cancer 50: 1021–1032.
179. Begueret H, Galateau-Salle F, Guillou L et al. (2005). Primary intrathoracic synovial sarcoma: a clinicopathologic study of 40 t(X;18)-positive cases from the French Sarcoma Group and the Mesopath Group. Am J Surg Pathol 29: 339–346.
180. Beham A, Fletcher CD (1991). Intramuscular angioma: a clinicopathological analysis of 74 cases. Histopathology 18: 53–59.
180A. Behery RE, Bedrnicek J, Lazenby A et al. (2012). Translocation t(12;17)(q24.1;q21) as the sole anomaly in a nasal chondromesenchymal hamartoma arising in a patient with pleuropulmonary blastoma. Pediatr Dev Pathol. 15:249–253.
181. Behrens GM, Stoll M, Schmidt RE (2000). Lipodystrophy syndrome in HIV infection: what is it, what causes it and how can it be managed? Drug Saf 23: 57–76.
182. Bejarano PA, Padhya TA, Smith R et al. (2000). Hyalinizing spindle cell tumor with giant rosettes—a soft tissue tumor with mesenchymal and neuroendocrine features. An immunohistochemical, ultrastructural, and cytogenetic analysis. Arch Pathol Lab Med 124: 1179–1184.
183. Bella GP, Manivel JC, Thompson RC, Jr. et al. (2007). Intramuscular hemangioma: recurrence risk related to surgical margins. Clin Orthop Relat Res 459: 186–191.
184. Bellini C, Rutigliani M, Boccardo FM et al. (2009). Nuchal translucency and lymphatic system maldevelopment. J Perinat Med 37: 673–676.
185. Ben-Izhak O, Elmalach I, Kerner H et al. (1996). Pericardial myolipoma: a tumour presenting as a mediastinal mass and containing oestrogen receptors. Histopathology 29: 184–186.
186. Bendl BJ, Asano K, Lewis RJ (1977). Nodular angioblastic hyperplasia with eosinophilia and lymphofolliculosis. Cutis 19: 327–329.
187. Beneteau C, Cave H, Moncla A et al. (2009). SOS1 and PTPN11 mutations in five cases of Noonan syndrome with multiple giant cell lesions. Eur J Hum Genet 17: 1216–1221.
188. Bengesser K, Cooper DN, Steinmann K et al. (2010). A novel third type of recurrent NF1 microdeletion mediated by nonallelic homologous recombination between LRRC37B-containing low-copy repeats in 17q11.2. Hum Mutat 31: 742–751.
189. Benisch B, Peison B, Marquet E et al. (1983). Pre-elastofibroma and elastofibroma (the continuum of elastic-producing fibrous tumors). A light and ultrastructural study. Am J Clin Pathol 80: 88–92.
190. Bennicelli JL, Advani S, Schafer BW et al. (1999). PAX3 and PAX7 exhibit conserved cis-acting transcription repression domains and utilize a common gain of function mechanism in alveolar rhabdomyosarcoma. Oncogene 18: 4348–4356.
191. Berber O, wson-Bowling S, Jalgaonkar A et al. (2011). Bizarre parosteal osteochondromatous proliferation of bone: clinical management of a series of 22 cases. J Bone Joint Surg Br 93: 1118–1121.
192. Bergh P, Meis-Kindblom JM, Gherlinzoni F et al. (1999). Synovial sarcoma: identification of low and high risk groups. Cancer 85: 2596–2607.
193. Berlin O, Angervall L, Kindblom LG et al. (1987). Primary leiomyosarcoma of bone. A clinical, radiographic, pathologic-anatomic, and prognostic study of 16 cases. Skeletal Radiol

16: 364–376.
194. Berlin O, Stener B, Kindblom LG et al. (1984). Leiomyosarcomas of venous origin in the extremities. A correlated clinical, roentgenologic, and morphologic study with diagnostic and surgical implications. Cancer 54: 2147–2159.
195. Bernado L, Admella C, Lucaya J et al. (1987). Infantile fibrosarcoma of femur. Pediatr Pathol 7: 201–207.
196. Bernal K, Nelson M, Neff JR et al. (2004). Translocation (2;11)(q31;q12) is recurrent in collagenous fibroma (desmoplastic fibroblastoma). Cancer Genet Cytogenet 149: 161–163.
197. Bernard MA, Hall CE, Hogue DA et al. (2001). Diminished levels of the putative tumor suppressor proteins EXT1 and EXT2 in exostosis chondrocytes. Cell Motil Cytoskeleton 48: 149–162.
198. Bernard SA, Murphey MD, Flemming DJ et al. (2010). Improved differentiation of benign osteochondromas from secondary chondrosarcomas with standardized measurement of cartilage cap at CT and MR imaging. Radiology 255: 857–865.
199. Berner JM, Sorlie T, Mertens F et al. (1999). Chromosome band 9p21 is frequently altered in malignant peripheral nerve sheath tumors: studies of CDKN2A and other genes of the pRB pathway. Genes Chromosomes Cancer 26: 151–160.
200. Bernstein KE, Lattes R (1982). Nodular (pseudosarcomatous) fasciitis, a nonrecurrent lesion: clinicopathologic study of 134 cases. Cancer 49: 1668–1678.
201. Bernstein R, Zeltzer PM, Lin F et al. (1994). Trisomy 11 and other nonrandom trisomies in congenital fibrosarcoma. Cancer Genet Cytogenet 78: 82–86.
202. Berti E, Roncaroli F (1994). Fibrolipomatous hamartoma of a cranial nerve. Histopathology 24: 391–392.
203. Bertoni F, Bacchini P, Capanna R et al. (1993). Solid variant of aneurysmal bone cyst. Cancer 71: 729–734.
204. Bertoni F, Bacchini P, Donati D et al. (1993). Osteoblastoma-like osteosarcoma. The Rizzoli Institute experience. Mod Pathol 6: 707–716.
205. Bertoni F, Bacchini P, Fabbri N et al. (1993). Osteosarcoma. Low-grade intraosseous-type osteosarcoma, histologically resembling parosteal osteosarcoma, fibrous dysplasia, and desmoplastic fibroma. Cancer 71: 338–345.
206. Bertoni F, Bacchini P, Staals EL (2003). Giant cell-rich osteosarcoma. Orthopedics 26: 179–181.
207. Bertoni F, Bacchini P, Staals EL et al. (2005). Dedifferentiated parosteal osteosarcoma: the experience of the Rizzoli Institute. Cancer 103: 2373–2382.
208. Bertoni F, Boriani S, Laus M et al. (1982). Periosteal chondrosarcoma and periosteal osteosarcoma. Two distinct entities. J Bone Joint Surg Br 64: 370–376.
209. Bertoni F, Calderoni P, Bacchini P et al. (1986). Benign fibrous histiocytoma of bone. J Bone Joint Surg Am 68: 1225–1230.
210. Bertoni F, Capanna R, Calderoni P et al. (1984). Primary central (medullary) fibrosarcoma of bone. Semin Diagn Pathol 1: 185–198.
211. Bertoni F, Picci P, Bacchini P et al. (1983). Mesenchymal chondrosarcoma of bone and soft tissues. Cancer 52: 533–541.
212. Bertoni F, Present D, Bacchini P et al. (1989). The Istituto Rizzoli experience with small cell osteosarcoma. Cancer 64: 2591–2599.
213. Bertoni F, Present D, Hudson T et al. (1985). The meaning of radiolucencies in parosteal osteosarcoma. J Bone Joint Surg Am 67: 901–910.
214. Bertoni F, Unni KK, Beabout JW et al. (1987). Chondroblastoma of the skull and facial bones. Am J Clin Pathol 88: 1–9.
215. Bertoni F, Unni KK, Beabout JW et al. (1995). Parosteal osteoma of bones other than of the skull and face. Cancer 75: 2466–2473.
216. Bertoni F, Unni KK, Beabout JW et al. (1997). Malignant giant cell tumor of the tendon sheaths and joints (malignant pigmented villonodular synovitis). Am J Surg Pathol 21: 153–163.
217. Betts DR, Avoledo P, von der Weid N et al. (2005). Cytogenetic characterization of Ewing tumors with high-ploidy. Cancer Genet Cytogenet 159: 160–163.
218. Bhagavathi S, Micale MA, Les K et al. (2009). Primary bone diffuse large B-cell lymphoma: clinicopathologic study of 21 cases and review of literature. Am J Surg Pathol 33: 1463–1469.
219. Bhattacharya B, Dilworth HP, Iacobuzio-Donahue C et al. (2005). Nuclear beta-catenin expression distinguishes deep fibromatosis from other benign and malignant fibroblastic and myofibroblastic lesions. Am J Surg Pathol 29: 653–659.
220. Bhawan J, Bacchetta C, Joris I et al. (1979). A myofibroblastic tumor. Infantile digital fibroma (recurrent digital fibrous tumor of childhood). Am J Pathol 94: 19–36.
221. Bhutoria B, Konar A, Chakrabarti S et al. (2009). Retiform hemangioendothelioma with lymph node metastasis: a rare entity. Indian J Dermatol Venereol Leprol 75: 60–62.
222. Bianco P, Riminucci M, Majolagbe A et al. (2000). Mutations of the GNAS1 gene, stromal cell dysfunction, and osteomalacic changes in non-McCune-Albright fibrous dysplasia of bone. J Bone Miner Res 15: 120–128.
223. Bianco P, Wientroub S (2011). Fibrous dysplasia. In: Pediatric Bone - Biology and Disease 2nd edition Edition. Glorieux FH, Pettifor J, Juppner H Elsevier: New York: pp 589–624.
224. Bibbo C, Warren AM (1994). Fibrolipomatous hamartoma of nerve. J Foot Ankle Surg 33: 64–71.
225. Biegel JA, Conard K, Brooks JJ (1993). Translocation (11;22)(p13;q12): primary change in intra-abdominal desmoplastic small round cell tumor. Genes Chromosomes Cancer 7: 119–121.
226. Biegel JA, Meek RS, Parmiter AH et al. (1991). Chromosomal translocation t(1;13)(p36;q14) in a case of rhabdomyosarcoma. Genes Chromosomes Cancer 3: 483–484.
227. Biegel JA, Tan L, Zhang F et al. (2002). Alterations of the hSNF5/INI1 gene in central nervous system atypical teratoid/rhabdoid tumors and renal and extrarenal rhabdoid tumors. Clin Cancer Res 8: 3461–3467.
228. Biegel JA, Zhou JY, Rorke LB et al. (1999). Germ-line and acquired mutations of INI1 in atypical teratoid and rhabdoid tumors. Cancer Res 59: 74–79.
229. Bielack SS, Kempf-Bielack B, Delling G et al. (2002). Prognostic factors in high-grade osteosarcoma of the extremities or trunk: an analysis of 1,702 patients treated on neoadjuvant cooperative osteosarcoma study group protocols. J Clin Oncol 20: 776–790.
230. Bielack SS, Schroeders A, Fuchs N et al. (1999). Malignant fibrous histiocytoma of bone: a retrospective EMSOS study of 125 cases. European Musculo-Skeletal Oncology Society. Acta Orthop Scand 70: 353–360.
231. Bigby SM, Symmans PJ, Miller MV et al. (2011). Aggressive angiomyxoma [corrected] of the female genital tract and pelvis—clinicopathologic features with immunohistochemical analysis. Int J Gynecol Pathol 30: 505–513.
232. Biggar RJ (2001). AIDS-related cancers in the era of highly active antiretroviral therapy. Oncology (Williston Park) 15: 439–448.
233. Bijlsma EK, Merel P, Bosch DA et al. (1994). Analysis of mutations in the SCH gene in schwannomas. Genes Chromosomes Cancer 11: 7–14.
234. Billeret L, V (1999). [Granular cell tumor. Epidemiology of 263 cases]. Arch Anat Cytol Pathol 47: 26–30.
235. Billings SD, Folpe AL, Weiss SW (2001). Do leiomyomas of deep soft tissue exist? An analysis of highly differentiated smooth muscle tumors of deep soft tissue supporting two distinct subtypes. Am J Surg Pathol 25: 1134–1142.
236. Billings SD, Folpe AL, Weiss SW (2003). Epithelioid sarcoma-like hemangioendothelioma. Am J Surg Pathol 27: 48–57.
237. Billings SD, Giblen G, Fanburg-Smith JC (2005). Superficial low-grade fibromyxoid sarcoma (Evans tumor): a clinicopathologic analysis of 19 cases with a unique observation in the pediatric population. Am J Surg Pathol 29: 204–210.
238. Binder H, Eng GD, Gaiser JF et al. (1987). Congenital muscular torticollis: results of conservative management with long-term follow-up in 85 cases. Arch Phys Med Rehabil 68: 222–225.
239. Binh MB, Sastre-Garau X, Guillou L et al. (2005). MDM2 and CDK4 immunostainings are useful adjuncts in diagnosing well-differentiated and dedifferentiated liposarcoma subtypes: a comparative analysis of 559 soft tissue neoplasms with genetic data. Am J Surg Pathol 29: 1340–1347.
240. Birch JM (1994). Li-Fraumeni syndrome. Eur J Cancer 30A: 1935–1941.
241. Birdsall SH, Shipley JM, Summersgill BM et al. (1995). Cytogenetic findings in a case of nodular fasciitis of the breast. Cancer Genet Cytogenet 81: 166–168.
242. Bisceglia M, Cammisa M, Suster S et al. (2003). Erdheim-Chester disease: clinical and pathologic spectrum of four cases from the Arkadi M. Rywlin slide seminars. Adv Anat Pathol 10: 160–171.
243. Bisceglia M, Cardone M, Fantasia L et al. (2001). Mixed tumors, myoepitheliomas, and oncocytomas of the soft tissues are likely members of the same family: a clinicopathologic and ultrastructural study. Ultrastruct Pathol 25: 399–418.
244. Bisceglia M, Magro G (1999). Low-grade myofibroblastic sarcoma of the salivary gland. Am J Surg Pathol 23: 1435–1436.
245. Bisceglia M, Spagnolo D, Galliani C et al. (2006). Tumoral, quasitumoral and pseudotumoral lesions of the superficial and somatic soft tissue: new entities and new variants of old entities recorded during the last 25 years. Part XII: appendix. Pathologica 98: 239–298.
246. Biselli R, Boldrini R, Ferlini C et al. (1999). Myofibroblastic tumours: neoplasias with divergent behaviour. Ultrastructural and flow cytometric analysis. Pathol Res Pract 195: 619–632.
247. Bispo Junior RZ, Guedes AV (2007). Parosteal lipoma of the femur with hyperostosis: case report and literature review. Clinics (Sao Paulo) 62: 647–652.
248. Bixby SD, Hettmer S, Taylor GA et al. (2010). Synovial sarcoma in children: imaging features and common benign mimics. AJR Am J Roentgenol 195: 1026–1032.
249. Bjerregaard P, Hagen K, Daugaard S et al. (1989). Intramuscular lipoma of the lower limb. Long-term follow-up after local resection. J Bone Joint Surg Br 71: 812–815.
250. Bjornsson J, McLeod RA, Unni KK et al. (1998). Primary chondrosarcoma of long bones and limb girdles. Cancer 83: 2105–2119.
251. Bjornsson J, Unni KK, Dahlin DC et al. (1984). Clear cell chondrosarcoma of bone. Observations in 47 cases. Am J Surg Pathol 8: 223–230.
252. Bjornsson J, Wold LE, Ebersold MJ et al. (1993). Chordoma of the mobile spine. A clinicopathologic analysis of 40 patients. Cancer 71: 735–740.
253. Blauvelt A (1999). The role of human herpesvirus 8 in the pathogenesis of Kaposi's sarcoma. Adv Dermatol 14: 167–206.
254. Blazo MA, Lewis RA, Chintagumpala MM et al. (2004). Outcomes of systematic screening for optic pathway tumors in children with Neurofibromatosis Type 1. Am J Med Genet A 127A: 224–229.
255. Bleiweiss IJ, Klein MJ (1990). Chondromyxoid fibroma: report of six cases with immunohistochemical studies. Mod Pathol 3: 664–666.
256. Blocker S, Koenig J, Ternberg J (1987). Congenital fibrosarcoma. J Pediatr Surg 22: 665–670.
257. Bloem JL, Mulder JD (1985). Chondroblastoma: a clinical and radiological study of 104 cases. Skeletal Radiol 14: 1–9.
258. Bloem JL, van der Heul RO, Schuttevaer HM et al. (1991). Fibrous dysplasia vs adamantinoma of the tibia: differentiation based on discriminant analysis of clinical and plain film findings. AJR Am J Roentgenol 156: 1017–1023.
259. Blumberg AK, Kay S, Adelaar RS (1989). Nerve sheath myxoma of digital nerve. Cancer 63: 1215–1218.
260. Bode-Lesniewska B, Frigerio S, Exner U et al. (2007). Relevance of translocation type in myxoid liposarcoma and identification of a novel EWSR1-DDIT3 fusion. Genes Chromosomes Cancer 46: 961–971.
261. Bode-Lesniewska B, Zhao J, Speel EJ et al. (2001). Gains of 12q13-14 and overexpression of mdm2 are frequent findings in intimal sarcomas of the pulmonary artery. Virchows Arch 438: 57–65.
262. Bohm P, Krober S, Greschniok A et al. (1996). Desmoplastic fibroma of the bone. A report of two patients, review of the literature, and therapeutic implications. Cancer 78: 1011–1023.
263. Boland JM, Folpe AL, Hornick JL et al. (2009). Clusterin is expressed in normal synoviocytes and in tenosynovial giant cell tumors of localized and diffuse types: diagnostic and histogenetic implications. Am J Surg Pathol 33: 1225–1229.
264. Boland JM, Weiss SW, Oliveira AM et al. (2010). Liposarcomas with mixed well-differentiated and pleomorphic features: a clinicopathologic study of 12 cases. Am J Surg Pathol 34: 837–843.
265. Bolen JW, Thorning D (1980). Benign lipoblastoma and myxoid liposarcoma: a comparative light- and electron-microscopic study. Am J Surg Pathol 4: 163–174.

266. Bond GL, Hirshfield KM, Kirchhoff T et al. (2006). MDM2 SNP309 accelerates tumor formation in a gender-specific and hormone-dependent manner. Cancer Res 66: 5104–5110.

267. Bonetti F, Martignoni G, Colato C et al. (2001). Abdominopelvic sarcoma of perivascular epithelioid cells. Report of four cases in young women, one with tuberous sclerosis. Mod Pathol 14: 563–568.

268. Bonvalot S, Miceli R, Berselli M et al. (2010). Aggressive surgery in retroperitoneal soft tissue sarcoma carried out at high-volume centers is safe and is associated with improved local control. Ann Surg Oncol 17: 1507–1514.

269. Bonvalot S, Rivoire M, Castaing M et al. (2009). Primary retroperitoneal sarcomas: a multivariate analysis of surgical factors associated with local control. J Clin Oncol 27: 31–37.

270. Bookstein R, Lee EY, To H et al. (1988). Human retinoblastoma susceptibility gene: genomic organization and analysis of heterozygous intragenic deletion mutants. Proc Natl Acad Sci U S A 85: 2210–2214.

271. Boon LM, Brouillard P, Irrthum A et al. (1999). A gene for inherited cutaneous venous anomalies ("glomangiomas") localizes to chromosome 1p21-22. Am J Hum Genet 65: 125–133.

272. Bos GD, Pritchard DJ, Reiman HM et al. (1988). Epithelioid sarcoma. An analysis of fifty-one cases. J Bone Joint Surg Am 70: 862–870.

273. Bottillo I, Ahlquist T, Brekke H et al. (2009). Germline and somatic NF1 mutations in sporadic and NF1-associated malignant peripheral nerve sheath tumours. J Pathol 217: 693–701.

274. Boue DR, Parham DM, Webber B et al. (2000). Clinicopathologic study of ectomesenchymomas from Intergroup Rhabdomyosarcoma Study Groups III and IV. Pediatr Dev Pathol 3: 290–300.

275. Boufassa F, Dulioust A, Lascaux AS et al. (2001). Lipodystrophy in 685 HIV-1-treated patients: influence of antiretroviral treatment and immunovirological response. HIV Clin Trials 2: 339–345.

276. Bourdeaut F, Freneaux P, Thuille B et al. (2008). Extra-renal non-cerebral rhabdoid tumours. Pediatr Blood Cancer 51: 363–368.

277. Bourdeaut F, Lequin D, Brugieres L et al. (2011). Frequent hSNF5/INI1 germline mutations in patients with rhabdoid tumor. Clin Cancer Res 17: 31–38.

278. Bourgeois JM, Knezevich SR, Mathers JA et al. (2000). Molecular detection of the ETV6-NTRK3 gene fusion differentiates congenital fibrosarcoma from other childhood spindle cell tumors. Am J Surg Pathol 24: 937–946.

279. Bouron-Dal SD, Rougemont AL, Absi R et al. (2009). SNP genotyping of a sclerosing rhabdomyosarcoma: reveals highly aneuploid profile and a specific MDM2/HMGA2 amplification. Hum Pathol 40: 1347–1352.

280. Bousdras K, O'Donnell P, Vujovic S et al. (2007). Chondroblastomas but not chondromyxoid fibromas express cytokeratins: an unusual presentation of a chondroblastoma in the metaphyseal cortex of the tibia. Histopathology 51: 414–416.

280A. Bovee JV. (2010). EXTra hit for mouse osteochondroma. Proc Natl Acad Sci U S A. 107:1813–1814.

281. Bovee JV, Cleton-Jansen AM, Kuipers-Dijkshoorn NJ et al. (1999). Loss of heterozygosity and DNA ploidy point to a diverging genetic mechanism in the origin of peripheral and central chondrosarcoma. Genes Chromosomes Cancer 26: 237–246.

282. Bovee JV, Cleton-Jansen AM, Rosenberg C et al. (1999). Molecular genetic characterization of both components of a dedifferentiated chondrosarcoma, with implications for its histogenesis. J Pathol 189: 454–462.

283. Bovee JV, Cleton-Jansen AM, Wuyts W et al. (1999). EXT-mutation analysis and loss of heterozygosity in sporadic and hereditary osteochondromas and secondary chondrosarcomas. Am J Hum Genet 65: 689–698.

284. Bovee JV, Hogendoorn PC, Wunder JS et al. (2010). Cartilage tumours and bone development: molecular pathology and possible therapeutic targets. Nat Rev Cancer 10: 481–488.

285. Bovee JV, Sakkers RJ, Geirnaerdt MJ et al. (2002). Intermediate grade osteosarcoma and chondrosarcoma arising in an osteochondroma. A case report of a patient with hereditary multiple exostoses. J Clin Pathol 55: 226–229.

286. Bovee JV, Sciot R, Dal Cin P et al. (2001). Chromosome 9 alterations and trisomy 22 in central chondrosarcoma: a cytogenetic and DNA flow cytometric analysis of chondrosarcoma subtypes. Diagn Mol Pathol 10: 228–235.

287. Bovee JV, van den Broek LJ, Cleton-Jansen AM et al. (2000). Up-regulation of PTHrP and Bcl-2 expression characterizes the progression of osteochondroma towards peripheral chondrosarcoma and is a late event in central chondrosarcoma. Lab Invest 80: 1925–1934.

288. Bovee JV, van den Broek LJ, de Boer WI et al. (1998). Expression of growth factors and their receptors in adamantinoma of long bones and the implication for its histogenesis. J Pathol 184: 24–30.

289. Bovee JV, van der Heul RO, Taminiau AH et al. (1999). Chondrosarcoma of the phalanx: a locally aggressive lesion with minimal metastatic potential: a report of 35 cases and a review of the literature. Cancer 86: 1724–1732.

290. Bovee JV, van Royen M, Bardoel AF et al. (2000). Near-haploidy and subsequent polyploidization characterize the progression of peripheral chondrosarcoma. Am J Pathol 157: 1587–1595.

291. Bowe AE, Finnegan R, Jan de Beur SM et al. (2001). FGF-23 inhibits renal tubular phosphate transport and is a PHEX substrate. Biochem Biophys Res Commun 284: 977–981.

292. Bowen ME, Boyden ED, Holm IA et al. (2011). Loss-of-function mutations in PTPN11 cause metachondromatosis, but not Ollier disease or Maffucci syndrome. PLoS Genet 7: e1002050

293. Bowne WB, Antonescu CR, Leung DH et al. (2000). Dermatofibrosarcoma protuberans: A clinicopathologic analysis of patients treated and followed at a single institution. Cancer 88: 2711–2720.

293A. Boyce AM, Chong WH, Shawker TH et al. (2012). Characterization and management of testicular pathology in McCune-Albright syndrome. J Clin Endocrinol Metab 97:1782–1790.

294. Braatz B, Evans R, Kelman A et al. (2010). Perinatal evolution of mesenchymal hamartoma of the chest wall. J Pediatr Surg 45: e37–e40.

295. Brady MS, Gaynor JJ, Brennan MF (1992). Radiation-associated sarcoma of bone and soft tissue. Arch Surg 127: 1379–1385.

296. Brainard JA, Goldblum JR (1997). Stromal tumors of the jejunum and ileum: a clinicopathologic study of 39 cases. Am J Surg Pathol 21: 407–416.

297. Bramwell V, Rouesse J, Steward W et al. (1994). Adjuvant CYVADIC chemotherapy for adult soft tissue sarcoma—reduced local recurrence but no improvement in survival: a study of the European Organization for Research and Treatment of Cancer Soft Tissue and Bone Sarcoma Group. J Clin Oncol 12: 1137–1149.

298. Bramwell VH, Steward WP, Nooij M et al. (1999). Neoadjuvant chemotherapy with doxorubicin and cisplatin in malignant fibrous histiocytoma of bone: A European Osteosarcoma Intergroup study. J Clin Oncol 17: 3260–3269.

299. Brandal P, Bjerkehagen B, Heim S (2006). Rearrangement of chromosomal region 8q11-13 in lipomatous tumours: correlation with lipoblastoma morphology. J Pathol 208: 388–394.

300. Brandal P, Panagopoulos I, Bjerkehagen B et al. (2008). Detection of a t(1;22)(q23;q12) translocation leading to an EWSR1-PBX1 fusion gene in a myoepithelioma. Genes Chromosomes Cancer 47: 558–564.

301. Brandal P, Panagopoulos I, Bjerkehagen B et al. (2009). t(19;22)(q13;q12) Translocation leading to the novel fusion gene EWSR1-ZNF444 in soft tissue myoepithelial carcinoma. Genes Chromosomes Cancer 48: 1051–1056.

302. Brandser EA, Goree JC, El-Khoury GY (1998). Elastofibroma dorsi: prevalence in an elderly patient population as revealed by CT. AJR Am J Roentgenol 171: 977–980.

303. Brassesco MS, Valera ET, Engel EE et al. (2010). Clonal complex chromosome aberration in non-ossifying fibroma. Pediatr Blood Cancer 54: 764–767.

304. Braunstein EM, White SJ (1980). Non-Hodgkin lymphoma of bone. Radiology 135: 59–63.

305. Bredella MA, Torriani M, Hornicek F et al. (2007). Value of PET in the assessment of patients with neurofibromatosis type 1. AJR Am J Roentgenol 189: 928–935.

306. Breiner JA, Nelson M, Bredthauer BD et al. (1999). Trisomy 8 and trisomy 14 in plantar fibromatosis. Cancer Genet Cytogenet 108: 176–177.

307. Brekke HR, Kolberg M, Skotheim RI et al. (2009). Identification of p53 as a strong predictor of survival for patients with malignant peripheral nerve sheath tumors. Neuro Oncol 11: 514–528.

308. Brekke HR, Ribeiro FR, Kolberg M et al. (2010). Genomic changes in chromosomes 10, 16, and X in malignant peripheral nerve sheath tumors identify a high-risk patient group. J Clin Oncol 28: 1573–1582.

309. Brems H, Beert E, de Ravel T et al. (2009). Mechanisms in the pathogenesis of malignant tumours in neurofibromatosis type 1. Lancet Oncol 10: 508–515.

310. Brems H, Chmara M, Sahbatou M et al. (2007). Germline loss-of-function mutations in SPRED1 cause a neurofibromatosis 1-like phenotype. Nat Genet 39: 1120–1126.

311. Brems H, Park C, Maertens O et al. (2009). Glomus tumors in neurofibromatosis type 1: genetic, functional, and clinical evidence of a novel association. Cancer Res 69: 7393–7401.

312. Bridge JA, Bhatia PS, Anderson JR et al. (1993). Biologic and clinical significance of cytogenetic and molecular cytogenetic abnormalities in benign and malignant cartilaginous lesions. Cancer Genet Cytogenet 69: 79–90.

313. Bridge JA, DeBoer J, Travis J et al. (1994). Simultaneous interphase cytogenetic analysis and fluorescence immunophenotyping of dedifferentiated chondrosarcoma. Implications for histopathogenesis. Am J Pathol 144: 215–220.

314. Bridge JA, DeBoer J, Walker CW et al. (1995). Translocation t(3;12)(q28;q14) in parosteal lipoma. Genes Chromosomes Cancer 12: 70–72.

315. Bridge JA, Dembinski A, DeBoer J et al. (1994). Clonal chromosomal abnormalities in osteofibrous dysplasia. Implications for histopathogenesis and its relationship with adamantinoma. Cancer 73: 1746–1752.

316. Bridge JA, Fidler ME, Neff JR et al. (1999). Adamantinoma-like Ewing's sarcoma: genomic confirmation, phenotypic drift. Am J Surg Pathol 23: 159–165.

317. Bridge JA, Kanamori M, Ma Z et al. (2001). Fusion of the ALK gene to the clathrin heavy chain gene, CLTC, in inflammatory myofibroblastic tumor. Am J Pathol 159: 411–415.

318. Bridge JA, Liu J, Qualman SJ et al. (2002). Genomic gains and losses are similar in genetic and histologic subsets of rhabdomyosarcoma, whereas amplification predominates in embryonal with anaplasia and alveolar subtypes. Genes Chromosomes Cancer 33: 310–321.

319. Bridge JA, Neff JR, Mouron BJ (1992). Giant cell tumor of bone. Chromosomal analysis of 48 specimens and review of the literature. Cancer Genet Cytogenet 58: 2–13.

320. Bridge JA, Nelson M, McComb E et al. (1997). Cytogenetic findings in 73 osteosarcoma specimens and a review of the literature. Cancer Genet Cytogenet 95: 74–87.

321. Bridge JA, Nelson M, Orndal C et al. (1998). Clonal karyotypic abnormalities of the hereditary multiple exostoses chromosomal loci 8q24.1 (EXT1) and 11p11-12 (EXT2) in patients with sporadic and hereditary osteochondromas. Cancer 82: 1657–1663.

322. Bridge JA, Swarts SJ, Buresh C et al. (1999). Trisomies 8 and 20 characterize a subgroup of benign fibrous lesions arising in both soft tissue and bone. Am J Pathol 154: 729–733.

323. Brien EW, Mirra JM, Luck JV, Jr. (1999). Benign and malignant cartilage tumors of bone and joint: their anatomic and theoretical basis with an emphasis on radiology, pathology and clinical biology. II. Juxtacortical cartilage tumors. Skeletal Radiol 28: 1–20.

324. Briggs TA, Rice GI, Daly S et al. (2011). Tartrate-resistant acid phosphatase deficiency causes a bone dysplasia with autoimmunity and a type I interferon expression signature. Nat Genet 43: 127–131.

325. Broberg K, Zhang M, Strombeck B et al. (2002). Fusion of RDC1 with HMGA2 in lipomas as the result of chromosome aberrations involving 2q35-37 and 12q13-15. Int J Oncol 21: 321–326.

326. Brock JE, Perez-Atayde AR, Kozakewich HP et al. (2005). Cytogenetic aberrations in perineurioma: variation with subtype. Am J Surg Pathol 29: 1164–1169.

327. Brouillard P, Boon LM, Mulliken JB et al. (2002). Mutations in a novel factor, glomulin, are responsible for glomuvenous malformations ("glomangiomas"). Am J Hum Genet 70: 866–874.

328. Brown KT, Kattapuram SV, Rosenthal DI (1986). Computed tomography analysis of bone tumors: patterns of cortical destruction and soft tissue extension. Skeletal Radiol 15: 448–451.

329. Brown RE, Boyle JL (2003).

Mesenchymal chondrosarcoma: molecular characterization by a proteomic approach, with morphogenic and therapeutic implications. Ann Clin Lab Sci 33: 131–141.

330. Brown RJ, Kelly MH, Collins MT (2010). Cushing syndrome in the McCune-Albright syndrome. J Clin Endocrinol Metab 95: 1508–1515.

331. Browne DS, Frazer MI (1990). Abdominoperineal urethral suspension: a report of 20 cases. Aust N Z J Obstet Gynaecol 30: 366–369.

332. Browne TJ, Fletcher CD (2006). Haemosiderotic fibrolipomatous tumour (so-called haemosiderotic fibrohistiocytic lipomatous tumour): analysis of 13 new cases in support of a distinct entity. Histopathology 48: 453–461.

333. Brtko J, Knopp J, Scherberg NH (1990). Anterior pituitary: triiodothyronine and/or dexamethasone induced changes in protein formation in thyroidectomized and/or adrenalectomized rats. Endocrinol Exp 24: 97–104.

334. Bruder E, Zanetti M, Boos N et al. (1999). Chondromyxoid fibroma of two thoracic vertebrae. Skeletal Radiol 28: 286–289.

335. Brun AL, Touitou-Gottenberg D, Haroche J et al. (2010). Erdheim-Chester disease: CT findings of thoracic involvement. Eur Radiol 20: 2579–2587.

336. Brunnemann RB, Ro JY, Ordonez NG et al. (1999). Extrapleural solitary fibrous tumor: a clinicopathologic study of 24 cases. Mod Pathol 12: 1034–1042.

337. Buccoliero AM, Castiglione F, Rossi Degl'Innocenti D et al. (2008). Congenital/Infantile fibrosarcoma of the colon: morphologic, immunohistochemical, molecular, and ultrastructural features of a relatively rare tumor in an extraordinary localization. J Pediatr Hematol Oncol 30: 723–727.

338. Buchkovich K, Duffy LA, Harlow E (1989). The retinoblastoma protein is phosphorylated during specific phases of the cell cycle. Cell 58: 1097–1105.

339. Buddingh EP, Krallman P, Neff JR et al. (2003). Chromosome 6 abnormalities are recurrent in synovial chondromatosis. Cancer Genet Cytogenet 140: 18–22.

340. Buddingh EP, Naumann S, Nelson M et al. (2003). Cytogenetic findings in benign cartilaginous neoplasms. Cancer Genet Cytogenet 141: 164–168.

341. Bui KL, Ilaslan H, Bauer TW et al. (2009). Cortical scalloping and cortical penetration by small eccentric chondroid lesions in the long tubular bones: not a sign of malignancy? Skeletal Radiol 38: 791–796.

342. Buiting K, Kanber D, Horsthemke B et al. (2010). Imprinting of RB1 (the new kid on the block). Brief Funct Genomics 9: 347–353.

343. Buresh CJ, Seemayer TA, Nelson M et al. (1999). t(X;4)(q22;q31.3) in giant cell reparative granuloma. Cancer Genet Cytogenet 115: 80–81.

344. Burge PD (2004). Dupuytren's disease. J Bone Joint Surg Br 86: 1088–1089.

345. Burger B, Hershkovitz D, Indelman M et al. (2010). Buschke-Ollendorff syndrome in a three-generation family: influence of a novel LEMD3 mutation to tropoelastin expression. Eur J Dermatol 20: 693–697.

346. Burke A, Virami R (1996). Tumors of the great vessels. In: Tumors of the Heart and Great Vessels. Burke A, Virami R AFIP Atlas of Tumor Pathology. AFIP: Washington, DC: pp 211–227.

347. Burke AP, Virmani R (1993). Sarcomas of the great vessels. A clinicopathologic study. Cancer 71: 1761–1773.

348. Burke FD, Proud G, Lawson IJ et al. (2007). An assessment of the effects of exposure to vibration, smoking, alcohol and diabetes on the prevalence of Dupuytren's disease in 97,537 miners. J Hand Surg Eur Vol 32: 400–406.

349. Burkhart DL, Sage J (2008). Cellular mechanisms of tumour suppression by the retinoblastoma gene. Nat Rev Cancer 8: 671–682.

350. Busson-Le Coniat M, Boucher N, Blanche H et al. (2002). Chromosome studies of in vitro senescent lymphocytes: nonrandom trisomy 2. Ann Genet 45: 193–196.

351. Byrne J, Blanc WA, Warburton D et al. (1984). The significance of cystic hygroma in fetuses. Hum Pathol 15: 61–67.

352. Caballes RL (1982). Enchondroma protuberans masquerading as osteochondroma. Hum Pathol 13: 734–739.

353. Cahlon O, Brennan MF, Jia X et al. (2012). A postoperative nomogram for local recurrence risk in extremity soft tissue sarcomas after limb-sparing surgery without adjuvant radiation. Ann Surg 255: 343–347.

354. Cai YC, McMenamin ME, Rose G et al. (2001). Primary liposarcoma of the orbit: a clinicopathologic study of seven cases. Ann Diagn Pathol 5: 255–266.

355. Caillaud JM, Gerard-Marchant R, Marsden HB et al. (1989). Histopathological classification of childhood rhabdomyosarcoma: a report from the International Society of Pediatric Oncology pathology panel. Med Pediatr Oncol 17: 391–400.

356. Cale AE, Freedman PD, Kerpel SM et al. (1989). Benign fibrous histiocytoma of the maxilla. Oral Surg Oral Med Oral Pathol 68: 444–450.

357. Callahan KS, Eberhardt SC, Fechner RE et al. (2006). Desmoplastic fibroma of bone with extensive cartilaginous metaplasia. Ann Diagn Pathol 10: 343–346.

358. Callister MD, Ballo MT, Pisters PW et al. (2001). Epithelioid sarcoma: results of conservative surgery and radiotherapy. Int J Radiat Oncol Biol Phys 51: 384–391.

359. Calonje E, Fletcher CD (1995). Cutaneous intraneural glomus tumor. Am J Dermatopathol 17: 395–398.

360. Calonje E, Fletcher CD (1996). Myoid differentiation in dermatofibrosarcoma protuberans and its fibrosarcomatous variant: clinicopathologic analysis of 5 cases. J Cutan Pathol 23: 30–36.

361. Calonje E, Fletcher CD, Wilson-Jones E et al. (1994). Retiform hemangioendothelioma. A distinctive form of low-grade angiosarcoma delineated in a series of 15 cases. Am J Surg Pathol 18: 115–125.

362. Calonje E, Wadden C, Wilson-Jones E et al. (1993). Spindle-cell non-pleomorphic atypical fibroxanthoma: analysis of a series and delineation of a distinctive variant. Histopathology 22: 247–254.

363. Cameron D, Ong TH, Borzi P (2001). Conservative management of mesenchymal hamartomas of the chest wall. J Pediatr Surg 36: 1346–1349.

364. Camp MD, Tompkins RK, Spanier SS et al. (2008). Best cases from the AFIP: Adamantinoma of the tibia and fibula with cytogenetic analysis. Radiographics 28: 1215–1220.

365. Campanacci M, Enneking WF (1999). Peripheral chondrosarcoma. In: Bone and Soft Tissue Tumors: Clinical Features, Imaging, Pathology and Treatment2 EditionSpringer-Verlag: New York: pp 335–361.

366. Campanacci DA, Matera D, Franchi A et al. (2008). Synovial chondrosarcoma of the hip: report of two cases and literature review. Chir Organi Mov 92: 139–144.

367. Campanacci M, Baldini N, Boriani S et al. (1987). Giant-cell tumor of bone. J Bone Joint Surg Am 69: 106–114.

368. Campanacci M, Boriani S, Giunti A (1980). Hemangioendothelioma of bone: a study of 29 cases. Cancer 46: 804–814.

369. Campanacci M, Laus M (1981). Osteofibrous dysplasia of the tibia and fibula. J Bone Joint Surg Am 63: 367–375.

370. Campanacci M, Laus M, Boriani S (1983). Multiple non-ossifying fibromata with extraskeletal anomalies: a new syndrome? J Bone Joint Surg Br 65: 627–632.

371. Campbell RS, Grainger AJ, Mangham DC et al. (2003). Intraosseous lipoma: report of 35 new cases and a review of the literature. Skeletal Radiol 32: 209–222.

372. Candeliere GA, Glorieux FH, Prud'homme J et al. (1995). Increased expression of the c-fos proto-oncogene in bone from patients with fibrous dysplasia. N Engl J Med 332: 1546–1551.

373. Candeliere GA, Roughley PJ, Glorieux FH (1997). Polymerase chain reaction-based technique for the selective enrichment and analysis of mosaic arg201 mutations in G alpha s from patients with fibrous dysplasia of bone. Bone 21: 201–206.

374. Canter RJ, Qin LX, Maki RG et al. (2008). A synovial sarcoma-specific preoperative nomogram supports a survival benefit to ifosfamide-based chemotherapy and improves risk stratification for patients. Clin Cancer Res 14: 8191–8197.

375. Cantwell CP, Obyrne J, Eustace S (2004). Current trends in treatment of osteoid osteoma with an emphasis on radiofrequency ablation. Eur Radiol 14: 607–617.

376. Cao W, Goolsby CL, Nelson BP et al. (2008). Instability of immunophenotype in plasma cell myeloma. Am J Clin Pathol 129: 926–933.

377. Capanna R, Dal Monte A, Gitelis S et al. (1982). The natural history of unicameral bone cyst after steroid injection. Clin Orthop Relat Res 204–211.

378. Carlson JW, Fletcher CD (2007). Immunohistochemistry for beta-catenin in the differential diagnosis of spindle cell lesions: analysis of a series and review of the literature. Histopathology 51: 509–514.

379. Carneiro A, Francis P, Bendahl PO et al. (2009). Indistinguishable genomic profiles and shared prognostic markers in undifferentiated pleomorphic sarcoma and leiomyosarcoma: different sides of a single coin? Lab Invest 89: 668–675.

380. Carney JA (1990). Psammomatous melanotic schwannoma. A distinctive, heritable tumor with special associations, including cardiac myxoma and the Cushing syndrome. Am J Surg Pathol 14: 206–222.

381. Carney JA (1999). Gastric stromal sarcoma, pulmonary chondroma, and extra-adrenal paraganglioma (Carney Triad): natural history, adrenocortical component, and possible familial occurrence. Mayo Clin Proc 74: 543–552.

382. Carney JA, Boccon-Gibod L, Jarka DE et al. (2001). Osteochondromyxoma of bone: a congenital tumor associated with lentigines and other unusual disorders. Am J Surg Pathol 25: 164–176.

383. Carney JA, Gordon H, Carpenter PC et al. (1985). The complex of myxomas, spotty pigmentation, and endocrine overactivity. Medicine (Baltimore) 64: 270–283.

384. Carney JA, Hruska LS, Beauchamp GD et al. (1986). Dominant inheritance of the complex of myxomas, spotty pigmentation, and endocrine overactivity. Mayo Clin Proc 61: 165–172.

385. Carpintero P, Leon F, Zafra M et al. (2003). Fractures of osteochondroma during physical exercise. Am J Sports Med 31: 1003–1006.

386. Carretto E, Dall'Igna P, Alaggio R et al. (2006). Fibrous hamartoma of infancy: an Italian multi-institutional experience. J Am Acad Dermatol 54: 800–803.

387. Carroll MB, Higgs JB (2007). Synovial haemangioma presenting as a recurrent monoarticular haemarthrosis. Arch Dis Child 92: 623–624.

388. Carron JD, Darrow DH, Karakla DW (2001). Fetal rhabdomyoma of the posterior cervical triangle. Int J Pediatr Otorhinolaryngol 61: 77–81.

389. Carter JM, O'Hara C, Dundas G et al. (2012). Epithelioid malignant peripheral nerve sheath tumor arising in a schwannoma, in a patient with "neuroblastoma-like" schwannomatosis and a novel germline SMARCB1 mutation. Am J Surg Pathol 36: 154–160.

390. Carvalho Silva E, Carvalho Silva GC, Vieira TC (2007). Cherubism: clinicoradiographic features, treatment, and long-term follow-up of 8 cases. Journal of Oral and Maxillofacial Surgery 65: 517–522.

391. Carvalho VM, Perdigao PF, Amaral FR et al. (2009). Novel mutations in the SH3BP2 gene associated with sporadic central giant cell lesions and cherubism. Oral Dis 15: 106–110.

392. Carvalho VM, Perdigao PF, Pimenta FJ et al. (2008). A novel mutation of the SH3BP2 gene in an aggressive case of cherubism. Oral Oncol 44: 153–155.

393. Casadei GP, Komori T, Scheithauer BW et al. (1993). Intracranial parenchymal schwannoma. A clinicopathological and neuroimaging study of nine cases. J Neurosurg 79: 217–222.

394. Casadei GP, Scheithauer BW, Hirose T et al. (1995). Cellular schwannoma. A clinicopathologic, DNA flow cytometric, and proliferation marker study of 70 patients. Cancer 75: 1109–1119.

395. Casadei R, Ricci M, Ruggieri P et al. (1991). Chondrosarcoma of the soft tissues. Two different sub-groups. J Bone Joint Surg Br 73: 162–168.

396. Casali PG, Blay JY (2010). Soft tissue sarcomas: ESMO Clinical Practice Guidelines for diagnosis, treatment and follow-up. Ann Oncol 21 Suppl 5: v198–v203.

397. Casanova M, Ferrari A, Collini P et al. (2006). Epithelioid sarcoma in children and adolescents: a report from the Italian Soft Tissue Sarcoma Committee. Cancer 106: 708–717.

398. Castro C, Winkelmann RK (1974). Angiolymphoid hyperplasia with eosinophilia in the skin. Cancer 34: 1696–1705.

399. Catalfamo L, Lombardo G, Siniscalchi EN et al. (2010). Rhabdomyomas of the submandibular and sublingual glands. J Craniofac Surg 21: 927–930.

400. Cates JM, Rosenberg AE, O'Connell JX et al. (2001). Chondroblastoma-like chondroma of soft tissue: an underrecognized variant and

its differential diagnosis. Am J Surg Pathol 25: 661–666.
401. Cavazzana AO, Schmidt D, Ninfo V et al. (1992). Spindle cell rhabdomyosarcoma. A prognostically favorable variant of rhabdomyosarcoma. Am J Surg Pathol 16: 229–235.
402. Cavenee WK, Dryja TP, Phillips RA et al. (1983). Expression of recessive alleles by chromosomal mechanisms in retinoblastoma. Nature 305: 779–784.
403. Cavenee WK, Hansen MF, Nordenskjold M et al. (1985). Genetic origin of mutations predisposing to retinoblastoma. Science 228: 501–503.
404. Cavenee WK, Murphree AL, Shull MM et al. (1986). Prediction of familial predisposition to retinoblastoma. N Engl J Med 314: 1201–1207.
405. Cawthon RM, Weiss R, Xu GF et al. (1990). A major segment of the neurofibromatosis type 1 gene: cDNA sequence, genomic structure, and point mutations. Cell 62: 193–201.
406. Cecchetto G, Carli M, Alaggio R et al. (2001). Fibrosarcoma in pediatric patients: results of the Italian Cooperative Group studies (1979-1995). J Surg Oncol 78: 225–231.
407. Cecchi R, Pavesi M, Apicella P (2011). Malignant glomus tumor of the trunk treated with Mohs micrographic surgery. J Dtsch Dermatol Ges 9: 391–392.
408. Cesari M, Alberghini M, Vanel D et al. (2011). Periosteal osteosarcoma: a single-institution experience. Cancer 117: 1731–1735.
409. Cesari M, Bertoni F, Bacchini P et al. (2007). Mesenchymal chondrosarcoma. An analysis of patients treated at a single institution. Tumori 93: 423–427.
410. Cessna MH, Zhou H, Perkins SL et al. (2001). Are myogenin and myoD1 expression specific for rhabdomyosarcoma? A study of 150 cases, with emphasis on spindle cell mimics. Am J Surg Pathol 25: 1150–1157.
411. Cessna MH, Zhou H, Sanger WG et al. (2002). Expression of ALK1 and p80 in inflammatory myofibroblastic tumor and its mesenchymal mimics: a study of 135 cases. Mod Pathol 15: 931–938.
412. Chaabane S, Bouaziz MC, Drissi C et al. (2009). Periosteal chondrosarcoma. AJR Am J Roentgenol 192: W1–W6.
413. Chadwick EG, Connor EJ, Hanson IC et al. (1990). Tumors of smooth-muscle origin in HIV-infected children. JAMA 263: 3182–3184.
414. Chaljub G, Johnson PR (1996). In vivo MRI characteristics of lipoma arborescens utilizing fat suppression and contrast administration. J Comput Assist Tomogr 20: 85–87.
415. Chan JA, McMenamin ME, Fletcher CD (2003). Synovial sarcoma in older patients: clinicopathological analysis of 32 cases with emphasis on unusual histological features. Histopathology 43: 72–83.
416. Chan JK (1997). Solitary fibrous tumour—everywhere, and a diagnosis in vogue. Histopathology 31: 568–576.
417. Chan JK, Cheuk W, Shimizu M (2001). Anaplastic lymphoma kinase expression in inflammatory pseudotumors. Am J Surg Pathol 25: 761–768.
418. Chan JK, Frizzera G, Fletcher CD et al. (1992). Primary vascular tumors of lymph nodes other than Kaposi's sarcoma. Analysis of 39 cases and delineation of two new entities. Am J Surg Pathol 16: 335–350.
419. Chan JK, Rosai J (1991). Tumors of the neck showing thymic or related branchial pouch differentiation: a unifying concept. Hum Pathol 22: 349–367.
420. Chan JK, Tsang WY, Seneviratne S et al. (1995). The MIC2 antibody 013. Practical application for the study of thymic epithelial tumors. Am J Surg Pathol 19: 1115–1123.
421. Chan YM, Hon E, Ngai SW et al. (2000). Aggressive angiomyxoma in females: is radical resection the only option? Acta Obstet Gynecol Scand 79: 216–220.
422. Chang H, Jiang A, Qi C et al. (2010). Impact of genomic aberrations including chromosome 1 abnormalities on the outcome of patients with relapsed or refractory multiple myeloma treated with lenalidomide and dexamethasone. Leuk Lymphoma 51: 2084–2091.
423. Chang JY, Wang S, Hung CC et al. (2002). Multiple Epstein-Barr virus-associated subcutaneous angioleiomyomas in a patient with acquired immunodeficiency syndrome. Br J Dermatol 147: 563–567.
424. Chang SE, Choi JH, Sung KJ et al. (2001). A case of cutaneous low-grade myofibroblastic sarcoma. J Dermatol 28: 383–387.
425. Chang Y, Cesarman E, Pessin MS et al. (1994). Identification of herpesvirus-like DNA sequences in AIDS-associated Kaposi's sarcoma. Science 266: 1865–1869.
426. Chapman AD, Pritchard SC, Yap WW et al. (2001). Primary pulmonary osteosarcoma: case report and molecular analysis. Cancer 91: 779–784.
427. Chapurlat RD, Meunier PJ (2000). Fibrous dysplasia of bone. Baillieres Best Pract Res Clin Rheumatol 14: 385–398.
428. Charrier JB, Leboulanger N, Roger G et al. (2006). [Nasal glial heterotopia: embryological and clinical approaches]. Rev Stomatol Chir Maxillofac 107: 44–49.
429. Chase DR, Enzinger FM (1985). Epithelioid sarcoma. Diagnosis, prognostic indicators, and treatment. Am J Surg Pathol 9: 241–263.
430. Chaudhry IH, Kazakov DV, Michal M et al. (2010). Fibro-osseous pseudotumor of the digit: a clinicopathological study of 17 cases. J Cutan Pathol 37: 323–329.
431. Chbani L, Guillou L, Terrier P et al. (2009). Epithelioid sarcoma: a clinicopathologic and immunohistochemical analysis of 106 cases from the French sarcoma group. Am J Clin Pathol 131: 222–227.
432. Chen CL, Chen WC, Chiang JH et al. (2011). Interscapular hibernoma: case report and literature review. Kaohsiung J Med Sci 27: 348–352.
433. Chen CW, Chang WC, Lee HS et al. (2010). MRI features of lipoblastoma: differentiating from other palpable lipomatous tumor in pediatric patients. Clin Imaging 34: 453–457.
434. Chen E, Fletcher CD (2010). Cellular angiofibroma with atypia or sarcomatous transformation: clinicopathologic analysis of 13 cases. Am J Surg Pathol 34: 707–714.
435. Chen E, O'Connell F, Fletcher CD (2011). Dedifferentiated leiomyosarcoma: clinicopathological analysis of 18 cases. Histopathology 59: 1135–1143.
436. Chen KT (1980). Atypical fibroxanthoma of the skin with osteoid production. Arch Dermatol 116: 113–114.
437. Chen KT (2003). Familial peritoneal multifocal calcifying fibrous tumor. Am J Clin Pathol 119: 811–815.
438. Chen ST, Lee JC (2008). An inflammatory myofibroblastic tumor in liver with ALK and RANBP2 gene rearrangement: combination of distinct morphologic, immunohistochemical, and genetic features. Hum Pathol 39: 1854–1858.
439. Cheng H, Dodge J, Mehl E et al. (2009). Validation of immature adipogenic status and identification of prognostic biomarkers in myxoid liposarcoma using tissue microarrays. Hum Pathol 40: 1244–1251.
440. Chervenak FA, Isaacson G, Blakemore KJ et al. (1983). Fetal cystic hygroma. Cause and natural history. N Engl J Med 309: 822–825.
441. Chetritt J, Paradis V, Dargere D et al. (1999). Chester-Erdheim disease: a neoplastic disorder. Hum Pathol 30: 1093–1096.
442. Cheung FM, Ma L, Wu WC et al. (2006). Oncogenic osteomalacia associated with an occult phosphaturic mesenchymal tumour: clinico-radiologico-pathological correlation and ultrastructural studies. Hong Kong Med J 12: 319–321.
443. Chibon F, Lagarde P, Salas S et al. (2010). Validated prediction of clinical outcome in sarcomas and multiple types of cancer on the basis of a gene expression signature related to genome complexity. Nat Med 16: 781–787.
444. Chibon F, Mairal A, Freneaux P et al. (2000). The RB1 gene is the target of chromosome 13 deletions in malignant fibrous histiocytoma. Cancer Res 60: 6339–6345.
445. Chibon F, Mariani O, Derre J et al. (2004). ASK1 (MAP3K5) as a potential therapeutic target in malignant fibrous histiocytomas with 12q14-q15 and 6q23 amplifications. Genes Chromosomes Cancer 40: 32–37.
446. Chibon F, Mariani O, Derre J et al. (2002). A subgroup of malignant fibrous histiocytomas is associated with genetic changes similar to those of well-differentiated liposarcomas. Cancer Genet Cytogenet 139: 24–29.
447. Chien AJ, Freeby JA, Win TT et al. (1998). Aggressive angiomyxoma of the female pelvis: sonographic, CT, and MR findings. AJR Am J Roentgenol 171: 530–531.
448. Chiles MC, Parham DM, Qualman SJ et al. (2004). Sclerosing rhabdomyosarcomas in children and adolescents: a clinicopathologic review of 13 cases from the Intergroup Rhabdomyosarcoma Study Group and Children's Oncology Group. Pediatr Dev Pathol 7: 583–594.
449. Chilosi M, Adami F, Lestani M et al. (1999). CD138/syndecan-1: a useful immunohistochemical marker of normal and neoplastic plasma cells on routine trephine bone marrow biopsies. Mod Pathol 12: 1101–1106.
450. Chinnam M, Goodrich DW (2011). RB1, development, and cancer. Curr Top Dev Biol 94: 129–169.
451. Cho JH, Joo YH, Kim MS et al. (2011). Venous hemangioma of parapharyngeal space with calcification. Clin Exp Otorhinolaryngol 4: 207–209.
452. Chomette G, Auriol M, Guilbert F et al. (1988). Cherubism. Histo-enzymological and ultrastructural study. Int J Oral Maxillofac Surg 17: 219–223.
453. Chompret A, Brugieres L, Ronsin M et al. (2000). P53 germline mutations in childhood cancers and cancer risk for carrier individuals. Br J Cancer 82: 1932–1937.
454. Chong Y, Eom M, Min HJ et al. (2009). Symplastic glomus tumor: a case report. Am J Dermatopathol 31: 71–73.
455. Choong PF, Pritchard DJ, Rock MG et al. (1996). Low grade central osteogenic sarcoma. A long-term followup of 20 patients. Clin Orthop Relat Res 198–206.
456. Chou AJ, Geller DS, Gorlick R (2008). Therapy for osteosarcoma: where do we go from here? Paediatr Drugs 10: 315–327.
457. Choufani S, Shuman C, Weksberg R (2010). Beckwith-Wiedemann syndrome. Am J Med Genet C Semin Med Genet 154C: 343–354.
458. Chowdhry M, Hughes C, Grimer RJ et al. (2009). Bone sarcomas arising in patients with neurofibromatosis type 1. J Bone Joint Surg Br 91: 1223–1226.
459. Christensen DR, Ramsamooj R, Gilbert TJ (1997). Sclerosing epithelioid fibrosarcoma: short T2 on MR imaging. Skeletal Radiol 26: 619–621.
460. Christensen WN, Strong EW, Bains MS et al. (1988). Neuroendocrine differentiation in the glandular peripheral nerve sheath tumor. Pathologic distinction from the biphasic synovial sarcoma with glands. Am J Surg Pathol 12: 417–426.
461. Chu PG, Arber DA, Weiss LM (2003). Expression of T/NK-cell and plasma cell antigens in nonhematopoietic epithelioid neoplasms. An immunohistochemical study of 447 cases. Am J Clin Pathol 120: 64–70.
462. Chun YS, Wang L, Nascimento AG et al. (2005). Pediatric inflammatory myofibroblastic tumor: anaplastic lymphoma kinase (ALK) expression and prognosis. Pediatr Blood Cancer 45: 796–801.
463. Chunder N, Basu D, Roy A et al. (2003). Prediction of retinoblastoma and osteosarcoma: linkage analysis of families by using polymorphic markers around RB1 locus. J BUON 8: 365–369.
464. Chung EB (1985). Pitfalls in diagnosing benign soft tissue tumors in infancy and childhood. Pathol Annu 20 Pt 2: 323–386.
465. Chung EB, Enzinger FM (1973). Benign lipoblastomatosis. An analysis of 35 cases. Cancer 32: 482–492.
466. Chung EB, Enzinger FM (1975). Proliferative fasciitis. Cancer 36: 1450–1458.
467. Chung EB, Enzinger FM (1976). Infantile fibrosarcoma. Cancer 38: 729–739.
468. Chung EB, Enzinger FM (1978). Chondroma of soft parts. Cancer 41: 1414–1424.
469. Chung EB, Enzinger FM (1979). Fibroma of tendon sheath. Cancer 44: 1945–1954.
470. Chung EB, Enzinger FM (1983). Malignant melanoma of soft parts. A reassessment of clear cell sarcoma. Am J Surg Pathol 7: 405–413.
471. Chung EB, Enzinger FM (1987). Extraskeletal osteosarcoma. Cancer 60: 1132–1142.
472. Ciatti R, Mariani PP (2009). Fibroma of tendon sheath located within the ankle joint capsule. J Orthop Traumatol 10: 147–150.
473. Cibull TL, Gleason BC, O'Malley DP et al. (2008). Malignant cutaneous glomus tumor presenting as a rapidly growing leg mass in a pregnant woman. J Cutan Pathol 35: 765–769.
474. Ackerman LV (1958). Extra-osseous localized non-neoplastic bone and cartilage formation (so-called myositis ossificans): clinical and pathological confusion with malignant neoplasms. J Bone Joint Surg Am 40-A: 279–298.
475. Clark SK, Smith TG, Katz DE et al. (1998). Identification and progression of a desmoid precursor lesion in patients with familial adenomatous polyposis. Br J Surg 85: 970–973.
476. Clark TD, Stelling CB, Fechner RE (1985). Benign fibrous histiocytoma of the left 8th rib. Case report 328. Skeletal Radiol 14:

149–151.
477. Clarke BE, Xipell JM, Thomas DP (1985). Benign fibrous histiocytoma of bone. Am J Surg Pathol 9: 806–815.
478. Clement A, Wiweger M, von der Hardt S et al. (2008). Regulation of zebrafish skeletogenesis by ext2/dackel and papst1/pinscher. PLoS Genet 4: e1000136
479. Clements SE, Mellerio JE, Holden ST et al. (2009). PORCN gene mutations and the protean nature of focal dermal hypoplasia. Br J Dermatol 160: 1103–1109.
480. Cleton-Jansen AM, Timmerman MC, Van de Vijver MJ et al. (2004). A distinct phenotype characterizes tumors from a putative genetic trait involving chondrosarcoma and breast cancer occurring in the same patient. Lab Invest 84: 191–202.
481. Clines GA, Ashley JA, Shah S et al. (1997). The structure of the human multiple exostoses 2 gene and characterization of homologs in mouse and Caenorhabditis elegans. Genome Res 7: 359–367.
482. Coffin CM, Dehner LP (1991). Fibroblastic-myofibroblastic tumors in children and adolescents: a clinicopathologic study of 108 examples in 103 patients. Pediatr Pathol 11: 569–588.
483. Coffin CM, Hornick JL, Fletcher CD (2007). Inflammatory myofibroblastic tumor: comparison of clinicopathologic, histologic, and immunohistochemical features including ALK expression in atypical and aggressive cases. Am J Surg Pathol 31: 509–520.
484. Coffin CM, Hornick JL, Zhou H et al. (2007). Gardner fibroma: a clinicopathologic and immunohistochemical analysis of 45 patients with 57 fibromas. Am J Surg Pathol 31: 410–416.
485. Coffin CM, Humphrey PA, Dehner LP (1998). Extrapulmonary inflammatory myofibroblastic tumor: a clinical and pathological survey. Semin Diagn Pathol 15: 85–101.
486. Coffin CM, Jaszcz W, O'Shea PA et al. (1994). So-called congenital-infantile fibrosarcoma: does it exist and what is it? Pediatr Pathol 14: 133–150.
487. Coffin CM, Lowichik A, Putnam A (2009). Lipoblastoma (LPB): a clinicopathologic and immunohistochemical analysis of 59 cases. Am J Surg Pathol 33: 1705–1712.
488. Coffin CM, Patel A, Perkins S et al. (2001). ALK1 and p80 expression and chromosomal rearrangements involving 2p23 in inflammatory myofibroblastic tumor. Mod Pathol 14: 569–576.
489. Coffin CM, Watterson J, Priest JR et al. (1995). Extrapulmonary inflammatory myofibroblastic tumor (inflammatory pseudotumor). A clinicopathologic and immunohistochemical study of 84 cases. Am J Surg Pathol 19: 859–872.
490. Cohen MC, Drut R, Garcia C et al. (1992). Mesenchymal hamartoma of the chest wall: a cooperative study with review of the literature. Pediatr Pathol 12: 525–534.
491. Cohen MM, Jr. (2001). Fibrous dysplasia is a neoplasm. Am J Med Genet 98: 290–293.
492. Cohen MM, Jr., Gorlin RJ (1991). Noonan-like/multiple giant cell lesion syndrome. Am J Med Genet 40: 159–166.
492A. Cohen MM, Jr. , Howell RE (1999). Etiology of fibrous dysplasia and McCune-Albright syndrome. Int J Oral Maxillofac Surg 28: 366–371.
493. Cohn BA, Wheeler CE, Jr., Briggaman RA (1970). Scleredema adultorum of Buschke and diabetes mellitus. Arch Dermatol 101: 27–35.
494. Coindre JM (2006). Grading of soft tissue sarcomas: review and update. Arch Pathol Lab Med 130: 1448–1453.
495. Coindre JM, de Mascarel A, Trojani M et al. (1988). Immunohistochemical study of rhabdomyosarcoma. Unexpected staining with S100 protein and cytokeratin. J Pathol 155: 127–132.
496. Coindre JM, Hostein I, Maire G et al. (2004). Inflammatory malignant fibrous histiocytomas and dedifferentiated liposarcomas: histological review, genomic profile, and MDM2 and CDK4 status favour a single entity. J Pathol 203: 822–830.
497. Coindre JM, Hostein I, Terrier P et al. (2006). Diagnosis of clear cell sarcoma by real-time reverse transcriptase-polymerase chain reaction analysis of paraffin embedded tissues: clinicopathologic and molecular analysis of 44 patients from the French sarcoma group. Cancer 107: 1055–1064.
498. Coindre JM, Mariani O, Chibon F et al. (2003). Most malignant fibrous histiocytomas developed in the retroperitoneum are dedifferentiated liposarcomas: a review of 25 cases initially diagnosed as malignant fibrous histiocytoma. Mod Pathol 16: 256–262.
499. Coindre JM, Pelmus M, Hostein I et al. (2003). Should molecular testing be required for diagnosing synovial sarcoma? A prospective study of 204 cases. Cancer 98: 2700–2707.
500. Coindre JM, Terrier P, Guillou L et al. (2001). Predictive value of grade for metastasis development in the main histologic types of adult soft tissue sarcomas: a study of 1240 patients from the French Federation of Cancer Centers Sarcoma Group. Cancer 91: 1914–1926.
501. Colby RS, Saul RA (2003). Is Jaffe-Campanacci syndrome just a manifestation of neurofibromatosis type 1? Am J Med Genet A 123A: 60–63.
502. Collins DH (1956). Paget's disease of bone; incidence and subclinical forms. Lancet 271: 51–57.
503. Collins MH, Chatten J (1997). Lipoblastoma/lipoblastomatosis: a clinicopathologic study of 25 tumors. Am J Surg Pathol 21: 1131–1137.
504. Collinson M, Leonard SJ, Charlton J et al. (2010). Symmetrical enchondromatosis is associated with duplication of 12p11.23 to 12p11.22 including PTHLH. Am J Med Genet A 152A: 3124–3128.
505. Colman SD, Williams CA, Wallace MR (1995). Benign neurofibromas in type 1 neurofibromatosis (NF1) show somatic deletions of the NF1 gene. Nat Genet 11: 90–92.
506. Comin CE, Novelli L, Tornaboni D et al. (2007). Clear cell sarcoma of the ileum: report of a case and review of literature. Virchows Arch 451: 839–845.
507. Cook JR, Dehner LP, Collins MH et al. (2001). Anaplastic lymphoma kinase (ALK) expression in the inflammatory myofibroblastic tumor: a comparative immunohistochemical study. Am J Surg Pathol 25: 1364–1371.
508. Cooper CL, Sindler P, Varol C et al. (2007). Paratesticular rhabdomyoma. Pathology 39: 367–369.
509. Cooper KL, Beabout JW, Dahlin DC (1984). Giant cell tumor: ossification in soft-tissue implants. Radiology 153: 597–602.
510. Cordon-Cardo C, Latres E, Drobnjak M et al. (1994). Molecular abnormalities of mdm2 and p53 genes in adult soft tissue sarcomas. Cancer Res 54: 794–799.
511. Corless CL, Barnett CM, Heinrich MC (2011). Gastrointestinal stromal tumours: origin and molecular oncology. Nat Rev Cancer 11: 865–878.
512. Cossarizza A, Mussini C, Vigano A (2001). Mitochondria in the pathogenesis of lipodystrophy induced by anti-HIV antiretroviral drugs: actors or bystanders? Bioessays 23: 1070–1080.
513. Costa J, Wesley RA, Glatstein E et al. (1984). The grading of soft tissue sarcomas. Results of a clinicohistopathologic correlation in a series of 163 cases. Cancer 53: 530–541.
514. Costa MJ, Weiss SW (1990). Angiomatoid malignant fibrous histiocytoma. A follow-up study of 108 cases with evaluation of possible histologic predictors of outcome. Am J Surg Pathol 14: 1126–1132.
515. Costes V, Magen V, Legouffe E et al. (1999). The Mi15 monoclonal antibody (anti-syndecan-1) is a reliable marker for quantifying plasma cells in paraffin-embedded bone marrow biopsy specimens. Hum Pathol 30: 1405–1411.
516. Coulibaly B, Barel E, Soulier M et al. (2008). Prenatal diagnosis of infantile fibrosarcoma with diffuse metastases. Prenat Diagn 28: 773–775.
517. Covinsky M, Gong S, Rajaram V et al. (2005). EWS-ATF1 fusion transcripts in gastrointestinal tumors previously diagnosed as malignant melanoma. Hum Pathol 36: 74–81.
518. Cowell JK, Bia B, Akoulitchev A (1996). A novel mutation in the promotor region in a family with a mild form of retinoblastoma indicates the location of a new regulatory domain for the RB1 gene. Oncogene 12: 431–436.
519. Craig WD, Fanburg-Smith JC, Henry LR et al. (2009). Fat-containing lesions of the retroperitoneum: radiologic-pathologic correlation. Radiographics 29: 261–290.
520. Cranshaw IM, Gikas PD, Fisher C et al. (2009). Clinical outcomes of extra-thoracic solitary fibrous tumours. Eur J Surg Oncol 35: 994–998.
521. Craver RD, Correa H, Kao YS et al. (1995). Aggressive giant cell fibroblastoma with a balanced 17;22 translocation. Cancer Genet Cytogenet 80: 20–22.
522. Craver RD, Henrich S, Kao YS (2006). Fibrous lipoblastoma with 8q11.2 abnormality. Cancer Genet Cytogenet 171: 112–114.
523. Crawford EA, Brooks JS, Ogilvie CM (2009). Osteosarcoma of the proximal part of the radius in Mazabraud syndrome. A case report. J Bone Joint Surg Am 91: 955–960.
524. Crawford SC, Harnsberger HR, Johnson L et al. (1988). Fibromatosis colli of infancy: CT and sonographic findings. AJR Am J Roentgenol 151: 1183–1184.
525. Cribier B, Noacco G, Peltre B et al. (2002). Stromelysin 3 expression: a useful marker for the differential diagnosis dermatofibroma versus dermatofibrosarcoma protuberans. J Am Acad Dermatol 46: 408–413.
526. Croes R, Debiec-Rychter M, Cokelaere K et al. (2005). Adult sclerosing rhabdomyosarcoma: cytogenetic link with embryonal rhabdomyosarcoma. Virchows Arch 446: 64–67.
527. Crotty PL, Nakhleh RE, Dehner LP (1993). Juvenile rhabdomyoma. An intermediate form of skeletal muscle tumor in children. Arch Pathol Lab Med 117: 43–47.
528. Crowson AN, Carlson-Sweet K, Macinnis C et al. (2002). Clear cell atypical fibroxanthoma:a clinicopathologic study. J Cutan Pathol 29: 374–381.
529. Crowther D (1997). Adjuvant chemotherapy for localised resectable soft-tissue sarcoma of adults: meta-analysis of individual data. Sarcoma Meta-analysis Collaboration. Lancet 350: 1647–1654.
530. Crozat A, Aman P, Mandahl N et al. (1993). Fusion of CHOP to a novel RNA-binding protein in human myxoid liposarcoma. Nature 363: 640–644.
531. Cruz-Mojarrieta J, Navarro S, Gomez-Cabrera E et al. (2001). Malignant granular cell tumor of soft tissues: a study of two new cases. Int J Surg Pathol 9: 255–259.
531A. Culver JE, Sweet DE, McCue FC. (1975)Chondrosarcoma of the hand arising from a pre-existent benign solitary enchondrom. Clin Orthop Relat Res.Nov-Dec;113:128-131.
532. Cummings OW, Ulbright TM, Young RH et al. (1997). Desmoplastic small round cell tumors of the paratesticular region. A report of six cases. Am J Surg Pathol 21: 219–225.
533. Cupp JS, Miller MA, Montgomery KD et al. (2007). Translocation and expression of CSF1 in pigmented villonodular synovitis, tenosynovial giant cell tumor, rheumatoid arthritis and other reactive synovitides. Am J Surg Pathol 31: 970–976.
534. Curran-Melendez SM, Dasher DA, Groben P et al. (2011). Case report: Meningothelial hamartoma of the scalp in a 9-year-old child. Pediatr Dermatol 28: 677–680.
535. D'Adamo DR (2011). Appraising the current role of chemotherapy for the treatment of sarcoma. Semin Oncol 38 Suppl 3: S19–S29.
536. D'Ercole C, Boubli L, Potier A et al. (1994). Fetal chest wall hamartoma: a case report. Fetal Diagn Ther 9: 261–263.
537. Dabska M (1969). Malignant endovascular papillary angioendothelioma of the skin in childhood. Clinicopathologic study of 6 cases. Cancer 24: 503–510.
538. Dabska M (1977). Parachordoma: a new clinicopathologic entity. Cancer 40: 1586–1592.
539. Dabska M, Huvos AG (1983). Mesenchymal chondrosarcoma in the young. Virchows Arch A Pathol Anat Histopathol 399: 89–104.
540. Daffner RH, Kirks DR, Gehweiler JA, Jr. et al. (1982). Computed tomography of fibrous dysplasia. AJR Am J Roentgenol 139: 943–948.
541. Dahl I, Angervall L (1974). Cutaneous and subcutaneous leiomyosarcoma. A clinicopathologic study of 47 patients. Pathol Eur 9: 307–315.
542. Dahl I, Save-Soderbergh J, Angervall L (1973). Fibrosarcoma in early infancy. Pathol Eur 8: 193–209.
543. Dahlen A, Debiec-Rychter M, Pedeutour F et al. (2003). Clustering of deletions on chromosome 13 in benign and low-malignant lipomatous tumors. Int J Cancer 103: 616–623.
544. Dahlen A, Fletcher CD, Mertens F et al. (2004). Activation of the GLI oncogene through fusion with the beta-actin gene (ACTB) in a group of distinctive pericytic neoplasms: pericytoma with t(7;12). Am J Pathol 164: 1645–1653.
545. Dahlen A, Mertens F, Mandahl N et al. (2004). Molecular genetic characterization of the genomic ACTB-GLI fusion in pericytoma with t(7;12). Biochem Biophys Res Commun 325: 1318–1323.
546. Dahlen A, Mertens F, Rydholm A et al. (2003). Fusion, disruption, and expression of HMGA2 in bone and soft tissue chondromas. Mod Pathol 16: 1132–1140.
547. Dahlin DC (1982). Case report 189. Infantile fibrosarcoma (congenital fibrosarco-

ma-like fibromatosis). Skeletal Radiol 8: 77–78.
548. Dahlin DC, Beabout JW (1971). Dedifferentiation of low-grade chondrosarcomas. Cancer 28: 461–466.
549. Dahlin DC, Coventry MB (1967). Osteogenic sarcoma. A study of six hundred cases. J Bone Joint Surg Am 49: 101–110.
550. Daimaru Y, Hashimoto H, Tsuneyoshi M et al. (1987). Epithelial profile of epithelioid sarcoma. An immunohistochemical analysis of eight cases. Cancer 59: 134–141.
551. Dakin MC, Leppard B, Theaker JM (1992). The palisaded, encapsulated neuroma (solitary circumscribed neuroma). Histopathology 20: 405–410.
552. Dal Cin P, Brock P, Casteels-Van Daele M et al. (1991). Cytogenetic characterization of congenital or infantile fibrosarcoma. Eur J Pediatr 150: 579–581.
553. Dal Cin P, De Smet L, Sciot R et al. (1999). Trisomy 7 and trisomy 8 in dividing and non-dividing tumor cells in Dupuytren's disease. Cancer Genet Cytogenet 108: 137–140.
554. Dal Cin P, Kozakewich HP, Goumnerova L et al. (2000). Variant translocations involving 16q22 and 17p13 in solid variant and extraosseous forms of aneurysmal bone cyst. Genes Chromosomes Cancer 28: 233–234.
555. Dal Cin P, Pauwels P, Poldermans LJ et al. (1999). Clonal chromosome abnormalities in a so-called Dupuytren's subungual exostosis. Genes Chromosomes Cancer 24: 162–164.
556. Dal Cin P, Pauwels P, Sciot R et al. (1996). Multiple chromosome rearrangements in a fibrosarcoma. Cancer Genet Cytogenet 87: 176–178.
557. Dal Cin P, Sciot R, Brys P et al. (2000). Recurrent chromosome aberrations in fibrous dysplasia of the bone: a report of the CHAMP study group. Chromosomes and Morphology. Cancer Genet Cytogenet 122: 30–32.
558. Dal Cin P, Sciot R, De Smet L et al. (1998). Translocation 2;11 in a fibroma of tendon sheath. Histopathology 32: 433–435.
559. Dal Cin P, Sciot R, De Wever I et al. (1996). Cytogenetic and immunohistochemical evidence that giant cell fibroblastoma is related to dermatofibrosarcoma protuberans. Genes Chromosomes Cancer 15: 73–75.
560. Dal Cin P, Sciot R, Polito P et al. (1997). Lesions of 13q may occur independently of deletion of 16q in spindle cell/pleomorphic lipomas. Histopathology 31: 222–225.
561. Dal Cin P, Sciot R, Samson I et al. (1998). Osteoid osteoma and osteoblastoma with clonal chromosome changes. Br J Cancer 78: 344–348.
562. Dalal KM, Kattan MW, Antonescu CR et al. (2006). Subtype specific prognostic nomogram for patients with primary liposarcoma of the retroperitoneum, extremity, or trunk. Ann Surg 244: 381–391.
563. Daluiski A, Seeger LL, Doberneck SA et al. (1995). A case of juxta-articular myxoma of the knee. Skeletal Radiol 24: 389–391.
564. Damato S, Alorjani M, Bonar F et al. (2012). IDH1 mutations are not found in cartilaginous tumours other than central and periosteal chondrosarcomas and enchondromas. Histopathology 60: 363–365.
565. Dancer JY, Henry SP, Bondaruk J et al. (2010). Expression of master regulatory genes controlling skeletal development in benign cartilage and bone forming tumors. Hum Pathol 41: 1788–1793.
566. Danielson LS, Menendez S, Attolini CS et al. (2010). A differentiation-based microRNA signature identifies leiomyosarcoma as a mesenchymal stem cell-related malignancy. Am J Pathol 177: 908–917.
567. Dantonello TM, Int-Veen C, Leuschner I et al. (2008). Mesenchymal chondrosarcoma of soft tissues and bone in children, adolescents, and young adults: experiences of the CWS and COSS study groups. Cancer 112: 2424–2431.
568. Dar P, Karmin I, Einstein MH (2008). Arteriovenous malformations of the uterus: long-term follow-up. Gynecol Obstet Invest 66: 157–161.
569. Darby AJ, Cassar-Pullicino VN, McCall IW et al. (1999). Vertebral intra-osseous chordoma or giant notochordal rest? Skeletal Radiol 28: 342–346.
570. Dargent JL, Delplace J, Roufosse C et al. (1999). Development of a calcifying fibrous pseudotumour within a lesion of Castleman disease, hyaline-vascular subtype. J Clin Pathol 52: 547–549.
571. Darilek S, Wicklund C, Novy D et al. (2005). Hereditary multiple exostosis and pain. J Pediatr Orthop 25: 369–376.
572. Daroca PJ, Jr., Pulitzer DR, LoCicero J, III (1982). Ossifying fasciitis. Arch Pathol Lab Med 106: 682–685.
573. Daroszewska A, Ralston SH (2005). Genetics of Paget's disease of bone. Clin Sci (Lond) 109: 257–263.
574. Darwish BS, Balakrishnan V, Maitra R (2002). Intramedullary ancient schwannoma of the cervical spinal cord: case report and review of literature. J Clin Neurosci 9: 321–323.
575. Daston MM, Scrable H, Nordlund M et al. (1992). The protein product of the neurofibromatosis type 1 gene is expressed at highest abundance in neurons, Schwann cells, and oligodendrocytes. Neuron 8: 415–428.
576. Datta V, Rawal YB, Mincer HH et al. (2007). Myopericytoma of the oral cavity. Head Neck 29: 605–608.
577. Davicioni E, Anderson MJ, Finckenstein FG et al. (2009). Molecular classification of rhabdomyosarcoma—genotypic and phenotypic determinants of diagnosis: a report from the Children's Oncology Group. Am J Pathol 174: 550–564.
578. Davidson JS, Demsey D (2011). Atypical fibroxanthoma: Clinicopathologic determinants for recurrence and implications for surgical management. J Surg Oncol 105:559-562.
579. Davies B, Noh P, Smaldone MC et al. (2007). Paratesticular rhabdomyoma in a young adult: case study and review of the literature. J Pediatr Surg 42: E5–E7.
580. Davies JD, Rees GJ, Mera SL (1983). Angiosarcoma in irradiated post-mastectomy chest wall. Histopathology 7: 947–956.
581. Davis DA, Sanchez RL (1998). Atrophic and plaquelike dermatofibrosarcoma protuberans. Am J Dermatopathol 20: 498–501.
582. Davis IJ, Kim JJ, Ozsolak F et al. (2006). Oncogenic MITF dysregulation in clear cell sarcoma: defining the MiT family of human cancers. Cancer Cell 9: 473–484.
583. Davis RI, Hamilton A, Biggart JD (1998). Primary synovial chondromatosis: a clinicopathologic review and assessment of malignant potential. Hum Pathol 29: 683–688.
584. Davis RJ, Barr FG (1997). Fusion genes resulting from alternative chromosomal translocations are overexpressed by gene-specific mechanisms in alveolar rhabdomyosarcoma. Proc Natl Acad Sci U S A 94: 8047–8051.
585. Davis RJ, D'Cruz CM, Lovell MA et al. (1994). Fusion of PAX7 to FKHR by the variant t(1;13)(p36;q14) translocation in alveolar rhabdomyosarcoma. Cancer Res 54: 2869–2872.
586. de Alava E, Antonescu CR, Panizo A et al. (2000). Prognostic impact of P53 status in Ewing sarcoma. Cancer 89: 783–792.
587. de Alava E, Ladanyi M, Rosai J et al. (1995). Detection of chimeric transcripts in desmoplastic small round cell tumor and related developmental tumors by reverse transcriptase polymerase chain reaction. A specific diagnostic assay. Am J Pathol 147: 1584–1591.
588. de Andrea CE, Kroon HM, Wolterbeek R et al. (2012). Interobserver reliability in the histopathological diagnosis of cartilaginous tumors in patients with multiple osteochondromas. Mod Pathol
589. de Andrea CE, Prins FA, Wiweger MI et al. (2011). Growth plate regulation and osteochondroma formation: insights from tracing proteoglycans in zebrafish models and human cartilage. J Pathol 224: 160–168.
590. de Andrea CE, Reijnders CM, Kroon HM et al. (2011). Secondary peripheral chondrosarcoma evolving from osteochondroma as a result of outgrowth of cells with functional EXT. Oncogene
591. de Andrea CE, Wiweger M, Prins F et al. (2010). Primary cilia organization reflects polarity in the growth plate and implies loss of polarity and mosaicism in osteochondroma. Lab Invest 90: 1091–1101.
592. de Andrea CE, Wiweger MI, Bovee JV et al. (2012). Peripheral chondrosarcoma progression is associated with increased type X collagen and vascularisation. Virchows Arch 460: 95–102.
593. de Baere T, Vanel D, Shapeero LG et al. (1992). Osteosarcoma after chemotherapy: evaluation with contrast material-enhanced subtraction MR imaging. Radiology 185: 587–592.
593A. de Berg JC, Pattynama PM, Obermann WR et al. (1995). Percutaneous computed-tomography-guided thermocoagulation for osteoid osteomas. Lancet 346:350–351.
594. de Beuckeleer LH, De Schepper AM, Vandevenne JE et al. (2000). MR imaging of clear cell sarcoma (malignant melanoma of the soft parts): a multicenter correlative MRI-pathology study of 21 cases and literature review. Skeletal Radiol 29: 187–195.
595. de Beur SM, Finnegan RB, Vassiliadis J et al. (2002). Tumors associated with oncogenic osteomalacia express genes important in bone and mineral metabolism. J Bone Miner Res 17: 1102–1110.
596. de Boeck G, Forsyth RG, Praet M et al. (2009). Telomere-associated proteins: cross-talk between telomere maintenance and telomere-lengthening mechanisms. J Pathol 217: 327–344.
597. de Bree E, Zoetmulder FA, Keus RB et al. (2004). Incidence and treatment of recurrent plantar fibromatosis by surgery and postoperative radiotherapy. Am J Surg 187: 33–38.
598. de Feraudy S, Fletcher CD (2010). Intradermal nodular fasciitis: a rare lesion analyzed in a series of 24 cases. Am J Surg Pathol 34: 1377–1381.
599. de Feraudy S, Mar N, McCalmont TH (2008). Evaluation of CD10 and procollagen 1 expression in atypical fibroxanthoma and dermatofibroma. Am J Surg Pathol 32: 1111–1122.
600. de Lange J, van Maarle MC, van den Akker HP et al. (2007). A new mutation in the SH3BP2 gene showing reduced penetrance in a family affected with cherubism. Oral Surg Oral Med Oral Pathol Oral Radiol Endod 103: 378–381.
601. de Leval L, Braaten KM, Ancukiewicz M et al. (2003). Diffuse large B-cell lymphoma of bone: an analysis of differentiation-associated antigens with clinical correlation. Am J Surg Pathol 27: 1269–1277.
602. de Maeseneer M, Jaovisidha S, Lenchik L et al. (1997). Fibrolipomatous hamartoma: MR imaging findings. Skeletal Radiol 26: 155–160.
603. de Raedt T, Brems H, Wolkenstein P et al. (2003). Elevated risk for MPNST in NF1 microdeletion patients. Am J Hum Genet 72: 1288–1292.
604. de Saint Aubain Somerhausen N, Coindre JM, Debiec-Rychter M et al. (2008). Lipoblastoma in adolescents and young adults: report of six cases with FISH analysis. Histopathology 52: 294–298.
605. de Saint Aubain Somerhausen N, Fletcher CD (1999). Leiomyosarcoma of soft tissue in children: clinicopathologic analysis of 20 cases. Am J Surg Pathol 23: 755–763.
606. de Santos LA, Murray JA (1978). Evaluation of giant cell tumour by computerized tomography.Skeletal Radiol 2:205–212.
607. de Silva MV, McMahon AD, Paterson L et al. (2003). Identification of poorly differentiated synovial sarcoma: a comparison of clinicopathological and cytogenetic features with those of typical synovial sarcoma. Histopathology 43: 220–230.
608. de Silva MV, Reid R (2003). Myositis ossificans and fibroosseous pseudotumor of digits: a clinicopathological review of 64 cases with emphasis on diagnostic pitfalls. Int J Surg Pathol 11: 187–195.
609. de Smet L, Sciot R, Legius E (2002). Multifocal glomus tumours of the fingers in two patients with neurofibromatosis type 1. J Med Genet 39: e45
610. de Vreeze RS, van Coevorden F, Boerrigter L et al. (2011). Delineation of chondroid lipoma: an immunohistochemical and molecular biological analysis. Sarcoma. In Press.
611. de Wever I, Dal Cin P, Fletcher CD et al. (2000). Cytogenetic, clinical, and morphologic correlations in 78 cases of fibromatosis: a report from the CHAMP Study Group. CHromosomes And Morphology. Mod Pathol 13: 1080–1085.
612. deBaun MR, Tucker MA (1998). Risk of cancer during the first four years of life in children from The Beckwith-Wiedemann Syndrome Registry. J Pediatr 132: 398–400.
613. Debelenko LV, Arthur DC, Pack SD et al. (2003). Identification of CARS-ALK fusion in primary and metastatic lesions of an inflammatory myofibroblastic tumor. Lab Invest 83: 1255–1265.
614. DeCaprio JA, Ludlow JW, Figge J et al. (1988). SV40 large tumor antigen forms a specific complex with the product of the retinoblastoma susceptibility gene. Cell 54: 275–283.
615. DeCaprio JA, Ludlow JW, Lynch D et al. (1989). The product of the retinoblastoma susceptibility gene has properties of a cell cycle regulatory element. Cell 58: 1085–1095.
616. Decaux O, Lode L, Magrangeas F et al. (2008). Prediction of survival in multiple myeloma based on gene expression profiles reveals cell cycle and chromosomal instability signatures in high-risk patients and hyperdiploid signatures in low-risk patients: a study of the Intergroupe Francophone du Myelome. J Clin Oncol 26: 4798–4805.
617. Deckert M, Rottapel R (2006). The adapter 3BP2: how it plugs into leukocyte signaling. Adv Exp Med Biol 584: 107–114.

618. Deenik W, Mooi WJ, Rutgers EJ et al. (1999). Clear cell sarcoma (malignant melanoma) of soft parts: A clinicopathologic study of 30 cases. Cancer 86: 969–975.

619. Deepti AN, Madhuri V, Walter NM et al. (2008). Lipofibromatosis: report of a rare paediatric soft tissue tumour. Skeletal Radiol 37: 555–558.

620. Degreef I, Sciot R, De Smet L (2007). Intraarticular fibroma of the tendon sheath in the wrist. J Hand Surg Eur Vol 32: 723

621. Dehner LP, Enzinger FM, Font RL (1972). Fetal rhabdomyoma. An analysis of nine cases. Cancer 30: 160–166.

622. Dei Tos AP (2000). Liposarcoma: new entities and evolving concepts. Ann Diagn Pathol 4: 252–266.

623. Dei Tos AP, Doglioni C, Piccinin S et al. (1997). Molecular abnormalities of the p53 pathway in dedifferentiated liposarcoma. J Pathol 181: 8–13.

624. Dei Tos AP, Doglioni C, Piccinin S et al. (2000). Coordinated expression and amplification of the MDM2, CDK4, and HMGI-C genes in atypical lipomatous tumours. J Pathol 190: 531–536.

625. Dei Tos AP, Maestro R, Doglioni C et al. (1994). Ultraviolet-induced p53 mutations in atypical fibroxanthoma. Am J Pathol 145: 11–17.

626. Dei Tos AP, Maestro R, Doglioni C et al. (1996). Tumor suppressor genes and related molecules in leiomyosarcoma. Am J Pathol 148: 1037–1045.

627. Dei Tos AP, Mentzel T, Fletcher CD (1998). Primary liposarcoma of the skin: a rare neoplasm with unusual high grade features. Am J Dermatopathol 20: 332–338.

628. Dei Tos AP, Mentzel T, Newman PL et al. (1994). Spindle cell liposarcoma, a hitherto unrecognized variant of liposarcoma. Analysis of six cases. Am J Surg Pathol 18: 913–921.

629. Dei Tos AP, Wadden C, Fletcher CD (1996). S-100 protein staining in liposarcoma. Its diagnostic utility in the high grade myxoid (round cell) variant. Appl Immunohistochem 4: 95–101.

630. Delaney D, Diss TC, Presneau N et al. (2009). GNAS1 mutations occur more commonly than previously thought in intramuscular myxoma. Mod Pathol 22: 718–724.

631. Delattre O, Zucman J, Plougastel B et al. (1992). Gene fusion with an ETS DNA-binding domain caused by chromosome translocation in human tumours. Nature 359: 162–165.

632. Delling G, Werner M (2003). [Pathomorphology of parosteal osteosarcoma. Experience with 125 cases in the Hamburg Register of Bone Tumors]. Orthopade 32: 74–81.

633. Dembinski A, Bridge JA, Neff JR et al. (1992). Trisomy 2 in proliferative fasciitis. Cancer Genet Cytogenet 60: 27–30.

634. Demicco EG, Deshpande V, Nielsen GP et al. (2010). Well-differentiated osteosarcoma of the jaw bones: a clinicopathologic study of 15 cases. Am J Surg Pathol 34: 1647–1655.

635. Demicco EG, Rosenberg AE, Bjornsson J et al. (2010). Primary Rosai-Dorfman disease of bone: a clinicopathologic study of 15 cases. Am J Surg Pathol 34: 1324–1333.

636. Demicco EG, Torres KE, Ghadimi MP et al. (2011). Involvement of the PI3K/Akt pathway in myxoid/round cell liposarcoma. Mod Pathol 25:212-221.

637. Demiralp B, Kose O, Oguz E et al. (2009). Benign fibrous histiocytoma of the lumbar vertebrae. Skeletal Radiol 38: 187–191.

638. Deng FM, Galvan K, de la Roza G et al. (2011). Molecular characterization of an EWSR1-POU5F1 fusion associated with a t(6;22) in an undifferentiated soft tissue sarcoma. Cancer Genet 204: 423–429.

639. Derkinderen DJ, Koten JW, Wolterbeek R et al. (1987). Non-ocular cancer in hereditary retinoblastoma survivors and relatives. Ophthalmic Paediatr Genet 8: 23–25.

640. Derre J, Lagace R, Nicolas A et al. (2001). Leiomyosarcomas and most malignant fibrous histiocytomas share very similar comparative genomic hybridization imbalances: an analysis of a series of 27 leiomyosarcomas. Lab Invest 81: 211–215.

641. Deruaz JP, Janzer RC, Costa J (1993). Cellular schwannomas of the intracranial and intraspinal compartment: morphological and immunological characteristics compared with classical benign schwannomas. J Neuropathol Exp Neurol 52: 114–118.

642. Desai P, Perino G, Present D et al. (1996). Sarcoma in association with bone infarcts. Report of five cases. Arch Pathol Lab Med 120: 482–489.

643. Deshpande V, Nielsen GP, Rosenthal DI et al. (2007). Intraosseous benign notochord cell tumors (BNCT): further evidence supporting a relationship to chordoma. Am J Surg Pathol 31: 1573–1577.

644. Deshpande V, Rosenberg AE, O'Connell JX et al. (2003). Epithelioid angiosarcoma of the bone: a series of 10 cases. Am J Surg Pathol 27: 709–716.

645. Desikan KR, Dhodapkar MV, Hough A et al. (1997). Incidence and impact of light chain associated (AL) amyloidosis on the prognosis of patients with multiple myeloma treated with autologous transplantation. Leuk Lymphoma 27: 315–319.

646. Destouet JM, Kyriakos M, Gilula LA (1980). Fibrous histiocytoma (fibroxanthoma) of a cervical vertebra. A report with a review of the literature. Skeletal Radiol 5: 241–246.

647. Devaney K, Vinh TN, Sweet DE (1993). Small cell osteosarcoma of bone: an immunohistochemical study with differential diagnostic considerations. Hum Pathol 24: 1211–1225.

648. Devaney K, Vinh TN, Sweet DE (1993). Synovial hemangioma: a report of 20 cases with differential diagnostic considerations. Hum Pathol 24: 737–745.

649. Devaney K, Vinh TN, Sweet DE (1994). Skeletal-extraskeletal angiomatosis. A clinicopathological study of fourteen patients and nosologic considerations. J Bone Joint Surg Am 76: 878–891.

650. Devesa SS (1975). The incidence of retinoblastoma. Am J Ophthalmol 80: 263–265.

651. Devoe K, Weidner N (2000). Immunohistochemistry of small round-cell tumors. Semin Diagn Pathol 17: 216–224.

652. Dewaele B, Floris G, Finalet-Ferreiro J et al. (2010). Coactivated platelet-derived growth factor receptor {alpha} and epidermal growth factor receptor are potential therapeutic targets in intimal sarcoma. Cancer Res 70: 7304–7314.

653. DeYoung BR, Swanson PE, Argenyi ZB et al. (1995). CD31 immunoreactivity in mesenchymal neoplasms of the skin and subcutis: report of 145 cases and review of putative immunohistologic markers of endothelial differentiation. J Cutan Pathol 22: 215–222.

654. Deyrup AT, Lee VK, Hill CE et al. (2006). Epstein-Barr virus-associated smooth muscle tumors are distinctive mesenchymal tumors reflecting multiple infection events: a clinicopathologic and molecular analysis of 29 tumors from 19 patients. Am J Surg Pathol 30: 75–82.

655. Deyrup AT, Miettinen M, North PE et al. (2009). Angiosarcomas arising in the viscera and soft tissue of children and young adults: a clinicopathologic study of 15 cases. Am J Surg Pathol 33: 264–269.

656. Deyrup AT, Montag AG, Inwards CY et al. (2007). Sarcomas arising in Paget disease of bone: a clinicopathologic analysis of 70 cases. Arch Pathol Lab Med 131: 942–946.

657. Deyrup AT, Tighiouart M, Montag AG et al. (2008). Epithelioid hemangioendothelioma of soft tissue: a proposal for risk stratification based on 49 cases. Am J Surg Pathol 32: 924–927.

658. Deyrup AT, Weiss SW (2006). Grading of soft tissue sarcomas: the challenge of providing precise information in an imprecise world. Histopathology 48: 42–50.

659. di Sant'Agnese PA, Knowles DM (1980). Extracardiac rhabdomyoma: a clinicopathologic study and review of the literature. Cancer 46: 780–789.

660. Di Tommaso L, Magrini E, Consales A et al. (2002). Malignant granular cell tumor of the lateral femoral cutaneous nerve: report of a case with cytogenetic analysis. Hum Pathol 33: 1237–1240.

661. Diaz-Cascajo C, Weyers W, Borghi S (2003). Pigmented atypical fibroxanthoma: a tumor that may be easily mistaken for malignant melanoma. Am J Dermatopathol 25: 1–5.

662. DiCaprio MR, Enneking WF (2005). Fibrous dysplasia. Pathophysiology, evaluation, and treatment. J Bone Joint Surg Am 87: 1848–1864.

663. Dickersin GR, Rosenberg AE (1991). The ultrastructure of small-cell osteosarcoma, with a review of the light microscopy and differential diagnosis. Hum Pathol 22: 267–275.

664. Dickey GE, Sotelo-Avila C (1999). Fibrous hamartoma of infancy: current review. Pediatr Dev Pathol 2: 236–243.

665. Dickey ID, Rose PS, Fuchs B et al. (2004). Dedifferentiated chondrosarcoma: the role of chemotherapy with updated outcomes. J Bone Joint Surg Am 86-A: 2412–2418.

666. Dickman PS, Triche TJ (1986). Extraosseous Ewing's sarcoma versus primitive rhabdomyosarcoma: diagnostic criteria and clinical correlation. Hum Pathol 17: 881–893.

667. Dickson BC, Gortzak Y, Bell RS et al. (2011). p63 expression in adamantinoma. Virchows Arch 459: 109–113.

668. Dimopoulos MA, Moulopoulos LA, Maniatis A et al. (2000). Solitary plasmacytoma of bone and asymptomatic multiple myeloma. Blood 96: 2037–2044.

669. Ding Y, Cai YB, Zhang Q (2003). [Parosteal osteosarcoma: a clinical study of 48 cases]. Zhonghua Wai Ke Za Zhi 41: 832–836.

670. Dini M, Lo Russo G, Colafranceschi M (1998). So-called nasal glioma: case report with immunohistochemical study. Tumori 84: 398–402.

671. Dion E, Graef C, Miquel A et al. (2006). Bone involvement in Erdheim-Chester disease: imaging findings including periostitis and partial epiphyseal involvement. Radiology 238: 632–639.

672. Dishop MK, O'Connor WN, Abraham S et al. (2001). Primary cardiac lipoblastoma. Pediatr Dev Pathol 4: 276–280.

673. Dispenzieri A (2011). POEMS syndrome: 2011 update on diagnosis, risk-stratification, and management. Am J Hematol 86: 591–601.

674. Diwadkar GB, Barber MD (2009). Vulvar mammary-type myofibroblastoma: a case report. J Reprod Med 54: 404–406.

675. Dixon AY, McGregor DH, Lee SH (1981). Angiolipomas: an ultrastructural and clinicopathological study. Hum Pathol 12: 739–747.

676. Domont J, Salas S, Lacroix L et al. (2010). High frequency of beta-catenin heterozygous mutations in extra-abdominal fibromatosis: a potential molecular tool for disease management. Br J Cancer 102: 1032–1036.

677. Donahoo JS, Miller JA, Lal B et al. (1996). Chest wall hamartoma in an adult: an unusual chest wall tumor. Thorac Cardiovasc Surg 44: 110–111.

678. Donato M, Vanel D, Alberghini M et al. (2009). Muscle fibers inside a fat tumor: a nonspecific imaging finding of benignancy. Eur J Radiol 72: 27–29.

679. Donmez FY, Tuzun U, Basaran C et al. (2008). MRI findings in parosteal osteosarcoma: correlation with histopathology. Diagn Interv Radiol 14: 142–152.

680. Donner LR, Clawson K, Dobin SM (2000). Sclerosing epithelioid fibrosarcoma: a cytogenetic, immunohistochemical, and ultrastructural study of an unusual histological variant. Cancer Genet Cytogenet 119: 127–131.

681. Donner LR, Silva T, Dobin SM (2002). Clonal rearrangement of 15p11.2, 16p11.2, and 16p13.3 in a case of nodular fasciitis: additional evidence favoring nodular fasciitis as a benign neoplasm and not a reactive tumefaction. Cancer Genet Cytogenet 139: 138–140.

682. Dorfman HD (2010). New knowledge of fibro-osseous lesions of bone. Int J Surg Pathol 18: 62S–65S.

683. Dorfman HD, Czerniak B (1998). Vascular lesions. In: Dorfman HD, Czerniak B eds, Bone tumors. Mosby: St Louis: pp 559-608.

684. Dorfman HD, Czerniak B (1998). Vascular lesions. In: Dorfman HD, Czerniak B eds, Bone tumors. Mosby: St Louis: pp 729–814.

685. Dorfman HD, Weiss SW (1984). Borderline osteoblastic tumors: problems in the differential diagnosis of aggressive osteoblastoma and low-grade osteosarcoma. Semin Diagn Pathol 1: 215–234.

686. Dorfman RF (1991). Multiple myeloma showing signet-ring cell change. Histopathology 18: 577–578.

687. Dorwart RH, Genant HK, Johnston WH et al. (1984). Pigmented villonodular synovitis of synovial joints: clinical, pathologic, and radiologic features. AJR Am J Roentgenol 143: 877–885.

688. dos Santos NR, de Bruijn DR, van Kessel AG (2001). Molecular mechanisms underlying human synovial sarcoma development. Genes Chromosomes Cancer 30: 1–14.

689. Dotsch J, Kiess W, Hanze J et al. (1996). Gs alpha mutation at codon 201 in pituitary adenoma causing gigantism in a 6-year-old boy with McCune-Albright syndrome. J Clin Endocrinol Metab 81: 3839–3842.

690. Douglass EC, Rowe ST, Valentine M et al. (1990). A second nonrandom translocation, der(16)t(1;16)(q21;q13), in Ewing sarcoma and peripheral neuroectodermal tumor. Cytogenet Cell Genet 53: 87–90.

691. Douglass EC, Valentine M, Green AA et al. (1986). t(11;22) and other chromosomal rearrangements in Ewing's sarcoma. J Natl Cancer Inst 77: 1211–1215.

692. Dounies R, Chwals WJ, Lally KP et al. (1994). Hamartomas of the chest wall in infants.

Ann Thorac Surg 57: 868–875.
693. Doussis IA, Puddle B, Athanasou NA (1992). Immunophenotype of multinucleated and mononuclear cells in giant cell lesions of bone and soft tissue. J Clin Pathol 45: 398–404.
694. Dowling O, Difeo A, Ramirez MC et al. (2003). Mutations in capillary morphogenesis gene-2 result in the allelic disorders juvenile hyaline fibromatosis and infantile systemic hyalinosis. Am J Hum Genet 73: 957–966.
695. Downes KA, Goldblum JR, Montgomery EA et al. (2001). Pleomorphic liposarcoma: a clinicopathologic analysis of 19 cases. Mod Pathol 14: 179–184.
696. Doyle LA, Wang W, Dal Cin P, et al. (2012) MUC4 is a sensitive and extremely useful marker for sclerosing epithelioid fibrosarcoma: association with FUS gene rearrangement. Am J Surg Pathol 36: 1444–1451.
697. Draper GJ, Sanders BM, Kingston JE (1986). Second primary neoplasms in patients with retinoblastoma. Br J Cancer 53: 661–671.
698. Dray MS, McCarthy SW, Palmer AA et al. (2006). Myopericytoma: a unifying term for a spectrum of tumours that show overlapping features with myofibroma. A review of 14 cases. J Clin Pathol 59: 67–73.
699. Dreux N, Marty M, Chibon F et al. (2010). Value and limitation of immunohistochemical expression of HMGA2 in mesenchymal tumors: about a series of 1052 cases. Mod Pathol 23: 1657–1666.
700. Drier A, Haroche J, Savatovsky J et al. (2010). Cerebral, facial, and orbital involvement in Erdheim-Chester disease: CT and MR imaging findings. Radiology 255: 586–594.
701. Drilon AD, Popat S, Bhuchar G et al. (2008). Extraskeletal myxoid chondrosarcoma: a retrospective review from 2 referral centers emphasizing long-term outcomes with surgery and chemotherapy. Cancer 113: 3364–3371.
702. Drut R (1988). Ossifying fibrolipomatous hamartoma of the ulnar nerve. Pediatr Pathol 8: 179–184.
703. Drut R, Pedemonte L, Rositto A (2005). Noninclusion-body infantile digital fibromatosis: a lesion heralding terminal osseous dysplasia and pigmentary defects syndrome. Int J Surg Pathol 13: 181–184.
704. Dryja TP, Cavenee W, White R et al. (1984). Homozygosity of chromosome 13 in retinoblastoma. N Engl J Med 310: 550–553.
705. Dubus P, Coindre JM, Groppi A et al. (2001). The detection of Tel-TrkC chimeric transcripts is more specific than TrkC immunoreactivity for the diagnosis of congenital fibrosarcoma. J Pathol 193: 88–94.
706. Ducatman BS, Scheithauer BW, Piepgras DG et al. (1984). Malignant peripheral nerve sheath tumors in childhood. J Neurooncol 2: 241–248.
707. Ducatman BS, Scheithauer BW, Piepgras DG et al. (1986). Malignant peripheral nerve sheath tumors. A clinicopathologic study of 120 cases. Cancer 57: 2006–2021.
708. Dudgeon J, Lee WR (1983). The trilateral retinoblastoma syndrome. Trans Ophthalmol Soc U K 103 (Pt 5): 523–529.
709. Duhamel LA, Ye H, Halai D et al. (2012). Frequency of Mouse Double Minute 2 (MDM2) and Mouse Double Minute 4 (MDM4) amplification in parosteal and conventional osteosarcoma subtypes. Histopathology 60: 357–359.
710. Dujardin F, Binh MB, Bouvier C et al. (2011). MDM2 and CDK4 immunohistochemistry is a valuable tool in the differential diagnosis of low-grade osteosarcomas and other primary fibro-osseous lesions of the bone. Mod Pathol 24: 624–637.
711. Duke D, Dvorak A, Harris TJ et al. (1996). Multiple retiform hemangioendotheliomas. A low-grade angiosarcoma. Am J Dermatopathol 18: 606–610.
712. Dumitrescu CE, Collins MT (2008). McCune-Albright syndrome. Orphanet J Rare Dis 3: 12
713. Dumont C, Monforte M, Flandrin A et al. (2011). Prenatal management of congenital infantile fibrosarcoma: unexpected outcome. Ultrasound Obstet Gynecol 37: 733–735.
714. Dunlap JB, Magenis RE, Davis C et al. (2009). Cytogenetic analysis of a primary bone angiosarcoma. Cancer Genet Cytogenet 194: 1–3.
715. Dunn JM, Phillips RA, Zhu X et al. (1989). Mutations in the RB1 gene and their effects on transcription. Mol Cell Biol 9: 4596–4604.
716. Durroux R, Ducoin H, Gaubert J (1993). [Adamantinoma of the tibia and osteofibrodysplasia. Report of a case]. Ann Pathol 13: 336–340.
717. Dymock RB, Allen PW, Stirling JW et al. (1987). Giant cell fibroblastoma. A distinctive, recurrent tumor of childhood. Am J Surg Pathol 11: 263–271.
718. Dyson N, Howley PM, Munger K et al. (1989). The human papilloma virus-16 E7 oncoprotein is able to bind to the retinoblastoma gene product. Science 243: 934–937.
719. Eaton KW, Tooke LS, Wainwright LM et al. (2011). Spectrum of SMARCB1/INI1 mutations in familial and sporadic rhabdoid tumors. Pediatr Blood Cancer 56: 7–15.
720. Ebhardt H, Kosmehl H, Katenkamp D (2001). [Acral myxoinflammatory fibroblastic sarcoma. Six cases of a tumor entity]. Pathologe 22: 157–161.
721. Eckardt JJ, Pritchard DJ, Soule EH (1983). Clear cell sarcoma. A clinicopathologic study of 27 cases. Cancer 52: 1482–1488.
722. Edge SB, Byrd DR, ComptonCC et al. (2010). AJCC cancer staging manual, seventh edition. Springer-Verlag: New York.
723. Edris B, Espinosa I, Muhlenberg T et al. (2012). ROR2 is a novel prognostic biomarker and a potential therapeutic target in leiomyosarcoma and gastrointestinal stromal tumour. J Pathol 227:223-233.
724. Edwards V, Tse G, Doucet J et al. (1999). Rhabdomyosarcoma metastasizing as a malignant ectomesenchymoma. Ultrastruct Pathol 23: 267–273.
725. Eefting D, Schrage YM, Geirnaerdt MJ et al. (2009). Assessment of interobserver variability and histologic parameters to improve reliability in classification and grading of central cartilaginous tumors. Am J Surg Pathol 33: 50–57.
726. Eeles RA (1995). Germline mutations in the TP53 gene. Cancer Surv 25: 101–124.
727. Efem SE, Ekpo MD (1993). Clinicopathological features of untreated fibrous hamartoma of infancy. J Clin Pathol 46: 522–524.
728. Eich GF, Hoeffel JC, Tschappeler H et al. (1998). Fibrous tumours in children: imaging features of a heterogeneous group of disorders. Pediatr Radiol 28: 500–509.
729. Eilber FC, Brennan MF, Eilber FR et al. (2004). Validation of the postoperative nomogram for 12-year sarcoma-specific mortality. Cancer 101: 2270–2275.
730. Eilber FC, Brennan MF, Eilber FR et al. (2007). Chemotherapy is associated with improved survival in adult patients with primary extremity synovial sarcoma. Ann Surg 246: 105–113.
731. Eilber FC, Eilber FR, Eckardt J et al. (2004). The impact of chemotherapy on the survival of patients with high-grade primary extremity liposarcoma. Ann Surg 240: 686–695.
732. el-Jabbour JN, Bennett MH, Burke MM et al. (1991). Proliferative myositis. An immunohistochemical and ultrastructural study. Am J Surg Pathol 15: 654–659.
733. el-Naggar AK, Hurr K, Tu ZN et al. (1995). DNA and RNA content analysis by flow cytometry in the pathobiologic assessment of bone tumors. Cytometry 19: 256–262.
734. el-Naggar AK, Ro JY, Ayala AG et al. (1989). Angiomatoid malignant fibrous histiocytoma: flow cytometric DNA analysis of six cases. J Surg Oncol 40: 201–204.
735. El-Rifai W, Sarlomo-Rikala M, Andersson LC et al. (2000). DNA sequence copy number changes in gastrointestinal stromal tumors: tumor progression and prognostic significance. Cancer Res 60: 3899–3903.
736. Elco CP, Marino-Enriquez A, Abraham JA et al. (2010). Hybrid myxoinflammatory fibroblastic sarcoma/hemosiderotic fibrolipomatous tumor: report of a case providing further evidence for a pathogenetic link. Am J Surg Pathol 34: 1723–1727.
737. Eldridge R (1981). Central neurofibromatosis with bilateral acoustic neuroma. Adv Neurol 29: 57–65.
738. Elefteriou F, Kolanczyk M, Schindeler A et al. (2009). Skeletal abnormalities in neurofibromatosis type 1: approaches to therapeutic options. Am J Med Genet A 149A: 2327–2338.
739. Elgar F, Goldblum JR (1997). Well-differentiated liposarcoma of the retroperitoneum: a clinicopathologic analysis of 20 cases, with particular attention to the extent of low-grade dedifferentiation. Mod Pathol 10: 113–120.
740. Elkins CT, Wakely PE, Jr. (2011). Sclerosing epithelioid fibrosarcoma of the oral cavity. Head Neck Pathol 5: 428–431.
741. Elliott M, Bayly R, Cole T et al. (1994). Clinical features and natural history of Beckwith-Wiedemann syndrome: presentation of 74 new cases. Clin Genet 46: 168–174.
742. Emberger M, Laimer M, Steiner H et al. (2009). Retiform hemangioendothelioma: presentation of a case expressing D2-40. J Cutan Pathol 36: 987–990.
743. Emile JF, Wechsler J, Brousse N et al. (1995). Langerhans' cell histiocytosis. Definitive diagnosis with the use of monoclonal antibody O10 on routinely paraffin-embedded samples. Am J Surg Pathol 19: 636–641.
744. Emory TS, Scheithauer BW, Hirose T et al. (1995). Intraneural perineurioma. A clonal neoplasm associated with abnormalities of chromosome 22. Am J Clin Pathol 103: 696–704.
745. Endo M, Hasegawa T, Tashiro T et al. (2005). Bizarre parosteal osteochondromatous proliferation with a t(1;17) translocation. Virchows Arch 447: 99–102.
746. Eng C, Li FP, Abramson DH et al. (1993). Mortality from second tumors among long-term survivors of retinoblastoma. J Natl Cancer Inst 85: 1121–1128.
747. Ensoli B, Sgadari C, Barillari G et al. (2001). Biology of Kaposi's sarcoma. Eur J Cancer 37: 1251–1269.
748. Enzinger FM (1965). Clear-cell sarcoma of tendons and aponeuroses. An analysis of 21 cases. Cancer 18: 1163–1174.
749. Enzinger FM (1965). Fibrous hamartoma of infancy. Cancer 18: 241–248.
750. Enzinger FM (1965). Intramuscular myxoma; a review and follow-up study of 34 cases. Am J Clin Pathol 43: 104–113.
751. Enzinger FM (1979). Angiomatoid malignant fibrous histiocytoma: a distinct fibrohistiocytic tumor of children and young adults simulating a vascular neoplasm. Cancer 44: 2147–2157.
752. Enzinger FM, Dulcey F (1967). Proliferative myositis. Report of thirty-three cases. Cancer 20: 2213–2223.
753. Enzinger FM, Harvey DA (1975). Spindle cell lipoma. Cancer 36: 1852–1859.
754. Enzinger FM, Shiraki M (1972). Extraskeletal myxoid chondrosarcoma. An analysis of 34 cases. Hum Pathol 3: 421–435.
755. Enzinger FM, Weiss SW (1988). Benign tumors and tumor-like lesions of fibrous tissue. In: Soft tissue tumors. Second edition. C.V. Mosby: St. Louis.
756. Enzinger FM, Weiss SW (1988). Soft tissue tumors. Second edition. C.V. Mosby: St Louis.
757. Enzinger FM, Weiss SW, Liang CY (1989). Ossifying fibromyxoid tumor of soft parts. A clinicopathological analysis of 59 cases. Am J Surg Pathol 13: 817–827.
758. Enzinger FM, Winslow DJ (1962). Liposarcoma. A study of 103 cases. Virchows Arch Pathol Anat Physiol Klin Med 335: 367–388.
759. Enzinger FM, Zhang RY (1988). Plexiform fibrohistiocytic tumor presenting in children and young adults. An analysis of 65 cases. Am J Surg Pathol 12: 818–826.
760. Eppley BL, Harruff R, Shah M et al. (1994). Fibrous hamartomas of the scalp in infancy. Plast Reconstr Surg 94: 195–197.
761. Eppsteiner RW, DeYoung BR, Milhem MM et al. (2011). Leiomyosarcoma of the head and neck: a population-based analysis. Arch Otolaryngol Head Neck Surg 137: 921–924.
762. Epstein CJ, Martin GM, Schultz AL et al. (1966). Werner's syndrome a review of its symptomatology, natural history, pathologic features, genetics and relationship to the natural aging process. Medicine (Baltimore) 45: 177–221.
763. Epstein DS, Pashaei S, Hunt E Jr et al. (2007). Pustulo-ovoid bodies of Milian in granular cell tumors. J Cutan Pathol 34: 405–409.
764. Erickson-Johnson MR, Chou MM, Evers BR et al. (2011). Nodular fasciitis: a novel model of transient neoplasia induced by MYH9-USP6 gene fusion. Lab Invest 91: 1427–1433.
765. Erickson-Johnson MR, Seys AR, Roth CW et al. (2009). Carboxypeptidase M: a biomarker for the discrimination of well-differentiated liposarcoma from lipoma. Mod Pathol 22: 1541–1547.
766. Eriksson M, Hardell L, Adami HO (1990). Exposure to dioxins as a risk factor for soft tissue sarcoma: a population-based case-control study. J Natl Cancer Inst 82: 486–490.
767. Erlandson RA (1985). Melanotic schwannoma of spinal nerve origin. Ultrastruct Pathol 9: 123–129.
768. Erlandson RA (1987). The ultrastructural distinction between rhabdomyosarcoma and other undifferentiated "sarcomas". Ultrastruct Pathol 11: 83–101.
769. Erlandson RA, Woodruff JM (1982). Peripheral nerve sheath tumors: an electron microscopic study of 43 cases. Cancer 49: 273–287.
770. Errani C, Kreshak J, Ruggieri P et al. (2011). Imaging of bone tumors for the musculoskeletal oncologic surgeon. Eur J Radiol

771. Errani C, Sung YS, Zhang L et al. (2012). Monoclonality of multifocal epithelioid hemangioendothelioma of the liver by analysis of WWTR1-CAMTA1 Breakpoints. Cancer Genetics 205: 12–17.
772. Errani C, Zhang L, Panicek DM et al. (2011). Epithelioid hemangioma of bone and soft tissue: A reappraisal of a controversial entity. Clin Orthop Relat Res 470:1498-1506.
773. Errani C, Zhang L, Sung YS et al. (2011). A novel WWTR1-CAMTA1 gene fusion is a consistent abnormality in epithelioid hemangioendothelioma of different anatomic sites. Genes Chromosomes Cancer 50: 644–653.
774. Escobar C, Munker R, Thomas JO et al. (2011). Update on desmoid tumors. Ann Onco 23:562-569.l
775. Espinosa I, Lee CH, Kim MK et al. (2008). A novel monoclonal antibody against DOG1 is a sensitive and specific marker for gastrointestinal stromal tumors. Am J Surg Pathol 32: 210–218.
776. Eulderink F, de Graaf PW (1998). Ectopic hamartomatous thymoma located presternally. Eur J Surg 164: 629–630.
777. Evans DG, Baser ME, McGaughran J et al. (2002). Malignant peripheral nerve sheath tumours in neurofibromatosis 1. J Med Genet 39: 311–314.
778. Evans HL (1979). Liposarcoma: a study of 55 cases with a reassessment of its classification. Am J Surg Pathol 3: 507–523.
779. Evans HL (1980). Synovial sarcoma. A study of 23 biphasic and 17 probable monophasic examples. Pathol Annu 15: 309–331.
780. Evans HL (1985). Alveolar soft-part sarcoma. A study of 13 typical examples and one with a histologically atypical component. Cancer 55: 912–917.
781. Evans HL (1987). Low-grade fibromyxoid sarcoma. A report of two metastasizing neoplasms having a deceptively benign appearance. Am J Clin Pathol 88: 615–619.
782. Evans HL (1988). Liposarcoma and atypical lipomatous tumors: a study of 66 cases followed for a minimum of 10 years. Surg Pathol 1: 41–54.
783. Evans HL (1993). Low-grade fibromyxoid sarcoma. A report of 12 cases. Am J Surg Pathol 17: 595–600.
784. Evans HL (1995). Desmoplastic fibroblastoma. A report of seven cases. Am J Surg Pathol 19: 1077–1081.
785. Evans HL (2006). Expert commentary 1. Int J Surg Pathol 14: 16
786. Evans HL (2007). Atypical lipomatous tumor, its variants, and its combined forms: a study of 61 cases, with a minimum follow-up of 10 years. Am J Surg Pathol 31: 1–14.
787. Evans HL (2011). Low-grade fibromyxoid sarcoma: a clinicopathologic study of 33 cases with long-term follow-up. Am J Surg Pathol 35: 1450–1462.
788. Evans HL, Ayala AG, Romsdahl MM (1977). Prognostic factors in chondrosarcoma of bone: a clinicopathologic analysis with emphasis on histologic grading. Cancer 40: 818–831.
789. Evans HL, Baer SC (1993). Epithelioid sarcoma: a clinicopathologic and prognostic study of 26 cases. Semin Diagn Pathol 10: 286–291.
790. Evans HL, Raymond AK, Ayala AG (2003). Vascular tumors of bone: A study of 17 cases other than ordinary hemangioma, with an evaluation of the relationship of hemangioendothelioma of bone to epithelioid hemangioma, epithelioid hemangioendothelioma, and high-grade angiosarcoma. Hum Pathol 34: 680–689.
791. Evans HL, Soule EH, Winkelmann RK (1979). Atypical lipoma, atypical intramuscular lipoma, and well differentiated retroperitoneal liposarcoma: a reappraisal of 30 cases formerly classified as well differentiated liposarcoma. Cancer 43: 574–584.
792. Eversole LR (2009). Cellular angiofibroma of oral mucosa: report of two cases. Head Neck Pathol 3: 136–139.
793. Eyden BP, Banerjee SS (1990). Multiple myeloma showing signet-ring cell change. Histopathology 17: 170–172.
794. Eyden BP, Manson C, Banerjee SS et al. (1998). Sclerosing epithelioid fibrosarcoma: a study of five cases emphasizing diagnostic criteria. Histopathology 33: 354–360.
795. Eyzaguirre E, Liqiang W, Karla GM et al. (2007). Intraosseous lipoma. A clinical, radiologic, and pathologic study of 5 cases. Ann Diagn Pathol 11: 320–325.
796. Fadare O, Bonvicino A, Martel M et al. (2010). Pleomorphic rhabdomyosarcoma of the uterine corpus: a clinicopathologic study of 4 cases and a review of the literature. Int J Gynecol Pathol 29: 122–134.
797. Faircloth WJ, Jr., Edwards RC, Farhood VW (1991). Cherubism involving a mother and daughter: case reports and review of the literature. J Oral Maxillofac Surg 49: 535–542.
798. Faivre L, Nivelon-Chevallier A, Kottler ML et al. (2001). Mazabraud syndrome in two patients: clinical overlap with McCune-Albright syndrome. Am J Med Genet 99: 132–136.
799. Falco NA, Upton J (1995). Infantile digital fibromas. J Hand Surg Am 20: 1014–1020.
800. Falini B, Fizzotti M, Pucciarini A et al. (2000). A monoclonal antibody (MUM1p) detects expression of the MUM1/IRF4 protein in a subset of germinal center B cells, plasma cells, and activated T cells. Blood 95: 2084–2092.
801. Falk S, Schmidts HL, Muller H et al. (1987). Autopsy findings in AIDS—a histopathological analysis of fifty cases. Klin Wochenschr 65: 654–663.
802. Falleti J, De Cecio R, Mentone A et al. (2009). Extraskeletal chondroma of the masseter muscle: a case report with review of the literature. Int J Oral Maxillofac Surg 38: 895–899.
803. Fanburg JC, Meis-Kindblom JM, Rosenberg AE (1995). Multiple enchondromas associated with spindle-cell hemangioendotheliomas. An overlooked variant of Maffucci's syndrome. Am J Surg Pathol 19: 1029–1038.
804. Fanburg JC, Rosenberg AE, Weaver DL et al. (1997). Osteocalcin and osteonectin immunoreactivity in the diagnosis of osteosarcoma. Am J Clin Pathol 108: 464–473.
805. Fanburg-Smith JC, Auerbach A, Marwaha JS et al. (2010). Reappraisal of mesenchymal chondrosarcoma: novel morphologic observations of the hyaline cartilage and endochondral ossification and beta-catenin, Sox9, and osteocalcin immunostaining of 22 cases. Hum Pathol 41: 653–662.
806. Fanburg-Smith JC, Auerbach A, Marwaha JS et al. (2010). Immunoprofile of mesenchymal chondrosarcoma: aberrant desmin and EMA expression, retention of INI1, and negative estrogen receptor in 22 female-predominant central nervous system and musculoskeletal cases. Ann Diagn Pathol 14: 8–14.
807. Fanburg-Smith JC, Bratthauer GL, Miettinen M (1999). Osteocalcin and osteonectin immunoreactivity in extraskeletal osteosarcoma: a study of 28 cases. Hum Pathol 30: 32–38.
808. Fanburg-Smith JC, Devaney KO, Miettinen M et al. (1998). Multiple spindle cell lipomas: a report of 7 familial and 11 nonfamilial cases. Am J Surg Pathol 22: 40–48.
809. Fanburg-Smith JC, Hengge M, Hengge UR et al. (1998). Extrarenal rhabdoid tumors of soft tissue: a clinicopathologic and immunohistochemical study of 18 cases. Ann Diagn Pathol 2: 351–362.
810. Fanburg-Smith JC, Meis-Kindblom JM, Fante R et al. (1998). Malignant granular cell tumor of soft tissue: diagnostic criteria and clinicopathologic correlation. Am J Surg Pathol 22: 779–794.
811. Fanburg-Smith JC, Michal M, Partanen TA et al. (1999). Papillary intralymphatic angioendothelioma (PILA): a report of twelve cases of a distinctive vascular tumor with phenotypic features of lymphatic vessels. Am J Surg Pathol 23: 1004–1010.
812. Fanburg-Smith JC, Miettinen M (1998). Liposarcoma with meningothelial-like whorls: a study of 17 cases of a distinctive histological pattern associated with dedifferentiated liposarcoma. Histopathology 33: 414–424.
813. Fanburg-Smith JC, Miettinen M (1999). Angiomatoid "malignant" fibrous histiocytoma: a clinicopathologic study of 158 cases and further exploration of the myoid phenotype. Hum Pathol 30: 1336–1343.
814. Fanburg-Smith JC, Miettinen M, Folpe AL et al. (2004). Lingual alveolar soft part sarcoma; 14 cases: novel clinical and morphological observations. Histopathology 45: 526–537.
815. Fandridis EM, Kiriako AS, Spyridonos SG et al. (2009). Lipomatosis of the sciatic nerve: report of a case and review of the literature. Microsurgery 29: 66–71.
816. Farnebo M, Bykov VJ, Wiman KG (2010). The p53 tumor suppressor: a master regulator of diverse cellular processes and therapeutic target in cancer. Biochem Biophys Res Commun 396: 85–89.
817. Farshid G, Pradhan M, Goldblum J et al. (2002). Leiomyosarcoma of somatic soft tissues: a tumor of vascular origin with multivariate analysis of outcome in 42 cases. Am J Surg Pathol 26: 14–24.
818. Fayette J, Martin E, Piperno-Neumann S et al. (2007). Angiosarcomas, a heterogeneous group of sarcomas with specific behavior depending on primary site: a retrospective study of 161 cases. Ann Oncol 18: 2030–2036.
819. Feany MB, Anthony DC, Fletcher CD (1998). Nerve sheath tumours with hybrid features of neurofibroma and schwannoma: a conceptual challenge. Histopathology 32: 405–410.
820. Fechner RE and Mills SE. (1993). Tumors of the bones and joint. Atlas of Tumor Pathology. AFIP
821. Feely MG, Boehm AK, Bridge RS et al. (2002). Cytogenetic and molecular cytogenetic evidence of recurrent 8q24.1 loss in osteochondroma. Cancer Genet Cytogenet 137: 102–107.
822. Fehr A, Loning T, Stenman G (2011). Mammary analogue secretory carcinoma of the salivary glands with ETV6-NTRK3 gene fusion. Am J Surg Pathol 35: 1600–1602.
823. Feldman F, Vanheertum R, Saxena C (2006). 18Fluoro-deoxyglucose positron emission tomography evaluation of benign versus malignant osteochondromas: preliminary observations. J Comput Assist Tomogr 30: 858–864.
824. Feldmann R, Denecke J, Grenzebach M et al. (2003). Neurofibromatosis type 1: motor and cognitive function and T2-weighted MRI hyperintensities. Neurology 61: 1725–1728.
825. Fergusson IL (1972). Haemangiomata of skeletal muscle. Br J Surg 59: 634–637.
826. Ferner RE, Golding JF, Smith M et al. (2008). [18F]2-fluoro-2-deoxy-D-glucose positron emission tomography (FDG PET) as a diagnostic tool for neurofibromatosis 1 (NF1) associated malignant peripheral nerve sheath tumours (MPNSTs): a long-term clinical study. Ann Oncol 19: 390–394.
827. Ferner RE, Huson SM, Thomas N et al. (2007). Guidelines for the diagnosis and management of individuals with neurofibromatosis 1. J Med Genet 44: 81–88.
828. Ferrari A, Sultan I, Huang TT et al. (2011). Soft tissue sarcoma across the age spectrum: a population-based study from the Surveillance Epidemiology and End Results database. Pediatr Blood Cancer 57: 943–949.
829. Ferrari S, Smeland S, Mercuri M et al. (2005). Neoadjuvant chemotherapy with high-dose Ifosfamide, high-dose methotrexate, cisplatin, and doxorubicin for patients with localized osteosarcoma of the extremity: a joint study by the Italian and Scandinavian Sarcoma Groups. J Clin Oncol 23: 8845–8852.
830. Ferreiro JA, Nascimento AG (1995). Hyaline-cell rich chondroid syringoma. A tumor mimicking malignancy. Am J Surg Pathol 19: 912–917.
831. Fetsch JF, Laskin WB, Hallman JR et al. (2007). Neurothekeoma: an analysis of 178 tumors with detailed immunohistochemical data and long-term patient follow-up information. Am J Surg Pathol 31: 1103–1114.
832. Fetsch JF, Laskin WB, Lefkowitz M et al. (1996). Aggressive angiomyxoma: a clinicopathologic study of 29 female patients. Cancer 78: 79–90.
833. Fetsch JF, Laskin WB, Michal M et al. (2004). Ectopic hamartomatous thymoma: a clinicopathologic and immunohistochemical analysis of 21 cases with data supporting reclassification as a branchial anlage mixed tumor. Am J Surg Pathol 28: 1360–1370.
834. Fetsch JF, Laskin WB, Miettinen M (2001). Superficial acral fibromyxoma: a clinicopathologic and immunohistochemical analysis of 37 cases of a distinctive soft tissue tumor with a predilection for the fingers and toes. Hum Pathol 32: 704–714.
835. Fetsch JF, Laskin WB, Miettinen M (2005). Nerve sheath myxoma: a clinicopathologic and immunohistochemical analysis of 57 morphologically distinctive, S-100 protein- and GFAP-positive, myxoid peripheral nerve sheath tumors with a predilection for the extremities and a high local recurrence rate. Am J Surg Pathol 29: 1615–1624.
836. Fetsch JF, Laskin WB, Miettinen M (2005). Palmar-plantar fibromatosis in children and preadolescents: a clinicopathologic study of 56 cases with newly recognized demographics and extended follow-up information. Am J Surg Pathol 29: 1095–1105.
837. Fetsch JF, Michal M, Miettinen M (2000). Pigmented (melanotic) neurofibroma: a clinicopathologic and immunohistochemical analysis of 19 lesions from 17 patients. Am J Surg Pathol 24: 331–343.
838. Fetsch JF, Miettinen M (1997). Sclerosing perineurioma: a clinicopathologic study of 19 cases of a distinctive soft tissue lesion with a predilection for the fingers and palms of young adults. Am J Surg Pathol 21: 1433–1442.
839. Fetsch JF, Miettinen M (1998). Calcifying aponeurotic fibroma: a clinicopatho-

logic study of 22 cases arising in uncommon sites. Hum Pathol 29: 1504–1510.

840. Fetsch JF, Miettinen M, Laskin WB et al. (2000). A clinicopathologic study of 45 pediatric soft tissue tumors with an admixture of adipose tissue and fibroblastic elements, and a proposal for classification as lipofibromatosis. Am J Surg Pathol 24: 1491–1500.

841. Fetsch JF, Montgomery EA, Meis JM (1993). Calcifying fibrous pseudotumor. Am J Surg Pathol 17: 502–508.

842. Fetsch JF, Sesterhenn IA, Miettinen M et al. (2004). Epithelioid hemangioma of the penis: a clinicopathologic and immunohistochemical analysis of 19 cases, with special reference to exuberant examples often confused with epithelioid hemangioendothelioma and epithelioid angiosarcoma. Am J Surg Pathol 28: 523–533.

843. Fetsch JF, Vinh TN, Remotti F et al. (2003). Tenosynovial (extraarticular) chondromatosis: an analysis of 37 cases of an underrecognized clinicopathologic entity with a strong predilection for the hands and feet and a high local recurrence rate. Am J Surg Pathol 27: 1260–1268.

844. Fetsch JF, Weiss SW (1990). Ectopic hamartomatous thymoma: clinicopathologic, immunohistochemical, and histogenetic considerations in four new cases. Hum Pathol 21: 662–668.

845. Fetsch JF, Weiss SW (1991). Observations concerning the pathogenesis of epithelioid hemangioma (angiolymphoid hyperplasia). Mod Pathol 4: 449–455.

846. Feugeas O, Guriec N, Babin-Boilletot A et al. (1996). Loss of heterozygosity of the RB gene is a poor prognostic factor in patients with osteosarcoma. J Clin Oncol 14: 467–472.

847. Filie AC, Lage JM, Azumi N (1996). Immunoreactivity of S100 protein, alpha-1-antitrypsin, and CD68 in adult and congenital granular cell tumors. Mod Pathol 9: 888–892.

848. Fine BA, Munoz AK, Litz CE et al. (2001). Primary medical management of recurrent aggressive angiomyxoma of the vulva with a gonadotropin-releasing hormone agonist. Gynecol Oncol 81: 120–122.

849. Fiore M, Rimareix F, Mariani L et al. (2009). Desmoid-type fibromatosis: a front-line conservative approach to select patients for surgical treatment. Ann Surg Oncol 16: 2587–2593.

850. Fisher C (1986). Synovial sarcoma: ultrastructural and immunohistochemical features of epithelial differentiation in monophasic and biphasic tumors. Hum Pathol 17: 996–1008.

851. Fisher C (1988). Epithelioid sarcoma: the spectrum of ultrastructural differentiation in seven immunohistochemically defined cases. Hum Pathol 19: 265–275.

852. Fisher C, Folpe AL, Hashimoto H et al. (2004). Intra-abdominal synovial sarcoma: a clinicopathological study. Histopathology 45: 245–253.

853. Fisher C, Hedges M, Weiss SW (1994). Ossifying fibromyxoid tumor of soft parts with stromal cyst formation and ribosome-lamella complexes. Ultrastruct Pathol 18: 593–600.

854. Flanagan AM, Delaney D, O'Donnell P (2010). Benefits of molecular pathology in the diagnosis of musculoskeletal disease : Part II of a two-part review: bone tumors and metabolic disorders. Skeletal Radiol 39: 213–224.

855. Fleischmajer R, Faludi G, Krol S (1970). Scleredema and diabetes mellitus. Arch Dermatol 101: 21–26.

856. Fletcher CD (1989). Solitary circumscribed neuroma of the skin (so-called palisaded, encapsulated neuroma). A clinicopathologic and immunohistochemical study. Am J Surg Pathol 13: 574–580.

857. Fletcher CD (1990). Benign fibrous histiocytoma of subcutaneous and deep soft tissue: a clinicopathologic analysis of 21 cases. Am J Surg Pathol 14: 801–809.

858. Fletcher CD (1992). Pleomorphic malignant fibrous histiocytoma: fact or fiction? A critical reappraisal based on 159 tumors diagnosed as pleomorphic sarcoma. Am J Surg Pathol 16: 213–228.

859. Fletcher CD (2000). Soft tissue tumors. In: Diagnostic histopathology of tumors, 2nd edition. Fletcher CD Churchill Livingstone: London: pp

860. Fletcher CD (2007). Soft tissue tumors. In: Diagnostic histopathology of tumors, third editionChurchill Livingstone Elsevier: Edinburgh: pp 1527–1592.

861. Fletcher CD (2008). Undifferentiated sarcomas: what to do? And does it matter? A surgical pathology perspective. Ultrastruct Pathol 32: 31–36.

862. Fletcher CD, Akerman M, Dal Cin P et al. (1996). Correlation between clinicopathological features and karyotype in lipomatous tumors. A report of 178 cases from the Chromosomes and Morphology (CHAMP) Collaborative Study Group. Am J Pathol 148: 623–630.

863. Fletcher CD, Beham A, Bekir S et al. (1991). Epithelioid angiosarcoma of deep soft tissue: a distinctive tumor readily mistaken for an epithelial neoplasm. Am J Surg Pathol 15: 915–924.

864. Fletcher CD, Dal Cin P, De Wever I et al. (1999). Correlation between clinicopathological features and karyotype in spindle cell sarcomas. A report of 130 cases from the CHAMP study group. Am J Pathol 154: 1841–1847.

865. Fletcher CD, Davies SE, McKee PH (1987). Cellular schwannoma: a distinct pseudosarcomatous entity. Histopathology 11: 21–35.

866. Fletcher CD, Gustafson P, Rydholm A et al. (2001). Clinicopathologic re-evaluation of 100 malignant fibrous histiocytomas: prognostic relevance of subclassification. J Clin Oncol 19: 3045–3050.

867. Fletcher CD, Martin-Bates E (1987). Spindle cell lipoma: a clinicopathological study with some original observations. Histopathology 11: 803–817.

868. Fletcher CD, Martin-Bates E (1988). Intramuscular and intermuscular lipoma: neglected diagnoses. Histopathology 12: 275–287.

869. Fletcher CD, Powell G, van Noorden S et al. (1988). Fibrous hamartoma of infancy: a histochemical and immunohistochemical study. Histopathology 12: 65–74.

870. Fletcher CD, Tsang WY, Fisher C et al. (1992). Angiomyofibroblastoma of the vulva. A benign neoplasm distinct from aggressive angiomyxoma. Am J Surg Pathol 16: 373–382.

870A. Fletcher CD, Unni KK, Mertens F (eds) (2002) Tumours of soft tissue and bone. Third edition. World Health Organization: Geneva.

871. Fletcher JA, Gebhardt MC, Kozakewich HP (1994). Cytogenetic aberrations in osteosarcomas. Nonrandom deletions, rings, and double-minute chromosomes. Cancer Genet Cytogenet 77: 81–88.

872. Fletcher JA, Naeem R, Xiao S et al. (1995). Chromosome aberrations in desmoid tumors. Trisomy 8 may be a predictor of recurrence. Cancer Genet Cytogenet 79: 139–143.

873. Fletcher JA, Rubin BP (2007). KIT mutations in GIST. Curr Opin Genet Dev 17: 3–7.

874. Floris G, Debiec-Rychter M, Wozniak A et al. (2007). Malignant ectomesenchymoma: genetic profile reflects rhabdomyosarcomatous differentiation. Diagn Mol Pathol 16: 243–248.

875. Floris G, Deraedt K, Samson I et al. (2006). Epithelioid hemangioma of bone: a potentially metastasizing tumor? Int J Surg Pathol 14: 9–15.

876. Flucke U, Hulsebos TJ, van Krieken JH et al. (2010). Myxoid epithelioid sarcoma: a diagnostic challenge. A report on six cases. Histopathology 57: 753–759.

877. Flucke U, van Krieken JH, Mentzel T (2011). Cellular angiofibroma: analysis of 25 cases emphasizing its relationship to spindle cell lipoma and mammary-type myofibroblastoma. Mod Pathol 24: 82–89.

878. Folk GS, Williams SB, Foss RB et al. (2007). Oral and maxillofacial sclerosing epithelioid fibrosarcoma: report of five cases. Head Neck Pathol 1: 13–20.

879. Folpe AL (2002). MyoD1 and myogenin expression in human neoplasia: a review and update. Adv Anat Pathol 9: 198–203.

880. Folpe AL, Agoff SN, Willis J et al. (1999). Parachordoma is immunohistochemically and cytogenetically distinct from axial chordoma and extraskeletal myxoid chondrosarcoma. Am J Surg Pathol 23: 1059–1067.

881. Folpe AL, Billings SD, McKenney JK et al. (2002). Expression of claudin-1, a recently described tight junction-associated protein, distinguishes soft tissue perineurioma from potential mimics. Am J Surg Pathol 26: 1620–1626.

882. Folpe AL, Chand EM, Goldblum JR et al. (2001). Expression of Fli-1, a nuclear transcription factor, distinguishes vascular neoplasms from potential mimics. Am J Surg Pathol 25: 1061–1066.

883. Folpe AL, Devaney K, Weiss SW (1999). Lipomatous hemangiopericytoma: a rare variant of hemangiopericytoma that may be confused with liposarcoma. Am J Surg Pathol 23: 1201–1207.

884. Folpe AL, Fanburg-Smith JC, Billings SD et al. (2004). Most osteomalacia-associated mesenchymal tumors are a single histopathologic entity: an analysis of 32 cases and a comprehensive review of the literature. Am J Surg Pathol 28: 1–30.

885. Folpe AL, Fanburg-Smith JC, Miettinen M et al. (2001). Atypical and malignant glomus tumors: analysis of 52 cases, with a proposal for the reclassification of glomus tumors. Am J Surg Pathol 25: 1–12.

886. Folpe AL, Goodman ZD, Ishak KG et al. (2000). Clear cell myomelanocytic tumor of the falciform ligament/ligamentum teres: a novel member of the perivascular epithelioid clear cell family of tumors with a predilection for children and young adults. Am J Surg Pathol 24: 1239–1246.

887. Folpe AL, Kwiatkowski DJ (2010). Perivascular epithelioid cell neoplasms: pathology and pathogenesis. Hum Pathol 41: 1–15.

888. Folpe AL, Lane KL, Paull G et al. (2000). Low-grade fibromyxoid sarcoma and hyalinizing spindle cell tumor with giant rosettes: a clinicopathologic study of 73 cases supporting their identity and assessing the impact of high-grade areas. Am J Surg Pathol 24: 1353–1360.

889. Folpe AL, McKenney JK, Bridge JA et al. (2002). Sclerosing rhabdomyosarcoma in adults: report of four cases of a hyalinizing, matrix-rich variant of rhabdomyosarcoma that may be confused with osteosarcoma, chon-

drosarcoma, or angiosarcoma. Am J Surg Pathol 26: 1175–1183.

890. Folpe AL, Mentzel T, Lehr HA et al. (2005). Perivascular epithelioid cell neoplasms of soft tissue and gynecologic origin: a clinicopathologic study of 26 cases and review of the literature. Am J Surg Pathol 29: 1558–1575.

891. Folpe AL, Morris RJ, Weiss SW (1999). Soft tissue giant cell tumor of low malignant potential: a proposal for the reclassification of malignant giant cell tumor of soft parts. Mod Pathol 12: 894–902.

892. Folpe AL, Weiss SW (2003). Ossifying fibromyxoid tumor of soft parts: a clinicopathologic study of 70 cases with emphasis on atypical and malignant variants. Am J Surg Pathol 27: 421–431.

893. Folpe AL, Weiss SW (2004). Pleomorphic hyalinizing angiectatic tumor: analysis of 41 cases supporting evolution from a distinctive precursor lesion. Am J Surg Pathol 28: 1417–1425.

894. Folpe AL, Weiss SW, Fletcher CD et al. (1998). Tenosynovial giant cell tumors: evidence for a desmin-positive dendritic cell subpopulation. Mod Pathol 11: 939–944.

895. Fonseca R, Blood E, Rue M et al. (2003). Clinical and biologic implications of recurrent genomic aberrations in myeloma. Blood 101: 4569–4575.

896. Fonseca R, Blood EA, Oken MM et al. (2002). Myeloma and the t(11;14)(q13;q32); evidence for a biologically defined unique subset of patients. Blood 99: 3735–3741.

897. Fonseca R, Oken MM, Greipp PR (2001). The t(4;14)(p16.3;q32) is strongly associated with chromosome 13 abnormalities in both multiple myeloma and monoclonal gammopathy of undetermined significance. Blood 98: 1271–1272.

898. Font RL, Blanco G, Soparkar CN et al. (2003). Giant cell reparative granuloma of the orbit associated with cherubism. Ophthalmology 110: 1846–1849.

899. Font RL, Truong LD (1984). Melanotic schwannoma of soft tissues. Electron-microscopic observations and review of literature. Am J Surg Pathol 8: 129–138.

900. Foo WC, Cruise MW, Wick MR et al. (2011). Immunohistochemical staining for TLE1 distinguishes synovial sarcoma from histologic mimics. Am J Clin Pathol 135: 839–844.

901. Forghieri F, Morselli M, Potenza L et al. (2011). Chronic eosinophilic leukaemia with ETV6-NTRK3 fusion transcript in an elderly patient affected with pancreatic carcinoma. Eur J Haematol 86: 352–355.

902. Forsyth RG, De Boeck G, Bekaert S et al. (2008). Telomere biology in giant cell tumour of bone. J Pathol 214: 555–563.

903. Foucar E, Rosai J, Dorfman R (1990). Sinus histiocytosis with massive lymphadenopathy (Rosai-Dorfman disease): review of the entity. Semin Diagn Pathol 7: 19–73.

904. Foulkes WD, Bahubeshi A, Hamel N et al. (2011). Extending the phenotypes associated with DICER1 mutations. Hum Mutat 32: 1381–1384.

905. Francke U (1976). Retinoblastoma and chromosome 13. Birth Defects Orig Artic Ser 12: 131–134.

906. Francke U, Kung F (1976). Sporadic bilateral retinoblastoma and 13q- chromosomal deletion. Med Pediatr Oncol 2: 379–385.

907. Francois J (1978). Differential diagnosis of leukokoria in children. Ann Ophthalmol 10: 1375–2.

908. Frassica FJ, Unni KK, Beabout JW et al. (1986). Dedifferentiated chondrosarcoma. A report of the clinicopathological features and treatment of seventy-eight cases. J Bone Joint Surg Am 68: 1197–1205.
909. Frassica FJ, Waltrip RL, Sponseller PD et al. (1996). Clinicopathologic features and treatment of osteoid osteoma and osteoblastoma in children and adolescents. Orthop Clin North Am 27: 559–574.
910. Frau DV, Erdas E, Caria P et al. (2010). Deep fibrous histiocytoma with a clonal karyotypic alteration: molecular cytogenetic characterization of a t(16;17)(p13.3;q21.3). Cancer Genet Cytogenet 202: 17–21.
911. Freeburn AM, McAloon J (2001). Infantile chest hamartoma—case outcome aged 11. Arch Dis Child 85: 244–245.
912. French CA, Mentzel T, Kutzner H et al. (2000). Intradermal spindle cell/pleomorphic lipoma: a distinct subset. Am J Dermatopathol 22: 496–502.
913. Friedman L, Patel M, Lew E et al. (1989). Benign histiocytic fibroma of rib with CT correlation. Can Assoc Radiol J 40: 114–116.
914. Friedrich K, Lee L, Leistritz DF et al. (2010). WRN mutations in Werner syndrome patients: genomic rearrangements, unusual intronic mutations and ethnic-specific alterations. Hum Genet 128: 103–111.
915. Friend SH, Bernards R, Rogelj S et al. (1986). A human DNA segment with properties of the gene that predisposes to retinoblastoma and osteosarcoma. Nature 323: 643–646.
916. Frierson HF, Jr., Fechner RE, Stallings RG et al. (1987). Malignant fibrous histiocytoma in bone infarct. Association with sickle cell trait and alcohol abuse. Cancer 59: 496–500.
916A. Fritz A, Percy C, Jack A et al. (eds) (2000). International classification of diseases for oncology (ICD-O). Third edition. World Health Organization: Geneva.
917. Fritz B, Schubert F, Wrobel G et al. (2002). Microarray-based copy number and expression profiling in dedifferentiated and pleomorphic liposarcoma. Cancer Res 62: 2993–2998.
918. Frustaci S, Gherlinzoni F, De Paoli A et al. (2001). Adjuvant chemotherapy for adult soft tissue sarcomas of the extremities and girdles: results of the Italian randomized cooperative trial. J Clin Oncol 19: 1238–1247.
919. Fukuda T, Ishikawa H, Ohnishi Y et al. (1986). Extraskeletal myxoid chondrosarcoma arising from the retroperitoneum. Am J Clin Pathol 85: 514–519.
920. Fukuda W, Morohashi S, Fukuda I (2011). Intimal sarcoma of the pulmonary artery—diagnostic challenge. Acta Cardiol 66: 539–541.
921. Fukuda Y, Miyake H, Masuda Y et al. (1987). Histogenesis of unique elastinophilic fibers of elastofibroma: ultrastructural and immunohistochemical studies. Hum Pathol 18: 424–429.
922. Fukunaga M (2005). Expression of D2-40 in lymphatic endothelium of normal tissues and in vascular tumours. Histopathology 46: 396–402.
923. Fukunaga M, Endo Y, Masui F et al. (1996). Retiform haemangioendothelioma. Virchows Arch 428: 301–304.
924. Fukunaga M, Naganuma H, Nikaido T et al. (1997). Extrapleural solitary fibrous tumor: a report of seven cases. Mod Pathol 10: 443–450.
925. Fukunaga M, Naganuma H, Ushigome S et al. (1996). Malignant solitary fibrous tumour of the peritoneum. Histopathology 28: 463–466.
926. Fukunaga M, Suzuki K, Saegusa N et al. (2007). Composite hemangioendothelioma: report of 5 cases including one with associated Maffucci syndrome. Am J Surg Pathol 31: 1567–1572.
927. Fukunaga M, Ushigome S (1998). Periosteal Ewing-like adamantinoma. Virchows Arch 433: 385–389.
928. Fung YK, Murphree AL, T'Ang A et al. (1987). Structural evidence for the authenticity of the human retinoblastoma gene. Science 236: 1657–1661.
929. Furlong MA, Fanburg-Smith JC (2001). Pleomorphic rhabdomyosarcoma in children: four cases in the pediatric age group. Ann Diagn Pathol 5: 199–206.
930. Furlong MA, Fanburg-Smith JC, Childers EL (2004). Lipoma of the oral and maxillofacial region: Site and subclassification of 125 cases. Oral Surg Oral Med Oral Pathol Oral Radiol Endod 98: 441–450.
931. Furlong MA, Fanburg-Smith JC, Miettinen M (2001). The morphologic spectrum of hibernoma: a clinicopathologic study of 170 cases. Am J Surg Pathol 25: 809–814.
932. Furlong MA, Mentzel T, Fanburg-Smith JC (2001). Pleomorphic rhabdomyosarcoma in adults: a clinicopathologic study of 38 cases with emphasis on morphologic variants and recent skeletal muscle-specific markers. Mod Pathol 14: 595–603.
933. Furusato E, Valenzuela IA, Fanburg-Smith JC et al. (2011). Orbital solitary fibrous tumor: encompassing terminology for hemangiopericytoma, giant cell angiofibroma, and fibrous histiocytoma of the orbit: reappraisal of 41 cases. Hum Pathol 42: 120–128.
934. Gaal J, Stratakis CA, Carney JA et al. (2011). SDHB immunohistochemistry: a useful tool in the diagnosis of Carney-Stratakis and Carney triad gastrointestinal stromal tumors. Mod Pathol 24: 147–151.
935. Gad A, Eusebi V (1975). Rhabdomyoma of the vagina. J Pathol 115: 179–181.
936. Gaertner EM, Steinberg DM, Huber M et al. (2000). Pulmonary and mediastinal glomus tumors—report of five cases including a pulmonary glomangiosarcoma: a clinicopathologic study with literature review. Am J Surg Pathol 24: 1105–1114.
937. Gailani MR, Bale SJ, Leffell DJ et al. (1992). Developmental defects in Gorlin syndrome related to a putative tumor suppressor gene on chromosome 9. Cell 69: 111–117.
938. Gaitonde S (2007). Multifocal, extranodal sinus histiocytosis with massive lymphadenopathy: an overview. Arch Pathol Lab Med 131: 1117–1121.
939. Galili N, Davis RJ, Fredericks WJ et al. (1993). Fusion of a fork head domain gene to PAX3 in the solid tumour alveolar rhabdomyosarcoma. Nat Genet 5: 230–235.
940. Gallager RL, Helwig EB (1980). Neurothekeoma—a benign cutaneous tumor of neural origin. Am J Clin Pathol 74: 759–764.
941. Galli SJ, Weintraub HP, Proppe KH (1978). Malignant fibrous histiocytoma and pleomorphic sarcoma in association with medullary bone infarcts. Cancer 41: 607–619.
942. Ganem D, Ziegelbauer J (2008). MicroRNAs of Kaposi's sarcoma-associated herpes virus. Semin Cancer Biol 18: 437–440.
943. Gao SJ, Kingsley L, Hoover DR et al. (1996). Seroconversion to antibodies against Kaposi's sarcoma-associated herpesvirus-related latent nuclear antigens before the development of Kaposi's sarcoma. N Engl J Med 335: 233–241.
944. Garand R, Avet-Loiseau H, Accard F et al. (2003). t(11;14) and t(4;14) translocations correlated with mature lymphoplasmacytoid and immature morphology, respectively, in multiple myeloma. Leukemia 17: 2032–2035.
945. Garber JE, Offit K (2005). Hereditary cancer predisposition syndromes. J Clin Oncol 23: 276–292.
946. Garcia CA, Spencer RP (2002). Bone and In-111 octreotide imaging in oncogenic osteomalacia: a case report. Clin Nucl Med 27: 582–583.
947. Garcia RA, Inwards CY, Unni KK (2011). Benign bone tumors—recent developments. Semin Diagn Pathol 28: 73–85.
948. Gardiner GA, Linda L (1974). Clavicular nonosteogenic fibroma. An old tumor in a new location. Am J Dis Child 127: 734–735.
949. Garraway LA, Sellers WR (2006). Lineage dependency and lineage-survival oncogenes in human cancer. Nat Rev Cancer 6: 593–602.
950. Garritano S, Gemignani F, Palmero EI et al. (2010). Detailed haplotype analysis at the TP53 locus in p.R337H mutation carriers in the population of Southern Brazil: evidence for a founder effect. Hum Mutat 31: 143–150.
951. Gascoyne RD, Lamant L, Martin-Subero JI et al. (2003). ALK-positive diffuse large B-cell lymphoma is associated with Clathrin-ALK rearrangements: report of 6 cases. Blood 102: 2568–2573.
952. Gasparini P, Facchinetti F, Boeri M et al. (2011). Prognostic determinants in epithelioid sarcoma. Eur J Cancer 47: 287–295.
953. Gatta G, van der Zwan JM, Casali PG et al. (2011). Rare cancers are not so rare: the rare cancer burden in Europe. Eur J Cancer 47: 2493–2511.
954. Gatter KM, Olson S, Lawce H et al. (2005). Trisomy 8 as the sole cytogenetic abnormality in a case of extraskeletal mesenchymal chondrosarcoma. Cancer Genet Cytogenet 159: 151–154.
955. Gebhard S, Coindre JM, Michels JJ et al. (2002). Pleomorphic liposarcoma: clinicopathologic, immunohistochemical, and follow-up analysis of 63 cases: a study from the French Federation of Cancer Centers Sarcoma Group. Am J Surg Pathol 26: 601–616.
956. Gebre-Medhin S, Broberg K, Jonson T et al. (2009). Telomeric associations correlate with telomere length reduction and clonal chromosome aberrations in giant cell tumor of bone. Cytogenet Genome Res 124: 121–127.
956A. Gebre-Medhin S, Nord KH, Möller E et al. (2012). Recurrent rearrangement of the PHF1 gene in ossifying fibromyxoid tumors. Am J Pathol. 181:1069-77.
957. Geirnaerdt MJ, Hogendoorn PC, Bloem JL et al. (2000). Cartilaginous tumors: fast contrast-enhanced MR imaging. Radiology 214: 539–546.
958. Geissmann F, Lepelletier Y, Fraitag S et al. (2001). Differentiation of Langerhans cells in Langerhans cell histiocytosis. Blood 97: 1241–1248.
959. Gelderblom H, Hogendoorn PC, Dijkstra SD et al. (2008). The clinical approach towards chondrosarcoma. Oncologist 13: 320–329.
960. Gengler C, Letovanec I, Taminelli L et al. (2006). Desmin and myogenin reactivity in mesenchymal chondrosarcoma: a potential diagnostic pitfall. Histopathology 48: 201–203.
961. Gerald WL, Haber DA (2005). The EWS-WT1 gene fusion in desmoplastic small round cell tumor. Semin Cancer Biol 15: 197–205.
962. Gerald WL, Ladanyi M, de Alava E et al. (1998). Clinical, pathologic, and molecular spectrum of tumors associated with t(11;22)(p13;q12): desmoplastic small round-cell tumor and its variants. J Clin Oncol 16: 3028–3036.
963. Gerald WL, Miller HK, Battifora H et al. (1991). Intra-abdominal desmoplastic small round-cell tumor. Report of 19 cases of a distinctive type of high-grade polyphenotypic malignancy affecting young individuals. Am J Surg Pathol 15: 499–513.
964. Gerald WL, Rosai J, Ladanyi M (1995). Characterization of the genomic breakpoint and chimeric transcripts in the EWS-WT1 gene fusion of desmoplastic small round cell tumor. Proc Natl Acad Sci U S A 92: 1028–1032.
965. Gherlinzoni F, Rock M, Picci P (1983). Chondromyxoid fibroma. The experience at the Istituto Ortopedico Rizzoli. J Bone Joint Surg Am 65: 198–204.
966. Ghosal N, Furtado SV, Saikiran NA et al. (2011). Angiolipoma in sellar, suprasellar and parasellar region: report on two new cases and review of literature. Clin Neuropathol 30: 118–121.
967. Ghosh AK, Rossi ML, Singh DK et al. (2012). RECQL4, the protein mutated in Rothmund-Thomson syndrome, functions in telomere maintenance. J Biol Chem 287: 196–209.
968. Ghosh S, Sinha R, Bandyopadhyay R et al. (2009). Oncogenous osteomalacia. J Cancer Res Ther 5: 210–212.
969. Giacchero D, Maire G, Nuin PA et al. (2010). No correlation between the molecular subtype of COL1A1-PDGFB fusion gene and the clinico-histopathological features of dermatofibrosarcoma protuberans. J Invest Dermatol 130: 904–907.
970. Gianelli U, Patriarca C, Moro A et al. (2002). Lymphomas of the bone: a pathological and clinical study of 54 cases. Int J Surg Pathol 10: 257–266.
971. Giannico G, Holt GE, Homlar KC et al. (2009). Osteoblastoma characterized by a three-way translocation: report of a case and review of the literature. Cancer Genet Cytogenet 195: 168–171.
972. Giannini C, Scheithauer BW, Jenkins RB et al. (1997). Soft-tissue perineurioma. Evidence for an abnormality of chromosome 22, criteria for diagnosis, and review of the literature. Am J Surg Pathol 21: 164–173.
973. Giannini C, Scheithauer BW, Wenger DE et al. (1996). Pigmented villonodular synovitis of the spine: a clinical, radiological, and morphological study of 12 cases. J Neurosurg 84: 592–597.
974. Gibas Z, Miettinen M (1992). Recurrent parapharyngeal rhabdomyoma. Evidence of neoplastic nature of the tumor from cytogenetic study. Am J Surg Pathol 16: 721–728.
975. Gibault L, Perot G, Chibon F et al. (2011). New insights in sarcoma oncogenesis: a comprehensive analysis of a large series of 160 soft tissue sarcomas with complex genomics. J Pathol 223: 64–71.
976. Gill AJ, Chou A, Vilain R et al. (2010). Immunohistochemistry for SDHB divides gastrointestinal stromal tumors (GISTs) into 2 distinct types. Am J Surg Pathol 34: 636–644.
977. Gill R, O'Donnell RJ, Horvai A (2009). Utility of immunohistochemistry for endothelial markers in distinguishing epithelioid hemangioendothelioma from carcinoma metastatic to bone. Arch Pathol Lab Med 133: 967–972.
978. Gillespie WJ, Frampton CM, Henderson

RJ et al. (1988). The incidence of cancer following total hip replacement. J Bone Joint Surg Br 70: 539–542.

979. Giovannini M, Selleri L, Biegel JA et al. (1992). Interphase cytogenetics for the detection of the t(11;22)(q24;q12) in small round cell tumors. J Clin Invest 90: 1911–1918.

980. Gisselsson D, Andreasson P, Meis-Kindblom JM et al. (1998). Amplification of 12q13 and 12q15 sequences in a sclerosing epithelioid fibrosarcoma. Cancer Genet Cytogenet 107: 102–106.

981. Gisselsson D, Hibbard MK, Dal Cin P et al. (2001). PLAG1 alterations in lipoblastoma: involvement in varied mesenchymal cell types and evidence for alternative oncogenic mechanisms. Am J Pathol 159: 955–962.

982. Gisselsson D, Hoglund M, Mertens F et al. (1999). Hibernomas are characterized by homozygous deletions in the multiple endocrine neoplasia type I region. Metaphase fluorescence in situ hybridization reveals complex rearrangements not detected by conventional cytogenetics. Am J Pathol 155: 61–66.

983. Gisselsson D, Hoglund M, Mertens F et al. (1999). The structure and dynamics of ring chromosomes in human neoplastic and non-neoplastic cells. Hum Genet 104: 315–325.

984. Gisselsson D, Hoglund M, Mertens F et al. (1998). Chromosomal organization of amplified chromosome 12 sequences in mesenchymal tumors detected by fluorescence in situ hybridization. Genes Chromosomes Cancer 23: 203–212.

985. Gisselsson D, Palsson E, Hoglund M et al. (2002). Differentially amplified chromosome 12 sequences in low- and high-grade osteosarcoma. Genes Chromosomes Cancer 33: 133–140.

986. Giunti A, Laus M (1978). Malignant tumours in chronic osteomyelitis. (A report of thirty nine cases, twenty six with long term follow up). Ital J Orthop Traumatol 4: 171–182.

987. Gladdy RA, Qin LX, Moraco N et al. (2010). Do radiation-associated soft tissue sarcomas have the same prognosis as sporadic soft tissue sarcomas? J Clin Oncol 28: 2064–2069.

988. Gleason BC, Calder KB, Cibull TL et al. (2009). Utility of p63 in the differential diagnosis of atypical fibroxanthoma and spindle cell squamous cell carcinoma. J Cutan Pathol 36: 543–547.

989. Gleason BC, Fletcher CD (2007). Myoepithelial carcinoma of soft tissue in children: an aggressive neoplasm analyzed in a series of 29 cases. Am J Surg Pathol 31: 1813–1824.

990. Gleason BC, Fletcher CD (2008). Deep "benign" fibrous histiocytoma: clinicopathologic analysis of 69 cases of a rare tumor indicating occasional metastatic potential. Am J Surg Pathol 32: 354–362.

991. Gleason BC, Hornick JL (2008). Inflammatory myofibroblastic tumours: where are we now? J Clin Pathol 61: 428–437.

992. Gleason BC, Liegl-Atzwanger B, Kozakewich HP et al. (2008). Osteofibrous dysplasia and adamantinoma in children and adolescents: a clinicopathologic reappraisal. Am J Surg Pathol 32: 363–376.

993. Gleason BC, Nascimento AF (2007). HMB-45 and Melan-A are useful in the differential diagnosis between granular cell tumor and malignant melanoma. Am J Dermatopathol 29: 22–27.

994. Glowacki M, Ignys-O'Byrne A, Ignys I et al. (2010). Evaluation of volume and solitary

bone cyst remodeling using conventional radiological examination. Skeletal Radiol 39: 251–259.

995. Glowacki M, Ignys-O'Byrne A, Ignys I et al. (2011). Limb shortening in the course of solitary bone cyst treatment—a comparative study. Skeletal Radiol 40: 173–179.

996. Goedert JJ (2000). The epidemiology of acquired immunodeficiency syndrome malignancies. Semin Oncol 27: 390–401.

997. Goetz SP, Robinson RA, Landas SK (1992). Extraskeletal myxoid chondrosarcoma of the pleura. Report of a case clinically simulating mesothelioma. Am J Clin Pathol 97: 498–502.

998. Gold JS, Antonescu CR, Hajdu C et al. (2002). Clinicopathologic correlates of solitary fibrous tumors. Cancer 94: 1057–1068.

999. Goldberg J, Azizad S, Bandovic J et al. (2009). Primary mediastinal giant cell tumor. Rare Tumors 1: e45

1000. Goldblum JR, Appelman HD (1995). Stromal tumors of the duodenum. A histologic and immunohistochemical study of 20 cases. Am J Surg Pathol 19: 71–80.

1001. Goldblum JR, Reith JD, Weiss SW (2000). Sarcomas arising in dermatofibrosarcoma protuberans: a reappraisal of biologic behavior in eighteen cases treated by wide local excision with extended clinical follow up. Am J Surg Pathol 24: 1125–1130.

1002. Goldblum JR, Rice TW (1995). Epithelioid angiosarcoma of the pulmonary artery. Hum Pathol 26: 1275–1277.

1003. Gologorsky Y, Gologorsky D, Yarygina AS et al. (2007). Familial multiple lipomatosis: report of a new family. Cutis 79: 227–232.

1004. Gomez-Brouchet A, Soulie M, Delisle MB et al. (2001). Mesenchymal chondrosarcoma of the kidney. J Urol 166: 2305

1005. Gong L, Liu W, Sun X et al. (2012). Histological and clinical characteristics of malignant giant cell tumor of bone. Virchows Arch 460: 327–334.

1006. Gonin-Laurent N, Gibaud A, Huygue M et al. (2006). Specific TP53 mutation pattern in radiation-induced sarcomas. Carcinogenesis 27: 1266–1272.

1007. Gonin-Laurent N, Hadj-Hamou NS, Vogt N et al. (2007). RB1 and TP53 pathways in radiation-induced sarcomas. Oncogene 26: 6106–6112.

1008. Gonzalez KD, Noltner KA, Buzin CH et al. (2009). Beyond Li Fraumeni Syndrome: clinical characteristics of families with p53 germline mutations. J Clin Oncol 27: 1250–1256.

1009. Gonzalez-Crussi F, Chou P, Crawford SE (1991). Congenital, infiltrating giant-cell angioblastoma. A new entity? Am J Surg Pathol 15: 175–183.

1010. Gonzalez-Vasconcellos I, Domke T, Kuosaite V et al. (2011). Differential effects of genes of the Rb1 signalling pathway on osteosarcoma incidence and latency in alpha-particle irradiated mice. Radiat Environ Biophys 50: 135–141.

1011. Good DA, Busfield F, Fletcher BH et al. (2002). Linkage of Paget disease of bone to a novel region on human chromosome 18q23. Am J Hum Genet 70: 517–525.

1012. Goodlad JR, Mentzel T, Fletcher CD (1995). Low grade fibromyxoid sarcoma: clinicopathological analysis of eleven new cases in support of a distinct entity. Histopathology 26: 229–237.

1013. Gordon A, McManus A, Anderson J et al. (2003). Chromosomal imbalances in pleomorphic rhabdomyosarcomas and identification of

the alveolar rhabdomyosarcoma-associated PAX3-FOXO1A fusion gene in one case. Cancer Genet Cytogenet 140: 73–77.

1014. Gordon T, McManus A, Anderson J et al. (2001). Cytogenetic abnormalities in 42 rhabdomyosarcoma: a United Kingdom Cancer Cytogenetics Group Study. Med Pediatr Oncol 36: 259–267.

1015. Gorlin RJ (1995). Nevoid basal cell carcinoma syndrome. Dermatol Clin 13: 113–125.

1016. Gorunova L, Vult von Steyern F, Storlazzi CT et al. (2009). Cytogenetic analysis of 101 giant cell tumors of bone: nonrandom patterns of telomeric associations and other structural aberrations. Genes Chromosomes Cancer 48: 583–602.

1017. Goto M (1997). Hierarchical deterioration of body systems in Werner's syndrome: implications for normal ageing. Mech Ageing Dev 98: 239–254.

1018. Goto M, Miller RW, Ishikawa Y et al. (1996). Excess of rare cancers in Werner syndrome (adult progeria). Cancer Epidemiol Biomarkers Prev 5: 239–246.

1019. Goto M, Yamabe Y, Shiratori M et al. (1999). Immunological diagnosis of Werner syndrome by down-regulated and truncated gene products. Hum Genet 105: 301–307.

1020. Goutagny S, Kalamarides M (2010). Meningiomas and neurofibromatosis. J Neurooncol 99: 341–347.

1021. Graadt van Roggen JF, McMenamin ME, Belchis DA et al. (2001). Reticular perineurioma: a distinctive variant of soft tissue perineurioma. Am J Surg Pathol 25: 485–493.

1022. Grabellus F, Konik MJ, Worm K et al. (2010). MET overexpressing chordomas frequently exhibit polysomy of chromosome 7 but no MET activation through sarcoma-specific gene fusions. Tumour Biol 31: 157–163.

1023. Graham C, Chilton-MacNeill S, Zielenska M et al. (2012). The CIC-DUX4 fusion transcript is present in a subgroup of pediatric primitive round cell sarcomas. Hum Pathol 43: 180–189.

1024. Graham RP, Dry S, Li X et al. (2011). Ossifying fibromyxoid tumor of soft parts: a clinicopathologic, proteomic, and genomic study. Am J Surg Pathol 35: 1615–1625.

1025. Graham RP, Hodge JC, Folpe AL et al. (2012). A cytogenetic analysis of two cases of phosphaturic mesenchymal tumor mixed connective tissue type. Am J Surg Pathol. 43:1334-1338.

1026. Granter SR, Badizadegan K, Fletcher CD (1998). Myofibromatosis in adults, glomangiopericytoma, and myopericytoma: a spectrum of tumors showing perivascular myoid differentiation. Am J Surg Pathol 22: 513–525.

1027. Granter SR, Nucci MR, Fletcher CD (1997). Aggressive angiomyxoma: reappraisal of its relationship to angiomyofibroblastoma in a series of 16 cases. Histopathology 30: 3–10.

1028. Granter SR, Renshaw AA, Fletcher CD et al. (1996). CD99 reactivity in mesenchymal chondrosarcoma. Hum Pathol 27: 1273–1276.

1029. Green P, Whittaker RP (1975). Benign chondroblastoma. Case report with pulmonary metastasis. J Bone Joint Surg Am 57: 418–420.

1030. Greene AK, Karnes J, Padua HM et al. (2009). Diffuse lipofibromatosis of the lower extremity masquerading as a vascular anomaly. Ann Plast Surg 62: 703–706.

1031. Greene AK, Liu AS, Mulliken JB et al. (2011). Vascular anomalies in 5,621 patients: guidelines for referral. J Pediatr Surg 46: 1784–1789.

1032. Greenspan A, Azouz EM, Matthews J et

al. (1995). Synovial hemangioma: imaging features in eight histologically proven cases, review of the literature, and differential diagnosis. Skeletal Radiol 24: 583–590.

1033. Gregory PA, Bert AG, Paterson EL et al. (2008). The miR-200 family and miR-205 regulate epithelial to mesenchymal transition by targeting ZEB1 and SIP1. Nat Cell Biol 10: 593–601.

1034. Greiss ME, Williams DH (1991). Macrodystrophia lipomatosis in the foot. A case report and review of the literature. Arch Orthop Trauma Surg 110: 220–221.

1035. Grieten M, Buckwalter KA, Cardinal E et al. (1994). Case report 873: Lipoma arborescens (villous lipomatous proliferation of the synovial membrane). Skeletal Radiol 23: 652–655.

1036. Griffin CA, Hawkins AL, Dvorak C et al. (1999). Recurrent involvement of 2p23 in inflammatory myofibroblastic tumors. Cancer Res 59: 2776–2780.

1037. Grimer RJ, Bielack S, Flege S et al. (2005). Periosteal osteosarcoma—a European review of outcome. Eur J Cancer 41: 2806–2811.

1038. Grimer RJ, Briggs TW (2010). Earlier diagnosis of bone and soft-tissue tumours. J Bone Joint Surg Br 92: 1489–1492.

1039. Grimer RJ, Gosheger G, Taminiau A et al. (2007). Dedifferentiated chondrosarcoma: prognostic factors and outcome from a European group. Eur J Cancer 43: 2060–2065.

1040. Grimmett GM, Hall MG, Jr., Aird CC et al. (1973). Pelvic lipomatosis. Am J Surg 125: 347–349.

1041. Grochola LF, Zeron-Medina J, Meriaux S et al. (2010). Single-nucleotide polymorphisms in the p53 signaling pathway. Cold Spring Harb Perspect Biol 2: a001032

1042. Groen EJ, Roos A, Muntinghe FL et al. (2008). Extra-intestinal manifestations of familial adenomatous polyposis. Ann Surg Oncol 15: 2439–2450.

1043. Grogan TM, Spier CM (2001). The B cell immunoproliferative disorders, including multiple myeloma and amyloidosis. In: Neoplastic hematopathology. Knowles DM Lippincott Williams and Wilkins: Philadelphia: pp 1557-1587.

1044. Grohs JG, Nicolakis M, Kainberger F et al. (2002). Benign fibrous histiocytoma of bone: a report of ten cases and review of literature. Wien Klin Wochenschr 114: 56–63.

1045. Groisman G, Lichtig C (1991). Fibrous hamartoma of infancy: an immunohistochemical and ultrastructural study. Hum Pathol 22: 914–918.

1046. Gronchi A, Casali PG, Mariani L et al. (2005). Status of surgical margins and prognosis in adult soft tissue sarcomas of the extremities: a series of patients treated at a single institution. J Clin Oncol 23: 96–104.

1047. Gronchi A, Frustaci S, Mercuri M (2012). Short, full-dose adjuvant chemotherapy in high-risk adult soft tissue sarcomas (STS): a randomized clinical trial from the Italian Sarcoma Group (ISG) and the Spanish Sarcoma Group (GEIS). J Clin Oncol 30: 850–856.

1048. Gronchi A, Lo Vullo S, Colombo C et al. (2010). Extremity soft tissue sarcoma in a series of patients treated at a single institution: local control directly impacts survival. Ann Surg 251: 506–511.

1049. Gronchi A, Lo Vullo S, Fiore M et al. (2009). Aggressive surgical policies in a retrospectively reviewed single-institution case series of retroperitoneal soft tissue sarcoma

patients. J Clin Oncol 27: 24–30.
1050. Gronchi A, Miceli R, Colombo C et al. (2011). Frontline extended surgery is associated with improved survival in retroperitoneal low- to intermediate-grade soft tissue sarcomas. Ann Oncol 23:1067-1073.
1051. Groom KR, Murphey MD, Howard LM et al. (2002). Mesenchymal hamartoma of the chest wall: radiologic manifestations with emphasis on cross-sectional imaging and histopathologic comparison. Radiology 222: 205–211.
1052. Grosso F, Jones RL, Demetri GD et al. (2007). Efficacy of trabectedin (ecteinascidin-743) in advanced pretreated myxoid liposarcomas: a retrospective study. Lancet Oncol 8: 595–602.
1053. Gruber G, Giessauf C, Leithner A et al. (2008). Bizarre parosteal osteochondromatous proliferation (Nora lesion): a report of 3 cases and a review of the literature. Can J Surg 51: 486–489.
1054. Grunewald TG, von Luettichau I, Weirich G et al. (2010). Sclerosing epithelioid fibrosarcoma of the bone: a case report of high resistance to chemotherapy and a survey of the literature. Sarcoma 2010: 431627
1055. Grynspan D, Meir K, Senger C et al. (2007). Cutaneous changes in fibrous hamartoma of infancy. J Cutan Pathol 34: 39–43.
1056. Guarda-Nardini L, Piccotti F, Ferronato G et al. (2010). Synovial chondromatosis of the temporomandibular joint: a case description with systematic literature review. Int J Oral Maxillofac Surg 39: 745–755.
1057. Guccion JG, Font RL, Enzinger FM et al. (1973). Extraskeletal mesenchymal chondrosarcoma. Arch Pathol 95: 336–340.
1058. Guillou L, Benhattar J, Bonichon F et al. (2004). Histologic grade, but not SYT-SSX fusion type, is an important prognostic factor in patients with synovial sarcoma: a multicenter, retrospective analysis. J Clin Oncol 22: 4040–4050.
1059. Guillou L, Benhattar J, Gengler C et al. (2007). Translocation-positive low-grade fibromyxoid sarcoma: clinicopathologic and molecular analysis of a series expanding the morphologic spectrum and suggesting potential relationship to sclerosing epithelioid fibrosarcoma: a study from the French Sarcoma Group. Am J Surg Pathol 31: 1387–1402.
1060. Guillou L, Coindre JM, Bonichon F et al. (1997). Comparative study of the National Cancer Institute and French Federation of Cancer Centers Sarcoma Group grading systems in a population of 410 adult patients with soft tissue sarcoma. J Clin Oncol 15: 350–362.
1061. Guillou L, Gebhard S, Coindre JM (2000). Lipomatous hemangiopericytoma: a fat-containing variant of solitary fibrous tumor? Clinicopathologic, immunohistochemical, and ultrastructural analysis of a series in favor of a unifying concept. Hum Pathol 31: 1108–1115.
1062. Guillou L, Wadden C, Coindre JM et al. (1997). "Proximal-type" epithelioid sarcoma, a distinctive aggressive neoplasm showing rhabdoid features. Clinicopathologic, immunohistochemical, and ultrastructural study of a series. Am J Surg Pathol 21: 130–146.
1063. Gumus A, Yildirim SV, Kizilkilic O et al. (2007). Case report: seizures in a child caused by a large venous angioma. J Child Neurol 22: 787–789.
1064. Guo H, Garcia RA, Perle MA et al. (2005). Giant cell tumor of soft tissue with pulmonary metastases: pathologic and cytogenetic study. Pediatr Dev Pathol 8: 718–724.
1065. Guo T, Zhang L, Chang NE et al. (2011). Consistent MYC and FLT4 gene amplification in radiation-induced angiosarcoma but not in other radiation-associated atypical vascular lesions. Genes Chromosomes Cancer 50: 25–33.
1066. Gupta P, Babyn P (2008). Sinus histiocytosis with massive lymphadenopathy (Rosai-Dorfman disease): a clinicoradiological profile of three cases including two with skeletal disease. Pediatr Radiol 38: 721–728.
1067. Gurbuz AK, Giardiello FM, Petersen GM et al. (1994). Desmoid tumours in familial adenomatous polyposis. Gut 35: 377–381.
1068. Gurney JG, Davis S, Severson RK et al. (1996). Trends in cancer incidence among children in the U.S. Cancer 78: 532–541.
1069. Gustafson P (1994). Soft tissue sarcoma. Epidemiology and prognosis in 508 patients. Acta Orthop Scand Suppl 259: 1–31.
1070. Haase R, Merkel N, Milzsch M et al. (2007). Mesenchymal chest wall hamartoma – surgery is prefered. Archives of Perinatal Medicine 13: 56–61.
1071. Hachach-Haram N, Gerarchi P, Benyon SL et al. (2011). Multidisciplinary surgical management of cherubism complicated by neurofibromatosis type 1. J Craniofac Surg 22: 2318–2322.
1072. Hachisuga T, Hashimoto H, Enjoji M (1984). Angioleiomyoma. A clinicopathologic reappraisal of 562 cases. Cancer 54: 126–130.
1073. Hachitanda Y, Tsuneyoshi M, Daimaru Y et al. (1988). Extraskeletal myxoid chondrosarcoma in young children. Cancer 61: 2521–2526.
1074. Hacker U, Nybakken K, Perrimon N (2005). Heparan sulphate proteoglycans: the sweet side of development. Nat Rev Mol Cell Biol 6: 530–541.
1075. Hahn H, Wicking C, Zaphiropoulous PG et al. (1996). Mutations of the human homolog of Drosophila patched in the nevoid basal cell carcinoma syndrome. Cell 85: 841–851.
1076. Hahn HP, Fletcher CD (2007). Primary mediastinal liposarcoma: clinicopathologic analysis of 24 cases. Am J Surg Pathol 31: 1868–1874.
1077. Haibach H, Farrell C, Dittrich FJ (1985). Neoplasms arising in Paget's disease of bone: a study of 82 cases. Am J Clin Pathol 83: 594–600.
1078. Hajdu M, Singer S, Maki RG et al. (2010). IGF2 over-expression in solitary fibrous tumours is independent of anatomical location and is related to loss of imprinting. J Pathol 221: 300–307.
1079. Hallel T, Lew S, Bansal M (1988). Villous lipomatous proliferation of the synovial membrane (lipoma arborescens). J Bone Joint Surg Am 70: 264–270.
1080. Halling AC, Wollan PC, Pritchard DJ et al. (1996). Epithelioid sarcoma: a clinicopathologic review of 55 cases. Mayo Clin Proc 71: 636–642.
1081. Hallor KH, Heidenblad M, Brosjo O et al. (2007). Tiling resolution array comparative genomic hybridization analysis of a fibrosarcoma of bone. Cancer Genet Cytogenet 172: 80–83.
1082. Hallor KH, Mertens F, Jin Y et al. (2005). Fusion of the EWSR1 and ATF1 genes without expression of the MITF-M transcript in angiomatoid fibrous histiocytoma. Genes Chromosomes Cancer 44: 97–102.
1083. Hallor KH, Micci F, Meis-Kindblom JM et al. (2007). Fusion genes in angiomatoid fibrous histiocytoma. Cancer Lett 251: 158–163.
1084. Hallor KH, Sciot R, Staaf J et al. (2009). Two genetic pathways, t(1;10) and amplification of 3p11-12, in myxoinflammatory fibroblastic sarcoma, haemosiderotic fibrolipomatous tumour, and morphologically similar lesions. J Pathol 217: 716–727.
1085. Hallor KH, Staaf J, Bovee JV et al. (2009). Genomic profiling of chondrosarcoma: chromosomal patterns in central and peripheral tumors. Clin Cancer Res 15: 2685–2694.
1086. Hallor KH, Staaf J, Jonsson G et al. (2008). Frequent deletion of the CDKN2A locus in chordoma: analysis of chromosomal imbalances using array comparative genomic hybridisation. Br J Cancer 98: 434–442.
1087. Hallor KH, Teixeira MR, Fletcher CD et al. (2008). Heterogeneous genetic profiles in soft tissue myoepitheliomas. Mod Pathol 21: 1311–1319.
1088. Halperin EC, Greenberg MS, Suit HD (1984). Sarcoma of bone and soft tissue following treatment of Hodgkin's disease. Cancer 53: 232–236.
1089. Hamada T, Ito H, Araki Y et al. (1996). Benign fibrous histiocytoma of the femur: review of three cases. Skeletal Radiol 25: 25–29.
1090. Hamblen DL, Carter RL (1984). Sarcoma and joint replacement. J Bone Joint Surg Br 66: 625–627.
1091. Hameed M, Clarke K, Amer HZ et al. (2007). Cellular angiofibroma is genetically similar to spindle cell lipoma: a case report. Cancer Genet Cytogenet 177: 131–134.
1092. Hameed M, Ulger C, Yasar D et al. (2009). Genome profiling of chondrosarcoma using oligonucleotide array-based comparative genomic hybridization. Cancer Genet Cytogenet 192: 56–59.
1093. Hameetman L, Bovee JV, Taminiau AH et al. (2004). Multiple osteochondromas: clinicopathological and genetic spectrum and suggestions for clinical management. Hered Cancer Clin Pract 2: 161–173.
1094. Hameetman L, Rozeman LB, Lombaerts M et al. (2006). Peripheral chondrosarcoma progression is accompanied by decreased Indian Hedgehog signalling. J Pathol 209: 501–511.
1095. Hameetman L, Szuhai K, Yavas A et al. (2007). The role of EXT1 in nonhereditary osteochondroma: identification of homozygous deletions. J Natl Cancer Inst 99: 396–406.
1096. Hamlat A, Saikali S, Gueye EM et al. (2005). Primary liposarcoma of the thoracic spine: case report. Eur Spine J 14: 613–618.
1097. Hamre MR, Severson RK, Chuba P et al. (2002). Osteosarcoma as a second malignant neoplasm. Radiother Oncol 65: 153–157.
1098. Han HJ, Lim GY, You CY (2009). A large infiltrating fibrous hamartoma of infancy in the abdominal wall with rare associated tuberous sclerosis. Pediatr Radiol 39: 743–746.
1099. Haniball J, Sumathi VP, Kindblom LG et al. (2011). Prognostic factors and metastatic patterns in primary myxoid/round-cell liposarcoma. Sarcoma 2011: 538085
1100. Hanks S, Adams S, Douglas J et al. (2003). Mutations in the gene encoding capillary morphogenesis protein 2 cause juvenile hyaline fibromatosis and infantile systemic hyalinosis. Am J Hum Genet 73: 791–800.
1101. Hanna N, Parfait B, Talaat IM et al. (2009). SOS1: a new player in the Noonan-like/multiple giant cell lesion syndrome. Clin Genet 75: 568–571.
1102. Hansen MF, Koufos A, Gallie BL et al. (1985). Osteosarcoma and retinoblastoma: a shared chromosomal mechanism revealing recessive predisposition. Proc Natl Acad Sci U S A 82: 6216–6220.
1103. Hansen MF, Nellissery MJ, Bhatia P (1999). Common mechanisms of osteosarcoma and Paget's disease. J Bone Miner Res 14 Suppl 2: 39–44.
1104. Hansen T, Burg JE, Koutsimpelas D et al. (2005). Cervical adult rhabdomyoma presenting as a rapidly growing mass in a patient with diffuse large B-cell non-Hodgkin's lymphoma. Mund Kiefer Gesichtschir 9: 184–187.
1105. Happle R, Konig A (1999). Type 2 segmental manifestation of multiple glomus tumors: A review and reclassification of 5 case reports. Dermatology 198: 270–272.
1106. Harada H, Kawano MM, Huang N et al. (1993). Phenotypic difference of normal plasma cells from mature myeloma cells. Blood 81: 2658–2663.
1107. Harada K, Toyooka S, Maitra A et al. (2002). Aberrant promoter methylation and silencing of the RASSF1A gene in pediatric tumors and cell lines. Oncogene 21: 4345–4349.
1108. Harada K, Toyooka S, Shivapurkar N et al. (2002). Deregulation of caspase 8 and 10 expression in pediatric tumors and cell lines. Cancer Res 62: 5897–5901.
1109. Hardcastle P, Nade S, Arnold W (1986). Hereditary bone dysplasia with malignant change. Report of three families. J Bone Joint Surg Am 68: 1079–1089.
1110. Hardell L, Eriksson M (1988). The association between soft tissue sarcomas and exposure to phenoxyacetic acids. A new case-referent study. Cancer 62: 652–656.
1111. Harder A, Wesemann M, Hagel C et al. (2012). Hybrid neurofibroma/schwannoma is overrepresented among schwannomatosis and neurofibromatosis patients. Am J Surg Pathol 36: 702–709.
1112. Harik LR, Merino C, Coindre JM et al. (2006). Pseudosarcomatous myofibroblastic proliferations of the bladder: a clinicopathologic study of 42 cases. Am J Surg Pathol 30: 787–794.
1113. Harms D (1995). Alveolar rhabdomyosarcoma: a prognostically unfavorable rhabdomyosarcoma type and its necessary distinction from embryonal rhabdomyosarcoma. Curr Top Pathol 89: 273–296.
1114. Haroche J, Amoura Z, Dion E et al. (2004). Cardiovascular involvement, an overlooked feature of Erdheim-Chester disease: report of 6 new cases and a literature review. Medicine (Baltimore) 83: 371–392.
1114A. Haroche J, Charlotte F, Arnaud L et al. (2012). High prevalence of BRAF V600E mutations in Erdheim-Chester disease but not in other non-Langerhans cell histiocytoses.Blood 120: 2700–2703.
1115. Harris M, Coyne J, Tariq M et al. (2000). Extraskeletal myxoid chondrosarcoma with neuroendocrine differentiation: a pathologic, cytogenetic, and molecular study of a case with a novel translocation t(9;17)(q22;q11.2). Am J Surg Pathol 24: 1020–1026.
1116. Harris WH, Dudley HRJ, Barry RJ (1962). The natural history of fibrous dysplasia. An orthopaedic, pathological, and roentgenographic study. J Bone Joint Surg Am 44-A: 207–233.
1117. Harwood AR, Krajbich JI, Fornasier VL (1981). Mesenchymal chondrosarcoma: a report of 17 cases. Clin Orthop Relat Res 158:144–148.
1118. Hasegawa T, Hirose T, Kudo E et al.

(1991). Immunophenotypic heterogeneity in osteosarcomas. Hum Pathol 22: 583–590.

1119. Hasegawa T, Hirose T, Seki K et al. (1996). Solitary fibrous tumor of the soft tissue. An immunohistochemical and ultrastructural study. Am J Clin Pathol 106: 325–331.

1120. Hasegawa T, Matsuno Y, Niki T et al. (1998). Second primary rhabdomyosarcomas in patients with bilateral retinoblastoma: a clinicopathologic and immunohistochemical study. Am J Surg Pathol 22: 1351–1360.

1121. Hasegawa T, Matsuno Y, Shimoda T et al. (1999). Extrathoracic solitary fibrous tumors: their histological variability and potentially aggressive behavior. Hum Pathol 30: 1464–1473.

1122. Hasegawa T, Matsuno Y, Shimoda T et al. (2001). Proximal-type epithelioid sarcoma: a clinicopathologic study of 20 cases. Mod Pathol 14: 655–663.

1123. Hasegawa T, Seki K, Ono K et al. (2000). Angiomatoid (malignant) fibrous histiocytoma: a peculiar low-grade tumor showing immunophenotypic heterogeneity and ultrastructural variations. Pathol Int 50: 731–738.

1124. Hasegawa T, Shimoda T, Hirohashi S et al. (1998). Collagenous fibroma (desmoplastic fibroblastoma): report of four cases and review of the literature. Arch Pathol Lab Med 122: 455–460.

1125. Hasegawa T, Yamamoto S, Yokoyama R et al. (2002). Prognostic significance of grading and staging systems using MIB-1 score in adult patients with soft tissue sarcoma of the extremities and trunk. Cancer 95: 843–851.

1126. Hashimoto H (1995). Incidence of soft tissue sarcomas in adults. Curr Top Pathol 89: 1–16.

1127. Hashimoto H, Daimaru Y, Tsuneyoshi M et al. (1986). Leiomyosarcoma of the external soft tissues. A clinicopathologic, immunohistochemical, and electron microscopic study. Cancer 57: 2077–2088.

1128. Hashimoto H, Tsuneyoshi M, Daimaru Y et al. (1986). Intramuscular myxoma. A clinicopathologic, immunohistochemical, and electron microscopic study. Cancer 58: 740–747.

1129. Hashimoto H, Tsuneyoshi M, Enjoji M (1985). Malignant smooth muscle tumors of the retroperitoneum and mesentery: a clinicopathologic analysis of 44 cases. J Surg Oncol 28: 177–186.

1130. Hashimoto N, Ueda T, Joyama S et al. (2005). Extraskeletal mesenchymal chondrosarcoma: an imaging review of ten new patients. Skeletal Radiol 34: 785–792.

1131. Hatano H, Morita T, Ogose A et al. (2008). Clinicopathological features of lipomas with gene fusions involving HMGA2. Anticancer Res 28: 535–538.

1132. Hattinger CM, Potschger U, Tarkkanen M et al. (2002). Prognostic impact of chromosomal aberrations in Ewing tumours. Br J Cancer 86: 1763–1769.

1133. Hattinger CM, Rumpler S, Ambros IM et al. (1996). Demonstration of the translocation der(16)t(1;16)(q12;q11.2) in interphase nuclei of Ewing tumors. Genes Chromosomes Cancer 17: 141–150.

1134. Hattinger CM, Rumpler S, Strehl S et al. (1999). Prognostic impact of deletions at 1p36 and numerical aberrations in Ewing tumors. Genes Chromosomes Cancer 24: 243–254.

1135. Hattinger CM, Tarkkanen M, Benini S et al. (2004). Genetic analysis of fibrosarcoma of bone, a rare tumour entity closely related to osteosarcoma and malignant fibrous histiocytoma of bone. Eur J Cell Biol 83: 483–491.

1136. Hauben E, van den Broek LC, Van Marck E et al. (2001). Adamantinoma-like Ewing's sarcoma and Ewing's-like adamantinoma. The t(11; 22), t(21; 22) status. J Pathol 195: 218–221.

1137. Hauben EI, Jundt G, Cleton-Jansen AM et al. (2005). Desmoplastic fibroma of bone: an immunohistochemical study including beta-catenin expression and mutational analysis for beta-catenin. Hum Pathol 36: 1025–1030.

1138. Hauben EI, Weeden S, Pringle J et al. (2002). Does the histological subtype of high-grade central osteosarcoma influence the response to treatment with chemotherapy and does it affect overall survival? A study on 570 patients of two consecutive trials of the European Osteosarcoma Intergroup. Eur J Cancer 38: 1218–1225.

1139. Hawley IC, Krausz T, Evans DJ et al. (1994). Spindle cell lipoma—a pseudoangiomatous variant. Histopathology 24: 565–569.

1140. Hayashi M, Kitagawa Y, Kim Y et al. (2008). Malignant glomus tumor arising among multiple glomus tumors. J Orthop Sci 13: 472–475.

1141. Hayashi T, Tsuda N, Chowdhury PR et al. (1995). Infantile digital fibromatosis: a study of the development and regression of cytoplasmic inclusion bodies. Mod Pathol 8: 548–552.

1142. Hays DM, Donaldson SS, Shimada H et al. (1997). Primary and metastatic rhabdomyosarcoma in the breast: neoplasms of adolescent females, a report from the Intergroup Rhabdomyosarcoma Study. Med Pediatr Oncol 29: 181–189.

1143. Hays DM, Newton W, Jr., Soule EH et al. (1983). Mortality among children with rhabdomyosarcomas of the alveolar histologic subtype. J Pediatr Surg 18: 412–417.

1144. Hazelbag HM, Fleuren GJ, Cornelisse CJ et al. (1995). DNA aberrations in the epithelial cell component of adamantinoma of long bones. Am J Pathol 147: 1770–1779.

1145. Hazelbag HM, Fleuren GJ, van den Broek LJ et al. (1993). Adamantinoma of the long bones: keratin subclass immunoreactivity pattern with reference to its histogenesis. Am J Surg Pathol 17: 1225–1233.

1146. Hazelbag HM, Hogendoorn PC (2001). [Adamantinoma of the long bones: an anatomo-clinical review and its relationship with osteofibrous dysplasia]. Ann Pathol 21: 499–511.

1147. Hazelbag HM, Laforga JB, Roels HJ et al. (2003). Dedifferentiated adamantinoma with revertant mesenchymal phenotype. Am J Surg Pathol 27: 1530–1537.

1148. Hazelbag HM, Taminiau AH, Fleuren GJ et al. (1994). Adamantinoma of the long bones. A clinicopathological study of thirty-two patients with emphasis on histological subtype, precursor lesion, and biological behavior. J Bone Joint Surg Am 76: 1482–1499.

1149. Hazelbag HM, van den Broek LJ, Fleuren GJ et al. (1997). Distribution of extracellular matrix components in adamantinoma of long bones suggests fibrous-to-epithelial transformation. Hum Pathol 28: 183–188.

1150. Hazelbag HM, Wessels JW, Mollevangers P et al. (1997). Cytogenetic analysis of adamantinoma of long bones: further indications for a common histogenesis with osteofibrous dysplasia. Cancer Genet Cytogenet 97: 5–11.

1151. Healey JH, Ghelman B (1986). Osteoid osteoma and osteoblastoma. Current concepts and recent advances. Clin Orthop Relat Res 76–85.

1152. Hebert-Blouin MN, Scheithauer BW, Amrami KK et al. (2012). Fibromatosis: a potential sequela of neuromuscular choristoma. J Neurosurg 116: 399–408.

1153. Heenan PJ, Quirk CJ, Papadimitriou JM (1986). Epithelioid sarcoma. A diagnostic problem. Am J Dermatopathol 8: 95–104.

1154. Heerema-McKenney A, Wijnaendts LC, Pulliam JF et al. (2008). Diffuse myogenin expression by immunohistochemistry is an independent marker of poor survival in pediatric rhabdomyosarcoma: a tissue microarray study of 71 primary tumors including correlation with molecular phenotype. Am J Surg Pathol 32: 1513–1522.

1155. Hefti F, Jundt G (1995). [Langerhans cell histiocytosis]. Orthopade 24: 73–81.

1156. Heidenblad M, Hallor KH, Staaf J et al. (2006). Genomic profiling of bone and soft tissue tumors with supernumerary ring chromosomes using tiling resolution bacterial artificial chromosome microarrays. Oncogene 25: 7106–7116.

1157. Heimann P, El Housni H, Ogur G et al. (2001). Fusion of a novel gene, RCC17, to the TFE3 gene in t(X;17)(p11.2;q25.3)-bearing papillary renal cell carcinomas. Cancer Res 61: 4130–4135.

1158. Heinrich MC, Rubin BP, Longley BJ et al. (2002). Biology and genetic aspects of gastrointestinal stromal tumors: KIT activation and cytogenetic alterations. Hum Pathol 33: 484–495.

1159. Heinsohn S, Evermann U, Zur Stadt U et al. (2007). Determination of the prognostic value of loss of heterozygosity at the retinoblastoma gene in osteosarcoma. Int J Oncol 30: 1205–1214.

1160. Hemsrichart V, Charoenkwan P (2007). Fatal bilateral congenital mesenchymal hamartoma of the chest wall. J Med Assoc Thai 90: 2519–2523.

1161. Henderson CJ, Gupta L (2000). Ectopic hamartomatous thymoma: a case study and review of the literature. Pathology 32: 142–146.

1162. Henricks WH, Chu YC, Goldblum JR et al. (1997). Dedifferentiated liposarcoma: a clinicopathological analysis of 155 cases with a proposal for an expanded definition of dedifferentiation. Am J Surg Pathol 21: 271–281.

1163. Heo MS, Cho HJ, Kwon KJ et al. (2004). Benign fibrous histiocytoma in the mandible. Oral Surg Oral Med Oral Pathol Oral Radiol Endod 97: 276–280.

1164. Hernandez JL, Rodriguez-Parets JO, Valero JM et al. (2010). High-resolution genome-wide analysis of chromosomal alterations in elastofibroma. Virchows Arch 456: 681–687.

1165. Hertoghs M, Van Schil P, Rutsaert R et al. (2009). Intrathoracic hibernoma: report of two cases. Lung Cancer 64: 367–370.

1166. Herzberg AJ, Kerns BJ, Honkanen FA et al. (1992). DNA ploidy and proliferation index of soft tissue sarcomas determined by image cytometry of fresh frozen tissue. Am J Clin Pathol 97: S29–S37.

1167. Hethcote HW, Knudson AG, Jr. (1978). Model for the incidence of embryonal cancers: application to retinoblastoma. Proc Natl Acad Sci U S A 75: 2453–2457.

1168. Heymann S, Delaloge S, Rahal A et al. (2010). Radio-induced malignancies after breast cancer postoperative radiotherapy in patients with Li-Fraumeni syndrome. Radiat Oncol 5: 104

1169. Heyning FH, Hogendoorn PC, Kramer MH et al. (1999). Primary non-Hodgkin's lymphoma of bone: a clinicopathological investigation of 60 cases. Leukemia 13: 2094–2098.

1170. Heyning FH, Jansen PM, Hogendoorn PC et al. (2010). Array-based comparative genomic hybridisation analysis reveals recurrent chromosomal alterations in primary diffuse large B cell lymphoma of bone. J Clin Pathol 63: 1095–1100.

1171. Heyning FH, Kroon HM, Hogendoorn PC et al. (2007). MR imaging characteristics in primary lymphoma of bone with emphasis on non-aggressive appearance. Skeletal Radiol 36: 937–944.

1172. Heyns CF (1991). Pelvic lipomatosis: a review of its diagnosis and management. J Urol 146: 267–273.

1173. Hibbard MK, Kozakewich HP, Dal Cin P et al. (2000). PLAG1 fusion oncogenes in lipoblastoma. Cancer Res 60: 4869–4872.

1174. Hicks J, Dilley A, Patel D et al. (2001). Lipoblastoma and lipoblastomatosis in infancy and childhood: histopathologic, ultrastructural, and cytogenetic features. Ultrastruct Pathol 25: 321–333.

1175. Hicks MJ, Roth JR, Kozinetz CA et al. (2007). Clinicopathologic features of osteosarcoma in patients with Rothmund-Thomson syndrome. J Clin Oncol 25: 370–375.

1176. Hill DA, Pfeifer JD, Marley EF et al. (2000). WT1 staining reliably differentiates desmoplastic small round cell tumor from Ewing sarcoma/primitive neuroectodermal tumor. An immunohistochemical and molecular diagnostic study. Am J Clin Pathol 114: 345–353.

1177. Hill KA, Gonzalez-Crussi F, Chou PM (2001). Calcifying fibrous pseudotumor versus inflammatory myofibroblastic tumor: a histological and immunohistochemical comparison. Mod Pathol 14: 784–790.

1178. Hill S, Rademaker M (2009). A collection of rare anomalies: multiple digital glomuvenous malformations, epidermal naevus, temporal alopecia, heterochromia and abdominal lipoblastoma. Clin Exp Dermatol 34: e862–e864.

1179. Hirai K, Takeuchi S, Bessho R et al. (2010). Venous hemangioma of the anterior mediastinum. J Nihon Med Sch 77: 115–118.

1180. Hirose T, Hasegawa T, Seki K et al. (1996). Atypical glomus tumor in the mediastinum: a case report with immunohistochemical and ultrastructural studies. Ultrastruct Pathol 20: 451–456.

1181. Hirose T, Scheithauer BW, Sano T (1998). Perineurial malignant peripheral nerve sheath tumor (MPNST): a clinicopathologic, immunohistochemical, and ultrastructural study of seven cases. Am J Surg Pathol 22: 1368–1378.

1182. Hirose T, Tani T, Shimada T et al. (2003). Immunohistochemical demonstration of EMA/Glut1-positive perineurial cells and CD34-positive fibroblastic cells in peripheral nerve sheath tumors. Mod Pathol 16: 293–298.

1183. Hirsch MS, Dal Cin P, Fletcher CD (2006). ALK expression in pseudosarcomatous myofibroblastic proliferations of the genitourinary tract. Histopathology 48: 569–578.

1184. Hisada M, Garber JE, Fung CY et al. (1998). Multiple primary cancers in families with Li-Fraumeni syndrome. J Natl Cancer Inst 90: 606–611.

1185. Hisaoka M, Hashimoto H (2005). Extraskeletal myxoid chondrosarcoma: updated clinicopathological and molecular genetic characteristics. Pathol Int 55: 453–463.

1186. Hisaoka M, Hashimoto H (2006). Elastofibroma: clonal fibrous proliferation with predominant CD34-positive cells. Virchows Arch 448: 195–199.

1187. Hisaoka M, Ishida T, Imamura T et al. (2004). TFG is a novel fusion partner of NOR1 in extraskeletal myxoid chondrosarcoma. Genes Chromosomes Cancer 40: 325–328.

1188. Hisaoka M, Ishida T, Kuo TT et al. (2008). Clear cell sarcoma of soft tissue: a clinicopathologic, immunohistochemical, and molecular analysis of 33 cases. Am J Surg Pathol 32: 452–460.

1189. Hisaoka M, Kouho H, Aoki T et al. (1995). Angiomyofibroblastoma of the vulva: a clinicopathologic study of seven cases. Pathol Int 45: 487–492.

1190. Hisaoka M, Morimitsu Y, Hashimoto H et al. (1999). Retroperitoneal liposarcoma with combined well-differentiated and myxoid malignant fibrous histiocytoma-like myxoid areas. Am J Surg Pathol 23: 1480–1492.

1191. Hisaoka M, Okamoto S, Yokoyama K et al. (2004). Coexpression of NOR1 and SIX3 proteins in extraskeletal myxoid chondrosarcomas without detectable NR4A3 fusion genes. Cancer Genet Cytogenet 152: 101–107.

1192. Hisaoka M, Sheng WQ, Tanaka A et al. (2002). HMGIC alterations in smooth muscle tumors of soft tissues and other sites. Cancer Genet Cytogenet 138: 50–55.

1193. Ho YH, Cheng MH, Yap WM et al. (2011). Cytokeratin-, calponin-, and p63-positive chondroblastoma with extensive soft tissue involvement and vascular invasion: a potential diagnostic dilemma. Ann Diagn Pathol 15: 58–63.

1194. Hoang MP, Suarez PA, Donner LR et al. (2000). Mesenchymal chondrosarcoma: a small cell neoplasm with polyphenotypic differentiation. Int J Surg Pathol 8: 291–301.

1195. Hoch B, Montag A (2011). Reactive bone lesions mimicking neoplasms. Semin Diagn Pathol 28: 102–112.

1196. Hoeber I, Spillane AJ, Fisher C et al. (2001). Accuracy of biopsy techniques for limb and limb girdle soft tissue tumors. Ann Surg Oncol 8: 80–87.

1197. Hogenporn PC, Athanasou N, Bielack S et al. (2010). Bone sarcomas: ESMO Clinical Practice Guidelines for diagnosis, treatment and follow-up. Ann Oncol 21 Suppl 5: v204–v213.

1198. Hojo H, Newton WA, Jr., Hamoudi AB et al. (1995). Pseudosarcomatous myofibroblastic tumor of the urinary bladder in children: a study of 11 cases with review of the literature. An Intergroup Rhabdomyosarcoma Study. Am J Surg Pathol 19: 1224–1236.

1199. Holimon JL, Rosenblum WI (1971). "Gangliorhabdomyosarcoma": a tumor of ectomesenchyme. Case report. J Neurosurg 34: 417–422.

1200. Hollmann TJ, Bovee JV, Fletcher CD (2012). Digital fibromyxoma (superficial acral fibromyxoma): a detailed characterization of 124 cases. Am J Surg Pathol 36: 789–798.

1201. Hollmann TJ, Hornick JL (2011). INI1-deficient tumors: diagnostic features and molecular genetics. Am J Surg Pathol 35: e47–e63.

1202. Hollowood K, Holley MP, Fletcher CD (1991). Plexiform fibrohistiocytic tumour: clinicopathological, immunohistochemical and ultrastructural analysis in favour of a myofibroblastic lesion. Histopathology 19: 503–513.

1203. Holscher HC, Bloem JL, van der Woude HJ et al. (1995). Can MRI predict the histopathological response in patients with osteosarcoma after the first cycle of chemotherapy? Clin Radiol 50: 384–390.

1204. Holscher HC, Bloem JL, Vanel D et al. (1992). Osteosarcoma: chemotherapy-induced changes at MR imaging. Radiology 182: 839–844.

1205. Holzapfel BM, Geitner U, Diebold J et al. (2009). Synovial hemangioma of the knee joint with cystic invasion of the femur: a case report and review of the literature. Arch Orthop Trauma Surg 129: 143–148.

1206. Hondar Wu HT, Chen W, Lee O et al. (2006). Imaging and pathological correlation of soft-tissue chondroma: a serial five-case study and literature review. Clin Imaging 30: 32–36.

1207. Hoogerwerf WA, Hawkins AL, Perlman EJ et al. (1994). Chromosome analysis of nine osteosarcomas. Genes Chromosomes Cancer 9: 88–92.

1208. Hoot AC, Russo P, Judkins AR et al. (2004). Immunohistochemical analysis of hSNF5/INI1 distinguishes renal and extra-renal malignant rhabdoid tumors from other pediatric soft tissue tumors. Am J Surg Pathol 28: 1485–1491.

1209. Hopkins SM, Freitas EL (1965). Bilateral osteochondroma of the ribs in an infant: an unusual cause of cyanosis. J Thorac Cardiovasc Surg 49: 247–249.

1210. Hopyan S, Gokgoz N, Poon R et al. (2002). A mutant PTH/PTHrP type I receptor in enchondromatosis. Nat Genet 30: 306–310.

1211. Hopyan S, Nadesan P, Yu C et al. (2005). Dysregulation of hedgehog signalling predisposes to synovial chondromatosis. J Pathol 206: 143–150.

1212. Horii E, Sugiura Y, Nakamura R (1998). A syndrome of digital fibromas, facial pigmentary dysplasia, and metacarpal and metatarsal disorganization. Am J Med Genet 80: 1–5.

1213. Hornick JL, Bosenberg MW, Mentzel T et al. (2004). Pleomorphic liposarcoma: clinicopathologic analysis of 57 cases. Am J Surg Pathol 28: 1257–1267.

1214. Hornick JL, Bundock EA, Fletcher CD (2009). Hybrid schwannoma/perineurioma: clinicopathologic analysis of 42 distinctive benign nerve sheath tumors. Am J Surg Pathol 33: 1554–1561.

1215. Hornick JL, Dal Cin P, Fletcher CD (2009). Loss of INI1 expression is characteristic of both conventional and proximal-type epithelioid sarcoma. Am J Surg Pathol 33: 542–550.

1216. Hornick JL, Fletcher CD (2003). Myoepithelial tumors of soft tissue: a clinicopathologic and immunohistochemical study of 101 cases with evaluation of prognostic parameters. Am J Surg Pathol 27: 1183–1196.

1217. Hornick JL, Fletcher CD (2004). Cutaneous myoepithelioma: a clinicopathologic and immunohistochemical study of 14 cases. Hum Pathol 35: 14–24.

1218. Hornick JL, Fletcher CD (2005). Intestinal perineuriomas: clinicopathologic definition of a new anatomic subset in a series of 10 cases. Am J Surg Pathol 29: 859–865.

1219. Hornick JL, Fletcher CD (2005). Intraabdominal cystic lymphangiomas obscured by marked superimposed reactive changes: clinicopathological analysis of a series. Hum Pathol 36: 426–432.

1220. Hornick JL, Fletcher CD (2005). Soft tissue perineurioma: clinicopathologic analysis of 81 cases including those with atypical histologic features. Am J Surg Pathol 29: 845–858.

1221. Hornick JL, Fletcher CD (2006). PEComa: what do we know so far? Histopathology 48: 75–82.

1222. Hornick JL, Fletcher CD (2007). Cellular neurothekeoma: detailed characterization in a series of 133 cases. Am J Surg Pathol 31: 329–340.

1223. Hornick JL, Fletcher CD (2008). Sclerosing PEComa: clinicopathologic analysis of a distinctive variant with a predilection for the retroperitoneum. Am J Surg Pathol 32: 493–501.

1224. Hornick JL, Fletcher CD (2011). Pseudomyogenic hemangioendothelioma: a distinctive, often multicentric tumor with indolent behavior. Am J Surg Pathol 35: 190–201.

1225. Horowitz JM, Park SH, Bogenmann E et al. (1990). Frequent inactivation of the retinoblastoma anti-oncogene is restricted to a subset of human tumor cells. Proc Natl Acad Sci U S A 87: 2775–2779.

1226. Horsthemke B, Barnert HJ, Greger V et al. (1987). Early diagnosis in hereditary retinoblastoma by detection of molecular deletions at gene locus. Lancet 1: 511–512.

1227. Horvath A, Bertherat J, Groussin L et al. (2010). Mutations and polymorphisms in the gene encoding regulatory subunit type 1-alpha of protein kinase A (PRKAR1A): an update. Hum Mutat 31: 369–379.

1228. Hosalkar H, Greenberg J, Gaugler RL et al. (2007). Abnormal scarring with keloid formation after osteochondroma excision in children with multiple hereditary exostoses. J Pediatr Orthop 27: 333–337.

1229. Hoshi M, Matsumoto S, Manabe J et al. (2006). Malignant change secondary to fibrous dysplasia. Int J Clin Oncol 11: 229–235.

1230. Hostein I, Pelmus M, Aurias A et al. (2004). Evaluation of MDM2 and CDK4 amplification by real-time PCR on paraffin wax-embedded material: a potential tool for the diagnosis of atypical lipomatous tumours/well-differentiated liposarcomas. J Pathol 202: 95–102.

1231. Hottenrott G, Mentzel T, Peters A et al. (1999). Intravascular ("intimal") epithelioid angiosarcoma: clinicopathological and immunohistochemical analysis of three cases. Virchows Arch 435: 473–478.

1232. Howard GM, Ellsworth RM (1965). Differential diagnosis of retinoblastoma. A statistical survey of 500 children. I. Relative frequency of the lesions which simulate retinoblastoma. Am J Ophthalmol 60: 610–618.

1233. Howard GM, Ellsworth RM (1965). Differential diagnosis of retinoblastoma. A statistical survey of 500 children. II. Factors relating to the diagnosis of retinoblastoma. Am J Ophthalmol 60: 618–621.

1234. Howat AJ, Campbell PE (1987). Angiomatosis: a vascular malformation of infancy and childhood. Report of 17 cases. Pathology 19: 377–382.

1235. Howley S, Stack D, Morris T et al. (2012). Ectomesenchymoma with t(1;12)(p32;p13) evolving from embryonal rhabdomyosarcoma shows no rearrangement of ETV6. Hum Pathol 43: 299–302.

1236. Howman-Giles R, McCowage G, Kellie S et al. (2012). Extrarenal malignant rhabdoid tumor in childhood: application of 18F-FDG PET/CT. J Pediatr Hematol Oncol 34: 17–21.

1237. Hox V, Vander Poorten V, Delaere PR et al. (2009). Extramammary myofibroblastoma in the head and neck region. Head Neck 31: 1240–1244.

1238. Hoyer JD, Hanson CA, Fonseca R et al. (2000). The (11;14)(q13;q32) translocation in multiple myeloma. A morphologic and immunohistochemical study. Am J Clin Pathol 113: 831–837.

1239. Hsieh PP, Tseng HH, Chang ST et al. (2006). Primary non-Hodgkin's lymphoma of bone: a rare disorder with high frequency of T-cell phenotype in southern Taiwan. Leuk Lymphoma 47: 65–70.

1240. Huang D, Sumegi J, Dal Cin P et al. (2010). C11orf95-MKL2 is the resulting fusion oncogene of t(11;16)(q13;p13) in chondroid lipoma. Genes Chromosomes Cancer 49: 810–818.

1241. Huang HY, Hsieh MJ, Chen WJ et al. (2002). Primary mesenchymal chondrosarcoma of the lung. Ann Thorac Surg 73: 1960–1962.

1242. Huang HY, Illei PB, Zhao Z et al. (2005). Ewing sarcomas with p53 mutation or p16/p14ARF homozygous deletion: a highly lethal subset associated with poor chemoresponse. J Clin Oncol 23: 548–558.

1243. Huang HY, Lal P, Qin J et al. (2004). Low-grade myxofibrosarcoma: a clinicopathologic analysis of 49 cases treated at a single institution with simultaneous assessment of the efficacy of 3-tier and 4-tier grading systems. Hum Pathol 35: 612–621.

1244. Huang L, Teng XY, Cheng YY et al. (2004). Expression of preosteoblast markers and Cbfa-1 and Osterix gene transcripts in stromal tumour cells of giant cell tumour of bone. Bone 34: 393–401.

1245. Huebner-Chan D, Fernandes B, Yang G et al. (2001). An immunophenotypic and molecular study of primary large B-cell lymphoma of bone. Mod Pathol 14: 1000–1007.

1246. Hughes AE, Ralston SH, Marken J et al. (2000). Mutations in TNFRSF11A, affecting the signal peptide of RANK, cause familial expansile osteolysis. Nat Genet 24: 45–48.

1247. Huh WW, Yuen C, Munsell M et al. (2011). Liposarcoma in children and young adults: a multi-institutional experience. Pediatr Blood Cancer 57: 1142–1146.

1248. Hulsebos TJ, Plomp AS, Wolterman RA et al. (2007). Germline mutation of INI1/SMARCB1 in familial schwannomatosis. Am J Hum Genet 80: 805–810.

1249. Humphreys S, Pambakian H, McKee PH et al. (1986). Soft tissue chondroma—a study of 15 tumours. Histopathology 10: 147–159.

1250. Hunt SJ, Santa Cruz DJ, Barr RJ (1990). Cellular angiolipoma. Am J Surg Pathol 14: 75–81.

1251. Husein OF, Collins M, Kang DR (2008). Neuroglial heterotopia causing neonatal airway obstruction: presentation, management, and literature review. Eur J Pediatr 167: 1351–1355.

1252. Huson SM, Compston DA, Clark P et al. (1989). A genetic study of von Recklinghausen neurofibromatosis in south east Wales. I. Prevalence, fitness, mutation rate, and effect of parental transmission on severity. J Med Genet 26: 704–711.

1253. Hussong JW, Brown M, Perkins SL et al. (1999). Comparison of DNA ploidy, histologic, and immunohistochemical findings with clinical outcome in inflammatory myofibroblastic tumors. Mod Pathol 12: 279–286.

1254. Hutter G, Nowak D, Blau IW et al. (2009). Auer rod-like intracytoplasmic inclusions in multiple myeloma. A case report and review of the literature. Int J Lab Hematol 31: 236–240.

1255. Hutter RV, Stewart FW, Foote Jr FW (1962). Fasciitis. A report of 70 cases with follow-up proving the benignity of the lesion. Cancer 15: 992–1003.

1256. Huvos AG (1991). Bone tumors: diagnosis, treatment and prognosis. Second edition.

WB Saunders Company.

1257. Huvos AG (2001). Malignant surface lesions of bone. Curr Diag Path 7: 247–250.

1258. Huvos AG (1999). Bone tumors: diagnosis, treatment and prognosis. Second edition. WB Saunders Company.

1259. Huvos AG, Butler A, Bretsky SS (1983). Osteogenic sarcoma associated with Paget's disease of bone. A clinicopathologic study of 65 patients. Cancer 52: 1489–1495.

1260. Huvos AG, Heilweil M, Bretsky SS (1985). The pathology of malignant fibrous histiocytoma of bone. A study of 130 patients. Am J Surg Pathol 9: 853–871.

1261. Huvos AG, Higinbotham NL (1975). Primary fibrosarcoma of bone. A clinicopathologic study of 130 patients. Cancer 35: 837–847.

1262. Huvos AG, Marcove RC, Erlandson RA et al. (1972). Chondroblastoma of bone. A clinicopathologic and electron microscopic study. Cancer 29: 760–771.

1263. Huvos AG, Rosen G, Dabska M et al. (1983). Mesenchymal chondrosarcoma. A clinicopathologic analysis of 35 patients with emphasis on treatment. Cancer 51: 1230–1237.

1264. Huvos AG, Woodard HQ, Cahan WG et al. (1985). Postradiation osteogenic sarcoma of bone and soft tissues. A clinicopathologic study of 66 patients. Cancer 55: 1244–1255.

1265. Huvos AG, Woodard HQ, Heilweil M (1986). Postradiation malignant fibrous histiocytoma of bone. A clinicopathologic study of 20 patients. Am J Surg Pathol 10: 9–18.

1266. Huwait H, Meneghetti A, Nielsen TO (2011). Kaposi sarcoma of the adrenal gland resembling epithelioid angiosarcoma: a case report. Sarcoma 2011: 898257

1267. Hwang JS, Beebe KS, Rojas J et al. (2011). Malignant granular cell tumor of the thigh. Orthopedics 34: e428–e431.

1268. Hwang SJ, Lozano G, Amos CI et al. (2003). Germline p53 mutations in a cohort with childhood sarcoma: sex differences in cancer risk. Am J Hum Genet 72: 975–983.

1269. Hyman SL, Gill DS, Shores EA et al. (2007). T2 hyperintensities in children with neurofibromatosis type 1 and their relationship to cognitive functioning. J Neurol Neurosurg Psychiatry 78: 1088–1091.

1270. IARC (1999). Surgical implants and other foreign bodies. IARC Monogr Eval Carcinog Risks Hum 74: i–409.

1271. Ichinose H, Wickstrom JK, Hoerner HE et al. (1979). The early clinical presentation of synovial sarcoma. Clin Orthop Relat Res 142:185–189.

1272. Ida CM, Rolig KA, Hulshizer RL et al. (2007). Myxoinflammatory fibroblastic sarcoma showing t(2;6)(q31;p21.3) as a sole cytogenetic abnormality. Cancer Genet Cytogenet 177: 139–142.

1273. Ida CM, Wang X, Erickson-Johnson MR et al. (2008). Primary retroperitoneal lipoma: a soft tissue pathology heresy? Report of a case with classic histologic, cytogenetics, and molecular genetic features. Am J Surg Pathol 32: 951–954.

1274. Idbaih A, Coindre JM, Derre J et al. (2005). Myxoid malignant fibrous histiocytoma and pleomorphic liposarcoma share very similar genomic imbalances. Lab Invest 85: 176–181.

1275. Ide F, Mishima K, Yamada H et al. (2008). Perivascular myoid tumors of the oral region: a clinicopathologic re-evaluation of 35 cases. J Oral Pathol Med 37: 43–49.

1276. Ideguchi M, Kajiwara K, Yoshikawa K et al. (2009). Benign fibrous histiocytoma of the skull with increased intracranial pressure caused by cerebral venous sinus occlusion. J Neurosurg 111: 504–508.

1277. Idowu BD, Al-Adnani M, O'Donnell P et al. (2007). A sensitive mutation-specific screening technique for GNAS1 mutations in cases of fibrous dysplasia: the first report of a codon 227 mutation in bone. Histopathology 50: 691–704.

1278. Iezzoni JC, Fechner RE, Wong LS et al. (1995). Aggressive angiomyxoma in males. A report of four cases. Am J Clin Pathol 104: 391–396.

1279. Iiboshi Y, Azuma T, Kitayama Y et al. (2003). Successful excision of a congenital, prenatally diagnosed fibrosarcoma involving the entire right ovary. Pediatr Surg Int 19: 683–685.

1280. Ikediobi NI, Iyengar V, Hwang L et al. (2003). Infantile myofibromatosis: support for autosomal dominant inheritance. J Am Acad Dermatol 49: S148–S150.

1281. Insabato L, Siano M, Somma A et al. (2009). Extrapleural solitary fibrous tumor: a clinicopathologic study of 19 cases. Int J Surg Pathol 17: 250–254.

1282. International Myeloma Working Group (2003). Criteria for the classification of monoclonal gammopathies, multiple myeloma and related disorders: a report of the International Myeloma Working Group. Br J Haematol 121: 749–757.

1283. Ioachim HL, Adsay V, Giancotti FR et al. (1995). Kaposi's sarcoma of internal organs. A multiparameter study of 86 cases. Cancer 75: 1376–1385.

1284. Iolascon A, Faienza MF, Coppola B et al. (1996). Analysis of cyclin-dependent kinase inhibitor genes (CDKN2A, CDKN2B, and CDKN2C) in childhood rhabdomyosarcoma. Genes Chromosomes Cancer 15: 217–222.

1285. Ippolito E, Bray EW, Corsi A et al. (2003). Natural history and treatment of fibrous dysplasia of bone: a multicenter clinicopathologic study promoted by the European Pediatric Orthopaedic Society. J Pediatr Orthop B 12: 155–177.

1286. Iqbal CW, St Peter S, Ishitani MB (2011). Pediatric dermatofibrosarcoma protuberans: multi-institutional outcomes. J Surg Res 170: 69–72.

1287. Isaacs H, Jr. (1985). Perinatal (congenital and neonatal) neoplasms: a report of 110 cases. Pediatr Pathol 3: 165–216.

1288. Isaacs H, Jr. (2010). Fetal and neonatal rhabdoid tumor. J Pediatr Surg 45: 619–626.

1289. Ishida T, Iijima T, Kikuchi F et al. (1992). A clinicopathological and immunohistochemical study of osteofibrous dysplasia, differentiated adamantinoma, and adamantinoma of long bones. Skeletal Radiol 21: 493–502.

1290. Ishida T, Yamamoto M, Goto T et al. (1999). Clear cell chondrosarcoma of the pelvis in a skeletally immature patient. Skeletal Radiol 28: 290–293.

1291. Itakura E, Tamiya S, Morita K et al. (2001). Subcellular distribution of cytokeratin and vimentin in malignant rhabdoid tumor: three-dimensional imaging with confocal laser scanning microscopy and double immunofluorescence. Mod Pathol 14: 854–861.

1292. Itala A, Leerapun T, Inwards C et al. (2005). An institutional review of clear cell chondrosarcoma. Clin Orthop Relat Res 440: 209–212.

1293. Italiano A, Bianchini L, Gjernes E et al. (2009). Clinical and biological significance of CDK4 amplification in well-differentiated and dedifferentiated liposarcomas. Clin Cancer Res 15: 5696–5703.

1294. Italiano A, Bianchini L, Keslair F et al. (2008). HMGA2 is the partner of MDM2 in well-differentiated and dedifferentiated liposarcomas whereas CDK4 belongs to a distinct inconsistent amplicon. Int J Cancer 122: 2233–2241.

1295. Italiano A, Cardot N, Dupre F et al. (2007). Gains and complex rearrangements of the 12q13-15 chromosomal region in ordinary lipomas: the "missing link" between lipomas and liposarcomas? Int J Cancer 121: 308–315.

1296. Italiano A, Chambonniere ML, Attias R et al. (2008). Monosomy 7 and absence of 12q amplification in two cases of spindle cell liposarcomas. Cancer Genet Cytogenet 184: 99–104.

1297. Italiano A, Ebran N, Attias R et al. (2008). NFIB rearrangement in superficial, retroperitoneal, and colonic lipomas with aberrations involving chromosome band 9p22. Genes Chromosomes Cancer 47: 971–977.

1298. Italiano A, Maire G, Sirvent N et al. (2009). Variability of origin for the neocentromeric sequences in analphoid supernumerary marker chromosomes of well-differentiated liposarcomas. Cancer Lett 273: 323–330.

1299. Italiano A, Sung YS, Zhang L et al. (2012). High prevalence of CIC fusion with double-homeobox (DUX4) transcription factors in EWSR1-negative undifferentiated small blue round cell sarcomas. Genes Chromosomes Cancer 51: 207–218.

1300. Iversen UM (1996). Two cases of benign vaginal rhabdomyoma. Case reports. APMIS 104: 575–578.

1301. Iwasa Y, Fletcher CD (2004). Cellular angiofibroma: clinicopathologic and immunohistochemical analysis of 51 cases. Am J Surg Pathol 28: 1426–1435.

1302. Iwasaki H, Enjoji M (1979). Infantile and adult fibrosarcomas of the soft tissues. Acta Pathol Jpn 29: 377–388.

1303. Izquierdo FM, Ramos LR, Sanchez-Herraez S et al. (2010). Dedifferentiated classic adamantinoma of the tibia: a report of a case with eventual complete revertant mesenchymal phenotype. Am J Surg Pathol 34: 1388–1392.

1304. Izumi T, Oda Y, Hasegawa T et al. (2006). Prognostic significance of dysadherin expression in epithelioid sarcoma and its diagnostic utility in distinguishing epithelioid sarcoma from malignant rhabdoid tumor. Mod Pathol 19: 820–831.

1305. Jackson EM, Sievert AJ, Gai X et al. (2009). Genomic analysis using high-density single nucleotide polymorphism-based oligonucleotide arrays and multiplex ligation-dependent probe amplification provides a comprehensive analysis of INI1/SMARCB1 in malignant rhabdoid tumors. Clin Cancer Res 15: 1923–1930.

1306. Jackson RP, Reckling FW, Mants FA (1977). Osteoid osteoma and osteoblastoma. Similar histologic lesions with different natural histories. Clin Orthop Relat Res 128:303–313.

1307. Jacobs JL, Merriam JC, Chadburn A et al. (1994). Mesenchymal chondrosarcoma of the orbit. Report of three new cases and review of the literature. Cancer 73: 399–405.

1308. Jacoby LB, Jones D, Davis K et al. (1997). Molecular analysis of the NF2 tumor-suppressor gene in schwannomatosis. Am J Hum Genet 61: 1293–1302.

1309. Jacoby LB, MacCollin M, Barone R et al. (1996). Frequency and distribution of NF2 mutations in schwannomas. Genes Chromosomes Cancer 17: 45–55.

1310. Jacoby LB, MacCollin M, Louis DN et al. (1994). Exon scanning for mutation of the NF2 gene in schwannomas. Hum Mol Genet 3: 413–419.

1311. Jaffe H.L., Lichtenstein L. (1944). Eosinophilic granuloma of bone: a condition affecting one, several or many bones, but apparently limited to the skeleton and representing the mildest clinical expression of the peculiar inflammatory histiocytosis also underlying Letterer-Siwe disease and Schuller-Christian disease. Arch Pathol 37:99-118.

1312. Jaffe HL (1953). Osteoid-osteoma. Proc R Soc Med 46: 1007–1012.

1313. Jaffe HL, Lichtenstein L (1942). Non-osteogenic fibroma of bone. Am J Pathol 18: 205–221.

1314. Jaffe HL, Lichtenstein L, Sutro CJ (1941). Pigmented villonodular synovitis, bursitis and tenosynovitis: a discussion of the synovial and bursal equivalents of the tenosynovial lesion commonly denoted as xanthoma, xanthogranuloma, giant cell tumor or myeloplaxoma of the tendon sheath, with some consideration of this tendon sheath lesion itself. Arch Pathol 31: 731–765.

1315. Jager M, Westhoff B, Portier S et al. (2007). Clinical outcome and genotype in patients with hereditary multiple exostoses. J Orthop Res 25: 1541–1551.

1316. Jakowski JD, Wakely PE, Jr. (2008). Primary intrathoracic low-grade fibromyxoid sarcoma. Hum Pathol 39: 623–628.

1317. Jalali M, Netscher DT, Connelly JH (2002). Glomangiomatosis. Ann Diagn Pathol 6: 326–328.

1318. Janeway KA, Kim SY, Lodish M et al. (2011). Defects in succinate dehydrogenase in gastrointestinal stromal tumors lacking KIT and PDGFRA mutations. Proc Natl Acad Sci U S A 108: 314–318.

1319. Janoyer M, Reau AF, Pontallier JR et al. (1999). Congenital fibrous hamartoma of the hand: a case report. J Pediatr Orthop B 8: 129–131.

1320. Janzer RC, Makek M (1983). Intraoral malignant melanotic schwannoma. Ultrastructural evidence for melanogenesis by Schwann's cells. Arch Pathol Lab Med 107: 298–301.

1321. Jarvi OH, Lansimies PH (1975). Subclinical elastofibromas in the scapular region in an autopsy series. Acta Pathol Microbiol Scand A 83: 87–108.

1322. Jarvi OH, Saxen AE, Hopsu-Havu VK et al. (1969). Elastofibroma—a degenerative pseudotumor. Cancer 23: 42–63.

1323. Jebson PJ, Louis DS (1997). Fibrous hamartoma of infancy in the hand: a case report. J Hand Surg Am 22: 740–742.

1324. Jee WH, Choi KH, Choe BY et al. (1996). Fibrous dysplasia: MR imaging characteristics with radiopathologic correlation. AJR Am J Roentgenol 167: 1523–1527.

1325. Jelinek JS, Kransdorf MJ, Shmookler BM et al. (1994). Giant cell tumor of the tendon sheath: MR findings in nine cases. AJR Am J Roentgenol 162: 919–922.

1326. Jennes I, Pedrini E, Zuntini M et al. (2009). Multiple osteochondromas: mutation update and description of the multiple osteochondromas mutation database (MOdb). Hum Mutat 30: 1620–1627.

1327. Jennes I, Zuntini M, Mees K et al. (2012). Identification and functional characterization of the human EXT1 promoter region. Gene 492: 148–159.

1328. Jensen OA, Bretlau P (1990). Melanotic schwannoma of the orbit. Immunohistochemical and ultrastructural study of a case and survey of the literature. APMIS 98: 713–723.

1329. Jeon DG, Song WS, Kong CB et al. (2011). MFH of bone and osteosarcoma show similar survival and chemosensitivity. Clin Orthop Relat Res 469: 584–590.

1330. Jeon IS, Davis JN, Braun BS et al. (1995). A variant Ewing's sarcoma translocation (7;22) fuses the EWS gene to the ETS gene ETV1. Oncogene 10: 1229–1234.

1331. Jha P, Moosavi C, Fanburg-Smith JC (2007). Giant cell fibroblastoma: an update and addition of 86 new cases from the Armed Forces Institute of Pathology, in honor of Dr. Franz M. Enzinger. Ann Diagn Pathol 11: 81–88.

1332. Jhala D, Coventry S, Rao P et al. (2008). Juvenile juxtacortical chondromyxoid fibroma of bone: a case report. Hum Pathol 39: 960–965.

1333. Jhala DN, Eltoum I, Carroll AJ et al. (2003). Osteosarcoma in a patient with McCune-Albright syndrome and Mazabraud's syndrome: a case report emphasizing the cytological and cytogenetic findings. Hum Pathol 34: 1354–1357.

1334. Jin B, Saleh H (2009). Pitfalls in the diagnosis of adult rhabdomyoma by fine needle aspiration: report of a case and a brief literature review. Diagn Cytopathol 37: 483–486.

1335. Johnson L (1972). Congenital pseudoarthrosis, adamantinoma of long bone and intracortical fibrous dysplasia of the tibia. J Bone Joint Surg Am 54A: 1355

1336. Johnson MD, Glick AD, Davis BW (1988). Immunohistochemical evaluation of Leu-7, myelin basic-protein, S100-protein, glial-fibrillary acidic-protein, and LN3 immunoreactivity in nerve sheath tumors and sarcomas. Arch Pathol Lab Med 112: 155–160.

1337. Johnson RL, Rothman AL, Xie J et al. (1996). Human homolog of patched, a candidate gene for the basal cell nevus syndrome. Science 272: 1668–1671.

1338. Johnsson A, Collin A, Rydholm A et al. (2007). Unstable translocation (8;22) in a case of giant cell reparative granuloma. Cancer Genet Cytogenet 177: 59–63.

1339. Jokinen CH, Ragsdale BD, Argenyi ZB (2010). Expanding the clinicopathologic spectrum of palisaded encapsulated neuroma. J Cutan Pathol 37: 43–48.

1340. Jones D, Bhatia VK, Krausz T et al. (1999). Crystal-storing histiocytosis: a disorder occurring in plasmacytic tumors expressing immunoglobulin kappa light chain. Hum Pathol 30: 1441–1448.

1341. Jones EW, Bleehen SS (1969). Inflammatory angiomatous nodules with abnormal blood vessels occurring about the ears and scalp (pseudo or atypical pyogenic granuloma). Br J Dermatol 81: 804–816.

1342. Jones FE, Soule EH, Coventry MB (1969). Fibrous xanthoma of synovium (giant-cell tumor of tendon sheath, pigmented nodular synovitis). A study of one hundred and eighteen cases. J Bone Joint Surg Am 51: 76–86.

1343. Jones KB, Piombo V, Searby C et al. (2010). A mouse model of osteochondromagenesis from clonal inactivation of Ext1 in chondrocytes. Proc Natl Acad Sci U S A 107: 2054–2059.

1344. Jones WA (1933). Familial multilocular cystic disease of the jaws. Am J Ca 17: 946–950.

1345. Jones WA, Gerrie J, Pritchard J (1950). Cherubism—familial fibrous dysplasia of the jaws. J Bone Joint Surg Br 32-B: 334–347.

1346. Joshi D, Anderson JR, Paidas C et al. (2004). Age is an independent prognostic factor in rhabdomyosarcoma: a report from the Soft Tissue Sarcoma Committee of the Children's Oncology Group. Pediatr Blood Cancer 42: 64–73.

1347. Joste NE, Racz MI, Montgomery KD et al. (2004). Clonal chromosome abnormalities in a plexiform cellular schwannoma. Cancer Genet Cytogenet 150: 73–77.

1348. Joyama S, Ueda T, Shimizu K et al. (1999). Chromosome rearrangement at 17q25 and xp11.2 in alveolar soft-part sarcoma: A case report and review of the literature. Cancer 86: 1246–1250.

1349. Jundt G, Moll C, Nidecker A et al. (1994). Primary leiomyosarcoma of bone: report of eight cases. Hum Pathol 25: 1205–1212.

1350. Jundt G, Remberger K, Roessner A et al. (1995). Adamantinoma of long bones. A histopathological and immunohistochemical study of 23 cases. Pathol Res Pract 191: 112–120.

1351. Jung AL, Johnson DG, Condon VR et al. (1994). Congenital chest wall mesenchymal hamartoma. J Perinatol 14: 487–491.

1352. Jung GH, Kim JD, Cho Y et al. (2010). A 9-month-old phosphaturic mesenchymal tumor mimicking the intractable rickets. J Pediatr Orthop B 19: 127–132.

1353. Jung SM, Chang PY, Luo CC et al. (2005). Lipoblastoma/lipoblastomatosis: a clinicopathologic study of 16 cases in Taiwan. Pediatr Surg Int 21: 809–812.

1354. Jurcic V, Zidar A, Montiel MD et al. (2002). Myxoinflammatory fibroblastic sarcoma: a tumor not restricted to acral sites. Ann Diagn Pathol 6: 272–280.

1355. Kabasawa Y, Katsube K, Harada H et al. (2007). A male infant case of lipofibromatosis in the submental region exhibited the expression of the connective tissue growth factor. Oral Surg Oral Med Oral Pathol Oral Radiol Endod 103: 677–682.

1356. Kalil RK, Inwards CY, Unni KK et al. (2000). Dedifferentiated clear cell chondrosarcoma. Am J Surg Pathol 24: 1079–1086.

1357. Kalinina J, Carroll A, Wang L et al. (2012). Detection of "oncometabolite" 2-hydroxyglutarate by magnetic resonance analysis as a biomarker of IDH1/2 mutations in glioma. J Mol Med (Berl) 90: 1161–1171.

1358. Kamarashev J, French LE, Dummer R et al. (2009). Symplastic glomus tumor - a rare but distinct benign histological variant with analogy to other 'ancient' benign skin neoplasms. J Cutan Pathol 36: 1099–1102.

1359. Kambham N, Kong C, Longacre TA et al. (2005). Utility of syndecan-1 (CD138) expression in the diagnosis of undifferentiated malignant neoplasms: a tissue microarray study of 1,754 cases. Appl Immunohistochem Mol Morphol 13: 304–310.

1360. Kan AE, Rogers M (1989). Juvenile hyaline fibromatosis: an expanded clinicopathologic spectrum. Pediatr Dermatol 6: 68–75.

1361. Kanamori M, Antonescu CR, Scott M et al. (2001). Extra copies of chromosomes 7, 8, 12, 19, and 21 are recurrent in adamantinoma. J Mol Diagn 3: 16–21.

1362. Kanber D, Berulava T, Ammerpohl O et al. (2009). The human retinoblastoma gene is imprinted. PLoS Genet 5: e1000790SBD

1363. Kandil DH, Kida M, Laub DR et al. (2009). Sarcomatous transformation in a cellular angiofibroma: a case report. J Clin Pathol 62: 945–947.

1364. Kaneko T, Suzuki Y, Takata R et al. (2006). Extraskeletal mesenchymal chondrosarcoma of the kidney. Int J Urol 13: 285–286.

1365. Kaneko Y, Yoshida K, Handa M et al. (1996). Fusion of an ETS-family gene, EIAF, to EWS by t(17;22)(q12;q12) chromosome translocation in an undifferentiated sarcoma of infancy. Genes Chromosomes Cancer 15: 115–121.

1366. Kanik AB, Oh CH, Bhawan J (1995). Cellular angiolipoma. Am J Dermatopathol 17: 312–315.

1367. Kanner WA, Brill LB, Patterson JW et al. (2010). CD10, p63 and CD99 expression in the differential diagnosis of atypical fibroxanthoma, spindle cell squamous cell carcinoma and desmoplastic melanoma. J Cutan Pathol 37: 744–750.

1368. Kanter WR, Eldridge R, Fabricant R et al. (1980). Central neurofibromatosis with bilateral acoustic neuroma: genetic, clinical and biochemical distinctions from peripheral neurofibromatosis. Neurology 30: 851–859.

1369. Kanu A, Oermann CM, Malicki D et al. (2002). Pulmonary lipoblastoma in an 18-month-old child: a unique tumor in children. Pediatr Pulmonol 34: 150–154.

1370. Kapadia SB, Meis JM, Frisman DM et al. (1993). Fetal rhabdomyoma of the head and neck: a clinicopathologic and immunophenotypic study of 24 cases. Hum Pathol 24: 754–765.

1371. Kapukaya A, Subasi M, Dabak N et al. (2006). Osseous lipoma: eleven new cases and review of the literature. Acta Orthop Belg 72: 603–614.

1372. Karcioglu Z, Someren A, Mathes SJ (1977). Ectomesenchymoma. A malignant tumor of migratory neural crest (ectomesenchyme) remnants showing ganglionic, schwannian, melanocytic and rhabdomyoblastic differentiation. Cancer 39: 2486–2496.

1373. Karlsson L, Alpsten M, Appelgren KL et al. (1980). Intratumor distribution of vascular and extravascular spaces. Microvasc Res 19: 71–79.

1374. Karlsson P, Holmberg E, Samuelsson A et al. (1998). Soft tissue sarcoma after treatment for breast cancer—a Swedish population-based study. Eur J Cancer 34: 2068–2075.

1374A. Karol LA, Brown DS, Wise CA et al. (2005). Familial osteofibrous dysplasia. A case series. J Bone Joint Surg Am. 87:2297–2307.

1375. Karnak I, Senocak ME, Ciftci AO et al. (2001). Inflammatory myofibroblastic tumor in children: diagnosis and treatment. J Pediatr Surg 36: 908–912.

1376. Kashima TG, Dongre A, Flanagan AM et al. (2011). Podoplanin expression in adamantinoma of long bones and osteofibrous dysplasia. Virchows Arch 459: 41–46.

1377. Katodritou E, Dimopoulos MA, Zervas K et al. (2009). Update on the use of erythropoiesis-stimulating agents (ESAs) for the management of anemia of multiple myeloma and lymphoma. Cancer Treat Rev 35: 738–743.

1378. Katz JA, Mahoney DH, Shukla LW et al. (1988). Endovascular papillary angioendothelioma in the spleen. Pediatr Pathol 8: 185–193.

1379. Kaur S, Vauhkonen H, Bohling T et al. (2006). Gene copy number changes in dermatofibrosarcoma protuberans - a fine-resolution study using array comparative genomic hybridization. Cytogenet Genome Res 115: 283–288.

1380. Kawaguchi K, Oda Y, Saito T et al. (2003). Mechanisms of inactivation of the p16INK4a gene in leiomyosarcoma of soft tissue: decreased p16 expression correlates with promoter methylation and poor prognosis. J Pathol 201: 487–495.

1381. Kawaguchi K, Oda Y, Sakamoto A et al. (2002). Molecular analysis of p53, MDM2, and H-ras genes in osteosarcoma and malignant fibrous histiocytoma of bone in patients older than 40 years. Mod Pathol 15: 878–888.

1382. Kawamoto EH, Weidner N, Agostini RM, Jr. et al. (1987). Malignant ectomesenchymoma of soft tissue. Report of two cases and review of the literature. Cancer 59: 1791–1802.

1383. Kawamura-Saito M, Yamazaki Y, Kaneko K et al. (2006). Fusion between CIC and DUX4 up-regulates PEA3 family genes in Ewing-like sarcomas with t(4;19)(q35;q13) translocation. Hum Mol Genet 15: 2125–2137.

1384. Kawasaki G, Yanamoto S, Mizuno A et al. (2001). Juvenile hyaline fibromatosis complicated with oral squamous cell carcinoma: a case report. Oral Surg Oral Med Oral Pathol Oral Radiol Endod 91: 200–204.

1385. Kawashima A, Magid D, Fishman EK et al. (1993). Parosteal ossifying lipoma: CT and MR findings. J Comput Assist Tomogr 17: 147–150.

1386. Kawashima H, Ogose A, Umezu H et al. (2007). Ossifying fibromyxoid tumor of soft parts with clonal chromosomal aberrations. Cancer Genet Cytogenet 176: 156–160.

1387. Kaya H, Peressini B, Jawed I et al. (2012). Impact of age, race and decade of treatment on overall survival in a critical population analysis of 40,000 multiple myeloma patients. Int J Hematol 95: 64–70.

1388. Kazakov DV, Mukensnabl P, Hes O et al. (2004). 'Ectopic' ectopic hamartomatous thymoma. Histopathology 45: 202–204.

1389. Kazakov DV, Pitha J, Sima R et al. (2005). Hybrid peripheral nerve sheath tumors: Schwannoma-perineurioma and neurofibroma-perineurioma. A report of three cases in extradigital locations. Ann Diagn Pathol 9: 16–23.

1390. Kazmierczak B, Wanschura S, Meyer-Bolte K et al. (1995). Cytogenic and molecular analysis of an aggressive angiomyxoma. Am J Pathol 147: 580–585.

1391. Keasbey LE (1953). Juvenile aponeurotic fibroma (calcifying fibroma); a distinctive tumor arising in the palms and soles of young children. Cancer 6: 338–346.

1392. Keel SB, Jaffe KA, Petur Nielsen G et al. (2001). Orthopaedic implant-related sarcoma: a study of twelve cases. Mod Pathol 14: 969–977.

1393. Keel SB, Rosenberg AE (1999). Hemorrhagic epithelioid and spindle cell hemangioma: a newly recognized, unique vascular tumor of bone. Cancer 85: 1966–1972.

1394. Keeney GL, Unni KK, Beabout JW et al. (1989). Adamantinoma of long bones. A clinicopathologic study of 85 cases. Cancer 64: 730–737.

1395. Keller C, Arenkiel BR, Coffin CM et al. (2004). Alveolar rhabdomyosarcomas in conditional Pax3:Fkhr mice: cooperativity of Ink4a/ARF and Trp53 loss of function. Genes Dev 18: 2614–2626.

1396. Kelley MJ, Korczak JF, Sheridan E et al. (2001). Familial chordoma, a tumor of notochordal remnants, is linked to chromosome 7q33. Am J Hum Genet 69: 454–460.

1397. Kenan S, Floman Y, Robin GC et al. (1985). Aggressive osteoblastoma. A case report and review of the literature. Clin Orthop Relat Res 195:294–298.

1398. Kenan S, Klein M, Lewis MM (1989).

Juxtacortical liposarcoma. A case report and review of the literature. Clin Orthop Relat Res 243:225–229.

1399. Kenney B, Richkind KE, Friedlaender G et al. (2007). Chromosomal rearrangements in lipofibromatosis. Cancer Genet Cytogenet 179: 136–139.

1400. Kenney PJ, Gilula LA, Murphy WA (1981). The use of computed tomography to distinguish osteochondroma and chondrosarcoma. Radiology 139: 129–137.

1401. Kern WH (1960). Proliferative myositis; a pseudosarcomatous reaction to injury: a report of seven cases. Arch Pathol 69: 209–216.

1402. Keser G, Karabulut B, Oksel F et al. (1999). Two siblings with juvenile hyaline fibromatosis: case reports and review of the literature. Clin Rheumatol 18: 248–252.

1403. Kesserwan C, Sokolic R, Cowen EW et al. (2012). Multicentric dermatofibrosarcoma protuberans in patients with adenosine deaminase-deficient severe combined immune deficiency. J Allergy Clin Immunol 129: 762–769.

1404. Kevorkian J, Cento DP (1973). Leiomyosarcoma of large arteries and veins. Surgery 73: 390–400.

1404A. Keynan O, Fisher CG, O'Connell JX et al (2005). Mesenchymal hamartoma of the spine. A case report. J Bone Joint Surg Am 87:172–176.

1405. Khanna M, Delaney D, Tirabosco R et al. (2008). Osteofibrous dysplasia, osteofibrous dysplasia-like adamantinoma and adamantinoma: correlation of radiological imaging features with surgical histology and assessment of the use of radiology in contributing to needle biopsy diagnosis. Skeletal Radiol 37: 1077–1084.

1406. Khedhaier A, Maalla R, Ennouri K et al. (2007). Soft tissues chondromas of the hand: a report of five cases. Acta Orthop Belg 73: 458–461.

1407. Khoddami M, Bedard YC, Bell RS et al. (1996). Primary leiomyosarcoma of bone: report of seven cases and review of the literature. Arch Pathol Lab Med 120: 671–675.

1408. Kikuchi Y, Yamaguchi T, Kishi H et al. (2011). Pulmonary tumor with notochordal differentiation: report of 2 cases suggestive of benign notochordal cell tumor of extraosseous origin. Am J Surg Pathol 35: 1158–1164.

1409. Kilpatrick SE, Hitchcock MG, Kraus MD et al. (1997). Mixed tumors and myoepitheliomas of soft tissue: a clinicopathologic study of 19 cases with a unifying concept. Am J Surg Pathol 21: 13–22.

1410. Kilpatrick SE, Inwards CY, Fletcher CD et al. (1997). Myxoid chondrosarcoma (chordoid sarcoma) of bone: a report of two cases and review of the literature. Cancer 79: 1903–1910.

1411. Kilpatrick SE, Mentzel T, Fletcher CD (1994). Leiomyoma of deep soft tissue. Clinicopathologic analysis of a series. Am J Surg Pathol 18: 576–582.

1412. Kim B, Park SH, Min HS et al. (2004). Nasal chondromesenchymal hamartoma of infancy clinically mimicking meningoencephalocele. Pediatr Neurosurg 40: 136–140.

1413. Kim HS, Choi KH, Kim HO et al. (2009). A true chondroma cutis. J Eur Acad Dermatol Venereol 23: 612–613.

1414. Kim JY, Jung WH, Yoon CS et al. (2000). Mesenchymal hamartomas of the chest wall in infancy: radiologic and pathologic correlation. Yonsei Med J 41: 615–622.

1415. Kim S, Lee HJ, Jun HJ et al. (2008). The hTAF II 68-TEC fusion protein functions as a strong transcriptional activator. Int J Cancer 122: 2446–2453.

1416. Kim SH, Lee JH, Kim DC et al. (2007). Subcutaneous venous hemangioma of the breast. J Ultrasound Med 26: 1097–1100.

1417. Kim YH, Reiner L (1982). Ultrastructure of lipoma. Cancer 50: 102–106.

1418. Kimura Y, Morita T, Hayashi K et al. (2010). Myocardin functions as an effective inducer of growth arrest and differentiation in human uterine leiomyosarcoma cells. Cancer Res 70: 501–511.

1419. Kindblom LG, Angervall L, Fassina AS (1982). Atypical lipoma. Acta Pathol Microbiol Immunol Scand A 90: 27–36.

1420. Kindblom LG, Angervall L, Haglid K (1984). An immunohistochemical analysis of S-100 protein and glial fibrillary acidic protein in nasal glioma. Acta Pathol Microbiol Immunol Scand A 92: 387–389.

1421. Kindblom LG, Angervall L, Stener B et al. (1974). Intermuscular and intramuscular lipomas and hibernomas. A clinical, roentgenologic, histologic, and prognostic study of 46 cases. Cancer 33: 754–762.

1422. Kindblom LG, Lodding P, Angervall L (1983). Clear-cell sarcoma of tendons and aponeuroses. An immunohistochemical and electron microscopic analysis indicating neural crest origin. Virchows Arch A Pathol Anat Histopathol 401: 109–128.

1423. Kindblom LG, Meis-Kindblom JM (1995). Chondroid lipoma: an ultrastructural and immunohistochemical analysis with further observations regarding its differentiation. Hum Pathol 26: 706–715.

1424. Kindblom LG, Stener B, Angervall L (1974). Intramuscular myxoma. Cancer 34: 1737–1744.

1425. King DG, Saifuddin A, Preston HV et al. (1995). Magnetic resonance imaging of juxta-articular myxoma. Skeletal Radiol 24: 145–147.

1426. Kirkpatrick CJ, Alves A, Kohler H et al. (2000). Biomaterial-induced sarcoma: A novel model to study preneoplastic change. Am J Pathol 156: 1455–1467.

1427. Kirschner LS, Carney JA, Pack SD et al. (2000). Mutations of the gene encoding the protein kinase A type I-alpha regulatory subunit in patients with the Carney complex. Nat Genet 26: 89–92.

1428. Kirwan EO, Hutton PA, Pozo JL et al. (1984). Osteoid osteoma and benign osteoblastoma of the spine. Clinical presentation and treatment. J Bone Joint Surg Br 66: 21–26.

1429. Kitagawa Y, Wong F, Lo P et al. (1996). Overexpression of Bcl-2 and mutations in p53 and K-ras in resected human non-small cell lung cancers. Am J Respir Cell Mol Biol 15: 45–54.

1430. Kitao S, Shimamoto A, Goto M et al. (1999). Mutations in RECQL4 cause a subset of cases of Rothmund-Thomson syndrome. Nat Genet 22: 82–84.

1431. Kiuru-Kuhlefelt S, Sarlomo-Rikala M, Larramendy ML et al. (2000). FGF4 and INT2 oncogenes are amplified and expressed in Kaposi's sarcoma. Mod Pathol 13: 433–437.

1432. Kleer CG, Unni KK, McLeod RA (1996). Epithelioid hemangioendothelioma of bone. Am J Surg Pathol 20: 1301–1311.

1433. Kleihues P, Schauble B, zur Hausen A et al. (1997). Tumors associated with p53 germline mutations: a synopsis of 91 families. Am J Pathol 150: 1–13.

1434. Klein FA, Smith MJ, Kasenetz I (1988). Pelvic lipomatosis: 35-year experience. J Urol 139: 998–1001.

1435. Klein MJ, Bonar SF, Freemont T et al

(2011). Non-neoplastic diseases of bones and joints. Atlas of Nontumor Pathology. ARP: Washington.

1436. Kleinerman RA, Tucker MA, Tarone RE et al. (2005). Risk of new cancers after radiotherapy in long-term survivors of retinoblastoma: an extended follow-up. J Clin Oncol 23: 2272–2279.

1437. Kleinschmidt-DeMasters BK, Lovell MA, Donson AM et al. (2007). Molecular array analyses of 51 pediatric tumors shows overlap between malignant intracranial ectomesenchymoma and MPNST but not medulloblastoma or atypical teratoid rhabdoid tumor. Acta Neuropathol 113: 695–703.

1438. Kleinschmidt-DeMasters BK, Mierau GW, Sze CI et al. (1998). Unusual dural and skull-based mesenchymal neoplasms: a report of four cases. Hum Pathol 29: 240–245.

1439. Klijanienko J, Caillaud JM, Lagace R (2004). Fine-needle aspiration in liposarcoma: cytohistologic correlative study including well-differentiated, myxoid, and pleomorphic variants. Diagn Cytopathol 30: 307–312.

1440. Klopstock T, Naumann M, Seibel P et al. (1997). Mitochondrial DNA mutations in multiple symmetric lipomatosis. Mol Cell Biochem 174: 271–275.

1441. Kluin PM, Slootweg PJ, Schuurman HJ et al. (1984). Primary B-cell malignant lymphoma of the maxilla with a sarcomatous pattern and multilobated nuclei. Cancer 54: 1598–1605.

1442. Kluwe L, Siebert R, Gesk S et al. (2004). Screening 500 unselected neurofibromatosis 1 patients for deletions of the NF1 gene. Hum Mutat 23: 111–116.

1443. Knezevich SR, Garnett MJ, Pysher TJ et al. (1998). ETV6-NTRK3 gene fusions and trisomy 11 establish a histogenetic link between mesoblastic nephroma and congenital fibrosarcoma. Cancer Res 58: 5046–5048.

1444. Knezevich SR, McFadden DE, Tao W et al. (1998). A novel ETV6-NTRK3 gene fusion in congenital fibrosarcoma. Nat Genet 18: 184–187.

1445. Knight JC, Renwick PJ, Dal Cin P et al. (1995). Translocation t(12;16)(q13;p11) in myxoid liposarcoma and round cell liposarcoma: molecular and cytogenetic analysis. Cancer Res 55: 24–27.

1446. Knott PD, Gannon FH, Thompson LD (2003). Mesenchymal chondrosarcoma of the sinonasal tract: a clinicopathological study of 13 cases with a review of the literature. Laryngoscope 113: 783–790.

1447. Knowles DM, Pirog EC (2001). Pathology of AIDS-related lymphomas and other AIDS-defining neoplasms. Eur J Cancer 37: 1236–1250.

1448. Knudson AG, Jr. (1971). Mutation and cancer: statistical study of retinoblastoma. Proc Natl Acad Sci U S A 68: 820–823.

1449. Knutsen T, Gobu V, Knaus R et al. (2005). The interactive online SKY/M-FISH & CGH database and the Entrez cancer chromosomes search database: linkage of chromosomal aberrations with the genome sequence. Genes Chromosomes Cancer 44: 52–64.

1450. Kobayashi H, Kaneko G, Uchida A (2010). Retroperitoneal venous hemangioma. Int J Urol 17: 585–586.

1451. Kodet R, Kasthuri N, Marsden HB et al. (1986). Gangliorhabdomyosarcoma: a histopathological and immunohistochemical study of three cases. Histopathology 10: 181–193.

1452. Kodet R, Newton WA, Jr., Sachs N et al.

(1991). Rhabdoid tumors of soft tissues: a clinicopathologic study of 26 cases enrolled on the Intergroup Rhabdomyosarcoma Study. Hum Pathol 22: 674–684.

1453. Kodet R, Stejskal J, Pilat D et al. (1996). Congenital-infantile fibrosarcoma: a clinicopathological study of five patients entered on the Prague children's tumor registry. Pathol Res Pract 192: 845–853.

1454. Koga T, Iwasaki H, Ishiguro M et al. (2002). Losses in chromosomes 17, 19, and 22q in neurofibromatosis type 1 and sporadic neurofibromas: a comparative genomic hybridization analysis. Cancer Genet Cytogenet 136: 113–120.

1455. Kogon B, Shehata B, Katzenstein H et al. (2011). Primary congenital infantile fibrosarcoma of the heart: the first confirmed case. Ann Thorac Surg 91: 1276–1280.

1456. Kohashi K, Izumi T, Oda Y et al. (2009). Infrequent SMARCB1/INI1 gene alteration in epithelioid sarcoma: a useful tool in distinguishing epithelioid sarcoma from malignant rhabdoid tumor. Hum Pathol 40: 349–355.

1457. Koizumi H, Mikami M, Doi M et al. (2005). Clonality analysis of nodular fasciitis by HUMARA-methylation-specific PCR. Histopathology 47: 320–321.

1458. Kojimahara M, Baba Y, Nakajima T (1987). Ultrastructural study of hemangiomas. 5. Glomus tumor (Masson). Acta Pathol Jpn 37: 605–609.

1459. Kondo S, Yoshizaki T, Minato H et al. (2001). Myofibrosarcoma of the nasal cavity and paranasal sinus. Histopathology 39: 216–217.

1460. Konishi E, Kusuzaki K, Murata H et al. (2001). Extraskeletal osteosarcoma arising in myositis ossificans. Skeletal Radiol 30: 39–43.

1461. Konishi E, Nakashima Y, Iwasa Y et al. (2010). Immunohistochemical analysis for Sox9 reveals the cartilaginous character of chondroblastoma and chondromyxoid fibroma of the bone. Hum Pathol 41: 208–213.

1462. Konrad EA, Meister P, Hubner G (1982). Extracardiac rhabdomyoma: report of different types with light microscopic and ultrastructural studies. Cancer 49: 898–907.

1463. Konwaler BE, Keasbey L, Kaplan L (1955). Subcutaneous pseudosarcomatous fibromatosis (fasciitis). Am J Clin Pathol 25: 241–252.

1464. Kopelman JE, McLean IW, Rosenberg SH (1987). Multivariate analysis of risk factors for metastasis in retinoblastoma treated by enucleation. Ophthalmology 94: 371–377.

1465. Koscielniak E, Rodary C, Flamant F et al. (1992). Metastatic rhabdomyosarcoma and histologically similar tumors in childhood: a retrospective European multi-center analysis. Med Pediatr Oncol 20: 209–214.

1466. Koshy M, Paulino AC, Mai WY et al. (2005). Radiation-induced osteosarcomas in the pediatric population. Int J Radiat Oncol Biol Phys 63: 1169–1174.

1467. Koufos A, Hansen MF, Copeland NG et al. (1985). Loss of heterozygosity in three embryonal tumours suggests a common pathogenetic mechanism. Nature 316: 330–334.

1468. Kourea HP, Orlow I, Scheithauer BW et al. (1999). Deletions of the INK4A gene occur in malignant peripheral nerve sheath tumors but not in neurofibromas. Am J Pathol 155: 1855–1860.

1469. Koutlas IG, Scheithauer BW (2010). Palisaded encapsulated ("solitary circumscribed") neuroma of the oral cavity: a review of 55 cases. Head Neck Pathol 4: 15–26.

1470. Koutsimpelas D, Weber A, Lippert BM et al. (2008). Multifocal adult rhabdomyoma of the head and neck: a case report and literature review. Auris Nasus Larynx 35: 313–317.
1471. Kozakiewicz M, Perczynska-Partyka W, Kobos J (2001). Cherubism—clinical picture and treatment. Oral Dis 7: 123–130.
1472. Koziel L, Kunath M, Kelly OG et al. (2004). Ext1-dependent heparan sulfate regulates the range of Ihh signaling during endochondral ossification. Dev Cell 6: 801–813.
1473. Kralik JM, Kranewitter W, Boesmueller H et al. (2011). Characterization of a newly identified ETV6-NTRK3 fusion transcript in acute myeloid leukemia. Diagn Pathol 6: 19
1474. Kramer K, Hicks DG, Palis J et al. (1993). Epithelioid osteosarcoma of bone. Immunocytochemical evidence suggesting divergent epithelial and mesenchymal differentiation in a primary osseous neoplasm. Cancer 71: 2977–2982.
1475. Krane JF, Bertoni F, Fletcher CD (1999). Myxoid synovial sarcoma: an underappreciated morphologic subset. Mod Pathol 12: 456–462.
1476. Kransdorf MJ, Meis JM, Jelinek JS (1991). Myositis ossificans: MR appearance with radiologic-pathologic correlation. AJR Am J Roentgenol 157: 1243–1248.
1477. Kransdorf MJ, Moser RP, Jr., Jelinek JS et al. (1989). Intramuscular myxoma: MR features. J Comput Assist Tomogr 13: 836–839.
1478. Kransdorf MJ, Murphey MD, Sweet DE (1999). Liposclerosing myxofibrous tumor: a radiologic-pathologic-distinct fibro-osseous lesion of bone with a marked predilection for the intertrochanteric region of the femur. Radiology 212: 693–698.
1479. Kransdorf MJ, Sweet DE (1995). Aneurysmal bone cyst: concept, controversy, clinical presentation, and imaging. AJR Am J Roentgenol 164: 573–580.
1480. Kratz CP, Rapisuwon S, Reed H et al. (2011). Cancer in Noonan, Costello, cardiofaciocutaneous and LEOPARD syndromes. Am J Med Genet C Semin Med Genet 157: 83–89.
1481. Kraus MD, Guillou L, Fletcher CD (1997). Well-differentiated inflammatory liposarcoma: an uncommon and easily overlooked variant of a common sarcoma. Am J Surg Pathol 21: 518–527.
1482. Kravcik S (2000). HIV lipodystrophy: a review. HIV Clin Trials 1: 37–50.
1483. Kreiger PA, Judkins AR, Russo PA et al. (2009). Loss of INI1 expression defines a unique subset of pediatric undifferentiated soft tissue sarcomas. Mod Pathol 22: 142–150.
1484. Kresse SH, Berner JM, Meza-Zepeda LA et al. (2005). Mapping and characterization of the amplicon near APOA2 in 1q23 in human sarcomas by FISH and array CGH. Mol Cancer 4: 39
1485. Kresse SH, Ohnstad HO, Bjerkehagen B et al. (2010). DNA copy number changes in human malignant fibrous histiocytomas by array comparative genomic hybridisation. PLoS One 5: e15378
1486. Kresse SH, Ohnstad HO, Paulsen EB et al. (2009). LSAMP, a novel candidate tumor suppressor gene in human osteosarcomas, identified by array comparative genomic hybridization. Genes Chromosomes Cancer 48: 679–693.
1487. Krieg AH, Hefti F, Speth BM et al. (2011). Synovial sarcomas usually metastasize after >5 years: a multicenter retrospective analysis with minimum follow-up of 10 years for survivors. Ann Oncol 22: 458–467.
1488. Krishnan A, Shirkhoda A, Tehranzadeh J et al. (2003). Primary bone lymphoma: radiographic-MR imaging correlation. Radiographics 23: 1371–1383.
1489. Kubota T, Moritani S, Terasaki H (2012). Orbital venous hemangioma. Graefes Arch Clin Exp Ophthalmol 250: 157–158.
1490. Kuhnen C, Herter P, Leuschner I et al. (2006). Sclerosing pseudovascular rhabdomyosarcoma-immunohistochemical, ultrastructural, and genetic findings indicating a distinct subtype of rhabdomyosarcoma. Virchows Arch 449: 572–578.
1491. Kulkarni KR, Jambhekar NA (2003). Epithelioid hemangioendothelioma of bone—a clinicopathologic and immunohistochemical study of 7 cases. Indian J Pathol Microbiol 46: 600–604.
1492. Kumar B, Pradhan A (2011). Diagnosis of sternomastoid tumor of infancy by fine-needle aspiration cytology. Diagn Cytopathol 39: 13–17.
1493. Kumar R (1997). Phosphatonin—a new phosphaturetic hormone? (lessons from tumour-induced osteomalacia and X-linked hypophosphataemia). Nephrol Dial Transplant 12: 11–13.
1494. Kumar R (2002). New insights into phosphate homeostasis: fibroblast growth factor 23 and frizzled-related protein-4 are phosphaturic factors derived from tumors associated with osteomalacia. Curr Opin Nephrol Hypertens 11: 547–553.
1495. Kumar R, Deaver MT, Czerniak BA et al. (2011). Intraosseous hibernoma. Skeletal Radiol 40: 641–645.
1496. Kumar SK, Uno H, Jacobus SJ et al. (2011). Impact of gene expression profiling-based risk stratification in patients with myeloma receiving initial therapy with lenalidomide and dexamethasone. Blood 118: 4359–4362.
1497. Kumaratilake JS, Krishnan R, Lomax-Smith J et al. (1991). Elastofibroma: disturbed elastic fibrillogenesis by periosteal-derived cells? An immunoelectron microscopic and in situ hybridization study. Hum Pathol 22: 1017–1029.
1498. Kundangar R, Pandey V, Acharya KK et al. (2011). An intraarticular fibroma of the tendon sheath in the knee joint. Knee Surg Sports Traumatol Arthrosc 19: 1830–1833.
1499. Kuo TT, Chen TC, Lee LY (2009). Sclerosing angiomatoid nodular transformation of the spleen (SANT): clinicopathological study of 10 cases with or without abdominal disseminated calcifying fibrous tumors, and the presence of a significant number of IgG4+ plasma cells. Pathol Int 59: 844–850.
1500. Kurkchubasche AG, Halvorson EG, Forman EN et al. (2000). The role of preoperative chemotherapy in the treatment of infantile fibrosarcoma. J Pediatr Surg 35: 880–883.
1501. Kurt AM, Unni KK, McLeod RA et al. (1990). Low-grade intraosseous osteosarcoma. Cancer 65: 1418–1428.
1502. Kurtkaya-Yapicier O, Scheithauer BW, Woodruff JM et al. (2003). Schwannoma with rhabdomyoblastic differentiation: a unique variant of malignant triton tumor. Am J Surg Pathol 27: 848–853.
1503. Kurtycz DF, Logrono R, Hoerl HD et al. (2000). Diagnosis of fibromatosis colli by fine-needle aspiration. Diagn Cytopathol 23: 338–342.
1504. Kuruvath S, O'Donovan DG, Aspoas AR et al. (2006). Benign fibrous histiocytoma of the thoracic spine: case report and review of the literature. J Neurosurg Spine 4: 260–264.
1504A. Kuruvilla G, Steiner GC. (1998). Osteofibrous dysplasia-like adamantinoma of bone: a report of five cases with immunohistochemical and ultrastructural studies. Hum Pathol 29:809–14.
1505. Kurzrock EA, Busby JE, Gandour-Edwards R (2003). Paratesticular rhabdomyoma. J Pediatr Surg 38: 1546–1547.
1506. Kusafuka K, Muramatsu K, Yabuzaki T et al. (2008). Alveolar soft part sarcoma of the larynx: a case report of an unusual location with immunohistochemical and ultrastructural analyses. Head Neck 30: 1257–1263.
1507. Kushner BH, Hajdu SI, Helson L (1985). Synchronous neuroblastoma and von Recklinghausen's disease: a review of the literature. J Clin Oncol 3: 117–120.
1508. Kuttesch JF, Jr., Parham DM, Kaste SC et al. (1995). Embryonal malignancies of unknown primary origin in children. Cancer 75: 115–121.
1509. Kutzner H, Embacher G, Kutzner U et al. (1990). [Solitary encapsulated neuroma]. Hautarzt 41: 620–624.
1510. Kutzner H, Mentzel T, Kaddu S et al. (2001). Cutaneous myoepithelioma: an under-recognized cutaneous neoplasm composed of myoepithelial cells. Am J Surg Pathol 25: 348–355.
1511. Kutzner H, Mentzel T, Palmedo G et al. (2010). Plaque-like CD34-positive dermal fibroma ("medallion-like dermal dendrocyte hamartoma"): clinicopathologic, immunohistochemical, and molecular analysis of 5 cases emphasizing its distinction from superficial, plaque-like dermatofibrosarcoma protuberans. Am J Surg Pathol 34: 190–201.
1512. Kwittken J, Branche M (1969). Fasciitis ossificans. Am J Clin Pathol 51: 251–255.
1513. Kyle RA, Gertz MA (1995). Primary systemic amyloidosis: clinical and laboratory features in 474 cases. Semin Hematol 32: 45–59.
1514. Kyle RA, Gertz MA, Witzig TE et al. (2003). Review of 1027 patients with newly diagnosed multiple myeloma. Mayo Clin Proc 78: 21–33.
1515. Kynaston JA, Malcolm AJ, Craft AW et al. (1993). Chemotherapy in the management of infantile fibrosarcoma. Med Pediatr Oncol 21: 488–493.
1516. Kyriakos M (2011). Benign notochordal lesions of the axial skeleton: a review and current appraisal. Skeletal Radiol 40: 1141–1152.
1517. Labarre D, Aziza R, Filleron T et al. (2009). Detection of local recurrences of limb soft tissue sarcomas: is magnetic resonance imaging (MRI) relevant? Eur J Radiol 72: 50–53.
1518. Labelle Y, Bussieres J, Courjal F et al. (1999). The EWS/TEC fusion protein encoded by the t(9;22) chromosomal translocation in human chondrosarcomas is a highly potent transcriptional activator. Oncogene 18: 3303–3308.
1519. Labelle Y, Zucman J, Stenman G et al. (1995). Oncogenic conversion of a novel orphan nuclear receptor by chromosome translocation. Hum Mol Genet 4: 2219–2226.
1520. Lack EE, Worsham GF, Callihan MD et al. (1980). Granular cell tumor: a clinicopathologic study of 110 patients. J Surg Oncol 13: 301–316.
1521. Ladanyi M, Antonescu CR, Drobnjak M et al. (2002). The precrystalline cytoplasmic granules of alveolar soft part sarcoma contain monocarboxylate transporter 1 and CD147. Am J Pathol 160: 1215–1221.
1522. Ladanyi M, Antonescu CR, Leung DH et al. (2002). Impact of SYT-SSX fusion type on the clinical behavior of synovial sarcoma: a multi-institutional retrospective study of 243 patients. Cancer Res 62: 135–140.
1523. Ladanyi M, Gerald W (1994). Fusion of the EWS and WT1 genes in the desmoplastic small round cell tumor. Cancer Res 54: 2837–2840.
1524. Ladanyi M, Lui MY, Antonescu CR et al. (2001). The der(17)t(X;17)(p11;q25) of human alveolar soft part sarcoma fuses the TFE3 transcription factor gene to ASPL, a novel gene at 17q25. Oncogene 20: 48–57.
1525. Ladenstein R, Potschger U, Le Deley MC et al. (2010). Primary disseminated multifocal Ewing sarcoma: results of the Euro-EWING 99 trial. J Clin Oncol 28: 3284–3291.
1526. Ladhani S, Sundaram P, Joshi JM (2003). Sleep disordered breathing in an adult with cherubism. Thorax 58: 552
1527. Lagarde P, Perot G, Kauffmann A et al. (2012). Mitotic checkpoints and chromosome instability are strong predictors of clinical outcome in gastrointestinal stromal tumors. Clin Cancer Res 18: 826–838.
1528. Lahat G, Dhuka AR, Hallevi H et al. (2010). Angiosarcoma: clinical and molecular insights. Ann Surg 251: 1098–1106.
1529. Lakshminarayanan R, Konia T, Welborn J (2005). Fibrous hamartoma of infancy: a case report with associated cytogenetic findings. Arch Pathol Lab Med 129: 520–522.
1530. Lal DR, Su WT, Wolden SL et al. (2005). Results of multimodal treatment for desmoplastic small round cell tumors. J Pediatr Surg 40: 251–255.
1531. Lalloo F, Varley J, Moran A et al. (2006). BRCA1, BRCA2 and TP53 mutations in very early-onset breast cancer with associated risks to relatives. Eur J Cancer 42: 1143–1150.
1532. Lam PY, Sublett JE, Hollenbach AD et al. (1999). The oncogenic potential of the Pax3-FKHR fusion protein requires the Pax3 homeodomain recognition helix but not the Pax3 paired-box DNA binding domain. Mol Cell Biol 19: 594–601.
1533. Lamba G, Rafiyath SM, Kaur H et al. (2011). Malignant glomus tumor of kidney: the first reported case and review of literature. Hum Pathol 42: 1200–1203.
1534. Lambert I, Debiec-Rychter M, Guelinckx P et al. (2001). Acral myxoinflammatory fibroblastic sarcoma with unique clonal chromosomal changes. Virchows Arch 438: 509–512.
1535. Lamovec J, Spiler M, Jevtic V (1999). Osteosarcoma arising in a solitary osteochondroma of the fibula. Arch Pathol Lab Med 123: 832–834.
1536. Lane KL, Shannon RJ, Weiss SW (1997). Hyalinizing spindle cell tumor with giant rosettes: a distinctive tumor closely resembling low-grade fibromyxoid sarcoma. Am J Surg Pathol 21: 1481–1488.
1537. Lang FF, Macdonald OK, Fuller GN et al. (2000). Primary extradural meningiomas: a report on nine cases and review of the literature from the era of computerized tomography scanning. J Neurosurg 93: 940–950.
1538. Lang JE, Dodd L, Martinez S et al. (2006). Case reports: acral myxoinflammatory fibroblastic sarcoma: a report of five cases and literature review. Clin Orthop Relat Res 445: 254–260.
1539. Langer LO, Jr., Krassikoff N, Laxova R et al. (1984). The tricho-rhino-phalangeal syndrome with exostoses (or Langer-Giedion syndrome): four additional patients without mental retardation and review of the literature. Am J Med Genet 19: 81–112.

1540. Lapner PC, Chou S, Jimenez C (1997). Perianal fetal rhabdomyoma: case report. Pediatr Surg Int 12: 544–547.
1541. Lara C, Jurado P, Porras V et al. (2007). [Spermatic cord rhabdomyoma]. Arch Esp Urol 60: 695–697.
1542. Larizza L, Magnani I, Roversi G (2006). Rothmund-Thomson syndrome and RECQL4 defect: splitting and lumping. Cancer Lett 232: 107–120.
1543. Larizza L, Roversi G, Volpi L (2010). Rothmund-Thomson syndrome. Orphanet J Rare Dis 5: 2
1544. Larramendy ML, Gentile M, Soloneski S et al. (2008). Does comparative genomic hybridization reveal distinct differences in DNA copy number sequence patterns between leiomyosarcoma and malignant fibrous histiocytoma? Cancer Genet Cytogenet 187: 1–11.
1545. Larramendy ML, Mandahl N, Mertens F et al. (1999). Clinical significance of genetic imbalances revealed by comparative genomic hybridization in chondrosarcomas. Hum Pathol 30: 1247–1253.
1546. Larramendy ML, Tarkkanen M, Valle J et al. (1997). Gains, losses, and amplifications of DNA sequences evaluated by comparative genomic hybridization in chondrosarcomas. Am J Pathol 150: 685–691.
1547. Larrea-Oyarbide N, Valmaseda-Castellon E, Berini-Aytes L et al. (2008). Osteomas of the craniofacial region. Review of 106 cases. J Oral Pathol Med 37: 38–42.
1548. Larsson SE, Lorentzon R, Boquist L (1976). Fibrosarcoma of bone. A demographic, clinical and histopathological study of all cases recorded in the Swedish cancer registry from 1958 to 1968. J Bone Joint Surg Br 58-B: 412–417.
1549. Laskin WB, Fanburg-Smith JC, Burke AP et al. (2010). Leiomyosarcoma of the inferior vena cava: clinicopathologic study of 40 cases. Am J Surg Pathol 34: 873–881.
1550. Laskin WB, Fetsch JF, Miettinen M (2000). The "neurothekeoma": immunohistochemical analysis distinguishes the true nerve sheath myxoma from its mimics. Hum Pathol 31: 1230–1241.
1551. Laskin WB, Fetsch JF, Mostofi FK (1998). Angiomyofibroblastomalike tumor of the male genital tract: analysis of 11 cases with comparison to female angiomyofibroblastoma and spindle cell lipoma. Am J Surg Pathol 22: 6–16.
1552. Laskin WB, Fetsch JF, Tavassoli FA (1997). Angiomyofibroblastoma of the female genital tract: analysis of 17 cases including a lipomatous variant. Hum Pathol 28: 1046–1055.
1553. Laskin WB, Miettinen M (2003). Epithelioid sarcoma: new insights based on an extended immunohistochemical analysis. Arch Pathol Lab Med 127: 1161–1168.
1554. Laskin WB, Miettinen M, Fetsch JF (2009). Infantile digital fibroma/fibromatosis: a clinicopathologic and immunohistochemical study of 69 tumors from 57 patients with long-term follow-up. Am J Surg Pathol 33: 1–13.
1555. Laskin WB, Silverman TA, Enzinger FM (1988). Postradiation soft tissue sarcomas. An analysis of 53 cases. Cancer 62: 2330–2340.
1556. Lasota J, Fetsch JF, Wozniak A et al. (2001). The neurofibromatosis type 2 gene is mutated in perineurial cell tumors: a molecular genetic study of eight cases. Am J Pathol 158: 1223–1229.
1557. Lasota J, Miettinen M (2008). Clinical significance of oncogenic KIT and PDGFRA mutations in gastrointestinal stromal tumours. Histopathology 53: 245–266.
1558. Latronico AC, Pinto EM, Domenice S et al. (2001). An inherited mutation outside the highly conserved DNA-binding domain of the p53 tumor suppressor protein in children and adults with sporadic adrenocortical tumors. J Clin Endocrinol Metab 86: 4970–4973.
1559. Lau CC, Harris CP, Lu XY et al. (2004). Frequent amplification and rearrangement of chromosomal bands 6p12-p21 and 17p11.2 in osteosarcoma. Genes Chromosomes Cancer 39: 11–21.
1560. Lau K, Massad M, Pollak C et al. (2011). Clinical patterns and outcome in epithelioid hemangioendothelioma with or without pulmonary involvement: insights from an internet registry in the study of a rare cancer. Chest 140: 1312–1318.
1561. Lau N, Feldkamp MM, Roncari L et al. (2000). Loss of neurofibromin is associated with activation of RAS/MAPK and PI3-K/AKT signaling in a neurofibromatosis 1 astrocytoma. J Neuropathol Exp Neurol 59: 759–767.
1562. Lau PP, Wong OK, Lui PC et al. (2009). Myopericytoma in patients with AIDS: a new class of Epstein-Barr virus-associated tumor. Am J Surg Pathol 33: 1666–1672.
1563. Lau SK, Klein R, Jiang Z et al. (2010). Myopericytoma of the kidney. Hum Pathol 41: 1500–1504.
1564. Lau YS, Sabokbar A, Gibbons CL et al. (2005). Phenotypic and molecular studies of giant-cell tumors of bone and soft tissue. Hum Pathol 36: 945–954.
1565. Lauer DH, Enzinger FM (1980). Cranial fasciitis of childhood. Cancer 45: 401–406.
1565A. Lauper JM, Krause A, Vaughan TL (2012) Spectrum and risk of neoplasia in Werner syndrome: A systematic review. PLoS One (In Press).
1566. Laurin N, Brown JP, Morissette J et al. (2002). Recurrent mutation of the gene encoding sequestosome 1 (SQSTM1/p62) in Paget disease of bone. Am J Hum Genet 70: 1582–1588.
1567. Laurini JA, Zhang L, Goldblum JR et al. (2011). Low-grade fibromyxoid sarcoma of the small intestine: report of 4 cases with molecular cytogenetic confirmation. Am J Surg Pathol 35: 1069–1073.
1568. Lausch E, Janecke A, Bros M et al. (2011). Genetic deficiency of tartrate-resistant acid phosphatase associated with skeletal dysplasia, cerebral calcifications and autoimmunity. Nat Genet 43: 132–137.
1569. Lawlor ER, Mathers JA, Bainbridge T et al. (1998). Peripheral primitive neuroectodermal tumors in adults: documentation by molecular analysis. J Clin Oncol 16: 1150–1157.
1570. Lawrence B, Perez-Atayde A, Hibbard MK et al. (2000). TPM3-ALK and TPM4-ALK oncogenes in inflammatory myofibroblastic tumors. Am J Pathol 157: 377–384.
1571. Lawrence W, Jr., Donegan WL, Natarajan N et al. (1987). Adult soft tissue sarcomas. A pattern of care survey of the American College of Surgeons. Ann Surg 205: 349–359.
1572. Lawrence WT, Azizkhan RG (1989). Congenital muscular torticollis: a spectrum of pathology. Ann Plast Surg 23: 523–530.
1573. Layfield LJ, Emerson L, Crim JR et al. (2008). Squamous differentiation and cytokeratin expression in an osteosarcoma: a case report and review of the literature. Clin Med Pathol 1: 55–59.
1574. Lazar AJ, Tuvin D, Hajibashi S et al. (2008). Specific mutations in the beta-catenin gene (CTNNB1) correlate with local recurrence in sporadic desmoid tumors. Am J Pathol 173: 1518–1527.
1575. Lazarus SS, Trombetta LD (1978). Ultrastructural identification of a benign perineurial cell tumor. Cancer 41: 1823–1829.
1576. Le Deley MC, Delattre O, Schaefer KL et al. (2010). Impact of EWS-ETS fusion type on disease progression in Ewing's sarcoma/ peripheral primitive neuroectodermal tumor: prospective results from the cooperative Euro-E.W.I.N.G. 99 trial. J Clin Oncol 28: 1982–1988.
1577. Le Huu AR, Jokinen CH, Rubin BP et al. (2010). Expression of prox1, lymphatic endothelial nuclear transcription factor, in Kaposiform hemangioendothelioma and tufted angioma. Am J Surg Pathol 34: 1563–1573.
1578. Le Vu B, de Vathaire F, Shamsaldin A et al. (1998). Radiation dose, chemotherapy and risk of osteosarcoma after solid tumours during childhood. Int J Cancer 77: 370–377.
1579. Le LQ, Liu C, Shipman T et al. (2011). Susceptible stages in Schwann cells for NF1-associated plexiform neurofibroma development. Cancer Res 71: 4686–4695.
1580. Leake JF, Buscema J, Cho KR et al. (1991). Dermatofibrosarcoma protuberans of the vulva. Gynecol Oncol 41: 245–249.
1581. LeBoit PE, Gunter B, Weedon D, Sarasin A (2006). WHO classification of skin tumours, third edition. WHO Classification of Tumours. IARCPress: Lyon.
1582. Leclerc-Mercier S, Pedeutour F, Fabas T et al. (2011). Plexiform fibrohistiocytic tumor with molecular and cytogenetic analysis. Pediatr Dermatol 28: 26–29.
1583. Lee AF, Hayes MM, Lebrun D et al. (2011). FLI-1 distinguishes Ewing sarcoma from small cell osteosarcoma and mesenchymal chondrosarcoma. Appl Immunohistochem Mol Morphol 19: 233–238.
1584. Lee FY, Mankin HJ, Fondren G et al. (1999). Chondrosarcoma of bone: an assessment of outcome. J Bone Joint Surg Am 81: 326–338.
1585. Lee JC, Fletcher CD (2011). Malignant fat-forming solitary fibrous tumor (so-called "lipomatous hemangiopericytoma"): clinicopathologic analysis of 14 cases. Am J Surg Pathol 35: 1177–1185.
1586. Lee JS, Fetsch JF, Wasdhal DA et al. (1995). A review of 40 patients with extraskeletal osteosarcoma. Cancer 76: 2253–2259.
1587. Lee SK, Jung MS, Lee YH et al. (2007). Two distinctive subungual pathologies: subungual exostosis and subungual osteochondroma. Foot Ankle Int 28: 595–601.
1588. Lee WH, Bookstein R, Hong F et al. (1987). Human retinoblastoma susceptibility gene: cloning, identification, and sequence. Science 235: 1394–1399.
1589. Lee WH, Shew JY, Hong FD et al. (1987). The retinoblastoma susceptibility gene encodes a nuclear phosphoprotein associated with DNA binding activity. Nature 329: 642–645.
1590. Lee YF, John M, Edwards S et al. (2003). Molecular classification of synovial sarcomas, leiomyosarcomas and malignant fibrous histiocytomas by gene expression profiling. Br J Cancer 88: 510–515.
1591. Lee-Jones L, Aligianis I, Davies PA et al. (2004). Sacrococcygeal chordomas in patients with tuberous sclerosis complex show somatic loss of TSC1 or TSC2. Genes Chromosomes Cancer 41: 80–85.
1592. Legeai-Mallet L, Munnich A, Maroteaux P et al. (1997). Incomplete penetrance and expressivity skewing in hereditary multiple exostoses. Clin Genet 52: 12–16.
1593. Legius E, Marchuk DA, Collins FS et al. (1993). Somatic deletion of the neurofibromatosis type 1 gene in a neurofibrosarcoma supports a tumour suppressor gene hypothesis. Nat Genet 3: 122–126.
1594. Leithner A, Windhager R, Lang S et al. (1999). Aneurysmal bone cyst. A population based epidemiologic study and literature review. Clin Orthop Relat Res 363:176–179.
1595. Leone PG, Taylor HB (1973). Ultrastructure of a benign polypoid rhabdomyoma of the vagina. Cancer 31: 1414–1417.
1596. Leu HJ, Makek M (1986). Intramural venous leiomyosarcomas. Cancer 57: 1395–1400.
1597. Leuschner I, Newton WA, Jr., Schmidt D et al. (1993). Spindle cell variants of embryonal rhabdomyosarcoma in the paratesticular region. A report of the Intergroup Rhabdomyosarcoma Study. Am J Surg Pathol 17: 221–230.
1598. Levaot N, Voytyuk O, Dimitriou I et al. (2011). Loss of Tankyrase-mediated destruction of 3BP2 is the underlying pathogenic mechanism of cherubism. Cell 147: 1324–1339.
1599. Levesque S, Ahmed N, Nguyen VH et al. (2010). Neonatal Gardner fibroma: a sentinel presentation of severe familial adenomatous polyposis. Pediatrics 126: e1599–e1602.
1600. Lewis JJ, Brennan MF (1996). Soft tissue sarcomas. Curr Probl Surg 33: 817–872.
1601. Lewis JJ, Leung D, Woodruff JM et al. (1998). Retroperitoneal soft-tissue sarcoma: analysis of 500 patients treated and followed at a single institution. Ann Surg 228: 355–365.
1602. Lewis MM, Kenan S, Yabut SM et al. (1990). Periosteal chondroma. A report of ten cases and review of the literature. Clin Orthop Relat Res 256:185–192.
1603. Lewis VO, Raymond K, Mirza AN et al. (2006). Outcome of postradiation osteosarcoma does not correlate with chemotherapy response. Clin Orthop Relat Res 450: 60–66.
1604. Li CF, Wang JW, Huang WW et al. (2008). Malignant diffuse-type tenosynovial giant cell tumors: a series of 7 cases comparing with 24 benign lesions with review of the literature. Am J Surg Pathol 32: 587–599.
1605. Li CY, Yu SF (2006). A novel mutation in the SH3BP2 gene causes cherubism: case report. BMC Med Genet 7: 84
1606. Li FP, Fraumeni JF, Jr. (1969). Soft-tissue sarcomas, breast cancer, and other neoplasms. A familial syndrome? Ann Intern Med 71: 747–752.
1607. Li FP, Fraumeni JF, Jr., Mulvihill JJ et al. (1988). A cancer family syndrome in twenty-four kindreds. Cancer Res 48: 5358–5362.
1608. Li G, Ogose A, Kawashima H et al. (2009). Cytogenetic and real-time quantitative reverse-transcriptase polymerase chain reaction analyses in pleomorphic rhabdomyosarcoma. Cancer Genet Cytogenet 192: 1–9.
1609. Liang Q, Wei M, Hodge L et al. (2011). Quantitative analysis of activating alpha subunit of the G protein (Gsalpha) mutation by pyrosequencing in fibrous dysplasia and other bone lesions. J Mol Diagn 13: 137–142.
1610. Lidang Jensen M, Schumacher B, Myhre Jensen O et al. (1998). Extraskeletal osteosarcomas: a clinicopathologic study of 25 cases. Am J Surg Pathol 22: 588–594.
1611. Lieberman PH, Brennan MF, Kimmel M et al. (1989). Alveolar soft-part sarcoma. A clin-

ico-pathologic study of half a century. Cancer 63: 1–13.
1612. Lieberman PH, Jones CR, Steinman RM et al. (1996). Langerhans cell (eosinophilic) granulomatosis. A clinicopathologic study encompassing 50 years. Am J Surg Pathol 20: 519–552.
1613. Liegl B, Bennett MW, Fletcher CD (2008). Microcystic/reticular schwannoma: a distinct variant with predilection for visceral locations. Am J Surg Pathol 32: 1080–1087.
1614. Liegl B, Fletcher CD (2008). Ischemic fasciitis: analysis of 44 cases indicating an inconsistent association with immobility or debilitation. Am J Surg Pathol 32: 1546–1552.
1615. Liegl B, Hornick JL, Antonescu CR et al. (2009). Rhabdomyosarcomatous differentiation in gastrointestinal stromal tumors after tyrosine kinase inhibitor therapy: a novel form of tumor progression. Am J Surg Pathol 33: 218–226.
1616. Liegl B, Hornick JL, Fletcher CD (2008). Primary cutaneous PEComa: distinctive clear cell lesions of skin. Am J Surg Pathol 32: 608–614.
1617. Liegl B, Kepten I, Le C et al. (2008). Heterogeneity of kinase inhibitor resistance mechanisms in GIST. J Pathol 216: 64–74.
1618. Liess BD, Zitsch RP, III, Lane R et al. (2005). Multifocal adult rhabdomyoma: a case report and literature review. Am J Otolaryngol 26: 214–217.
1619. Lietman SA, Ding C, Levine MA (2005). A highly sensitive polymerase chain reaction method detects activating mutations of the GNAS gene in peripheral blood cells in McCune-Albright syndrome or isolated fibrous dysplasia. J Bone Joint Surg Am 87: 2489–2494.
1620. Lietman SA, Kalinchinko N, Deng X et al. (2006). Identification of a novel mutation of SH3BP2 in cherubism and demonstration that SH3BP2 mutations lead to increased NFAT activation. Hum Mutat 27: 717–718.
1621. Lietman SA, Schwindinger WF, Levine MA (2007). Genetic and molecular aspects of McCune-Albright syndrome. Pediatr Endocrinol Rev 4 Suppl 4: 380–385.
1622. Lillehei KO, Kleinschmidt-DeMasters B, Mitchell DH et al. (1993). Alveolar soft part sarcoma: an unusually long interval between presentation and brain metastasis. Hum Pathol 24: 1030–1034.
1623. Lima FP, Bousquet M, Gomez-Brouchet A et al. (2008). Primary diffuse large B-cell lymphoma of bone displays preferential rearrangements of the c-MYC or BCL2 gene. Am J Clin Pathol 129: 723–726.
1624. Limon J, Szadowska A, Iliszko M et al. (1998). Recurrent chromosome changes in two adult fibrosarcomas. Genes Chromosomes Cancer 21: 119–123.
1625. Lin GY, Sun X, Badve S (2002). Pathologic quiz case. Vaginal wall mass in a 47-year-old woman. Vaginal rhabdomyoma. Arch Pathol Lab Med 126: 1241–1242.
1626. Lin HK, Wang JD, Fu LS (2011). Recurrent hemarthrosis in a boy with synovial hemangioma: a case report. J Pediatr Orthop B 20: 81–83.
1627. Lin JJ, Lin F (1974). Two entities in angiolipoma. A study of 459 cases of lipoma with review of literature on infiltrating angiolipoma. Cancer 34: 720–727.
1628. Lin P, O'Brien JM (2009). Frontiers in the management of retinoblastoma. Am J Ophthalmol 148: 192–198.
1629. Lin P, Owens R, Tricot G et al. (2004). Flow cytometric immunophenotypic analysis of 306 cases of multiple myeloma. Am J Clin Pathol 121: 482–488.
1630. Linabery AM, Ross JA (2008). Childhood and adolescent cancer survival in the US by race and ethnicity for the diagnostic period 1975-1999. Cancer 113: 2575–2596.
1631. Lind T, Tufaro F, McCormick C et al. (1998). The putative tumor suppressors EXT1 and EXT2 are glycosyltransferases required for the biosynthesis of heparan sulfate. J Biol Chem 273: 26265–26268.
1632. Lindvall LE, Kormeili T, Chen E et al. (2008). Infantile systemic hyalinosis: Case report and review of the literature. J Am Acad Dermatol 58: 303–307.
1633. Linn SC, West RB, Pollack JR et al. (2003). Gene expression patterns and gene copy number changes in dermatofibrosarcoma protuberans. Am J Pathol 163: 2383–2395.
1634. Linos K, Sedivcova M, Cerna K et al. (2011). Extra nuchal-type fibroma associated with elastosis, traumatic neuroma, a rare APC gene missense mutation, and a very rare MUTYH gene polymorphism: a case report and review of the literature*. J Cutan Pathol 38: 911–918.
1635. Lisovsky M, Hoang MP, Dresser KA et al. (2008). Apolipoprotein D in CD34-positive and CD34-negative cutaneous neoplasms: a useful marker in differentiating superficial acral fibromyxoma from dermatofibrosarcoma protuberans. Mod Pathol 21: 31–38.
1636. Listernick R, Louis DN, Packer RJ et al. (1997). Optic pathway gliomas in children with neurofibromatosis 1: consensus statement from the NF1 Optic Pathway Glioma Task Force. Ann Neurol 41: 143–149.
1637. Littrell LA, Wenger DE, Wold LE et al. (2004). Radiographic, CT, and MR imaging features of dedifferentiated chondrosarcomas: a retrospective review of 174 de novo cases. Radiographics 24: 1397–1409.
1637A. Liu J, Guzman MA, Pezanowski D et al. (2011). FOXO1-FGFR1 fusion and amplification in a solid variant of alveolar rhabdomyosarcoma. Mod Pathol. 10:1327–35
1638. Liu J, Hudkins PG, Swee RG et al. (1987). Bone sarcomas associated with Ollier's disease. Cancer 59: 1376–1385.
1639. Liu Q, Schwaller J, Kutok J et al. (2000). Signal transduction and transforming properties of the TEL-TRKC fusions associated with t(12;15)(p13;q25) in congenital fibrosarcoma and acute myelogenous leukemia. EMBO J 19: 1827–1838.
1640. Liu Y (2010). Rothmund-Thomson syndrome helicase, RECQ4: on the crossroad between DNA replication and repair. DNA Repair (Amst) 9: 325–330.
1641. Livi L, Shah N, Paiar F et al. (2003). Treatment of epithelioid sarcoma at the royal marsden hospital. Sarcoma 7: 149–152.
1642. Llombart B, Monteagudo C, Sanmartin O et al. (2011). Dermatofibrosarcoma protuberans: a clinicopathological, immunohistochemical, genetic (COL1A1-PDGFB), and therapeutic study of low-grade versus high-grade (fibrosarcomatous) tumors. J Am Acad Dermatol 65: 564–575.
1643. Llombart B, Sanmartin O, Lopez-Guerrero JA et al. (2009). Dermatofibrosarcoma protuberans: clinical, pathological, and genetic (COL1A1-PDGFB) study with therapeutic implications. Histopathology 54: 860–872.
1644. Llombart-Bosch A, Machado I, Navarro S et al. (2009). Histological heterogeneity of Ewing's sarcoma/PNET: an immunohistochemical analysis of 415 genetically confirmed cases with clinical support. Virchows Arch 455: 397–411.
1645. Lo B, Faiyaz-Ul-Haque M, Kennedy S et al. (2003). Novel mutation in the gene encoding c-Abl-binding protein SH3BP2 causes cherubism. Am J Med Genet A 121A: 37–40.
1646. Lockwood WW, Stack D, Morris T et al. (2011). Cyclin E1 is amplified and overexpressed in osteosarcoma. J Mol Diagn 13: 289–296.
1647. Lodding P, Kindblom LG, Angervall L et al. (1990). Cellular schwannoma. A clinicopathologic study of 29 cases. Virchows Arch A Pathol Anat Histopathol 416: 237–248.
1648. Logan PM, Janzen DL, O'Connell JX et al. (1996). Chondroid lipoma: MRI appearances with clinical and histologic correlation. Skeletal Radiol 25: 592–595.
1649. Loh ML, Ahn P, Perez-Atayde AR et al. (2002). Treatment of infantile fibrosarcoma with chemotherapy and surgery: results from the Dana-Farber Cancer Institute and Children's Hospital, Boston. J Pediatr Hematol Oncol 24: 722–726.
1650. Lohmann DR, Brandt B, Hopping W et al. (1994). Distinct RB1 gene mutations with low penetrance in hereditary retinoblastoma. Hum Genet 94: 349–354.
1651. Lohmann DR, Gillessen-Kaesbach G (2000). Multiple subcutaneous granular-cell tumours in a patient with Noonan syndrome. Clin Dysmorphol 9: 301–302.
1652. Longacre TA, Smoller BR, Rouse RV (1993). Atypical fibroxanthoma. Multiple immunohistologic profiles. Am J Surg Pathol 17: 1199–1209.
1653. Longhi A, Benassi MS, Molendini L et al. (2001). Osteosarcoma in blood relatives. Oncol Rep 8: 131–136.
1654. Lopez DA, Silvers DN, Helwig EB (1974). Cutaneous meningiomas—a clinicopathologic study. Cancer 34: 728–744.
1655. Lopez-Barea F, Hardisson D, Rodriguez-Peralto JL et al. (1998). Intracortical hemangioma of bone. Report of two cases and review of the literature. J Bone Joint Surg Am 80: 1673–1678.
1656. Lopez-Barea F, Rodriguez-Peralto JL, Burgos-Lizaldez E et al. (1996). Primary aneurysmal cyst of soft tissue. Report of a case with ultrastructural and MRI studies. Virchows Arch 428: 125–129.
1657. Lopez-Ben R, Pitt MJ, Jaffe KA et al. (1999). Osteosarcoma in a patient with McCune-Albright syndrome and Mazabraud's syndrome. Skeletal Radiol 28: 522–526.
1658. Lopez-Correa C, Dorschner M, Brems H et al. (2001). Recombination hotspot in NF1 microdeletion patients. Hum Mol Genet 10: 1387–1392.
1659. Lopez-Guerrero JA, Lopez-Gines C, Pellin A et al. (2004). Deregulation of the G1 to S-phase cell cycle checkpoint is involved in the pathogenesis of human osteosarcoma. Diagn Mol Pathol 13: 81–91.
1660. Lorigan JG, O'Keeffe FN, Evans HL et al. (1989). The radiologic manifestations of alveolar soft-part sarcoma. AJR Am J Roentgenol 153: 335–339.
1661. Losi L, Choreutaki T, Nascetti D et al. (1995). [Recurrence in a case of rhabdomyoma of the vagina]. Pathologica 87: 704–708.
1662. Lothe RA, Karhu R, Mandahl N et al. (1996). Gain of 17q24-qter detected by comparative genomic hybridization in malignant tumors from patients with von Recklinghausen's neurofibromatosis. Cancer Res 56: 4778–4781.
1663. Lothe RA, Smith-Sorensen B, Hektoen M et al. (2001). Biallelic inactivation of TP53 rarely contributes to the development of malignant peripheral nerve sheath tumors. Genes Chromosomes Cancer 30: 202–206.
1664. Louis DN, Ramesh V, Gusella JF (1995). Neuropathology and molecular genetics of neurofibromatosis 2 and related tumors. Brain Pathol 5: 163–172.
1665. Lowry KC, Estroff JA, Rahbar R (2010). The presentation and management of fibromatosis colli. Ear Nose Throat J 89: E4–E8.
1666. Lu XY, Lu Y, Zhao YJ et al. (2008). Cell cycle regulator gene CDC5L, a potential target for 6p12-p21 amplicon in osteosarcoma. Mol Cancer Res 6: 937–946.
1667. Lualdi E, Modena P, Debiec-Rychter M et al. (2004). Molecular cytogenetic characterization of proximal-type epithelioid sarcoma. Genes Chromosomes Cancer 41: 283–290.
1668. Lubin J, Rywlin AM (1971). Lymphoma-like lymph node changes in Kaposi's sarcoma. Two additional cases. Arch Pathol 92: 338–341.
1669. Lucas DR, Fletcher CD, Adsay NV et al. (1999). High-grade extraskeletal myxoid chondrosarcoma: a high-grade epithelioid malignancy. Histopathology 35: 201–208.
1670. Lucas DR, Nascimento AG, Sanjay BK et al. (1994). Well-differentiated liposarcoma. The Mayo Clinic experience with 58 cases. Am J Clin Pathol 102: 677–683.
1671. Lucas DR, Nascimento AG, Sim FH (1992). Clear cell sarcoma of soft tissues. Mayo Clinic experience with 35 cases. Am J Surg Pathol 16: 1197–1204.
1672. Lucas DR, Unni KK, McLeod RA et al. (1994). Osteoblastoma: clinicopathologic study of 306 cases. Hum Pathol 25: 117–134.
1673. Ludecke HJ, Ahn J, Lin X et al. (1997). Genomic organization and promoter structure of the human EXT1 gene. Genomics 40: 351–354.
1674. Ludwig JA (2008). Ewing sarcoma: historical perspectives, current state-of-the-art, and opportunities for targeted therapy in the future. Curr Opin Oncol 20: 412–418.
1675. Lumbroso S, Paris F, Sultan C (2004). Activating Gsalpha mutations: analysis of 113 patients with signs of McCune-Albright syndrome—a European Collaborative Study. J Clin Endocrinol Metab 89: 2107–2113.
1676. Lundgren L, Kindblom LG, Willems J et al. (1992). Proliferative myositis and fasciitis. A light and electron microscopic, cytologic, DNA-cytometric and immunohistochemical study. APMIS 100: 437–448.
1677. Luo J, Melnick S, Rossi A et al. (2008). Primary cardiac alveolar soft part sarcoma. A report of the first observed case with molecular diagnostics corroboration. Pediatr Dev Pathol 11: 142–147.
1678. Luzar B, Antony F, Ramdial PK et al. (2007). Intravascular Kaposi's sarcoma - a hitherto unrecognized phenomenon. J Cutan Pathol 34: 861–864.
1679. Luzar B, Calonje E (2009). Superficial acral fibromyxoma: clinicopathological study of 14 cases with emphasis on a cellular variant. Histopathology 54: 375–377.
1680. Luzar B, Calonje E (2010). Morphological and immunohistochemical characteristics of atypical fibroxanthoma with a special emphasis on potential diagnostic pitfalls: a review. J Cutan Pathol 37: 301–309.
1681. Lyle PL, Amato CM, Fitzpatrick JE et al. (2008). Gastrointestinal melanoma or clear cell

sarcoma? Molecular evaluation of 7 cases previously diagnosed as malignant melanoma. Am J Surg Pathol 32: 858–866.

1682. Lyons LL, North PE, Mac-Moune Lai F et al. (2004). Kaposiform hemangioendothelioma: a study of 33 cases emphasizing its pathologic, immunophenotypic, and biologic uniqueness from juvenile hemangioma. Am J Surg Pathol 28: 559–568.

1683. Ma Z, Hill DA, Collins MH et al. (2003). Fusion of ALK to the Ran-binding protein 2 (RANBP2) gene in inflammatory myofibroblastic tumor. Genes Chromosomes Cancer 37: 98–105.

1684. Macarenco RS, Erickson-Johnson M, Wang X et al. (2009). Retroperitoneal lipomatous tumors without cytologic atypia: are they lipomas? A clinicopathologic and molecular study of 19 cases. Am J Surg Pathol 33: 1470–1476.

1685. Macchia G, Trombetta D, Moller E et al. (2012). FOSL1 as a candidate target gene for 11q12 rearrangements in desmoplastic fibroblastoma. Lab Invest 92:735-743.

1686. MacCollin M, Chiocca EA, Evans DG et al. (2005). Diagnostic criteria for schwannomatosis. Neurology 64: 1838–1845.

1687. Machado I, Alberghini M, Giner F et al. (2010). Histopathological characterization of small cell osteosarcoma with immunohistochemistry and molecular genetic support. A study of 10 cases. Histopathology 57: 162–167.

1688. Machado I, Noguera R, Mateos EA et al. (2011). The many faces of atypical Ewing's sarcoma. A true entity mimicking sarcomas, carcinomas and lymphomas. Virchows Arch 458: 281–290.

1689. Machen SK, Easley KA, Goldblum JR (1999). Synovial sarcoma of the extremities: a clinicopathologic study of 34 cases, including semi-quantitative analysis of spindled, epithelial, and poorly differentiated areas. Am J Surg Pathol 23: 268–275.

1690. Mackintosh C, Ordonez JL, Garcia-Dominguez DJ et al. (2012). 1q gain and CDT2 overexpression underlie an aggressive and highly proliferative form of Ewing sarcoma. Oncogene 31:1287-1298.

1691. Macmull S, Atkinson HD, Saso S et al. (2009). Primary intra-osseous liposarcoma of the femur: a case report. J Orthop Surg (Hong Kong) 17: 374–378.

1692. Madden NP, Spicer RD, Allibone EB et al. (1992). Spontaneous regression of neonatal fibrosarcoma. Br J Cancer Suppl 18: S72–S75.

1693. Maertens O, De Schepper S, Vandesompele J et al. (2007). Molecular dissection of isolated disease features in mosaic neurofibromatosis type 1. Am J Hum Genet 81: 243–251.

1694. Maertens O, Prenen H, Debiec-Rychter M et al. (2006). Molecular pathogenesis of multiple gastrointestinal stromal tumors in NF1 patients. Hum Mol Genet 15: 1015–1023.

1695. Maggiani F, Debiec-Rychter M, Vanbockrijck M et al. (2007). Cellular angiofibroma: another mesenchymal tumour with 13q14 involvement, suggesting a link with spindle cell lipoma and (extra)-mammary myofibroblastoma. Histopathology 51: 410–412.

1696. Maggiani F, Debiec-Rychter M, Verbeeck G et al. (2006). Extramammary myofibroblastoma is genetically related to spindle cell lipoma. Virchows Arch 449: 244–247.

1697. Maggiani F, Forsyth R, Hogendoorn PC et al. (2011). The immunophenotype of osteoclasts and macrophage polykaryons. J Clin Pathol 64: 701–705.

1698. Magro G (2008). Mammary myofibroblastoma: a tumor with a wide morphologic spectrum. Arch Pathol Lab Med 132: 1813–1820.

1699. Magro G, Caltabiano R, Kacerovska D et al. (2012). Vulvovaginal myofibroblastoma: expanding the morphological and immunohistochemical spectrum. A clinicopathologic study of 10 cases. Hum Pathol 43: 243–253.

1700. Mahajan A, Manchandia TC, Gould G et al. (2010). De novo arteriovenous malformations: case report and review of the literature. Neurosurg Rev 33: 115–119.

1701. Mahajan S, Juneja M, George T (2008). Osteosarcoma as a second neoplasm after chemotherapeutic treatment of hereditary retinoblastoma: a case report. Quintessence Int 39: 439–445.

1702. Maher CO, Spinner RJ, Giannini C et al. (2002). Neuromuscular choristoma of the sciatic nerve. Case report. J Neurosurg 96: 1123–1126.

1703. Mahima VG, Patil K, Srikanth HS (2011). Recurrent oral angioleiomyoma. Contemp Clin Dent 2: 102–105.

1704. Mahoney SE, Yao Z, Keyes CC et al. (2012). Genome-wide DNA methylation studies suggest distinct DNA methylation patterns in pediatric embryonal and alveolar rhabdomyosarcomas. Epigenetics 7:400-408.

1705. Maire G, Forus A, Foa C et al. (2003). 11q13 alterations in two cases of hibernoma: large heterozygous deletions and rearrangement breakpoints near GARP in 11q13.5. Genes Chromosomes Cancer 37: 389–395.

1706. Maire G, Yoshimoto M, Chilton-MacNeill S et al. (2009). Recurrent RECQL4 imbalance and increased gene expression levels are associated with structural chromosomal instability in sporadic osteosarcoma. Neoplasia 11: 260–268.

1707. Makek M (1980). Non ossifying fibroma of the mandible. A common lesion with unusual location. Arch Orthop Trauma Surg 96: 225–227.

1708. Maki M, Athanasou N (2004). Osteofibrous dysplasia and adamantinoma: correlation of proto-oncogene product and matrix protein expression. Hum Pathol 35: 69–74.

1709. Maki RG, Wathen JK, Patel SR et al. (2007). Randomized phase II study of gemcitabine and docetaxel compared with gemcitabine alone in patients with metastatic soft tissue sarcomas: results of sarcoma alliance for research through collaboration study 002 [corrected]. J Clin Oncol 25: 2755–2763.

1710. Malchoff CD, Reardon G, MacGillivray DC et al. (1994). An unusual presentation of McCune-Albright syndrome confirmed by an activating mutation of the Gs alpha-subunit from a bone lesion. J Clin Endocrinol Metab 78: 803–806.

1711. Malempati S, Rodeberg DA, Donaldson SS et al. (2011). Rhabdomyosarcoma in infants younger than 1 year: a report from the Children's Oncology Group. Cancer 117: 3493–3501.

1712. Malhas AM, Grimer RJ, Abudu A et al. (2011). The final diagnosis in patients with a suspected primary malignancy of bone. J Bone Joint Surg Br 93: 980–983.

1713. Malkin D, Li FP, Strong LC et al. (1990). Germ line p53 mutations in a familial syndrome of breast cancer, sarcomas, and other neoplasms. Science 250: 1233–1238.

1714. Mallet JF, Rigault P, Padovani JP et al. (1980). [Non-ossifying fibroma in children: a surgical condition?]. Chir Pediatr 21: 179–189.

1715. Man TK, Lu XY, Jaeweon K et al. (2004). Genome-wide array comparative genomic hybridization analysis reveals distinct amplifications in osteosarcoma. BMC Cancer 4: 45

1716. Mancini GM, Stojanov L, Willemsen R et al. (1999). Juvenile hyaline fibromatosis: clinical heterogeneity in three patients. Dermatology 198: 18–25.

1717. Mandahl N, Bartuma H, Magnusson L et al. (2011). HMGA2 and MDM2 expression in lipomatous tumors with partial, low-level amplification of sequences from the long arm of chromosome 12. Cancer Genet 204: 550–556.

1718. Mandahl N, Fletcher CD, Dal Cin P et al. (2000). Comparative cytogenetic study of spindle cell and pleomorphic leiomyosarcomas of soft tissues: a report from the CHAMP Study Group. Cancer Genet Cytogenet 116: 66–73.

1719. Mandahl N, Gustafson P, Mertens F et al. (2002). Cytogenetic aberrations and their prognostic impact in chondrosarcoma. Genes Chromosomes Cancer 33: 188–200.

1720. Mandahl N, Heim S, Kristoffersson U et al. (1985). Telomeric association in a malignant fibrous histiocytoma. Hum Genet 71: 321–324.

1721. Mandahl N, Heim S, Rydholm A et al. (1989). Structural chromosome aberrations in an adamantinoma. Cancer Genet Cytogenet 42: 187–190.

1722. Mandahl N, Heim S, Willen H et al. (1989). Characteristic karyotypic anomalies identify subtypes of malignant fibrous histiocytoma. Genes Chromosomes Cancer 1: 9–14.

1723. Mandahl N, Mertens F, Willen H et al. (1998). Nonrandom pattern of telomeric associations in atypical lipomatous tumors with ring and giant marker chromosomes. Cancer Genet Cytogenet 103: 25–34.

1724. Mangat KS, Jeys LM, Carter SR (2011). Latest developments in limb-salvage surgery in osteosarcoma. Expert Rev Anticancer Ther 11: 205–215.

1724A. Mangham DC and Athanasou NA (2011). Guidelines for histopathological specimen examination and diagnostic reporting of bone tumours. Clin Sarcoma Res. 1: 6.

1725. Mangion J, Rahman N, Edkins S et al. (1999). The gene for cherubism maps to chromosome 4p16.3. Am J Hum Genet 65: 151–157.

1726. Manieri M, Murano I, Fianchini A et al. (2010). Morphological and immunohistochemical features of brown adipocytes and preadipocytes in a case of human hibernoma. Nutr Metab Cardiovasc Dis 20: 567–574.

1727. Manivel JC, Wick MR, Dehner LP et al. (1987). Epithelioid sarcoma. An immunohistochemical study. Am J Clin Pathol 87: 319–326.

1728. Manner J, Radlwimmer B, Hohenberger P et al. (2010). MYC high level gene amplification is a distinctive feature of angiosarcomas after irradiation or chronic lymphedema. Am J Pathol 176: 34–39.

1729. Mansoor A, Fidda N, Himoe E et al. (2004). Myxoinflammatory fibroblastic sarcoma with complex supernumerary ring chromosomes composed of chromosome 3 segments. Cancer Genet Cytogenet 152: 61–65.

1730. Mantripragada KK, Diaz de Stahl T, Patridge C et al. (2009). Genome-wide high-resolution analysis of DNA copy number alterations in NF1-associated malignant peripheral nerve sheath tumors using 32K BAC array. Genes Chromosomes Cancer 48: 897–907.

1731. Margau R, Babyn P, Cole W et al. (2000). MR imaging of simple bone cysts in children: not so simple. Pediatr Radiol 30: 551–557.

1732. Mariani O, Brennetot C, Coindre JM et al. (2007). JUN oncogene amplification and overexpression block adipocytic differentiation in highly aggressive sarcomas. Cancer Cell 11: 361–374.

1733. Marino-Enriquez A, Fletcher CD, Dal Cin P et al. (2010). Dedifferentiated liposarcoma with "homologous" lipoblastic (pleomorphic liposarcoma-like) differentiation: clinicopathologic and molecular analysis of a series suggesting revised diagnostic criteria. Am J Surg Pathol 34: 1122–1131.

1734. Marino-Enriquez A, Wang WL, Roy A et al. (2011). Epithelioid inflammatory myofibroblastic sarcoma: An aggressive intra-abdominal variant of inflammatory myofibroblastic tumor with nuclear membrane or perinuclear ALK. Am J Surg Pathol 35: 135–144.

1735. Mark J, Wedell B, Dahlenfors R et al. (1992). Human benign chondroblastoma with a pseudodiploid stemline characterized by a complex and balanced translocation. Cancer Genet Cytogenet 58: 14–17.

1736. Marom EM, Helms CA (1999). Fibrolipomatous hamartoma: pathognomonic on MR imaging. Skeletal Radiol 28: 260–264.

1737. Marshall-Taylor C, Fanburg-Smith JC (2000). Hemosiderotic fibrohistiocytic lipomatous lesion: ten cases of a previously undescribed fatty lesion of the foot/ankle. Mod Pathol 13: 1192–1199.

1738. Martignetti JA, Desnick RJ, Aliprandis E et al. (1999). Diaphyseal medullary stenosis with malignant fibrous histiocytoma: a hereditary bone dysplasia/cancer syndrome maps to 9p21-22. Am J Hum Genet 64: 801–807.

1739. Martignetti JA, Gelb BD, Pierce H et al. (2000). Malignant fibrous histiocytoma: inherited and sporadic forms have loss of heterozygosity at chromosome bands 9p21-22-evidence for a common genetic defect. Genes Chromosomes Cancer 27: 191–195.

1740. Martignoni G, Pea M, Reghellin D et al. (2008). PEComas: the past, the present and the future. Virchows Arch 452: 119–132.

1741. Martin AJ, Summersgill BM, Fisher C et al. (2002). Chromosomal imbalances in meningeal solitary fibrous tumors. Cancer Genet Cytogenet 135: 160–164.

1742. Martin GA, Viskochil D, Bollag G et al. (1990). The GAP-related domain of the neurofibromatosis type 1 gene product interacts with ras p21. Cell 63: 843–849.

1743. Martin JW, Yoshimoto M, Ludkovski O et al. (2010). Analysis of segmental duplications, mouse genome synteny and recurrent cancer-associated amplicons in human chromosome 6p21-p12. Cytogenet Genome Res 128: 199–213.

1744. Martin JW, Zielenska M, Stein GS et al. (2011). The Role of RUNX2 in osteosarcoma oncogenesis. Sarcoma 2011: 282745

1745. Martin SE, Dwyer A, Kissane JM et al. (1982). Small-cell osteosarcoma. Cancer 50: 990–996.

1746. Martinez D, Millner PA, Coral A et al. (1992). Case report 745: Synovial lipoma arborescens. Skeletal Radiol 21: 393–395.

1747. Martinez JA, Quecedo E, Fortea JM et al. (1996). Pleomorphic angioleiomyoma. Am J Dermatopathol 18: 409–412.

1748. Martinez V, Sissons HA (1988). Aneurysmal bone cyst. A review of 123 cases including primary lesions and those secondary to other bone pathology. Cancer 61: 2291–2304.

1749. Martinsson T, Sjoberg RM, Hedborg F et al. (1997). Homozygous deletion of the neurofibromatosis-1 gene in the tumor of a patient with neuroblastoma. Cancer Genet Cytogenet 95: 183–189.

1750. Martorell M, Ortiz CM, Garcia JA (2010). Testicular fusocellular rhabdomyosarcoma as a metastasis of elbow sclerosing rhabdomyosarcoma: A clinicopathologic, immunohistochemical and molecular study of one case. Diagn Pathol 5: 52

1751. Mason WP, Krol GS, DeAngelis LM (1996). Low-grade oligodendroglioma responds to chemotherapy. Neurology 46: 203–207.

1752. Massi D, Beltrami G, Mela MM et al. (2004). Prognostic factors in soft tissue leiomyosarcoma of the extremities: a retrospective analysis of 42 cases. Eur J Surg Oncol 30: 565–572.

1753. Masson-Lecomte A, Rocher L, Ferlicot S et al. (2011). High-flow priapism due to a malignant glomus tumor (glomangiosarcoma) of the corpus cavernosum. J Sex Med 8: 3518–3522.

1754. Mastrangelo T, Modena P, Tornielli S et al. (2000). A novel zinc finger gene is fused to EWS in small round cell tumor. Oncogene 19: 3799–3804.

1755. Masui F, Ushigome S, Fujii K (1998). Giant cell tumor of bone: a clinicopathologic study of prognostic factors. Pathol Int 48: 723–729.

1756. Mathew J, Sen S, Chandi SM et al. (2001). Pulmonary lipoblastoma: a case report. Pediatr Surg Int 17: 543–544.

1757. Matsumoto K, Irie F, Mackem S et al. (2010). A mouse model of chondrocyte-specific somatic mutation reveals a role for Ext1 loss of heterozygosity in multiple hereditary exostoses. Proc Natl Acad Sci U S A 107: 10932–10937.

1758. Matsumoto K, Ishizawa M, Okabe H et al. (2000). Hemangioma of bone arising in the ulna: imaging findings with emphasis on MR. Skeletal Radiol 29: 231–234.

1759. Matsumura T, Yamaguchi T, Seki K et al. (2008). Advantage of FISH analysis using FKHR probes for an adjunct to diagnosis of rhabdomyosarcomas. Virchows Arch 452: 251–258.

1760. Matsumura T, Yamaguchi T, Tochigi N et al. (2010). Angiomatoid fibrous histiocytoma including cases with pleomorphic features analysed by fluorescence in situ hybridisation. J Clin Pathol 63: 124–128.

1761. Matsuno T (1990). Benign fibrous histiocytoma involving the ends of long bone. Skeletal Radiol 19: 561–566.

1762. Matsuno T, Unni KK, McLeod RA et al. (1976). Telangiectatic osteogenic sarcoma. Cancer 38: 2538–2547.

1763. Matsuoka K, Ueda M, Miyamoto Y (2011). Giant intramuscular haemangioma of the chest wall with osteolytic change. Eur J Cardiothorac Surg 41:1202-12-3.

1764. Matsuyama A, Hisaoka M, Hashimoto H (2007). Angioleiomyoma: a clinicopathologic and immunohistochemical reappraisal with special reference to the correlation with myopericytoma. Hum Pathol 38: 645–651.

1765. Matsuyama A, Hisaoka M, Shimajiri S et al. (2008). DNA-based polymerase chain reaction for detecting FUS-CREB3L2 in low-grade fibromyxoid sarcoma using formalin-fixed, paraffin-embedded tissue specimens. Diagn Mol Pathol 17: 237–240.

1766. Matyakhina L, Pack S, Kirschner LS et al. (2003). Chromosome 2 (2p16) abnormalities in Carney complex tumours. J Med Genet 40: 268–277.

1767. Maurici D, Perez-Atayde A, Grier HE et al. (1998). Frequency and implications of chro-

mosome 8 and 12 gains in Ewing sarcoma. Cancer Genet Cytogenet 100: 106–110.

1768. Mautner VF, Asuagbor FA, Dombi E et al. (2008). Assessment of benign tumor burden by whole-body MRI in patients with neurofibromatosis 1. Neuro Oncol 10: 593–598.

1769. Mavrogenis AF, Soucacos PN, Papagelopoulos PJ (2011). Heterotopic ossification revisited. Orthopedics 34: 177

1770. Mayer-da-Silva A, Poiares-Baptista A, Guerra Rodrigo F et al. (1988). Juvenile hyaline fibromatosis. A histologic and histochemical study. Arch Pathol Lab Med 112: 928–931.

1771. Mayr-Kanhauser S, Behmel A, Aberer W (2001). Multiple glomus tumors of the skin with male-to-male transmission over four generations. J Invest Dermatol 116: 475–476.

1772. Mazur MT, Shultz JJ, Myers JL (1990). Granular cell tumor. Immunohistochemical analysis of 21 benign tumors and one malignant tumor. Arch Pathol Lab Med 114: 692–696.

1773. Mc Auley G, Jagannathan J, O'Regan K et al. (2012). Extraskeletal osteosarcoma: spectrum of imaging findings. AJR Am J Roentgenol 198: W31–W37.

1774. McCahon E, Sorensen PH, Davis JH et al. (2003). Non-resectable congenital tumors with the ETV6-NTRK3 gene fusion are highly responsive to chemotherapy. Med Pediatr Oncol 40: 288–292.

1775. McCarron KF, Goldblum JR (1998). Plexiform neurofibroma with and without associated malignant peripheral nerve sheath tumor: a clinicopathologic and immunohistochemical analysis of 54 cases. Mod Pathol 11: 612–617.

1776. McCarthy DM, Dorr CA, Mackintosh CE (1969). Unilateral localised gigantism of the extremities with lipomatosis, arthropathy and psoriasis. J Bone Joint Surg Br 51: 348–353.

1777. McCarthy EF, Lietman S, Argani P et al. (1999). Endovascular papillary angioendothelioma (Dabska tumor) of bone. Skeletal Radiol 28: 100–103.

1778. McCarthy EF, Matsuno T, Dorfman HD (1979). Malignant fibrous histiocytoma of bone: a study of 35 cases. Hum Pathol 10: 57–70.

1779. McClain KL, Leach CT, Jenson HB et al. (1995). Association of Epstein-Barr virus with leiomyosarcomas in children with AIDS. N Engl J Med 332: 12–18.

1780. McCluggage WG, Connolly L, McBride HA (2010). HMGA2 is a sensitive but not specific immunohistochemical marker of vulvovaginal aggressive angiomyxoma. Am J Surg Pathol 34: 1037–1042.

1781. McCluggage WG, Ganesan R, Hirschowitz L et al. (2004). Cellular angiofibroma and related fibromatous lesions of the vulva: report of a series of cases with a morphological spectrum wider than previously described. Histopathology 45: 360–368.

1782. McCluggage WG, Jamieson T, Dobbs SP et al. (2006). Aggressive angiomyxoma of the vulva: Dramatic response to gonadotropin-releasing hormone agonist therapy. Gynecol Oncol 100: 623–625.

1783. McCluggage WG, Patterson A, Maxwell P (2000). Aggressive angiomyxoma of pelvic parts exhibits oestrogen and progesterone receptor positivity. J Clin Pathol 53: 603–605.

1784. McComb EN, Feely MG, Neff JR et al. (2001). Cytogenetic instability, predominantly involving chromosome 1, is characteristic of elastofibroma. Cancer Genet Cytogenet 126: 68–72.

1785. McComb EN, Neff JR, Johansson SL et

al. (1997). Chromosomal anomalies in a case of proliferative myositis. Cancer Genet Cytogenet 98: 142–144.

1786. McCormick C, Duncan G, Goutsos KT et al. (2000). The putative tumor suppressors EXT1 and EXT2 form a stable complex that accumulates in the Golgi apparatus and catalyzes the synthesis of heparan sulfate. Proc Natl Acad Sci U S A 97: 668–673.

1787. McCormick D, Mentzel T, Beham A et al. (1994). Dedifferentiated liposarcoma. Clinicopathologic analysis of 32 cases suggesting a better prognostic subgroup among pleomorphic sarcomas. Am J Surg Pathol 18: 1213–1223.

1788. McDowell HP (2003). Update on childhood rhabdomyosarcoma. Arch Dis Child 88: 354–357.

1789. McGowan J, Smith CD, Maize J, Jr. et al. (2011). Giant fibrous hamartoma of infancy: a report of two cases and review of the literature. J Am Acad Dermatol 64: 579–586.

1790. McGregor DB, Partensky C, Wilbourn J et al. (1998). An IARC evaluation of polychlorinated dibenzo-p-dioxins and polychlorinated dibenzofurans as risk factors in human carcinogenesis. Environ Health Perspect 106 Suppl 2: 755–760.

1791. McHugh JB, Mukherji SK, Lucas DR (2009). Sino-orbital osteoma: a clinicopathologic study of 45 surgically treated cases with emphasis on tumors with osteoblastoma-like features. Arch Pathol Lab Med 133: 1587–1593.

1792. McIntyre BA, Brouillard P, Aerts V et al. (2004). Glomulin is predominantly expressed in vascular smooth muscle cells in the embryonic and adult mouse. Gene Expr Patterns 4: 351–358.

1793. McKeen EA, Bodurtha J, Meadows AT et al. (1978). Rhabdomyosarcoma complicating multiple neurofibromatosis. J Pediatr 93: 992–993.

1794. McKenna RW, Kyle RA, Kuehl WM (2008). Plasma cell neoplasms. In: WHO classification of tumours of haematopoietic and lymphoid tissue. Swerdlow SH, Campo E, Harris NL International Agency for Research on Cancer: Lyon: pp 200–213.

1795. McKusick VA (2000). Online Mendelian Inheritance in Man, OMIM (TM). McKusick-Nathans Institute for Genetic Medicine, Johns Hopkins University (Baltimore, MD) and National Center for Biotechnology Information, World Wide Web URL. http://www.ncbi.nlm.nih.gov/omim/ :National Library of Medicine (Bethesda, MD)

1796. McLeod RA, Dahlin DC (1979). Hamartoma (mesenchymoma) of the chest wall in infancy. Radiology 131: 657–661.

1797. McMaster ML, Goldstein AM, Bromley CM et al. (2001). Chordoma: incidence and survival patterns in the United States, 1973-1995. Cancer Causes Control 12: 1–11.

1798. McMaster ML, Goldstein AM, Parry DM (2011). Clinical features distinguish childhood chordoma associated with tuberous sclerosis complex (TSC) from chordoma in the general paediatric population. J Med Genet 48: 444–449.

1799. McMenamin ME, Calonje E (2002). Intravascular myopericytoma. J Cutan Pathol 29: 557–561.

1800. McMenamin ME, Fletcher CD (2001). Expanding the spectrum of malignant change in schwannomas: epithelioid malignant change, epithelioid malignant peripheral nerve sheath tumor, and epithelioid angiosarcoma: a study of

17 cases. Am J Surg Pathol 25: 13–25.

1801. McMenamin ME, Fletcher CD (2001). Mammary-type myofibroblastoma of soft tissue: a tumor closely related to spindle cell lipoma. Am J Surg Pathol 25: 1022–1029.

1802. McMenamin ME, Fletcher CD (2002). Malignant myopericytoma: expanding the spectrum of tumours with myopericytic differentiation. Histopathology 41: 450–460.

1803. McMonagle B, Connor S, Gleeson M (2011). Venous haemangioma of the mandibular division of the trigeminal nerve. J Laryngol Otol 125: 649–650.

1804. Mechtersheimer G, Otano-Joos M, Ohl S et al. (1999). Analysis of chromosomal imbalances in sporadic and NF1-associated peripheral nerve sheath tumors by comparative genomic hybridization. Genes Chromosomes Cancer 25: 362–369.

1805. Medeiros F, Corless CL, Duensing A et al. (2004). KIT-negative gastrointestinal stromal tumors: proof of concept and therapeutic implications. Am J Surg Pathol 28: 889–894.

1806. Medeiros F, Erickson-Johnson MR, Keeney GL et al. (2007). Frequency and characterization of HMGA2 and HMGA1 rearrangements in mesenchymal tumors of the lower genital tract. Genes Chromosomes Cancer 46: 981–990.

1807. Mehnert F, Beschorner R, Kuker W et al. (2004). Retroclival ecchordosis physaliphora: MR imaging and review of the literature. AJNR Am J Neuroradiol 25: 1851–1855.

1808. Mehollin-Ray AR, Kozinetz CA, Schlesinger AE et al. (2008). Radiographic abnormalities in Rothmund-Thomson syndrome and genotype-phenotype correlation with RECQL4 mutation status. AJR Am J Roentgenol 191: W62–W66.

1809. Mehregan AH, Shapiro L (1971). Angiolymphoid hyperplasia with eosinophilia. Arch Dermatol 103: 50–57.

1810. Meijer D, Gelderblom H, Karperien M et al. (2011). Expression of aromatase and estrogen receptor alpha in chondrosarcoma, but no beneficial effect of inhibiting estrogen signaling both in vitro and in vivo. Clin Sarcoma Res 1: 5

1811. Meis JM, Enzinger FM (1991). Inflammatory fibrosarcoma of the mesentery and retroperitoneum. A tumor closely simulating inflammatory pseudotumor. Am J Surg Pathol 15: 1146–1156.

1812. Meis JM, Enzinger FM (1991). Myolipoma of soft tissue. Am J Surg Pathol 15: 121–125.

1813. Meis JM, Enzinger FM (1992). Juxta-articular myxoma: a clinical and pathologic study of 65 cases. Hum Pathol 23: 639–646.

1814. Meis JM, Enzinger FM (1992). Proliferative fasciitis and myositis of childhood. Am J Surg Pathol 16: 364–372.

1815. Meis JM, Enzinger FM (1993). Chondroid lipoma. A unique tumor simulating liposarcoma and myxoid chondrosarcoma. Am J Surg Pathol 17: 1103–1112.

1816. Meis-Kindblom JM, Bergh P, Gunterberg B et al. (1999). Extraskeletal myxoid chondrosarcoma: a reappraisal of its morphologic spectrum and prognostic factors based on 117 cases. Am J Surg Pathol 23: 636–650.

1817. Meis-Kindblom JM, Kindblom LG (1998). Acral myxoinflammatory fibroblastic sarcoma: a low-grade tumor of the hands and feet. Am J Surg Pathol 22: 911–924.

1818. Meis-Kindblom JM, Kindblom LG (1998). Angiosarcoma of soft tissue: a study of 80 cases. Am J Surg Pathol 22: 683–697.

1819. Meis-Kindblom JM, Kindblom LG,

Enzinger FM (1995). Sclerosing epithelioid fibrosarcoma. A variant of fibrosarcoma simulating carcinoma. Am J Surg Pathol 19: 979–993.
1820. Meis-Kindblom JM, Sjogren H, Kindblom LG et al. (2001). Cytogenetic and molecular genetic analyses of liposarcoma and its soft tissue simulators: recognition of new variants and differential diagnosis. Virchows Arch 439: 141–151.
1821. Meister P, Buckmann FW, Konrad E (1978). Nodular fasciitis (analysis of 100 cases and review of the literature). Pathol Res Pract 162: 133–165.
1822. Meister P, Konrad E, Hubner G (1979). Malignant tumor of humerus with features of "adamantinoma" and Ewing's sarcoma. Pathol Res Pract 166: 112–122.
1823. Mejia-Guerrero S, Quejada M, Gokgoz N et al. (2010). Characterization of the 12q15 MDM2 and 12q13-14 CDK4 amplicons and clinical correlations in osteosarcoma. Genes Chromosomes Cancer 49: 518–525.
1824. Mendenhall WM, Zlotecki RA, Scarborough MT (2004). Dermatofibrosarcoma protuberans. Cancer 101: 2503–2508.
1825. Mendlick MR, Nelson M, Pickering D et al. (2001). Translocation t(1;3)(p36.3;q25) is a nonrandom aberration in epithelioid hemangioendothelioma. Am J Surg Pathol 25: 684–687.
1826. Meneses MF, Unni KK, Swee RG (1993). Bizarre parosteal osteochondromatous proliferation of bone (Nora's lesion). Am J Surg Pathol 17: 691–697.
1827. Mentzel T, Bainbridge TC, Katenkamp D (1997). Solitary fibrous tumour: clinicopathological, immunohistochemical, and ultrastructural analysis of 12 cases arising in soft tissues, nasal cavity and nasopharynx, urinary bladder and prostate. Virchows Arch 430: 445–453.
1828. Mentzel T, Beham A, Calonje E et al. (1997). Epithelioid hemangioendothelioma of skin and soft tissues: clinicopathologic and immunohistochemical study of 30 cases. Am J Surg Pathol 21: 363–374.
1829. Mentzel T, Beham A, Katenkamp D et al. (1998). Fibrosarcomatous ("high-grade") dermatofibrosarcoma protuberans: clinicopathologic and immunohistochemical study of a series of 41 cases with emphasis on prognostic significance. Am J Surg Pathol 22: 576–587.
1830. Mentzel T, Brown LF, Dvorak HF et al. (2001). The association between tumour progression and vascularity in myxofibrosarcoma and myxoid/round cell liposarcoma. Virchows Arch 438: 13–22.
1831. Mentzel T, Calonje E, Fletcher CD (1993). Lipoblastoma and lipoblastomatosis: a clinicopathological study of 14 cases. Histopathology 23: 527–533.
1832. Mentzel T, Calonje E, Fletcher CD (1994). Leiomyosarcoma with prominent osteoclast-like giant cells. Analysis of eight cases closely mimicking the so-called giant cell variant of malignant fibrous histiocytoma. Am J Surg Pathol 18: 258–265.
1833. Mentzel T, Calonje E, Nascimento AG et al. (1994). Infantile hemangiopericytoma versus infantile myofibromatosis. Study of a series suggesting a continuous spectrum of infantile myofibroblastic lesions. Am J Surg Pathol 18: 922–930.
1834. Mentzel T, Calonje E, Wadden C et al. (1996). Myxofibrosarcoma. Clinicopathologic analysis of 75 cases with emphasis on the low-grade variant. Am J Surg Pathol 20: 391–405.
1835. Mentzel T, Dei Tos AP, Sapi Z et al. (2006). Myopericytoma of skin and soft tissues: clinicopathologic and immunohistochemical study of 54 cases. Am J Surg Pathol 30: 104–113.
1836. Mentzel T, Dry S, Katenkamp D et al. (1998). Low-grade myofibroblastic sarcoma: analysis of 18 cases in the spectrum of myofibroblastic tumors. Am J Surg Pathol 22: 1228–1238.
1837. Mentzel T, Katenkamp D (2000). Sclerosing, pseudovascular rhabdomyosarcoma in adults. Clinicopathological and immunohistochemical analysis of three cases. Virchows Arch 436: 305–311.
1838. Mentzel T, Kuhnen C (2006). Spindle cell rhabdomyosarcoma in adults: clinicopathological and immunohistochemical analysis of seven new cases. Virchows Arch 449: 554–560.
1839. Mentzel T, Kutzner H (2005). Reticular and plexiform perineurioma: clinicopathological and immunohistochemical analysis of two cases and review of perineurial neoplasms of skin and soft tissues. Virchows Arch 447: 677–682.
1840. Mentzel T, Mazzoleni G, Dei Tos AP et al. (1997). Kaposiform hemangioendothelioma in adults. Clinicopathologic and immunohistochemical analysis of three cases. Am J Clin Pathol 108: 450–455.
1841. Mentzel T, Palmedo G, Kuhnen C (2010). Well-differentiated spindle cell liposarcoma ('atypical spindle cell lipomatous tumor') does not belong to the spectrum of atypical lipomatous tumor but has a close relationship to spindle cell lipoma: clinicopathologic, immunohistochemical, and molecular analysis of six cases. Mod Pathol 23: 729–736.
1842. Mentzel T, Reisshauer S, Rutten A et al. (2005). Cutaneous clear cell myomelanocytic tumour: a new member of the growing family of perivascular epithelioid cell tumours (PEComas). Clinicopathological and immunohistochemical analysis of seven cases. Histopathology 46: 498–504.
1843. Mentzel T, Scharer L, Kazakov DV et al. (2007). Myxoid dermatofibrosarcoma protuberans: clinicopathologic, immunohistochemical, and molecular analysis of eight cases. Am J Dermatopathol 29: 443–448.
1844. Mentzel T, Schildhaus HU, Palmedo G et al. (2012). Postradiation cutaneous angiosarcoma after treatment of breast carcinoma is characterized by MYC amplification in contrast to atypical vascular lesions after radiotherapy and control cases: clinicopathological, immunohistochemical and molecular analysis of 66 cases. Mod Pathol 25: 75–85.
1845. Mentzel T, Stengel B, Katenkamp D (1997). [Retiform hemangioendothelioma. Clinico-pathologic case report and discussion of the group of low malignancy vascular tumors]. Pathologe 18: 390–394.
1846. Merchant A, Smielewska M, Patel N et al. (2009). Somatic mutations in SQSTM1 detected in affected tissues from patients with sporadic Paget's disease of bone. J Bone Miner Res 24: 484–494.
1847. Merchant NB, Lewis JJ, Woodruff JM et al. (1999). Extremity and trunk desmoid tumors: a multifactorial analysis of outcome. Cancer 86: 2045–2052.
1848. Merchant W, Calonje E, Fletcher CD (1995). Inflammatory leiomyosarcoma: a morphological subgroup within the heterogeneous family of so-called inflammatory malignant fibrous histiocytoma. Histopathology 27: 525–532.
1849. Merck C, Angervall L, Kindblom LG et al. (1983). Myxofibrosarcoma. A malignant soft tissue tumor of fibroblastic-histiocytic origin. A clinicopathologic and prognostic study of 110 cases using multivariate analysis. Acta Pathol Microbiol Immunol Scand Suppl 282: 1–40.
1850. Mertens F, Dal Cin P, De Wever I et al. (2000). Cytogenetic characterization of peripheral nerve sheath tumours: a report of the CHAMP study group. J Pathol 190: 31–38.
1851. Mertens F, Fletcher CD, Antonescu CR et al. (2005). Clinicopathologic and molecular genetic characterization of low-grade fibromyxoid sarcoma, and cloning of a novel FUS/CREB3L1 fusion gene. Lab Invest 85: 408–415.
1852. Mertens F, Fletcher CD, Dal Cin P et al. (1998). Cytogenetic analysis of 46 pleomorphic soft tissue sarcomas and correlation with morphologic and clinical features: a report of the CHAMP Study Group. Chromosomes and MorPhology. Genes Chromosomes Cancer 22: 16–25.
1853. Mertens F, Moller E, Mandahl N et al. (2011). The t(X;6) in subungual exostosis results in transcriptional deregulation of the gene for insulin receptor substrate 4. Int J Cancer 128: 487–491.
1854. Mertens F, Romeo S, Bovee JVMG et al. (2011). Reclassification and subtyping of so-called malignant fibrous histiocytoma of bone: comparison with cytogenetic features. Clinical Sarcoma Research 1: 10
1855. Mertens F, Rydholm A, Brosjo O et al. (1994). Hibernomas are characterized by rearrangements of chromosome bands 11q13-21. Int J Cancer 58: 503–505.
1856. Mertens F, Rydholm A, Kreicbergs A et al. (1994). Loss of chromosome band 8q24 in sporadic osteocartilaginous exostoses. Genes Chromosomes Cancer 9: 8–12.
1857. Mertens F, Willen H, Rydholm A et al. (1995). Trisomy 20 is a primary chromosome aberration in desmoid tumors. Int J Cancer 63: 527–529.
1858. Mervak TR, Unni KK, Pritchard DJ et al. (1991). Telangiectatic osteosarcoma. Clin Orthop Relat Res 135–139.
1859. Messiaen L, Yao S, Brems H et al. (2009). Clinical and mutational spectrum of neurofibromatosis type 1-like syndrome. JAMA 302: 2111–2118.
1860. Messiaen LM, Callens T, Mortier G et al. (2000). Exhaustive mutation analysis of the NF1 gene allows identification of 95% of mutations and reveals a high frequency of unusual splicing defects. Hum Mutat 15: 541–555.
1861. Meyer WH, Spunt SL (2004). Soft tissue sarcomas of childhood. Cancer Treat Rev 30: 269–280.
1862. Meyerding H, Broders A, Hargrave R (1936). Clinical aspects of fibrosarcoma of the soft tissues of the extremities. Surg Gynecol Obstet 62:
1863. Meyerson M, Pellman D (2011). Cancer genomes evolve by pulverizing single chromosomes. Cell 144: 9–10.
1864. Mezzelani A, Sozzi G, Nessling M et al. (2000). Low grade fibromyxoid sarcoma. a further low-grade soft tissue malignancy characterized by a ring chromosome. Cancer Genet Cytogenet 122: 144–148.
1865. Micci F, Panagopoulos I, Bjerkehagen B et al. (2006). Deregulation of HMGA2 in an aggressive angiomyxoma with t(11;12)(q23;q15). Virchows Arch 448: 838–842.
1866. Michal M (1994). Retroperitoneal myolipoma. A tumour mimicking retroperitoneal angiomyolipoma and liposarcoma with myosarcomatous differentiation. Histopathology 25: 86–88.
1867. Michal M (1998). Inflammatory myxoid tumor of the soft parts with bizarre giant cells. Pathol Res Pract 194: 529–533.
1868. Michal M, Fanburg-Smith JC, Lasota J et al. (2006). Minute synovial sarcomas of the hands and feet: a clinicopathologic study of 21 tumors less than 1 cm. Am J Surg Pathol 30: 721–726.
1869. Michal M, Fetsch JF, Hes O et al. (1999). Nuchal-type fibroma: a clinicopathologic study of 52 cases. Cancer 85: 156–163.
1870. Michal M, Kazakov DV, Belousova I et al. (2004). A benign neoplasm with histopathological features of both schwannoma and retiform perineurioma (benign schwannoma-perineurioma): a report of six cases of a distinctive soft tissue tumor with a predilection for the fingers. Virchows Arch 445: 347–353.
1871. Michal M, Miettinen M (1999). Myoepitheliomas of the skin and soft tissues. Report of 12 cases. Virchows Arch 434: 393–400.
1872. Michal M, Mukensnabl P, Chlumska A et al. (1992). Fibrous hamartoma of infancy. A study of eight cases with immunohistochemical and electron microscopical findings. Pathol Res Pract 188: 1049–1053.
1873. Michal M, Zamecnik M, Gogora M et al. (1996). Pitfalls in the diagnosis of ectopic hamartomatous thymoma. Histopathology 29: 549–555.
1874. Micheli A, Trapani S, Brizzi I et al. (2009). Myositis ossificans circumscripta: a paediatric case and review of the literature. Eur J Pediatr 168: 523–529.
1875. Michie BA, Reid RP, Fallowfield ME (1994). Aneuploidy in atypical fibroxanthoma: DNA content quantification of 10 cases by image analysis. J Cutan Pathol 21: 404–407.
1876. Miettinen M (1991). Ossifying fibromyxoid tumor of soft parts. Additional observations of a distinctive soft tissue tumor. Am J Clin Pathol 95: 142–149.
1877. Miettinen M, Enzinger FM (1999). Epithelioid variant of pleomorphic liposarcoma: a study of 12 cases of a distinctive variant of high-grade liposarcoma. Mod Pathol 12: 722–728.
1878. Miettinen M, Fanburg-Smith JC, Virolainen M et al. (1999). Epithelioid sarcoma: an immunohistochemical analysis of 112 classical and variant cases and a discussion of the differential diagnosis. Hum Pathol 30: 934–942.
1879. Miettinen M, Fetsch JF (1998). Collagenous fibroma (desmoplastic fibroblastoma): a clinicopathologic analysis of 63 cases of a distinctive soft tissue lesion with stellate-shaped fibroblasts. Hum Pathol 29: 676–682.
1880. Miettinen M, Fetsch JF (2000). Distribution of keratins in normal endothelial cells and a spectrum of vascular tumors: implications in tumor diagnosis. Hum Pathol 31: 1062–1067.
1881. Miettinen M, Fetsch JF, Sobin LH et al. (2006). Gastrointestinal stromal tumors in patients with neurofibromatosis 1: a clinicopathologic and molecular genetic study of 45 cases. Am J Surg Pathol 30: 90–96.
1882. Miettinen M, Finnell V, Fetsch JF (2008). Ossifying fibromyxoid tumor of soft parts—a clinicopathologic and immunohistochemical study of 104 cases with long-term follow-up and a critical review of the literature. Am J Surg Pathol 32: 996–1005.

1883. Miettinen M, Furlong M, Sarlomo-Rikala M et al. (2001). Gastrointestinal stromal tumors, intramural leiomyomas, and leiomyosarcomas in the rectum and anus: a clinicopathologic, immunohistochemical, and molecular genetic study of 144 cases. Am J Surg Pathol 25: 1121–1133.
1884. Miettinen M, Hockerstedt K, Reitamo J et al. (1985). Intramuscular myxoma—a clinicopathological study of twenty-three cases. Am J Clin Pathol 84: 265–272.
1885. Miettinen M, Lasota J (2006). Gastrointestinal stromal tumors: review on morphology, molecular pathology, prognosis, and differential diagnosis. Arch Pathol Lab Med 130: 1466–1478.
1886. Miettinen M, Lasota J, Sobin LH (2005). Gastrointestinal stromal tumors of the stomach in children and young adults: a clinicopathologic, immunohistochemical, and molecular genetic study of 44 cases with long-term follow-up and review of the literature. Am J Surg Pathol 29: 1373–1381.
1887. Miettinen M, Limon J, Niezabitowski A et al. (2000). Patterns of keratin polypeptides in 110 biphasic, monophasic, and poorly differentiated synovial sarcomas. Virchows Arch 437: 275–283.
1888. Miettinen M, Lindenmayer AE, Chaubal A (1994). Endothelial cell markers CD31, CD34, and BNH9 antibody to H- and Y-antigens—evaluation of their specificity and sensitivity in the diagnosis of vascular tumors and comparison with von Willebrand factor. Mod Pathol 7: 82–90.
1889. Miettinen M, Makhlouf H, Sobin LH et al. (2006). Gastrointestinal stromal tumors of the jejunum and ileum: a clinicopathologic, immunohistochemical, and molecular genetic study of 906 cases before imatinib with long-term follow-up. Am J Surg Pathol 30: 477–489.
1890. Miettinen M, Paal E, Lasota J et al. (2002). Gastrointestinal glomus tumors: a clinicopathologic, immunohistochemical, and molecular genetic study of 32 cases. Am J Surg Pathol 26: 301–311.
1891. Miettinen M, Rapola J (1989). Immunohistochemical spectrum of rhabdomyosarcoma and rhabdomyosarcoma-like tumors. Expression of cytokeratin and the 68-kD neurofilament protein. Am J Surg Pathol 13: 120–132.
1892. Miettinen M, Sarlomo-Rikala M, Wang ZF (2011). Claudin-5 as an immunohistochemical marker for angiosarcoma and hemangioendotheliomas. Am J Surg Pathol 35: 1848–1856.
1893. Miettinen M, Shekitka KM, Sobin LH (2001). Schwannomas in the colon and rectum: a clinicopathologic and immunohistochemical study of 20 cases. Am J Surg Pathol 25: 846–855.
1894. Miettinen M, Sobin LH, Lasota J (2005). Gastrointestinal stromal tumors of the stomach: a clinicopathologic, immunohistochemical, and molecular genetic study of 1765 cases with long-term follow-up. Am J Surg Pathol 29: 52–68.
1895. Miettinen M, Wang ZF (2012). Prox1 transcription factor as a marker for vascular tumors-evaluation of 314 vascular endothelial and 1086 nonvascular tumors. Am J Surg Pathol 36: 351–359.
1896. Miettinen M, Wang ZF, Lasota J (2009). DOG1 antibody in the differential diagnosis of gastrointestinal stromal tumors: a study of 1840 cases. Am J Surg Pathol 33: 1401–1408.
1897. Miettinen M, Wang ZF, Paetau A et al. (2011). ERG transcription factor as an immunohistochemical marker for vascular endothelial tumors and prostatic carcinoma. Am J Surg Pathol 35: 432–441.
1898. Miettinen M, Wang ZF, Sarlomo-Rikala M et al. (2011). Succinate dehydrogenase-deficient GISTs: a clinicopathologic, immunohistochemical, and molecular genetic study of 66 gastric GISTs with predilection to young age. Am J Surg Pathol 35: 1712–1721.
1899. Miettinen MM, El-Rifai W, Sarlomo-Rikala M et al. (1997). Tumor size-related DNA copy number changes occur in solitary fibrous tumors but not in hemangiopericytomas. Mod Pathol 10: 1194–1200.
1899A. Meyerson M, Pellman D. (2011). Cancer genomes evolve by pulverizing single chromosomes. Cell. 144:9-10.
1900. Mihic-Probst D, Zhao J, Saremaslani P et al. (2004). CGH analysis shows genetic similarities and differences in atypical fibroxanthoma and undifferentiated high grade pleomorphic sarcoma. Anticancer Res 24: 19–26.
1901. Milchgrub S, Ghandur-Mnaymneh L, Dorfman HD et al. (1993). Synovial sarcoma with extensive osteoid and bone formation. Am J Surg Pathol 17: 357–363.
1902. Miller KK, Daly PA, Sentochnik D et al. (1998). Pseudo-Cushing's syndrome in human immunodeficiency virus-infected patients. Clin Infect Dis 27: 68–72.
1903. Miller-Breslow A, Dorfman HD (1988). Dupuytren's (subungual) exostosis. Am J Surg Pathol 12: 368–378.
1904. Mills AM, Beck AH, Montgomery KD et al. (2011). Expression of subtype-specific group 1 leiomyosarcoma markers in a wide variety of sarcomas by gene expression analysis and immunohistochemistry. Am J Surg Pathol 35: 583–589.
1905. Min HS, Kang HG, Lee JH et al. (2010). Desmoplastic fibroma with malignant transformation. Ann Diagn Pathol 14: 50–55.
1906. Mirra JM (1989). Bone tumors: clinical, radiologic, and pathologic correlations. Lea & Febiger: Philadelphia: pp 692–735; 759–766.
1907. Mirra JM, Bauer FC, Grant TT (1981). Giant cell tumor with viral-like intranuclear inclusions associated with Paget's disease. Clin Orthop Relat Res 243–251.
1908. Mirra JM, Bullough PG, Marcove RC et al. (1974). Malignant fibrous histiocytoma and osteosarcoma in association with bone infarcts; report of four cases, two in caisson workers. J Bone Joint Surg Am 56: 932–940.
1909. Mirra JM, Gold R, Downs J et al. (1985). A new histologic approach to the differentiation of enchondroma and chondrosarcoma of the bones. A clinicopathologic analysis of 51 cases. Clin Orthop Relat Res 214–237.
1910. Mirra JM, Gold RH, Rand F (1982). Disseminated nonossifying fibromas in association with cafe-au-lait spots (Jaffe-Campanacci syndrome). Clin Orthop Relat Res 192–205.
1911. Mirra JM, Kessler S, Bhuta S et al. (1992). The fibroma-like variant of epithelioid sarcoma. A fibrohistiocytic/myoid cell lesion often confused with benign and malignant spindle cell tumors. Cancer 69: 1382–1395.
1912. Misago N, Ohkawa T, Yanai T et al. (2008). Superficial acral fibromyxoma on the tip of the big toe: expression of CD10 and nestin. J Eur Acad Dermatol Venereol 22: 255–257.
1913. Mitchell AD, Ayoub K, Mangham DC et al. (2000). Experience in the treatment of dedifferentiated chondrosarcoma. J Bone Joint Surg Br 82: 55–61.
1914. Mitchell ML, di Sant'Agnese PA, Gerber JE (1982). Fibrous hamartoma of infancy. Hum Pathol 13: 586–588.
1915. Mitelman F, Johansson B, Mertens F (2012). Mitelman Database of Chromosome Aberrations and Gene Fusions in Cancer. National Cancer Institute (http://cgap.nci.nih.gov/Chromosomes/Mitelman).
1916. Mittal S, Goswami C, Kanoria N et al. (2007). Post-irradiation angiosarcoma of bone. J Cancer Res Ther 3: 96–99.
1917. Miyajima K, Oda Y, Oshiro Y et al. (2002). Clinicopathological prognostic factors in soft tissue leiomyosarcoma: a multivariate analysis. Histopathology 40: 353–359.
1918. Miyake I, Tokumaru H, Sugino H et al. (1995). Juvenile hyaline fibromatosis. Case report with five years' follow-up. Am J Dermatopathol 17: 584–590.
1919. Miyaki M, Konishi M, Kikuchi-Yanoshita R et al. (1993). Coexistence of somatic and germ-line mutations of APC gene in desmoid tumors from patients with familial adenomatous polyposis. Cancer Res 53: 5079–5082.
1920. Miyamoto M, Tsunoda R, Gembun Y et al. (2010). Recurrence of fibrous hamartoma of infancy excised 14 years after the primary surgery. J Neurosurg Pediatr 5: 136–139.
1921. Mobley BC, McKenney JK, Bangs CD et al. (2010). Loss of SMARCB1/INI1 expression in poorly differentiated chordomas. Acta Neuropathol 120: 745–753.
1922. Modena P, Lualdi E, Facchinetti F et al. (2005). SMARCB1/INI1 tumor suppressor gene is frequently inactivated in epithelioid sarcomas. Cancer Res 65: 4012–4019.
1923. Mohamed AN, Zalupski MM, Ryan JR et al. (1997). Cytogenetic aberrations and DNA ploidy in soft tissue sarcoma. A Southwest Oncology Group Study. Cancer Genet Cytogenet 99: 45–53.
1924. Mohseny AB, Szuhai K, Romeo S et al. (2009). Osteosarcoma originates from mesenchymal stem cells in consequence of aneuploidization and genomic loss of Cdkn2. J Pathol 219: 294–305.
1925. Mohseny AB, Tieken C, van der Velden PA et al. (2010). Small deletions but not methylation underlie CDKN2A/p16 loss of expression in conventional osteosarcoma. Genes Chromosomes Cancer 49: 1095–1103.
1926. Molenaar WM, DeJong B, Buist J et al. (1989). Chromosomal analysis and the classification of soft tissue sarcomas. Lab Invest 60: 266–274.
1927. Moller E, Hornick JL, Magnusson L et al. (2011). FUS-CREB3L2/L1-positive sarcomas show a specific gene expression profile with upregulation of CD24 and FOXL1. Clin Cancer Res 17: 2646–2656.
1928. Momeni P, Glockner G, Schmidt O et al. (2000). Mutations in a new gene, encoding a zinc-finger protein, cause tricho-rhino-phalangeal syndrome type I. Nat Genet 24: 71–74.
1929. Monaghan H, Salter DM, Al-Nafussi A (2001). Giant cell tumour of tendon sheath (localised nodular tenosynovitis): clinicopathological features of 71 cases. J Clin Pathol 54: 404–407.
1930. Monda L, Wick MR (1985). S-100 protein immunostaining in the differential diagnosis of chondroblastoma. Hum Pathol 16: 287–293.
1931. Mondal SK (2010). Cytodiagnosis of benign fibrous histiocytoma of rib and diagnostic dilemma: a case report. Diagn Cytopathol 38: 457–460.
1932. Monnat RJ, Jr. (2001). Cancer pathogenesis in the human RecQ helicase deficiency syndromes. In: From Premature Gray Hair to Helicase: Werner Syndrome Implications for Aging and Cancer. Goto M, Miller RW GANN Monograph on Cancer Research. 83–94.
1933. Monnat RJ, Jr. (2010). Human RECQ helicases: roles in DNA metabolism, mutagenesis and cancer biology. Semin Cancer Biol 20: 329–339.
1934. Montgomery E, Goldblum JR, Fisher C (2001). Myofibrosarcoma: a clinicopathologic study. Am J Surg Pathol 25: 219–228.
1935. Montgomery E, Lee JH, Abraham SC et al. (2001). Superficial fibromatoses are genetically distinct from deep fibromatoses. Mod Pathol 14: 695–701.
1936. Montgomery E, Torbenson MS, Kaushal M et al. (2002). Beta-catenin immunohistochemistry separates mesenteric fibromatosis from gastrointestinal stromal tumor and sclerosing mesenteritis. Am J Surg Pathol 26: 1296–1301.
1937. Montgomery EA, Devaney KO, Giordano TJ et al. (1998). Inflammatory myxohyaline tumor of distal extremities with virocyte or Reed-Sternberg-like cells: a distinctive lesion with features simulating inflammatory conditions, Hodgkin's disease, and various sarcomas. Mod Pathol 11: 384–391.
1938. Montgomery EA, Meis JM (1991). Nodular fasciitis. Its morphologic spectrum and immunohistochemical profile. Am J Surg Pathol 15: 942–948.
1939. Montgomery EA, Meis JM, Mitchell MS et al. (1992). Atypical decubital fibroplasia. A distinctive fibroblastic pseudotumor occurring in debilitated patients. Am J Surg Pathol 16: 708–715.
1940. Moon NF (1994). Adamantinoma of the appendicular skeleton in children. Int Orthop 18: 379–388.
1941. Moon NF, Mori H (1986). Adamantinoma of the appendicular skeleton—updated. Clin Orthop Relat Res 215–237.
1942. Moore JR, Weiland AJ, Curtis RM (1984). Localized nodular tenosynovitis: experience with 115 cases. J Hand Surg Am 9: 412–417.
1943. Moore PS, Chang Y (1995). Detection of herpesvirus-like DNA sequences in Kaposi's sarcoma in patients with and without HIV infection. N Engl J Med 332: 1181–1185.
1944. Moosavi C, Jha P, Fanburg-Smith JC (2007). An update on plexiform fibrohistiocytic tumor and addition of 66 new cases from the Armed Forces Institute of Pathology, in honor of Franz M. Enzinger, MD. Ann Diagn Pathol 11: 313–319.
1945. Moosavi CA, Al-Nahar LA, Murphey MD et al. (2008). Fibroosseous [corrected] pseudotumor of the digit: a clinicopathologic study of 43 new cases. Ann Diagn Pathol 12: 21–28.
1946. Moreau LC, Turcotte R, Ferguson P et al. (2011). Myxoid\round cell liposarcoma (MRCLS) revisited: an analysis of 418 primarily managed cases. Ann Surg Oncol 19:1081-1088.
1947. Morel M, Taieb S, Penel N et al. (2011). Imaging of the most frequent superficial soft-tissue sarcomas. Skeletal Radiol 40: 271–284.
1948. Morerio C, Nozza P, Tassano E et al. (2009). Differential diagnosis of lipoma-like lipoblastoma. Pediatr Blood Cancer 52: 132–134.
1949. Morerio C, Rapella A, Rosanda C et al. (2005). PLAG1-HAS2 fusion in lipoblastoma with masked 8q intrachromosomal rearrangement. Cancer Genet Cytogenet 156: 183–184.
1950. Moretti VM, Brooks JS, Ogilvie CM (2010). Case report: hemosiderotic fibrohistiocytic lipomatous lesion: a clinicopathologic

characterization. Clin Orthop Relat Res 468: 2808–2813.

1951. Morimitsu Y, Nakajima M, Hisaoka M et al. (2000). Extrapleural solitary fibrous tumor: clinicopathologic study of 17 cases and molecular analysis of the p53 pathway. APMIS 108: 617–625.

1952. Morotti RA, Nicol KK, Parham DM et al. (2006). An immunohistochemical algorithm to facilitate diagnosis and subtyping of rhabdomyosarcoma: the Children's Oncology Group experience. Am J Surg Pathol 30: 962–968.

1953. Morris EJ, Dyson NJ SBD (2001). Retinoblastoma protein partners. Adv Cancer Res 82: 1–54.

1954. Morrison C, Radmacher M, Mohammed N et al. (2005). MYC amplification and polysomy 8 in chondrosarcoma: array comparative genomic hybridization, fluorescent in situ hybridization, and association with outcome. J Clin Oncol 23: 9369–9376.

1955. Morton K, Robertson AJ, Hadden W (1987). Angiolymphoid hyperplasia with eosinophilia: report of a case arising from the radial artery. Histopathology 11: 963–969.

1956. Moser MJ, Bigbee WL, Grant SG et al. (2000). Genetic instability and hematologic disease risk in Werner syndrome patients and heterozygotes. Cancer Res 60: 2492–2496.

1957. Moser MJ, Kamath-Loeb AS, Jacob JE et al. (2000). WRN helicase expression in Werner syndrome cell lines. Nucleic Acids Res 28: 648–654.

1958. Moser RP, Jr., Sweet DE, Haseman DB et al. (1987). Multiple skeletal fibroxanthomas: radiologic-pathologic correlation of 72 cases. Skeletal Radiol 16: 353–359.

1959. Moses AV, Jarvis MA, Raggo C et al. (2002). A functional genomics approach to Kaposi's sarcoma. Ann N Y Acad Sci 975: 180–191.

1960. Moskovszky L, Dezso K, Athanasou N et al. (2010). Centrosome abnormalities in giant cell tumour of bone: possible association with chromosomal instability. Mod Pathol 23: 359–366.

1961. Moskovszky L, Szuhai K, Krenacs T et al. (2009). Genomic instability in giant cell tumor of bone. A study of 52 cases using DNA ploidy, relocalization FISH, and array-CGH analysis. Genes Chromosomes Cancer 48: 468–479.

1962. Mosquera JM, Dal Cin P, Mertz KD et al. (2011). Validation of a TFE3 break-apart FISH assay for Xp11.2 translocation renal cell carcinomas. Diagn Mol Pathol 20: 129–137.

1963. Mosquera JM, Fletcher CD (2009). Expanding the spectrum of malignant progression in solitary fibrous tumors: a study of 8 cases with a discrete anaplastic component—is this dedifferentiated SFT? Am J Surg Pathol 33: 1314–1321.

1964. Motoi T, Kumagai A, Tsuji K et al. (2010). Diagnostic utility of dual-color break-apart chromogenic in situ hybridization for the detection of rearranged SS18 in formalin-fixed, paraffin-embedded synovial sarcoma. Hum Pathol 41: 1397–1404.

1965. Motoyama T, Ogose A, Watanabe H (1996). Ossifying fibromyxoid tumor of the retroperitoneum. Pathol Int 46: 79–83.

1966. Mouton SC, Rosenberg HS, Cohen MC et al. (1996). Malignant ectomesenchymoma in childhood. Pediatr Pathol Lab Med 16: 607–624.

1967. Muftuoglu M, Oshima J, von KC et al. (2008). The clinical characteristics of Werner syndrome: molecular and biochemical diagnosis. Hum Genet 124: 369–377.

1968. Mugneret F, Lizard S, Aurias A et al. (1988). Chromosomes in Ewing's sarcoma. II. Nonrandom additional changes, trisomy 8 and der(16)t(1;16). Cancer Genet Cytogenet 32: 239–245.

1969. Mukai M, Torikata C, Iri H et al. (1992). Immunohistochemical identification of aggregated actin filaments in formalin-fixed, paraffin-embedded sections. I. A study of infantile digital fibromatosis by a new pretreatment. Am J Surg Pathol 16: 110–115.

1970. Mukai M, Torikata C, Iri H et al. (1986). Infantile digital fibromatosis. An electron microscopic and immunohistochemical study. Acta Pathol Jpn 36: 1605–1615.

1971. Mukai M, Torikata C, Iri H et al. (1984). Histogenesis of clear cell sarcoma of tendons and aponeuroses. An electron-microscopic, biochemical, enzyme histochemical, and immunohistochemical study. Am J Pathol 114: 264–272.

1972. Mukai M, Torikata C, Iri H et al. (1984). Alveolar soft part sarcoma. An elaboration of a three-dimensional configuration of the crystalloids by digital image processing. Am J Pathol 116: 398–406.

1973. Mukherjee D, Chaichana KL, Gokaslan ZL et al. (2011). Survival of patients with malignant primary osseous spinal neoplasms: results from the Surveillance, Epidemiology, and End Results (SEER) database from 1973 to 2003. J Neurosurg Spine 14: 143–150.

1974. Mukonoweshuro P, McCormick F, Rachapalli V et al. (2007). Paratesticular mammary-type myofibroblastoma. Histopathology 50: 396–397.

1975. Mulder JD, Schutte HE, Kroon HM et al. (1993). Radiologic atlas of bone tumors. Elsevier: Amsterdam.

1976. Mulligan ME, McRae GA, Murphey MD (1999). Imaging features of primary lymphoma of bone. AJR Am J Roentgenol 173: 1691–1697.

1977. Mulliken JB, Glowacki J (1982). Hemangiomas and vascular malformations in infants and children: a classification based on endothelial characteristics. Plast Reconstr Surg 69: 412–422.

1978. Munshi NC, Anderson KC, Bergsagel PL et al. (2011). Consensus recommendations for risk stratification in multiple myeloma: report of the International Myeloma Workshop Consensus Panel 2. Blood 117: 4696–4700.

1979. Muramatsu K, Ihara K, Tani Y et al. (2008). Intramuscular hemangioma of the upper extremity in infants and children. J Pediatr Orthop 28: 387–390.

1980. Muroya K, Nishimura G, Douya H et al. (2002). Diaphyseal medullary stenosis with malignant fibrous histiocytoma: further evidence for loss of heterozygosity involving 9p21-22 in tumor tissue. Genes Chromosomes Cancer 33: 326–328.

1981. Murphey MD, Jelinek JS, Temple HT et al. (2004). Imaging of periosteal osteosarcoma: radiologic-pathologic comparison. Radiology 233: 129–138.

1982. Murphey MD, Nomikos GC, Flemming DJ et al. (2001). From the archives of AFIP. Imaging of giant cell tumor and giant cell reparative granuloma of bone: radiologic-pathologic correlation. Radiographics 21: 1283–1309.

1983. Murphey MD, Rhee JH, Lewis RB et al. (2008). Pigmented villonodular synovitis: radiologic-pathologic correlation. Radiographics 28: 1493–1518.

1984. Murphey MD, Ruble CM, Tyszko SM et al. (2009). From the archives of the AFIP: musculoskeletal fibromatoses: radiologic-pathologic correlation. Radiographics 29: 2143–2173.

1985. Murphey MD, Walker EA, Wilson AJ et al. (2003). From the archives of the AFIP: imaging of primary chondrosarcoma: radiologic-pathologic correlation. Radiographics 23: 1245–1278.

1986. Murphey MD, wan JS, Temple HT et al. (2003). Telangiectatic osteosarcoma: radiologic-pathologic comparison. Radiology 229: 545–553.

1987. Murphy BA, Kilpatrick SE, Panella MJ et al. (1996). Extra-acral calcifying aponeurotic fibroma: a distinctive case with 23-year follow-up. J Cutan Pathol 23: 369–372.

1988. Myers BW, Masi AT (1980). Pigmented villonodular synovitis and tenosynovitis: a clinical epidemiologic study of 166 cases and literature review. Medicine (Baltimore) 59: 223–238.

1989. Myhre-Jensen O (1981). A consecutive 7-year series of 1331 benign soft tissue tumours. Clinicopathologic data. Comparison with sarcomas. Acta Orthop Scand 52: 287–293.

1990. Myhre-Jensen O, Kaae S, Madsen EH et al. (1983). Histopathological grading in soft-tissue tumours. Relation to survival in 261 surgically treated patients. Acta Pathol Microbiol Immunol Scand A 91: 145–150.

1991. Mylona S, Patsoura S, Galani P et al. (2010). Osteoid osteomas in common and in technically challenging locations treated with computed tomography-guided percutaneous radiofrequency ablation. Skeletal Radiol 39: 443–449.

1992. Nagamine N, Nohara Y, Ito E (1982). Elastofibroma in Okinawa. A clinicopathologic study of 170 cases. Cancer 50: 1794–1805.

1993. Naka T, Fukuda T, Shinohara N et al. (1995). Osteosarcoma versus malignant fibrous histiocytoma of bone in patients older than 40 years. A clinicopathologic and immunohistochemical analysis with special reference to malignant fibrous histiocytoma-like osteosarcoma. Cancer 76: 972–984.

1994. Nakajima H, Sim FH, Bond JR et al. (1997). Small cell osteosarcoma of bone. Review of 72 cases. Cancer 79: 2095–2106.

1995. Nakanishi K, Yoshikawa H, Ueda T et al. (2001). Postradiation sarcomas of the pelvis after treatment for uterine cervical cancer: review of the CT and MR findings of five cases. Skeletal Radiol 30: 132–137.

1996. Nakashima Y, Unni KK, Shives TC et al. (1986). Mesenchymal chondrosarcoma of bone and soft tissue. A review of 111 cases. Cancer 57: 2444–2453.

1997. Nakashima Y, Yamamuro T, Fujiwara Y et al. (1983). Osteofibrous dysplasia (ossifying fibroma of long bones). A study of 12 cases. Cancer 52: 909–914.

1998. Nalbantoglu U, Gereli A, Kocaoglu B et al. (2008). Fibro-osseous pseudotumor of the digits: a rare tumor in an unusual location. J Hand Surg Am 33: 273–276.

1999. Naouri M, Michenet P, Chassaing N et al. (2007). Immunohistochemical characterization of elastofibroma and exclusion of ABCC6 as a predisposing gene. Br J Dermatol 156: 755–758.

2000. Narchi H (2001). Four half-siblings with infantile myofibromatosis: a case for autosomal-recessive inheritance. Clin Genet 59: 134–135.

2001. Narvaez JA, Martinez S, Dodd LG et al. (2007). Acral myxoinflammatory fibroblastic sarcomas: MRI findings in four cases. AJR Am J Roentgenol 188: 1302–1305.

2002. Nascimento AF, Bertoni F, Fletcher CD (2007). Epithelioid variant of myxofibrosarcoma: expanding the clinicomorphologic spectrum of myxofibrosarcoma in a series of 17 cases. Am J Surg Pathol 31: 99–105.

2003. Nascimento AF, Fletcher CD (2005). Spindle cell rhabdomyosarcoma in adults. Am J Surg Pathol 29: 1106–1113.

2004. Nascimento AF, Fletcher CD (2007). The controversial nosology of benign nerve sheath tumors: neurofilament protein staining demonstrates intratumoral axons in many sporadic schwannomas. Am J Surg Pathol 31: 1363–1370.

2005. Nascimento AF, McMenamin ME, Fletcher CD (2002). Liposarcomas/atypical lipomatous tumors of the oral cavity: a clinicopathologic study of 23 cases. Ann Diagn Pathol 6: 83–93.

2006. Nascimento AF, Ruiz R, Hornick JL et al. (2002). Calcifying fibrous 'pseudotumor': clinicopathologic study of 15 cases and analysis of its relationship to inflammatory myofibroblastic tumor. Int J Surg Pathol 10: 189–196.

2007. Nascimento AG, Huvos AG, Marcove RC (1979). Primary malignant giant cell tumor of bone: a study of eight cases and review of the literature. Cancer 44: 1393–1402.

2008. Nascimento AG, Keeney GL, Sciot R et al. (1997). Polymorphous hemangioendothelioma: a report of two cases, one affecting extranodal soft tissues, and review of the literature. Am J Surg Pathol 21: 1083–1089.

2009. Nascimento AG, Kurtin PJ, Guillou L et al. (1998). Dedifferentiated liposarcoma: a report of nine cases with a peculiar neurallike whorling pattern associated with metaplastic bone formation. Am J Surg Pathol 22: 945–955.

2010. Nasser H, Ahmed Y, Szpunar SM et al. (2011). Malignant granular cell tumor: a look into the diagnostic criteria. Pathol Res Pract 207: 164–168.

2011. Nasser H, Danforth RD, Jr., Sunbuli M et al. (2010). Malignant granular cell tumor: case report with a novel karyotype and review of the literature. Ann Diagn Pathol 14: 273–278.

2012. Naughton PA, Wandling M, Phade S et al. (2011). Intimal angiosarcoma causing abdominal aortic rupture. J Vasc Surg 53: 818–821.

2013. Naumann M, Schalke B, Klopstock T et al. (1995). Neurological multisystem manifestation in multiple symmetric lipomatosis: a clinical and electrophysiological study. Muscle Nerve 18: 693–698.

2014. Naumann S, Krallman PA, Unni KK et al. (2002). Translocation der(13;21)(q10;q10) in skeletal and extraskeletal mesenchymal chondrosarcoma. Mod Pathol 15: 572–576.

2015. Navarro M, Vilata J, Requena C et al. (2000). Palisaded encapsulated neuroma (solitary circumscribed neuroma) of the glans penis. Br J Dermatol 142: 1061–1062.

2016. Navas-Palacios JJ, Conde-Zurita JM (1984). Inclusion body myofibroblasts other than those seen in recurring digital fibroma of childhood. Ultrastruct Pathol 7: 109–121.

2017. Nayler SJ, Rubin BP, Calonje E et al. (2000). Composite hemangioendothelioma: a complex, low-grade vascular lesion mimicking angiosarcoma. Am J Surg Pathol 24: 352–361.

2018. Naylor MF, Nascimento AG, Sherrick AD et al. (1996). Elastofibroma dorsi: radiologic findings in 12 patients. AJR Am J Roentgenol 167: 683–687.

2019. NCCN (2011). NCCN clinical practice

guidelines in oncology: soft tissue sarcoma, version 2.2011. National Comprehensive Cancer Network Fort Washington, PA:National Comprehensive Cancer Network Inc. (http://www.nccn.org/professionals/physician_gls/pdf/sarcoma.pdf).
2020. NCI (2011). SEER Cancer statistics review, 1975-2008. National Cancer Institute, Bethesda Bethesda:National Cancer Institute (http://seer.cancer.gov/csr/1975_2008/).
2021. Negri T, Virdis E, Brich S et al. (2010). Functional mapping of receptor tyrosine kinases in myxoid liposarcoma. Clin Cancer Res 16: 3581–3593.
2022. Nelson M, Perry D, Ginsburg G et al. (2003). Translocation (1;4)(p31;q34) in nonossifying fibroma. Cancer Genet Cytogenet 142: 142–144.
2023. Nemoto O, Moser RP, Jr., Van Dam BE et al. (1990). Osteoblastoma of the spine. A review of 75 cases. Spine (Phila Pa 1976) 15: 1272–1280.
2024. Newton WA, Jr., Gehan EA, Webber BL et al. (1995). Classification of rhabdomyosarcomas and related sarcomas. Pathologic aspects and proposal for a new classification—an Intergroup Rhabdomyosarcoma Study. Cancer 76: 1073–1085.
2025. Newton WA, Jr., Meadows AT, Shimada H et al. (1991). Bone sarcomas as second malignant neoplasms following childhood cancer. Cancer 67: 193–201.
2026. Newton WA, Jr., Soule EH, Hamoudi AB et al. (1988). Histopathology of childhood sarcomas, Intergroup Rhabdomyosarcoma Studies I and II: clinicopathologic correlation. J Clin Oncol 6: 67–75.
2027. Ng TL, Gown AM, Barry TS et al. (2005). Nuclear beta-catenin in mesenchymal tumors. Mod Pathol 18: 68–74.
2028. Ng TL, O'Sullivan MJ, Pallen CJ et al. (2007). Ewing sarcoma with novel translocation t(2;16) producing an in-frame fusion of FUS and FEV. J Mol Diagn 9: 459–463.
2029. Niamba P, Leaute-Labreze C, Boralevi F et al. (2007). Further documentation of spontaneous regression of infantile digital fibromatosis. Pediatr Dermatol 24: 280–284.
2030. Nichols KE, Malkin D, Garber JE et al. (2001). Germ-line p53 mutations predispose to a wide spectrum of early-onset cancers. Cancer Epidemiol Biomarkers Prev 10: 83–87.
2031. Nicolaides A, Huang YQ, Li JJ et al. (1994). Gene amplification and multiple mutations of the K-ras oncogene in Kaposi's sarcoma. Anticancer Res 14: 921–926.
2032. Nicolas MM, Tamboli P, Gomez JA et al. (2010). Pleomorphic and dedifferentiated leiomyosarcoma: clinicopathologic and immunohistochemical study of 41 cases. Hum Pathol 41: 663–671.
2033. Nielsen AL, Kiaer T (1989). Malignant giant cell tumor of synovium and locally destructive pigmented villonodular synovitis: ultrastructural and immunohistochemical study and review of the literature. Hum Pathol 20: 765–771.
2034. Nielsen GP, Dickersin GR, Provenzal JM et al. (1995). Lipomatous hemangiopericytoma. A histologic, ultrastructural and immunohistochemical study of a unique variant of hemangiopericytoma. Am J Surg Pathol 19: 748–756.
2035. Nielsen GP, Fletcher CD, Smith MA et al. (2002). Soft tissue aneurysmal bone cyst: a clinicopathologic study of five cases. Am J Surg Pathol 26: 64–69.
2036. Nielsen GP, Keel SB, Dickersin GR et al. (1999). Chondromyxoid fibroma: a tumor showing myofibroblastic, myochondroblastic, and chondrocytic differentiation. Mod Pathol 12: 514–517.
2037. Nielsen GP, O'Connell JX, Dickersin GR et al. (1995). Chondroid lipoma, a tumor of white fat cells. A brief report of two cases with ultrastructural analysis. Am J Surg Pathol 19: 1272–1276.
2038. Nielsen GP, O'Connell JX, Dickersin GR et al. (1996). Collagenous fibroma (desmoplastic fibroblastoma): a report of seven cases. Mod Pathol 9: 781–785.
2039. Nielsen GP, O'Connell JX, Dickersin GR et al. (1997). Solitary fibrous tumor of soft tissue: a report of 15 cases, including 5 malignant examples with light microscopic, immunohistochemical, and ultrastructural data. Mod Pathol 10: 1028–1037.
2040. Nielsen GP, O'Connell JX, Rosenberg AE (1998). Intramuscular myxoma: a clinicopathologic study of 51 cases with emphasis on hypercellular and hypervascular variants. Am J Surg Pathol 22: 1222–1227.
2041. Nielsen GP, Oliva E, Young RH et al. (1995). Alveolar soft-part sarcoma of the female genital tract: a report of nine cases and review of the literature. Int J Gynecol Pathol 14: 283–292.
2042. Nielsen GP, Rosenberg AE, Young RH et al. (1996). Angiomyofibroblastoma of the vulva and vagina. Mod Pathol 9: 284–291.
2043. Nielsen GP, Srivastava A, Kattapuram S et al. (2009). Epithelioid hemangioma of bone revisited: a study of 50 cases. Am J Surg Pathol 33: 270–277.
2044. Nielsen GP, Stemmer-Rachamimov AO, Ino Y et al. (1999). Malignant transformation of neurofibromas in neurofibromatosis 1 is associated with CDKN2A/p16 inactivation. Am J Pathol 155: 1879–1884.
2045. Nielsen TO, West RB, Linn SC et al. (2002). Molecular characterisation of soft tissue tumours: a gene expression study. Lancet 359: 1301–1307.
2046. Niemeyer CM, Arico M, Basso G et al. (1997). Chronic myelomonocytic leukemia in childhood: a retrospective analysis of 110 cases. European Working Group on Myelodysplastic Syndromes in Childhood (EWOG-MDS). Blood 89: 3534–3543.
2047. Niemeyer P, Ludwig K, Werner M et al. (2004). Reconstruction of the pelvic ring using an autologous free non-vascularized fibula graft in a patient with benign fibrous histiocytoma. World J Surg Oncol 2: 38
2048. NIH (1988). Neurofibromatosis. Conference statement. National Institutes of Health Consensus Development Conference. Arch Neurol 45: 575–578.
2049. Niini T, Lopez-Guerrero JA, Ninomiya S et al. (2010). Frequent deletion of CDKN2A and recurrent coamplification of KIT, PDGFRA, and KDR in fibrosarcoma of bone—an array comparative genomic hybridization study. Genes Chromosomes Cancer 49: 132–143.
2050. Nilsson B, Bumming P, Meis-Kindblom JM et al. (2005). Gastrointestinal stromal tumors: the incidence, prevalence, clinical course, and prognostication in the preimatinib mesylate era—a population-based study in western Sweden. Cancer 103: 821–829.
2051. Nilsson M, Domanski HA, Mertens F et al. (2004). Molecular cytogenetic characterization of recurrent translocation breakpoints in bizarre parosteal osteochondromatous proliferation (Nora's lesion). Hum Pathol 35: 1063–1069.
2052. Nilsson M, Hoglund M, Panagopoulos I et al. (2002). Molecular cytogenetic mapping of recurrent chromosomal breakpoints in tenosynovial giant cell tumors. Virchows Arch 441: 475–480.
2053. Nilsson M, Mertens F, Hoglund M et al. (2006). Truncation and fusion of HMGA2 in lipomas with rearrangements of 5q32—>q33 and 12q14—>q15. Cytogenet Genome Res 112: 60–66.
2054. Nilsson M, Panagopoulos I, Mertens F et al. (2005). Fusion of the HMGA2 and NFIB genes in lipoma. Virchows Arch 447: 855–858.
2055. Nishida J, Sim FH, Wenger DE et al. (1997). Malignant fibrous histiocytoma of bone. A clinicopathologic study of 81 patients. Cancer 79: 482–493.
2056. Nishida N, Yutani C, Ishibashi-Ueda H et al. (2000). Histopathological characterization of aortic intimal sarcoma with multiple tumor emboli. Pathol Int 50: 923–927.
2057. Nishiguchi T, Mochizuki K, Tsujio T et al. (2010). Lumbar vertebral chordoma arising from an intraosseous benign notochordal cell tumour: radiological findings and histopathological description with a good clinical outcome. Br J Radiol 83: e49–e53.
2058. Nishijo K, Nakayama T, Aoyama T et al. (2004). Mutation analysis of the RECQL4 gene in sporadic osteosarcomas. Int J Cancer 111: 367–372.
2059. Nishio J, Akiho S, Iwasaki H et al. (2011). Translocation t(2;11) is characteristic of collagenous fibroma (desmoplastic fibroblastoma). Cancer Genet 204: 569–571.
2060. Nishio J, Althof PA, Bailey JM et al. (2006). Use of a novel FISH assay on paraffin-embedded tissues as an adjunct to diagnosis of alveolar rhabdomyosarcoma. Lab Invest 86: 547–556.
2061. Nishio J, Gentry JD, Neff JR et al. (2006). Monoallelic deletion of the p53 gene through chromosomal translocation in a small cell osteosarcoma. Virchows Arch 448: 852–856.
2062. Nishio J, Iwasaki H, Ohjimi Y et al. (2002). Ossifying fibromyxoid tumor of soft parts. Cytogenetic findings. Cancer Genet Cytogenet 133: 124–128.
2063. Nishio J, Iwasaki H, Ohjimi Y et al. (2004). Chromosomal imbalances in angioleiomyomas by comparative genomic hybridization. Int J Mol Med 13: 13–16.
2064. Nishio J, Reith JD, Ogose A et al. (2005). Cytogenetic findings in clear cell chondrosarcoma. Cancer Genet Cytogenet 162: 74–77.
2065. Nishio JN, Iwasaki H, Ohjimi Y et al. (2002). Gain of Xq detected by comparative genomic hybridization in elastofibroma. Int J Mol Med 10: 277–280.
2066. Nistal M, Paniagua R, Picazo ML et al. (1980). Granular changes in vascular leiomyosarcoma. Virchows Arch A Pathol Anat Histol 386: 239–248.
2067. Nixon HH, Scobie WG (1971). Congenital lipomatosis: a report of four cases. J Pediatr Surg 6: 742–745.
2067A. Noble-Topham SE, Burrow SR, Eppert Ket al. (1996). SAS is amplified predominantly in surface osteosarcoma.J Orthop Res 14: 700–705.
2068. Nofal A, Sanad M, Assaf M et al. (2009). Juvenile hyaline fibromatosis and infantile systemic hyalinosis: a unifying term and a proposed grading system. J Am Acad Dermatol 61: 695–700.
2069. Nojima T, Unni KK, McLeod RA et al. (1985). Periosteal chondroma and periosteal chondrosarcoma. Am J Surg Pathol 9: 666–677.
2070. Nonomura A, Kurumaya H, Kono N et al. (1988). Primary pulmonary artery sarcoma. Report of two autopsy cases studied by immunohistochemistry and electron microscopy, and review of 110 cases reported in the literature. Acta Pathol Jpn 38: 883–896.
2071. Nooij MA, Whelan J, Bramwell VH et al. (2005). Doxorubicin and cisplatin chemotherapy in high-grade spindle cell sarcomas of the bone, other than osteosarcoma or malignant fibrous histiocytoma: a European Osteosarcoma Intergroup Study. Eur J Cancer 41: 225–230.
2072. Nord KH, Magnusson L, Isaksson M et al. (2010). Concomitant deletions of tumor suppressor genes MEN1 and AIP are essential for the pathogenesis of the brown fat tumor hibernoma. Proc Natl Acad Sci U S A 107: 21122–21127.
2073. Norman A, Abdelwahab IF, Buyon J et al. (1986). Osteoid osteoma of the hip stimulating an early onset of osteoarthritis. Radiology 158: 417–420.
2074. North PE, Waner M, Mizeracki A et al. (2000). GLUT1: a newly discovered immunohistochemical marker for juvenile hemangiomas. Hum Pathol 31: 11–22.
2075. Norton KI, Wagreich JM, Granowetter L et al. (1996). Diaphyseal medullary stenosis (sclerosis) with bone malignancy (malignant fibrous histiocytoma): Hardcastle syndrome. Pediatr Radiol 26: 675–677.
2076. Nucci MR, Castrillon DH, Bai H et al. (2003). Biomarkers in diagnostic obstetric and gynecologic pathology: a review. Adv Anat Pathol 10: 55–68.
2077. Nucci MR, Granter SR, Fletcher CD (1997). Cellular angiofibroma: a benign neoplasm distinct from angiomyofibroblastoma and spindle cell lipoma. Am J Surg Pathol 21: 636–644.
2078. Nucci MR, Weremowicz S, Neskey DM et al. (2001). Chromosomal translocation t(8;12) induces aberrant HMGIC expression in aggressive angiomyxoma of the vulva. Genes Chromosomes Cancer 32: 172–176.
2079. Nunnery EW, Kahn LB, Guilford WB (1979). Locally aggressive fibrous histiocytoma of bone. A case report. S Afr Med J 55: 763–767.
2080. Nuovo M, Grimes M, Knowles D (1990). Glomus tumors: a clinicopathologic and immunohistochemical analysis of forty cases. Surgical Pathology 3: 31–45.
2081. Nuovo MA, Norman A, Chumas J et al. (1992). Myositis ossificans with atypical clinical, radiographic, or pathologic findings: a review of 23 cases. Skeletal Radiol 21: 87–101.
2082. Nussbeck W, Neureiter D, Soder S et al. (2004). Mesenchymal chondrosarcoma: an immunohistochemical study of 10 cases examining prognostic significance of proliferative activity and cellular differentiation. Pathology 36: 230–233.
2083. O'Connell FP, Pinkus JL, Pinkus GS (2004). CD138 (syndecan-1), a plasma cell marker immunohistochemical profile in hematopoietic and nonhematopoietic neoplasms. Am J Clin Pathol 121: 254–263.
2084. O'Connell JX, Kattapuram SV, Mankin HJ et al. (1993). Epithelioid hemangioma of bone. A tumor often mistaken for low-grade angiosarcoma or malignant hemangioendothelioma. Am J Surg Pathol 17: 610–617.
2085. O'Connell JX, Nielsen GP, Rosenberg AE (2001). Epithelioid vascular tumors of bone: a review and proposal of a classification

scheme. Adv Anat Pathol 8: 74–82.

2086. O'Connell JX, Wehrli BM, Nielsen GP et al. (2000). Giant cell tumors of soft tissue: a clinicopathologic study of 18 benign and malignant tumors. Am J Surg Pathol 24: 386–395.

2087. O'Malley DP, Opheim KE, Barry TS et al. (2001). Chromosomal changes in a dedifferentiated chondrosarcoma: a case report and review of the literature. Cancer Genet Cytogenet 124: 105–111.

2088. O'Regan EM, Vanguri V, Allen CM et al. (2009). Solitary fibrous tumor of the oral cavity: clinicopathologic and immunohistochemical study of 21 cases. Head Neck Pathol 3: 106–115.

2089. Ockner DM, Sayadi H, Swanson PE et al. (1997). Genital angiomyofibroblastoma. Comparison with aggressive angiomyxoma and other myxoid neoplasms of skin and soft tissue. Am J Clin Pathol 107: 36–44.

2090. Oda Y, Miyajima K, Kawaguchi K et al. (2001). Pleomorphic leiomyosarcoma: clinicopathologic and immunohistochemical study with special emphasis on its distinction from ordinary leiomyosarcoma and malignant fibrous histiocytoma. Am J Surg Pathol 25: 1030–1038.

2091. Oda Y, Sakamoto A, Saito T et al. (2001). Secondary malignant giant-cell tumour of bone: molecular abnormalities of p53 and H-ras gene correlated with malignant transformation. Histopathology 39: 629–637.

2092. Oda Y, Tamiya S, Oshiro Y et al. (2002). Reassessment and clinicopathological prognostic factors of malignant fibrous histiocytoma of soft parts. Pathol Int 52: 595–606.

2093. Oda Y, Tsuneyoshi M (2006). Extrarenal rhabdoid tumors of soft tissue: clinicopathological and molecular genetic review and distinction from other soft-tissue sarcomas with rhabdoid features. Pathol Int 56: 287–295.

2094. Oda Y, Yamamoto H, Takahira T et al. (2005). Frequent alteration of p16(INK4a)/p14(ARF) and p53 pathways in the round cell component of myxoid/round cell liposarcoma: p53 gene alterations and reduced p14(ARF) expression both correlate with poor prognosis. J Pathol 207: 410–421.

2095. Odink AE, van Asperen CJ, Vandenbroucke JP et al. (2001). An association between cartilaginous tumours and breast cancer in the national pathology registration in The Netherlands points towards a possible genetic trait. J Pathol 193: 190–192.

2096. Ogilvie CM, Crawford EA, Slotcavage RL et al. (2010). Treatment of adult rhabdomyosarcoma. Am J Clin Oncol 33: 128–131.

2097. Ognjanovic S, Linabery AM, Charbonneau B et al. (2009). Trends in childhood rhabdomyosarcoma incidence and survival in the United States, 1975-2005. Cancer 115: 4218–4226.

2098. Ognjanovic S, Olivier M, Bergemann TL et al. (2011). Sarcomas in TP53 germline mutation carriers: A review of the IARC TP53 database. Cancer

2099. Ogose A, Hotta T, Emura I et al. (2001). Recurrent malignant variant of phosphaturic mesenchymal tumor with oncogenic osteomalacia. Skeletal Radiol 30: 99–103.

2100. Ogose A, Kawashima H, Umezu H et al. (2004). Sclerosing epithelioid fibrosarcoma with der(10)t(10;17)(p11;q11). Cancer Genet Cytogenet 152: 136–140.

2101. Ogunsalu C, Smith NJ, Lewis A (1998). Fibrous dysplasia of the jaw bone: a review of 15 new cases and two cases of recurrence in Jamaica together with a case report. Aust Dent J 43: 390–394.

2102. Ogura K, Goto T, Nemoto T (2012). Painless giant angioleiomyoma in the subfascia of the lower leg. J Foot Ankle Surg 51: 99–102.

2103. Oh SD, Stephenson D, Schnall S et al. (2009). Malignant glomus tumor of the hand. Appl Immunohistochem Mol Morphol 17: 264–269.

2104. Ohali A, Avigad S, Cohen IJ et al. (2003). Association between telomerase activity and outcome in patients with nonmetastatic Ewing family of tumors. J Clin Oncol 21: 3836–3843.

2105. Ohjimi Y, Iwasaki H, Ishiguro M et al. (1994). Trisomy 2 found in proliferative myositis cultured cell. Cancer Genet Cytogenet 76: 157

2106. Ohsawa M, Naka N, Tomita Y et al. (1995). Use of immunohistochemical procedures in diagnosing angiosarcoma. Evaluation of 98 cases. Cancer 75: 2867–2874.

2107. Ohtani-Fujita N, Dryja TP, Rapaport JM et al. (1997). Hypermethylation in the retinoblastoma gene is associated with unilateral, sporadic retinoblastoma. Cancer Genet Cytogenet 98: 43–49.

2108. Okada K, Frassica FJ, Sim FH et al. (1994). Parosteal osteosarcoma. A clinicopathological study. J Bone Joint Surg Am 76: 366–378.

2109. Okada K, Hasegawa T, Yokoyama R et al. (2003). Osteosarcoma with cytokeratin expression: a clinicopathological study of six cases with an emphasis on differential diagnosis from metastatic cancer. J Clin Pathol 56: 742–746.

2110. Okada K, Unni KK, Swee RG et al. (1999). High grade surface osteosarcoma: a clinicopathologic study of 46 cases. Cancer 85: 1044–1054.

2111. Okada O, Demitsu T, Manabe M et al. (1999). A case of multiple subungual glomus tumors associated with neurofibromatosis type 1. J Dermatol 26: 535–537.

2112. Okamoto S, Hisaoka M, Ishida T et al. (2001). Extraskeletal myxoid chondrosarcoma: a clinicopathologic, immunohistochemical, and molecular analysis of 18 cases. Hum Pathol 32: 1116–1124.

2113. Okamoto S, Hisaoka M, Meis-Kindblom JM et al. (2002). Juxta-articular myxoma and intramuscular myxoma are two distinct entities. Activating Gs alpha mutation at Arg 201 codon does not occur in juxta-articular myxoma. Virchows Arch 440: 12–15.

2114. Okamoto S, Hisaoka M, Ushijima M et al. (2000). Activating Gs(alpha) mutation in intramuscular myxomas with and without fibrous dysplasia of bone. Virchows Arch 437: 133–137.

2115. Oliveira AM, Chou MM (2012). The TRE17/USP6 Oncogene: a riddle wrapped in a mystery inside an enigma. Front Biosci (Schol Ed) 4: 321–334.

2116. Oliveira AM, Dei Tos AP, Fletcher CD et al. (2000). Primary giant cell tumor of soft tissues: a study of 22 cases. Am J Surg Pathol 24: 248–256.

2117. Oliveira AM, Hsi BL, Weremowicz S et al. (2004). USP6 (Tre2) fusion oncogenes in aneurysmal bone cyst. Cancer Res 64: 1920–1923.

2118. Oliveira AM, Nascimento AG (2001). Pleomorphic liposarcoma. Semin Diagn Pathol 18: 274–285.

2119. Oliveira AM, Nascimento AG, Lloyd RV (2001). Leptin and leptin receptor mRNA are widely expressed in tumors of adipocytic differentiation. Mod Pathol 14: 549–555.

2120. Oliveira AM, Perez-Atayde AR, Dal Cin P et al. (2005). Aneurysmal bone cyst variant translocations upregulate USP6 transcription by promoter swapping with the ZNF9, COL1A1, TRAP150, and OMD genes. Oncogene 24: 3419–3426.

2121. Oliveira AM, Perez-Atayde AR, Inwards CY et al. (2004). USP6 and CDH11 oncogenes identify the neoplastic cell in primary aneurysmal bone cysts and are absent in so-called secondary aneurysmal bone cysts. Am J Pathol 165: 1773–1780.

2122. Oliveira AM, Sebo TJ, McGrory JE et al. (2000). Extraskeletal myxoid chondrosarcoma: a clinicopathologic, immunohistochemical, and ploidy analysis of 23 cases. Mod Pathol 13: 900–908.

2123. Olivier M, Goldgar DE, Sodha N et al. (2003). Li-Fraumeni and related syndromes: correlation between tumor type, family structure, and TP53 genotype. Cancer Res 63: 6643–6650.

2124. Olsen SH, Thomas DG, Lucas DR (2006). Cluster analysis of immunohistochemical profiles in synovial sarcoma, malignant peripheral nerve sheath tumor, and Ewing sarcoma. Mod Pathol 19: 659–668.

2125. Olsen TG, Helwig EB (1985). Angiolymphoid hyperplasia with eosinophilia. A clinicopathologic study of 116 patients. J Am Acad Dermatol 12: 781–796.

2126. Olsson L, Paulsson K, Bovee JV et al. (2011). Clonal evolution through loss of chromosomes and subsequent polyploidization in chondrosarcoma. PLoS One 6: e24977

2127. Onyango P, Feinberg AP (2011). A nucleolar protein, H19 opposite tumor suppressor (HOTS), is a tumor growth inhibitor encoded by a human imprinted H19 antisense transcript. Proc Natl Acad Sci U S A 108: 16759–16764.

2128. Oosthuizen SF, Barnetson J (1947). Two cases of lipomatosis involving bone. Br J Radiol 20: 426–432.

2129. Orbach D, Rey A, Cecchetto G et al. (2010). Infantile fibrosarcoma: management based on the European experience. J Clin Oncol 28: 318–323.

2130. Ordonez NG (1999). Alveolar soft part sarcoma: a review and update. Adv Anat Pathol 6: 125–139.

2131. Ordonez NG, Mackay B (1998). Alveolar soft-part sarcoma: a review of the pathology and histogenesis. Ultrastruct Pathol 22: 275–292.

2132. Orndal C, Rydholm A, Willen H et al. (1994). Cytogenetic intratumor heterogeneity in soft tissue tumors. Cancer Genet Cytogenet 78: 127–137.

2133. Orta L, Suprun U, Goldfarb A et al. (2006). Radiation-associated extraskeletal osteosarcoma of the chest wall. Arch Pathol Lab Med 130: 198–200.

2134. Oshima J, Martin GM, Hisama FM (1993). Werner syndrome. GeneReviewsTM [Internet] Seattle (WA): University of Seattle, Washington–[updated 2012 Feb 09].

2135. Oshiro Y, Fukuda T, Tsuneyoshi M (1995). Atypical fibroxanthoma versus benign and malignant fibrous histiocytoma. A comparative study of their proliferative activity using MIB-1, DNA flow cytometry, and p53 immunostaining. Cancer 75: 1128–1134.

2136. Oshiro Y, Shiratsuchi H, Tamiya S et al. (2000). Extraskeletal myxoid chondrosarcoma with rhabdoid features, with special reference to its aggressive behavior. Int J Surg Pathol 8: 145–152.

2137. Ostrowski ML, Inwards CY, Strickler JG et al. (1999). Osseous Hodgkin disease. Cancer 85: 1166–1178.

2138. Ostrowski ML, Spjut HJ (1997). Lesions of the bones of the hands and feet. Am J Surg Pathol 21: 676–690.

2139. Ote EL, Oriuchi N, Miyashita G et al. (2011). Pulmonary artery intimal sarcoma: the role of (1)F-fluorodeoxyglucose positron emission tomography in monitoring response to treatment. Jpn J Radiol 29: 279–282.

2140. Ottaviani G, Jaffe N (2009). The epidemiology of osteosarcoma. Cancer Treat Res 152: 3–13.

2141. Ottaviani S, Ayral X, Dougados M et al. (2011). Pigmented villonodular synovitis: a retrospective single-center study of 122 cases and review of the literature. Semin Arthritis Rheum 40: 539–546.

2142. Outwater EK, Marchetto BE, Wagner BJ et al. (1999). Aggressive angiomyxoma: findings on CT and MR imaging. AJR Am J Roentgenol 172: 435–438.

2143. Ozaki T, Paulussen M, Poremba C et al. (2001). Genetic imbalances revealed by comparative genomic hybridization in Ewing tumors. Genes Chromosomes Cancer 32: 164–171.

2144. Ozaki T, Schaefer KL, Wai D et al. (2002). Genetic imbalances revealed by comparative genomic hybridization in osteosarcomas. Int J Cancer 102: 355–365.

2145. Ozaki T, Wai D, Schafer KL et al. (2004). Comparative genomic hybridization in cartilaginous tumors. Anticancer Res 24: 1721–1725.

2146. Ozisik YY, Meloni AM, Peier A et al. (1994). Cytogenetic findings in 19 malignant bone tumors. Cancer 74: 2268–2275.

2147. Paal E, Miettinen M (2001). Retroperitoneal leiomyomas: a clinicopathologic and immunohistochemical study of 56 cases with a comparison to retroperitoneal leiomyosarcomas. Am J Surg Pathol 25: 1355–1363.

2148. Pack SD, Kirschner LS, Pak E et al. (2000). Genetic and histologic studies of somatomammotropic pituitary tumors in patients with the "complex of spotty skin pigmentation, myxomas, endocrine overactivity and schwannomas" (Carney complex). J Clin Endocrinol Metab 85: 3860–3865.

2149. Pagonidis K, Raissaki M, Gourtsoyiannis N (2005). Proliferative myositis: value of imaging. J Comput Assist Tomogr 29: 108–111.

2150. Paller AS, Gonzalez-Crussi F, Sherman JO (1989). Fibrous hamartoma of infancy. Eight additional cases and a review of the literature. Arch Dermatol 125: 88–91.

2151. Palmero EI, Achatz MI, Ashton-Prolla P et al. (2010). Tumor protein 53 mutations and inherited cancer: beyond Li-Fraumeni syndrome. Curr Opin Oncol 22: 64–69.

2152. Palmieri AJ, Kovarik JL (1962). Nonosteogenic fibroma of the rib. Am Surg 28: 794–798.

2153. Pan CC, Chung MY, Ng KF et al. (2008). Constant allelic alteration on chromosome 16p (TSC2 gene) in perivascular epithelioid cell tumour (PEComa): genetic evidence for the relationship of PEComa with angiomyolipoma. J Pathol 214: 387–393.

2154. Pan CC, Jong YJ, Chai CY et al. (2006). Comparative genomic hybridization study of perivascular epithelioid cell tumor: molecular genetic evidence of perivascular epithelioid cell tumor as a distinctive neoplasm. Hum Pathol 37: 606–612.

2155. Pan Z, Sanger WG, Bridge JA et al. (2012). A novel t(6;13)(q15;q34) translocation in a giant cell reparative granuloma (solid aneurysmal bone cyst). Hum Pathol 43:952-957.

2156. Panagopoulos I, Hoglund M, Mertens F et al. (1996). Fusion of the EWS and CHOP genes in myxoid liposarcoma. Oncogene 12: 489–494.

2157. Panagopoulos I, Mandahl N, Ron D et al. (1994). Characterization of the CHOP breakpoints and fusion transcripts in myxoid liposarcomas with the 12;16 translocation. Cancer Res 54: 6500–6503.

2158. Panagopoulos I, Mencinger M, Dietrich CU et al. (1999). Fusion of the RBP56 and CHN genes in extraskeletal myxoid chondrosarcomas with translocation t(9;17)(q22;q11). Oncogene 18: 7594–7598.

2159. Panagopoulos I, Mertens F, Debiec-Rychter M et al. (2002). Molecular genetic characterization of the EWS/ATF1 fusion gene in clear cell sarcoma of tendons and aponeuroses. Int J Cancer 99: 560–567.

2160. Panagopoulos I, Mertens F, Domanski HA et al. (2001). No EWS/FLI1 fusion transcripts in giant-cell tumors of bone. Int J Cancer 93: 769–772.

2161. Panagopoulos I, Mertens F, Isaksson M et al. (2002). Molecular genetic characterization of the EWS/CHN and RBP56/CHN fusion genes in extraskeletal myxoid chondrosarcoma. Genes Chromosomes Cancer 35: 340–352.

2162. Panagopoulos I, Storlazzi CT, Fletcher CD et al. (2004). The chimeric FUS/CREB3L2 gene is specific for low-grade fibromyxoid sarcoma. Genes Chromosomes Cancer 40: 218–228.

2163. Panoutsakopoulos G, Pandis N, Kyriazoglou I et al. (1999). Recurrent t(16;17)(q22;p13) in aneurysmal bone cysts. Genes Chromosomes Cancer 26: 265–266.

2164. Pansuriya TC, Kroon HM, Bovee JV (2010). Enchondromatosis: insights on the different subtypes. Int J Clin Exp Pathol 3: 557–569.

2165. Pansuriya TC, van Eijk R, d'Adamo P et al. (2011). Somatic mosaic IDH1 and IDH2 mutations are associated with enchondroma and spindle cell hemangioma in Ollier disease and Maffucci syndrome. Nat Genet 43: 1256–1261.

2166. Papachristou DJ, Palekar A, Surti U et al. (2009). Malignant granular cell tumor of the ulnar nerve with novel cytogenetic and molecular genetic findings. Cancer Genet Cytogenet 191: 46–50.

2167. Papadaki ME, Lietman SA, Levine MA et al. (2012). Review: Cherubism: best clinical practice. Orphanet Journal of Rare Diseases 7(Suppl 1):S6.

2168. Papadimitriou JC, Drachenberg CB (1994). Ultrastructural features of the matrix of small cell osteosarcoma. Hum Pathol 25: 430–431.

2169. Papagelopoulos PJ, Galanis E, Frassica FJ et al. (2000). Primary fibrosarcoma of bone. Outcome after primary surgical treatment. Clin Orthop Relat Res 373:88–103.

2170. Papagelopoulos PJ, Galanis EC, Mavrogenis AF et al. (2006). Survivorship analysis in patients with periosteal chondrosarcoma. Clin Orthop Relat Res 448: 199–207.

2171. Papagelopoulos PJ, Galanis EC, Sim FH et al. (2000). Clinicopathologic features, diagnosis, and treatment of malignant fibrous histiocytoma of bone. Orthopedics 23: 59–65.

2172. Papanastassiou I, Ioannou M, Papagelopoulos PJ et al. (2010). P53 expression as a prognostic marker in giant cell tumor

of bone: a pilot study. Orthopedics 33:

2173. Papaspyrou G, Werner JA, Roessler M et al. (2011). Adult rhabdomyoma in the parapharyngeal space: report of 2 cases and review of the literature. Am J Otolaryngol 32: 240–246.

2174. Parham DM, Bridge JA, Lukacs JL et al. (2004). Cytogenetic distinction among benign fibro-osseous lesions of bone in children and adolescents: value of karyotypic findings in differential diagnosis. Pediatr Dev Pathol 7: 148–158.

2175. Parham DM, Ellison DA (2006). Rhabdomyosarcomas in adults and children: an update. Arch Pathol Lab Med 130: 1454–1465.

2176. Parham DM, Hijazi Y, Steinberg SM et al. (1999). Neuroectodermal differentiation in Ewing's sarcoma family of tumors does not predict tumor behavior. Hum Pathol 30: 911–918.

2177. Parham DM, Reynolds AB, Webber BL (1995). Use of monoclonal antibody 1H1, anticortactin, to distinguish normal and neoplastic smooth muscle cells: comparison with anti-alpha-smooth muscle actin and antimuscle-specific actin. Hum Pathol 26: 776–783.

2178. Parham DM, Webber B, Holt H et al. (1991). Immunohistochemical study of childhood rhabdomyosarcomas and related neoplasms. Results of an Intergroup Rhabdomyosarcoma study project. Cancer 67: 3072–3080.

2179. Parikh SN, Crawford AH, Choudhury S (2004). Magnetic resonance imaging in the evaluation of infantile torticollis. Orthopedics 27: 509–515.

2180. Park CH, Kim KI, Lim YT et al. (2000). Ruptured giant intrathoracic lipoblastoma in a 4-month-old infant: CT and MR findings. Pediatr Radiol 30: 38–40.

2181. Park EA, Hong SH, Choi JY et al. (2005). Glomangiomatosis: magnetic resonance imaging findings in three cases. Skeletal Radiol 34: 108–111.

2182. Park HR, Jung WW, Bertoni F et al. (2004). Molecular analysis of p53, MDM2 and H-ras genes in low-grade central osteosarcoma. Pathol Res Pract 200: 439–445.

2183. Park SY, Jin SP, Yeom B et al. (2011). Multiple fibromas of tendon sheath: unusual presentation. Ann Dermatol 23 Suppl 1: S45–S47.

2184. Park YH, Choi SW, Cho BK et al. (1994). Solitary type of glomus tumor developed in multiple sites. Ann Dermatol 6: 225–229.

2185. Park YK, Cho CH, Chi SG et al. (2001). Low incidence of genetic alterations of the p16CDKN2a in clear cell chondrosarcoma. Int J Oncol 19: 749–753.

2186. Park YK, Park HR, Chi SG et al. (2001). Overexpression of p53 and absent genetic mutation in clear cell chondrosarcoma. Int J Oncol 19: 353–357.

2187. Park YK, Unni KK, Beabout JW et al. (1994). Oncogenic osteomalacia: a clinicopathologic study of 17 bone lesions. J Korean Med Sci 9: 289–298.

2188. Park YK, Unni KK, Kim YW et al. (1999). Primary alveolar soft part sarcoma of bone. Histopathology 35: 411–417.

2189. Parkin DM, Stiller CA, Draper GJ et al. (1988). The international incidence of childhood cancer. Int J Cancer 42: 511–520.

2190. Parkin DM, Whelan SL, Ferlay J et al.(1997). Cancer incidence in five continents. IARC Press: Lyon.

2191. Parsons A, Sheehan DJ, Sangueza OP (2008). Retiform hemangioendotheliomas usually do not express D2-40 and VEGFR-3. Am J Dermatopathol 30: 31–33.

2192. Pasic I, Shlien A, Durbin AD et al. (2010). Recurrent focal copy-number changes and loss of heterozygosity implicate two non-coding RNAs and one tumor suppressor gene at chromosome 3q13.31 in osteosarcoma. Cancer Res 70: 160–171.

2193. Pasini B, McWhinney SR, Bei T et al. (2008). Clinical and molecular genetics of patients with the Carney-Stratakis syndrome and germline mutations of the genes coding for the succinate dehydrogenase subunits SDHB, SDHC, and SDHD. Eur J Hum Genet 16: 79–88.

2194. Patchefsky AS, Enzinger FM (1981). Intravascular fasciitis: a report of 17 cases. Am J Surg Pathol 5: 29–36.

2195. Patel RM, Downs-Kelly E, Dandekar MN et al. (2011). FUS (16p11) gene rearrangement as detected by fluorescence in-situ hybridization in cutaneous low-grade fibromyxoid sarcoma: a potential diagnostic tool. Am J Dermatopathol 33: 140–143.

2196. Paterson DC (1970). Myositis ossificans circumscripta. Report of four cases without history of injury. J Bone Joint Surg Br 52: 296–301.

2197. Patil DT, Laskin WB, Fetsch JF et al. (2011). Inguinal smooth muscle tumors in women-a dichotomous group consisting of Mullerian-type leiomyomas and soft tissue leiomyosarcomas: an analysis of 55 cases. Am J Surg Pathol 35: 315–324.

2198. Patil S, Perry A, MacCollin M et al. (2008). Immunohistochemical analysis supports a role for INI1/SMARCB1 in hereditary forms of schwannomas, but not in solitary, sporadic schwannomas. Brain Pathol 18: 517–519.

2199. Paul SR, Hurford MT, Miettinen MM et al. (2008). Polymorphous hemangioendothelioma in a child with acquired immunodeficiency syndrome (AIDS). Pediatr Blood Cancer 50: 663–665.

2200. Paulson V, Chandler G, Rakheja D et al. (2011). High-resolution array CGH identifies common mechanisms that drive embryonal rhabdomyosarcoma pathogenesis. Genes Chromosomes Cancer 50: 397–408.

2201. Pauwels P, Sciot R, Croiset F et al. (2000). Myofibroblastoma of the breast: genetic link with spindle cell lipoma. J Pathol 191: 282–285.

2202. Pavel E, Nadella K, Towns WH et al. (2008). Mutation of Prkar1a causes osteoblast neoplasia driven by dysregulation of protein kinase A. Mol Endocrinol 22: 430–440.

2203. Pawel BR, Hamoudi AB, Asmar L et al. (1997). Undifferentiated sarcomas of children: pathology and clinical behavior—an Intergroup Rhabdomyosarcoma study. Med Pediatr Oncol 29: 170–180.

2204. Pea M, Martignoni G, Zamboni G et al. (1996). Perivascular epithelioid cell. Am J Surg Pathol 20: 1149–1153.

2205. Pedeutour F, Deville A, Steyaert H et al. (2012). Rearrangement of HMGA2 in a case of infantile lipoblastoma without Plag1 alteration. Pediatr Blood Cancer 58: 798–800.

2206. Pedeutour F, Forus A, Coindre JM et al. (1999). Structure of the supernumerary ring and giant rod chromosomes in adipose tissue tumors. Genes Chromosomes Cancer 24: 30–41.

2207. Pedeutour F, Simon MP, Minoletti F et al. (1995). Ring 22 chromosomes in dermatofibrosarcoma protuberans are low-level amplifiers of chromosome 17 and 22 sequences. Cancer Res 55: 2400–2403.

2208. Peimer CA, Schiller AL, Mankin HJ et al. (1980). Multicentric giant-cell tumor of bone. J

Bone Joint Surg Am 62: 652–656.

2209. Pellegrini AE, Drake RD, Qualman SJ (1995). Spindle cell hemangioendothelioma: a neoplasm associated with Maffucci's syndrome. J Cutan Pathol 22: 173–176.

2210. Pelmus M, Guillou L, Hostein I et al. (2002). Monophasic fibrous and poorly differentiated synovial sarcoma: immunohistochemical reassessment of 60 t(X;18)(SYT-SSX)-positive cases. Am J Surg Pathol 26: 1434–1440.

2211. Penel N, Bui BN, Bay JO et al. (2008). Phase II trial of weekly paclitaxel for unresectable angiosarcoma: the ANGIOTAX Study. J Clin Oncol 26: 5269–5274.

2212. Penel N, Taieb S, Ceugnart L et al. (2008). Report of eight recent cases of locally advanced primary pulmonary artery sarcomas: failure of Doxorubicin-based chemotherapy. J Thorac Oncol 3: 907–911.

2213. Penman HG, Ring PA (1984). Osteosarcoma in association with total hip replacement. J Bone Joint Surg Br 66: 632–634.

2214. Penn I (1979). Kaposi's sarcoma in organ transplant recipients: report of 20 cases. Transplantation 27: 8–11.

2215. Penner CR, Thompson L (2003). Nasal glial heterotopia: a clinicopathologic and immunophenotypic analysis of 10 cases with a review of the literature. Ann Diagn Pathol 7: 354–359.

2216. Penner CR, Thompson LD (2004). Nasal glial heterotopia. Ear Nose Throat J 83: 92–93.

2217. Pepper T, Falla L, Brennan PA (2010). Soft tissue giant cell tumour of low malignant potential arising in the masseter—a rare entity in the head and neck. Br J Oral Maxillofac Surg 48: 149–151.

2218. Perez-Alonso P, Sanchez-Simon R, Contreras F et al. (2000). Special feature: pathological case of the month. Denouement and discussion: fetal rhabdomyoma of the tongue (myxoid type). Arch Pediatr Adolesc Med 154: 1265–1266.

2219. Perez-Losada J, Pintado B, Gutierrez-Adan A et al. (2000). The chimeric FUS/TLS-CHOP fusion protein specifically induces liposarcomas in transgenic mice. Oncogene 19: 2413–2422.

2220. Perosio PM, Weiss SW (1993). Ischemic fasciitis: a juxta-skeletal fibroblastic proliferation with a predilection for elderly patients. Mod Pathol 6: 69–72.

2221. Perot G, Chibon F, Montero A et al. (2010). Constant p53 pathway inactivation in a large series of soft tissue sarcomas with complex genetics. Am J Pathol 177: 2080–2090.

2222. Perot G, Derre J, Coindre JM et al. (2009). Strong smooth muscle differentiation is dependent on myocardin gene amplification in most human retroperitoneal leiomyosarcomas. Cancer Res 69: 2269–2278.

2223. Perry A, Louis DN, Scheithauer BW et al. (20007). Meningiomas. In: WHO classification of tumours of the central nervous system. Louis DN, Ohgaki H, Wiestler OD, Cavenee WK IARC: Lyon: pp 164–172.

2224. Pervaiz N, Colterjohn N, Farrokhyar F et al. (2008). A systematic meta-analysis of randomized controlled trials of adjuvant chemotherapy for localized resectable soft-tissue sarcoma. Cancer 113: 573–581.

2225. Petek E, Jenne DE, Smolle J et al. (2003). Mitotic recombination mediated by the JJAZF1 (KIAA0160) gene causing somatic mosaicism and a new type of constitutional NF1 microdeletion in two children of a mosaic female with only few manifestations. J Med

Genet 40: 520–525.
2226. Peter M, Couturier J, Pacquement H et al. (1997). A new member of the ETS family fused to EWS in Ewing tumors. Oncogene 14: 1159–1164.
2227. Peterson Jr WC, Fusaro RM, Goltz RW (1964). Atypical pyogenic granuloma; a case of benign hemangioendotheliosis. Arch Dermatol 90: 197–201.
2228. Petersson F, Huang J (2011). Epstein-Barr virus—associated smooth muscle tumor mimicking cutaneous angioleiomyoma. Am J Dermatopathol 33: 407–409.
2229. Petit MM, Mols R, Schoenmakers EF et al. (1996). LPP, the preferred fusion partner gene of HMGIC in lipomas, is a novel member of the LIM protein gene family. Genomics 36: 118–129.
2230. Petit MM, Schoenmakers EF, Huysmans C et al. (1999). LHFP, a novel translocation partner gene of HMGIC in a lipoma, is a member of a new family of LHFP-like genes. Genomics 57: 438–441.
2231. Petit MM, Swarts S, Bridge JA et al. (1998). Expression of reciprocal fusion transcripts of the HMGIC and LPP genes in parosteal lipoma. Cancer Genet Cytogenet 106: 18–23.
2232. Petitjean A, Mathe E, Kato S et al. (2007). Impact of mutant p53 functional properties on TP53 mutation patterns and tumor phenotype: lessons from recent developments in the IARC TP53 database. Hum Mutat 28: 622–629.
2233. Petrik PK, Findlay JM, Sherlock RA (1993). Aneurysmal cyst, bone type, primary in an artery. Am J Surg Pathol 17: 1062–1066.
2234. Pettinato G, Manivel JC, De Rosa G et al. (1990). Angiomatoid malignant fibrous histiocytoma: cytologic, immunohistochemical, ultrastructural, and flow cytometric study of 20 cases. Mod Pathol 3: 479–487.
2235. Pettinato G, Manivel JC, De Rosa N et al. (1990). Inflammatory myofibroblastic tumor (plasma cell granuloma). Clinicopathologic study of 20 cases with immunohistochemical and ultrastructural observations. Am J Clin Pathol 94: 538–546.
2236. Pettit CK, Zukerberg LR, Gray MH et al. (1990). Primary lymphoma of bone. A B-cell neoplasm with a high frequency of multilobated cells. Am J Surg Pathol 14: 329–334.
2237. Pfeifer FM, Bridge JA, Neff JR et al. (1991). Cytogenetic findings in aneurysmal bone cysts. Genes Chromosomes Cancer 3: 416–419.
2238. Pham NS, Poirier B, Fuller SC et al. (2010). Pediatric lipoblastoma in the head and neck: a systematic review of 48 reported cases. Int J Pediatr Otorhinolaryngol 74: 723–728.
2239. Philippe-Chomette P, Kabbara N, Andre N et al. (2011). Desmoplastic small round cell tumors with EWS-WT1 fusion transcript in children and young adults. Pediatr Blood Cancer
2240. Pho LN, Coffin CM, Burt RW (2005). Abdominal desmoid in familial adenomatous polyposis presenting as a pancreatic cystic lesion. Fam Cancer 4: 135–138.
2241. Picci P, Vanel D, Briccoli A et al. (2001). Computed tomography of pulmonary metastases from osteosarcoma: the less poor technique. A study of 51 patients with histological correlation. Ann Oncol 12: 1601–1604.
2242. Pierron A, Fernandez C, Saada E et al. (2009). HMGA2-NFIB fusion in a pediatric intramuscular lipoma: a novel case of NFIB alteration in a large deep-seated adipocytic tumor. Cancer Genet Cytogenet 195: 66–70.
2243. Pierron G, Tirode F, Lucchesi C et al. (2012). A new subtype of bone sarcoma defined by BCOR-CCNB3 gene fusion. Nat Genet 44: 461–466.
2244. Pietschmann MF, Oliveira AM, Chou MM et al. (2011). Aneurysmal bone cysts of soft tissue represent true neoplasms: a report of two cases. J Bone Joint Surg Am 93: e45
2245. Pilotti S, Della Torre G, Lavarino C et al. (1997). Distinct mdm2/p53 expression patterns in liposarcoma subgroups: implications for different pathogenetic mechanisms. J Pathol 181: 14–24.
2246. Pineles SL, Liu GT, Acebes X et al. (2011). Presence of Erdheim-Chester disease and Langerhans cell histiocytosis in the same patient: a report of 2 cases. J Neuroophthalmol 31: 217–223.
2247. Pinkard NB, Wilson RW, Lawless N et al. (1996). Calcifying fibrous pseudotumor of pleura. A report of three cases of a newly described entity involving the pleura. Am J Clin Pathol 105: 189–194.
2247A. Pinto CH, Taminiau AH, Vanderschueren GM et al. (2002). Technical considerations in CT-guided radiofrequency thermal ablation of osteoid osteoma: tricks of the trade. Am J Roentgenol 179:1633–1642.
2248. Pinto EM, Billerbeck AE, Villares MC et al. (2004). Founder effect for the highly prevalent R337H mutation of tumor suppressor p53 in Brazilian patients with adrenocortical tumors. Arq Bras Endocrinol Metabol 48: 647–650.
2249. Pisciotto PT, Gray GF, Jr., Miller DR (1978). Abdominal plasma cell pseudotumor. J Pediatr 93: 628–630.
2250. Pisters PW, Pollock RE, Lewis VO et al. (2007). Long-term results of prospective trial of surgery alone with selective use of radiation for patients with T1 extremity and trunk soft tissue sarcomas. Ann Surg 246: 675–681.
2251. Pitchford CW, Schwartz HS, Atkinson JB et al. (2006). Soft tissue perineurioma in a patient with neurofibromatosis type 2: a tumor not previously associated with the NF2 syndrome. Am J Surg Pathol 30: 1624–1629.
2252. Pollock L, Malone M, Shaw DG (1995). Childhood soft tissue chondroma: a case report. Pediatr Pathol Lab Med 15: 437–441.
2253. Pollock M, Nicholson GI, Nukada H et al. (1988). Neuropathy in multiple symmetric lipomatosis. Madelung's disease. Brain 111 (Pt 5): 1157–1171.
2254. Pollock R, Lang A, Ge T et al. (1998). Wild-type p53 and a p53 temperature-sensitive mutant suppress human soft tissue sarcoma by enhancing cell cycle control. Clin Cancer Res 4: 1985–1994.
2255. Pomplun S, Goldstraw P, Davies SE et al. (2000). Calcifying fibrous pseudotumour arising within an inflammatory pseudotumour: evidence of progression from one lesion to the other? Histopathology 37: 380–382.
2256. Popek EJ, Montgomery EA, Fourcroy JL (1994). Fibrous hamartoma of infancy in the genital region: findings in 15 cases. J Urol 152: 990–993.
2257. Porter DE, Lonie L, Fraser M et al. (2004). Severity of disease and risk of malignant change in hereditary multiple exostoses. A genotype-phenotype study. J Bone Joint Surg Br 86: 1041–1046.
2258. Portera CA, Jr., Ho V, Patel SR et al. (2001). Alveolar soft part sarcoma: clinical course and patterns of metastasis in 70 patients treated at a single institution. Cancer 91: 585–591.
2259. Povysil C, Matejovsky Z (1979). Ultrastructural evidence of myofibroblasts in pseudomalignant myositis ossificans. Virchows Arch A Pathol Anat Histol 381: 189–203.
2260. Prakash S, Sarran L, Socci N et al. (2005). Gastrointestinal stromal tumors in children and young adults: a clinicopathologic, molecular, and genomic study of 15 cases and review of the literature. J Pediatr Hematol Oncol 27: 179–187.
2261. Prat J, Woodruff JM, Marcove RC (1978). Epithelioid sarcoma: an analysis of 22 cases indicating the prognostic significance of vascular invasion and regional lymph node metastasis. Cancer 41: 1472–1487.
2262. Premalata CS, Kumar RV, Saleem KM et al. (2009). Fetal rhabdomyoma of the lower extremity. Pediatr Blood Cancer 52: 881–883.
2263. Prescott RJ, Husain EA, Abdellaoui A et al. (2008). Superficial acral fibromyxoma: a clinicopathological study of new 41 cases from the U.K.: should myxoma (NOS) and fibroma (NOS) continue as part of 21st-century reporting? Br J Dermatol 159: 1315–1321.
2264. Present D, Bacchini P, Pignatti G et al. (1991). Clear cell chondrosarcoma of bone. A report of 8 cases. Skeletal Radiol 20: 187–191.
2265. Presneau N, Shalaby A, Idowu B et al. (2009). Potential therapeutic targets for chordoma: PI3K/AKT/TSC1/TSC2/mTOR pathway. Br J Cancer 100: 1406–1414.
2266. Presneau N, Shalaby A, Ye H et al. (2011). Role of the transcription factor T (brachyury) in the pathogenesis of sporadic chordoma: a genetic and functional-based study. J Pathol 223: 327–335.
2267. Prevot S, Bienvenu L, Vaillant JC et al. (1999). Benign schwannoma of the digestive tract: a clinicopathologic and immunohistochemical study of five cases, including a case of esophageal tumor. Am J Surg Pathol 23: 431–436.
2268. Price Jr EB, Silliphant WM, Shuman R (1961). Nodular fasciitis: a clinicopathologic analysis of 65 cases. Am J Clin Pathol 35: 122–136.
2269. Price AJ, Compson JP, Calonje E (1995). Fibrolipomatous hamartoma of nerve arising in the brachial plexus. J Hand Surg Br 20: 16–18.
2270. Prieur A, Tirode F, Cohen P et al. (2004). EWS/FLI-1 silencing and gene profiling of Ewing cells reveal downstream oncogenic pathways and a crucial role for repression of insulin-like growth factor binding protein 3. Mol Cell Biol 24: 7275–7283.
2271. Pritchard DJ, Soule EH, Taylor WF et al. (1974). Fibrosarcoma—a clinicopathologic and statistical study of 199 tumors of the soft tissues of the extremities and trunk. Cancer 33: 888–897.
2272. Pritchard-Jones K, Fleming S (1991). Cell types expressing the Wilms' tumour gene (WT1) in Wilms' tumours: implications for tumour histogenesis. Oncogene 6: 2211–2220.
2273. Pulford K, Morris SW, Mason DY (2001). Anaplastic lymphoma kinase proteins and malignancy. Curr Opin Hematol 8: 231–236.
2274. Pulitzer DR, Martin PC, Reed RJ (1989). Fibroma of tendon sheath. A clinicopathologic study of 32 cases. Am J Surg Pathol 13: 472–479.
2275. Pulitzer DR, Martin PC, Reed RJ (1995). Epithelioid glomus tumor. Hum Pathol 26: 1022–1027.
2276. Pummi KP, Aho HJ, Laato MK et al. (2006). Tight junction proteins and perineurial cells in neurofibromas. J Histochem Cytochem 54: 53–61.
2277. Puppala B, Mangurten HH, McFadden J et al. (1990). Nasal glioma. Presenting as neonatal respiratory distress. Definition of the tumor mass by MRI. Clin Pediatr (Phila) 29: 49–52.
2278. Purgina B, Rao UN, Miettinen M et al. (2011). AIDS-related EBV-associated smooth muscle tumors: a review of 64 published cases. Patholog Res Int 2011: 561548
2279. Pyakurel P, Montag U, Castanos-Velez E et al. (2006). CGH of microdissected Kaposi's sarcoma lesions reveals recurrent loss of chromosome Y in early and additional chromosomal changes in late tumour stages. AIDS 20: 1805–1812.
2280. Qiu X, Montgomery E, Sun B (2008). Inflammatory myofibroblastic tumor and low-grade myofibroblastic sarcoma: a comparative study of clinicopathologic features and further observations on the immunohistochemical profile of myofibroblasts. Hum Pathol 39: 846–856.
2281. Qualman S, Lynch J, Bridge J et al. (2008). Prevalence and clinical impact of anaplasia in childhood rhabdomyosarcoma : a report from the Soft Tissue Sarcoma Committee of the Children's Oncology Group. Cancer 113: 3242–3247.
2282. Quezado MM, Middleton LP, Bryant B et al. (1998). Allelic loss on chromosome 22q in epithelioid sarcomas. Hum Pathol 29: 604–608.
2283. Qureshi AA, Shott S, Mallin BA et al. (2000). Current trends in the management of adamantinoma of long bones. An international study. J Bone Joint Surg Am 82-A: 1122–1131.
2284. Rabbitts TH, Forster A, Larson R et al. (1993). Fusion of the dominant negative transcription regulator CHOP with a novel gene FUS by translocation t(12;16) in malignant liposarcoma. Nat Genet 4: 175–180.
2285. Raddaoui E, Donner LR, Panagopoulos I (2002). Fusion of the FUS and ATF1 genes in a large, deep-seated angiomatoid fibrous histiocytoma. Diagn Mol Pathol 11: 157–162.
2286. Radig K, Schneider-Stock R, Haeckel C et al. (1998). p53 gene mutations in osteosarcomas of low-grade malignancy. Hum Pathol 29: 1310–1316.
2287. Radio SJ, Wooldridge TN, Linder J (1988). Flow cytometric DNA analysis of malignant fibrous histiocytoma and related fibrohistiocytic tumors. Hum Pathol 19: 74–77.
2288. Raggo C, Ruhl R, McAllister S et al. (2005). Novel cellular genes essential for transformation of endothelial cells by Kaposi's sarcoma-associated herpesvirus. Cancer Res 65: 5084–5095.
2289. Rajani B, Smith TA, Reith JD et al. (1999). Retroperitoneal leiomyosarcomas unassociated with the gastrointestinal tract: a clinicopathologic analysis of 17 cases. Mod Pathol 12: 21–28.
2290. Ramachandra S, Hollowood K, Bisceglia M et al. (1995). Inflammatory pseudotumour of soft tissues: a clinicopathological and immunohistochemical analysis of 18 cases. Histopathology 27: 313–323.
2291. Ramani P, Cowell JK (1996). The expression pattern of Wilms' tumour gene (WT1) product in normal tissues and paediatric renal tumours. J Pathol 179: 162–168.
2292. Ramaswamy PV, Storm CA, Filiano JJ et al. (2010). Multiple granular cell tumors in a child with Noonan syndrome. Pediatr Dermatol 27: 209–211.
2293. Ramesh P, Annapureddy SR, Khan F et al. (2004). Angioleiomyoma: a clinical, pathological and radiological review. Int J Clin Pract 58: 587–591.

2294. Ramphal R, Manson D, Viero S et al. (2003). Retroperitoneal infantile fibrosarcoma: clinical, molecular, and therapeutic aspects of an unusual tumor. Pediatr Hematol Oncol 20: 635–642.

2295. Raney RB, Anderson JR, Barr FG et al. (2001). Rhabdomyosarcoma and undifferentiated sarcoma in the first two decades of life: a selective review of intergroup rhabdomyosarcoma study group experience and rationale for Intergroup Rhabdomyosarcoma Study V. J Pediatr Hematol Oncol 23: 215–220.

2296. Raney RB, Anderson JR, Brown KL et al. (2010). Treatment results for patients with localized, completely resected (Group I) alveolar rhabdomyosarcoma on Intergroup Rhabdomyosarcoma Study Group (IRSG) protocols III and IV, 1984-1997: a report from the Children's Oncology Group. Pediatr Blood Cancer 55: 612–616.

2297. Raney RB, Meza J, Anderson JR et al. (2002). Treatment of children and adolescents with localized parameningeal sarcoma: experience of the Intergroup Rhabdomyosarcoma Study Group protocols IRS-II through -IV, 1978-1997. Med Pediatr Oncol 38: 22–32.

2298. Raney RB, Walterhouse DO, Meza JL et al. (2011). Results of the Intergroup Rhabdomyosarcoma Study Group D9602 protocol, using vincristine and dactinomycin with or without cyclophosphamide and radiation therapy, for newly diagnosed patients with low-risk embryonal rhabdomyosarcoma: a report from the Soft Tissue Sarcoma Committee of the Children's Oncology Group. J Clin Oncol 29: 1312–1318.

2299. Ranger A, Szymczak A (2009). Do intracranial neoplasms differ in Ollier disease and maffucci syndrome? An in-depth analysis of the literature. Neurosurgery 65: 1106–1113.

2300. Rankine AJ, Filion PR, Platten MA et al. (2004). Perineurioma: a clinicopathological study of eight cases. Pathology 36: 309–315.

2301. Rao AS, Vigorita VJ (1984). Pigmented villonodular synovitis (giant-cell tumor of the tendon sheath and synovial membrane). A review of eighty-one cases. J Bone Joint Surg Am 66: 76–94.

2302. Rao L, Kini AC, Valiathan M et al. (2001). Infantile cartilaginous hamartoma of the rib. A case report. Acta Cytol 45: 69–73.

2303. Rao UN, Goodman M, Chung WW et al. (2005). Molecular analysis of primary and recurrent giant cell tumors of bone. Cancer Genet Cytogenet 158: 126–136.

2304. Rao VK, Weiss SW (1992). Angiomatosis of soft tissue. An analysis of the histologic features and clinical outcome in 51 cases. Am J Surg Pathol 16: 764–771.

2305. Rasalkar DD, Chow LT, Chu WC et al. (2011). Primary pleomorphic liposarcoma of bone in an adolescent: imaging features of a rare entity. Pediatr Radiol 41: 1342–1345.

2306. Rathi A, Virmani AK, Harada K et al. (2003). Aberrant methylation of the HIC1 promoter is a frequent event in specific pediatric neoplasms. Clin Cancer Res 9: 3674–3678.

2307. Rausch T, Jones DT, Zapatka M et al. (2012). Genome sequencing of pediatric medulloblastoma links catastrophic DNA rearrangements with TP53 mutations. Cell 148: 59–71.

2308. Rawlinson NJ, West WW, Nelson M et al. (2008). Aggressive angiomyxoma with t(12;21) and HMGA2 rearrangement: report of a case and review of the literature. Cancer Genet Cytogenet 181: 119–124.

2309. Reddick RL, Michelitch H, Triche TJ

(1979). Malignant soft tissue tumors (malignant fibrous histiocytoma, pleomorphic liposarcoma, and pleomorphic rhabdomyosarcoma): an electron microscopic study. Hum Pathol 10: 327–343.

2310. Redlich GC, Montgomery KD, Allgood GA et al. (1999). Plexiform fibrohistiocytic tumor with a clonal cytogenetic anomaly. Cancer Genet Cytogenet 108: 141–143.

2311. Reed RJ, Fine RM, Meltzer HD (1972). Palisaded, encapsulated neuromas of the skin. Arch Dermatol 106: 865–870.

2312. Reed RJ, Terazakis N (1972). Subcutaneous angioblastic lymphoid hyperplasia with eosinophilia (Kimura's disease). Cancer 29: 489–497.

2313. Regazzoli A, Pozzi A, Rossi G (1997). Pseudo-Gaucher plasma cells in the bone marrow of a patient with monoclonal gammopathy of undetermined significance. Haematologica 82: 727

2314. Rehring TF, Deutchman A, Cross JS (1999). Polymorphous hemangioendothelioma. Ann Thorac Surg 68: 1396–1397.

2315. Reichek JL, Duan F, Smith LM et al. (2011). Genomic and clinical analysis of amplification of the 13q31 chromosomal region in alveolar rhabdomyosarcoma: a report from the Children's Oncology Group. Clin Cancer Res 17: 1463–1473.

2315A. Reichenberger EJ, Levine MA, Olsen BR et al. 2012 The role of SH3BP2 in the pathophysiology of cherubism. Orphanet J Rare Dis 7 Suppl 1:S5.

2316. Reid R, de Silva MV, Paterson L et al. (2003). Low-grade fibromyxoid sarcoma and hyalinizing spindle cell tumor with giant rosettes share a common t(7;16)(q34;p11) translocation. Am J Surg Pathol 27: 1229–1236.

2317. Reijnders CM, Waaijer CJ, Hamilton A et al. (2010). No haploinsufficiency but loss of heterozygosity for EXT in multiple osteochondromas. Am J Pathol 177: 1946–1957.

2318. Reilly KE, Stern PJ, Dale JA (1999). Recurrent giant cell tumors of the tendon sheath. J Hand Surg Am 24: 1298–1302.

2319. Reimann JD, Fletcher CD (2007). Myxoid dermatofibrosarcoma protuberans: a rare variant analyzed in a series of 23 cases. Am J Surg Pathol 31: 1371–1377.

2320. Reis-Filho JS, Paiva ME, Lopes JM (2002). Congenital composite hemangioendothelioma: case report and reappraisal of the hemangioendothelioma spectrum. J Cutan Pathol 29: 226–231.

2321. Reiseter T, Nordshus T, Borthne A et al. (1999). Lipoblastoma: MRI appearances of a rare paediatric soft tissue tumour. Pediatr Radiol 29: 542–545.

2322. Reitamo JJ, Hayry P, Nykyri E et al. (1982). The desmoid tumor. I. Incidence, sex-, age- and anatomical distribution in the Finnish population. Am J Clin Pathol 77: 665–673.

2323. Rekhi B, Deshmukh M, Jambhekar NA (2011). Low-grade fibromyxoid sarcoma: a clinicopathologic study of 18 cases, including histopathologic relationship with sclerosing epithelioid fibrosarcoma in a subset of cases. Ann Diagn Pathol 15: 303–311.

2324. Rekhi B, Folpe AL, Deshmukh M et al. (2011). Sclerosing epithelioid fibrosarcoma - a report of two cases with cytogenetic analysis of FUS gene rearrangement by FISH technique. Pathol Oncol Res 17: 145–148.

2325. Rekhi B, Gorad BD, Chinoy RF (2008). Clinicopathological features with outcomes of a series of conventional and proximal-type epithelioid sarcomas, diagnosed over a period

of 10 years at a tertiary cancer hospital in India. Virchows Arch 453: 141–153.

2326. Rekhi B, Jambhekar NA (2010). Morphologic spectrum, immunohistochemical analysis, and clinical features of a series of granular cell tumors of soft tissues: a study from a tertiary referral cancer center. Ann Diagn Pathol 14: 162–167.

2327. Rekhi B, Kaur A, Puri A et al. (2011). Primary leiomyosarcoma of bone—a clinicopathologic study of 8 uncommon cases with immunohistochemical analysis and clinical outcomes. Ann Diagn Pathol 15: 147–156.

2328. Remstein ED, Arndt CA, Nascimento AG (1999). Plexiform fibrohistiocytic tumor: clinicopathologic analysis of 22 cases. Am J Surg Pathol 23: 662–670.

2329. Requena L, Luis DJ, Manzarbeitia F et al. (2008). Cutaneous composite hemangioendothelioma with satellitosis and lymph node metastases. J Cutan Pathol 35: 225–230.

2330. Reye RD (1965). Recurring digital fibrous tumors of childhood. Arch Pathol 80: 228–231.

2331. Ribeiro RC, Sandrini F, Figueiredo B et al. (2001). An inherited p53 mutation that contributes in a tissue-specific manner to pediatric adrenal cortical carcinoma. Proc Natl Acad Sci U S A 98: 9330–9335.

2332. Riccardi VM (1981). Von Recklinghausen neurofibromatosis. N Engl J Med 305: 1617–1627.

2333. Ricci A, Jr., Parham DM, Woodruff JM et al. (1984). Malignant peripheral nerve sheath tumors arising from ganglioneuromas. Am J Surg Pathol 8: 19–29.

2334. Richkind KE, Mortimer E, Mowery-Rushton P et al. (2002). Translocation (16;20)(p11.2;q13). sole cytogenetic abnormality in a unicameral bone cyst. Cancer Genet Cytogenet 137: 153–155.

2335. Richkind KE, Romansky SG, Finklestein JZ (1996). t(4;19)(q35;q13.1): a recurrent change in primitive mesenchymal tumors? Cancer Genet Cytogenet 87: 71–74.

2336. Riddell RJ, Louis CJ, Bromberger NA (1973). Pulmonary metastases from chondroblastoma of the tibia. Report of a case. J Bone Joint Surg Br 55: 848–853.

2337. Rieker RJ, Joos S, Bartsch C et al. (2002). Distinct chromosomal imbalances in pleomorphic and in high-grade dedifferentiated liposarcomas. Int J Cancer 99: 68–73.

2338. Rimareix F, Bardot J, Andrac L et al. (1997). Infantile digital fibroma—report on eleven cases. Eur J Pediatr Surg 7: 345–348.

2339. Riminucci M, Collins MT, Fedarko NS et al. (2003). FGF-23 in fibrous dysplasia of bone and its relationship to renal phosphate wasting. J Clin Invest 112: 683–692.

2340. Riminucci M, Fisher LW, Majolagbe A et al. (1999). A novel GNAS1 mutation, R201G, in McCune-albright syndrome. J Bone Miner Res 14: 1987–1989.

2341. Riminucci M, Kuznetsov SA, Cherman N et al. (2003). Osteoclastogenesis in fibrous dysplasia of bone: in situ and in vitro analysis of IL-6 expression. Bone 33: 434–442.

2342. Rimondi E, Mavrogenis AF, Rossi G et al. (2012). Radiofrequency ablation for non-spinal osteoid osteomas in 557 patients. Eur Radiol 22: 181–188.

2343. Rimondi E, Rossi G, Bartalena T et al. (2011). Percutaneous CT-guided biopsy of the musculoskeletal system: results of 2027 cases. Eur J Radiol 77: 34–42.

2344. Ringel MD, Schwindinger WF, Levine MA (1996). Clinical implications of genetic

defects in G proteins. The molecular basis of McCune-Albright syndrome and Albright hereditary osteodystrophy. Medicine (Baltimore) 75: 171–184.

2345. Rios-Martin JJ, Delgado MD, Moreno-Ramirez D et al. (2007). Granular cell atypical fibroxanthoma: report of two cases. Am J Dermatopathol 29: 84–87.

2346. Ritter J, Bielack SS (2010). Osteosarcoma. Ann Oncol 21 Suppl 7: vii320–vii325.

2347. Rivlin N, Brosh R, Oren M et al. (2011). Mutations in the p53 tumor suppressor gene: important milestones at the various steps of tumorigenesis. Genes Cancer 2: 466–474.

2348. Rizkalla H, Wildgrove H, Quinn F et al. (2011). Congenital fibrosarcoma of the ileum: case report with molecular confirmation and literature review. Fetal Pediatr Pathol 30: 156–160.

2349. Roarty JD, McLean IW, Zimmerman LE (1988). Incidence of second neoplasms in patients with bilateral retinoblastoma. Ophthalmology 95: 1583–1587.

2350. Roberts P, Burchill SA, Brownhill S et al. (2008). Ploidy and karyotype complexity are powerful prognostic indicators in the Ewing's sarcoma family of tumors: a study by the United Kingdom Cancer Cytogenetics and the Children's Cancer and Leukaemia Group. Genes Chromosomes Cancer 47: 207–220.

2351. Robillard N, Wuilleme S, Lode L et al. (2005). CD33 is expressed on plasma cells of a significant number of myeloma patients, and may represent a therapeutic target. Leukemia 19: 2021–2022.

2352. Rochanawutanon M, Praneetvatakul P, Laothamatas J et al. (2011). Extraskeletal giant cell tumor of the larynx: case report and review of the literature. Ear Nose Throat J 90: 226–230.

2353. Rodriguez E, Sreekantaiah C, Gerald W et al. (1993). A recurring translocation, t(11;22)(p13;q11.2), characterizes intra-abdominal desmoplastic small round-cell tumors. Cancer Genet Cytogenet 69: 17–21.

2354. Rodriguez HA, Berthrong M (1966). Multiple primary intracranial tumors in von Recklinghausen's neurofibromatosis. Arch Neurol 14: 467–475.

2355. Rodriguez-Peralto JL, Lopez-Barea F, Gonzalez-Lopez J et al. (1994). Case report 821: Parosteal ossifying lipoma of femur. Skeletal Radiol 23: 67–69.

2356. Roma AA, Yang B, Senior ME et al. (2005). TFE3 immunoreactivity in alveolar soft part sarcoma of the uterine cervix: case report. Int J Gynecol Pathol 24: 131–135.

2357. Romeo S, Bovee JV, Grogan SP et al. (2005). Chondromyxoid fibroma resembles in vitro chondrogenesis, but differs in expression of signalling molecules. J Pathol 206: 135–142.

2358. Romeo S, Bovee JVMG, Carrareno I et al. (2011). Malignant fibrous histiocytoma and fibrosarcoma of bone in 2011: what's new? Laboratory investigation 91: 20A–21A.

2358A. Romeo S, Bovée JVMG, Kroon HM et al. (2012). Malignant fibrous histiocytoma and fibrosarcoma of bone: a re-assessment in the light of currently employed morphological, immunohistochemical and molecular approaches. Virchows Arch 461:561-570.

2359. Romeo S, Duim RA, Bridge JA et al. (2010). Heterogeneous and complex rearrangements of chromosome arm 6q in chondromyxoid fibroma: delineation of breakpoints and analysis of candidate target genes. Am J Pathol 177: 1365–1376.

2360. Romeo S, Eyden B, Prins FA et al. (2006). TGF-beta1 drives partial myofibroblastic differentiation in chondromyxoid fibroma of bone. J Pathol 208: 26–34.

2361. Romeo S, Hogendoorn PC, Dei Tos AP (2009). Benign cartilaginous tumors of bone: from morphology to somatic and germ-line genetics. Adv Anat Pathol 16: 307–315.

2362. Romeo S, Oosting J, Rozeman LB et al. (2007). The role of noncartilage-specific molecules in differentiation of cartilaginous tumors: lessons from chondroblastoma and chondromyxoid fibroma. Cancer 110: 385–394.

2363. Romeo S, Szuhai K, Nishimori I et al. (2009). A balanced t(5;17) (p15;q22-23) in chondroblastoma: frequency of the re-arrangement and analysis of the candidate genes. BMC Cancer 9: 393

2364. Rosai J (1982). Angiolymphoid hyperplasia with eosinophilia of the skin. Its nosological position in the spectrum of histiocytoid hemangioma. Am J Dermatopathol 4: 175–184.

2365. Rosai J, Gold J, Landy R (1979). The histiocytoid hemangiomas. A unifying concept embracing several previously described entities of skin, soft tissue, large vessels, bone, and heart. Hum Pathol 10: 707–730.

2366. Rosai J, Limas C, Husband EM (1984). Ectopic hamartomatous thymoma. A distinctive benign lesion of lower neck. Am J Surg Pathol 8: 501–513.

2367. Rose B, Tamvakopoulos GS, Dulay K et al. (2011). The clinical significance of the FUS-CREB3L2 translocation in low-grade fibromyxoid sarcoma. J Orthop Surg Res 6: 15.

2368. Rose PS, Dickey ID, Wenger DE et al. (2006). Periosteal osteosarcoma: long-term outcome and risk of late recurrence. Clin Orthop Relat Res 453: 314–317.

2369. Rosenberg AE (2006). Expert commentary 2. Int J Surg Pathol 14: 17–20.

2370. Rosenberg AE (2008). Pseudosarcomas of soft tissue. Arch Pathol Lab Med 132: 579–586.

2371. Rosenberg HS, Stenback WA, Spjut HJ (1978). The fibromatoses of infancy and childhood. Perspect Pediatr Pathol 4: 269–348.

2372. Rosenthal DI (2006). Radiofrequency treatment. Orthop Clin North Am 37: 475–84.

2373. Rosenthal NS, Abdul-Karim FW (1988). Childhood fibrous tumor with psammoma bodies. Clinicopathologic features in two cases. Arch Pathol Lab Med 112: 798–800.

2374. Ross HM, Lewis JJ, Woodruff JM et al. (1997). Epithelioid sarcoma: clinical behavior and prognostic factors of survival. Ann Surg Oncol 4: 491–495.

2375. Rossi S, Orvieto E, Furlanetto A et al. (2004). Utility of the immunohistochemical detection of FLI-1 expression in round cell and vascular neoplasm using a monoclonal antibody. Mod Pathol 17: 547–552.

2376. Rossi S, Szuhai K, Ijszenga M et al. (2007). EWSR1-CREB1 and EWSR1-ATF1 fusion genes in angiomatoid fibrous histiocytoma. Clin Cancer Res 13: 7322–7328.

2377. Rougemont AL, Fetni R, Murthy S et al. (2006). A complex translocation (6;12;8) (q25;q24.3;q13) in a fibrous hamartoma of infancy. Cancer Genet Cytogenet 171: 115–118.

2378. Rouleau GA, Merel P, Lutchman M et al. (1993). Alteration in a new gene encoding a putative membrane-organizing protein causes neuro-fibromatosis type 2. Nature 363: 515–521.

2379. Rousseau A, Kujas M, van Effenterre R et al. (2005). Primary intracranial myopericytoma: report of three cases and review of the literature. Neuropathol Appl Neurobiol 31: 641–648.

2380. Rozeman LB, de Bruijn I, Bacchini P et al. (2009). Dedifferentiated peripheral chondrosarcomas: regulation of EXT-downstream molecules and differentiation-related genes. Mod Pathol 22: 1489–1498.

2381. Rozeman LB, Hameetman L, Cleton-Jansen AM et al. (2005). Absence of IHH and retention of PTHrP signalling in enchondromas and central chondrosarcomas. J Pathol 205: 476–482.

2382. Rozeman LB, Sangiorgi L, Briaire-de Bruijn I et al. (2004). Enchondromatosis (Ollier disease, Maffucci syndrome) is not caused by the PTHR1 mutation p.R150C. Hum Mutat 24: 466–473.

2383. Rozeman LB, Szuhai K, Schrage YM et al. (2006). Array-comparative genomic hybridization of central chondrosarcoma: identification of ribosomal protein S6 and cyclin-dependent kinase 4 as candidate target genes for genomic aberrations. Cancer 107: 380–388.

2384. Rozmaryn LM, Sadler AH, Dorfman HD (1987). Intraosseous glomus tumor in the ulna. A case report. Clin Orthop Relat Res 126–129.

2385. Rubin BP, Antonescu CR, Gannon FH et al. (2010). Protocol for the examination of specimens from patients with tumors of bone. Arch Pathol Lab Med 134: e1–e7.

2386. Rubin BP, Chen CJ, Morgan TW et al. (1998). Congenital mesoblastic nephroma t(12;15) is associated with ETV6-NTRK3 gene fusion: cytogenetic and molecular relationship to congenital (infantile) fibrosarcoma. Am J Pathol 153: 1451–1458.

2387. Rubin BP, Fletcher CD, Inwards C et al. (2006). Protocol for the examination of specimens from patients with soft tissue tumors of intermediate malignant potential, malignant soft tissue tumors, and benign/locally aggressive and malignant bone tumors. Arch Pathol Lab Med 130: 1616–1629.

2388. Rubin BP, Hasserjian RP, Singer S et al. (1998). Spindle cell rhabdomyosarcoma (so-called) in adults: report of two cases with emphasis on differential diagnosis. Am J Surg Pathol 22: 459–464.

2389. Ruckert RI, Fleige B, Rogalla P et al. (2000). Schwannoma with angiosarcoma. Report of a case and comparison with other types of nerve tumors with angiosarcoma. Cancer 89: 1577–1585.

2390. Rudisaile SN, Hurt MA, Santa Cruz DJ (2005). Granular cell atypical fibroxanthoma. J Cutan Pathol 32: 314–317.

2391. Rushing EJ, Armonda RA, Ansari Q et al. (1996). Mesenchymal chondrosarcoma: a clinicopathologic and flow cytometric study of 13 cases presenting in the central nervous system. Cancer 77: 1884–1891.

2392. Rusin LJ, Harrell ER (1976). Arteriovenous fistula. Cutaneous manifestations. Arch Dermatol 112: 1135–1138.

2393. Russell DS, Rubinstein LJ (2006). Pathology of tumours of the nervous system.Hodder Arnold: London: pp 663-764.

2394. Russell H, Hicks MJ, Bertuch AA et al. (2009). Infantile fibrosarcoma: clinical and histologic responses to cytotoxic chemotherapy. Pediatr Blood Cancer 53: 23–27.

2395. Russell WO, Cohen J, Enzinger F et al. (1977). A clinical and pathological staging system for soft tissue sarcomas. Cancer 40: 1562–1570.

2396. Ruszczak Z, Mayer da Silva A, Orfanos CE (1987). Angioproliferative changes in clinically noninvolved, perilesional skin in AIDS-associated Kaposi's sarcoma. Dermatologica 175: 270–279.

2397. Rutherfoord GS, Davies AG (1987). Chordomas—ultrastructure and immunohistochemistry: a report based on the examination of six cases. Histopathology 11: 775–787.

2398. Rydholm A (1983). Management of patients with soft-tissue tumors. Strategy developed at a regional oncology center. Acta Orthop Scand Suppl 203: 13–77.

2399. Rydholm A, Gustafson P, Rooser B et al. (1991). Limb-sparing surgery without radiotherapy based on anatomic location of soft tissue sarcoma. J Clin Oncol 9: 1757–1765.

2400. Ryman W, Bale P (1985). Recurring digital fibromas of infancy. Australas J Dermatol 26: 113–117.

2401. Saab ST, Hornick JL, Fletcher CD et al. (2011). IgG4 plasma cells in inflammatory myofibroblastic tumor: inflammatory marker or pathogenic link? Mod Pathol 24: 606–612.

2402. Sadikovic B, Thorner P, Chilton-MacNeill S et al. (2010). Expression analysis of genes associated with human osteosarcoma tumors shows correlation of RUNX2 overexpression with poor response to chemotherapy. BMC Cancer 10: 202

2403. Sadikovic B, Yoshimoto M, Chilton-MacNeill S et al. (2009). Identification of interactive networks of gene expression associated with osteosarcoma oncogenesis by integrated molecular profiling. Hum Mol Genet 18: 1962–1975.

2404. Saeed IT, Fletcher CD (1990). Ectopic hamartomatous thymoma containing myoid cells. Histopathology 17: 572–574.

2405. Sagerman RH, Cassady JR, Tretter P et al. (1969). Radiation induced neoplasia following external beam therapy for children with retinoblastoma. Am J Roentgenol Radium Ther Nucl Med 105: 529–535.

2406. Sahara N, Ohnishi K, Ono T et al. (2006). Clinicopathological and prognostic characteristics of CD33-positive multiple myeloma. Eur J Haematol 77: 14–18.

2407. Saito R, Caines MJ (1977). Atypical fibrous histiocytoma of the humerus: a light and electron microscopic study. Am J Clin Pathol 68: 409–415.

2408. Saito T (2000). Glomus tumor of the penis. Int J Urol 7: 115–117.

2409. Saito T, Mitomi H, Izumi H et al. (2011). A case of secondary malignant giant-cell tumor of bone with p53 mutation after long-term follow-up. Hum Pathol 42: 727–733.

2410. Sakaguchi N, Sano K, Ito M et al. (1996). A case of von Recklinghausen's disease with bilateral pheochromocytoma-malignant peripheral nerve sheath tumors of the adrenal and gastrointestinal autonomic nerve tumors. Am J Surg Pathol 20: 889–897.

2411. Sakai JN, Abe KT, Formigli LM et al. (2011). Cytogenetic findings in 14 benign cartilaginous neoplasms. Cancer Genet 204: 180–186.

2412. Sakaki M, Hirokawa M, Wakatsuki S et al. (2003). Acral myxoinflammatory fibroblastic sarcoma: a report of five cases and review of the literature. Virchows Arch 442: 25–30.

2413. Sakakibara N, Seki T, Maru A et al. (1989). Benign fibrous histiocytoma of the kidney. J Urol 142: 1558–1559.

2414. Sakamoto A, Akieda S, Oda Y et al. (2009). Mutation analysis of the Gadd45 gene at exon 4 in atypical fibroxanthoma. BMC Dermatol 9: 1

2415. Sakamoto A, Imamura S, Matsumoto Y et al. (2011). Bizarre parosteal osteochondromatous proliferation with an inversion of chromosome 7. Skeletal Radiol 40: 1487–1490.

2416. Sakamoto A, Oda Y, Itakura E et al. (2001). Immunoexpression of ultraviolet photoproducts and p53 mutation analysis in atypical fibroxanthoma and superficial malignant fibrous histiocytoma. Mod Pathol 14: 581–588.

2417. Sakamoto A, Oda Y, Itakura E et al. (2001). H-, K-, and N-ras gene mutation in atypical fibroxanthoma and malignant fibrous histiocytoma. Hum Pathol 32: 1225–1231.

2418. Sakamoto A, Oda Y, Iwamoto Y et al. (1999). A comparative study of fibrous dysplasia and osteofibrous dysplasia with regard to expressions of c-fos and c-jun products and bone matrix proteins: a clinicopathologic review and immunohistochemical study of c-fos, c-jun, type I collagen, osteonectin, osteopontin, and osteocalcin. Hum Pathol 30: 1418–1426.

2419. Sakamoto A, Tanaka K, Yoshida T et al. (2008). Nonossifying fibroma accompanied by pathological fracture in a 12-year-old runner. J Orthop Sports Phys Ther 38: 434–438.

2420. Sakamoto A, Yamamoto H, Yoshida T et al. (2007). Desmoplastic fibroblastoma (collagenous fibroma) with a specific breakpoint of 11q12. Histopathology 51: 859–860.

2421. Sakharpe A, Lahat G, Gulamhusein T et al. (2011). Epithelioid sarcoma and unclassified sarcoma with epithelioid features: clinicopathological variables, molecular markers, and a new experimental model. Oncologist 16: 512–522.

2422. Salamah MM, Hammoudi SM, Sadi AR (1988). Infantile myofibromatosis. J Pediatr Surg 23: 975–977.

2423. Salas S, Chibon F, Noguchi T et al. (2010). Molecular characterization by array comparative genomic hybridization and DNA sequencing of 194 desmoid tumors. Genes Chromosomes Cancer 49: 560–568.

2424. Salas S, Dufresne A, Bui B et al. (2011). Prognostic factors influencing progression-free survival determined from a series of sporadic desmoid tumors: a wait-and-see policy according to tumor presentation. J Clin Oncol 29: 3553–3558.

2425. Saleh G, Evans HL, Ro JY et al. (1992). Extraskeletal myxoid chondrosarcoma. A clinicopathologic study of ten patients with long-term follow-up. Cancer 70: 2827–2830.

2426. Salgado R, Llombart B, Pujol M et al. (2011). Molecular diagnosis of dermatofibrosarcoma protuberans: a comparison between reverse transcriptase-polymerase chain reaction and fluorescence in situ hybridization methodologies. Genes Chromosomes Cancer 50: 510–517.

2427. Salloum E, Caillaud JM, Flamant F et al. (1990). Poor prognosis infantile fibrosarcoma with pathologic features of malignant fibrous histiocytoma after local recurrence. Med Pediatr Oncol 18: 295–298.

2428. Salm R, Sissons HA (1972). Giant-cell tumours of soft tissues. J Pathol 107: 27–39.

2429. Samols MA, Skalsky RL, Maldonado AM et al. (2007). Identification of cellular genes targeted by KSHV-encoded microRNAs. PLoS Pathog 3: e65

2430. Sandberg AA (2004). Updates on the cytogenetics and molecular genetics of bone and soft tissue tumors: liposarcoma. Cancer Genet Cytogenet 155: 1–24.

2431. Sandberg AA, Bridge JA (2003). Updates on the cytogenetics and molecular genetics of bone and soft tissue tumors. Dermatofibrosarcoma protuberans and giant cell fibroblastoma. Cancer Genet Cytogenet

140: 1–12.
2432. Sanders BM, Draper GJ, Kingston JE (1988). Retinoblastoma in Great Britain 1969-80: incidence, treatment, and survival. Br J Ophthalmol 72: 576–583.
2433. Sanerkin NG, Mott MG, Roylance J (1983). An unusual intraosseous lesion with fibroblastic, osteoclastic, osteoblastic, aneurysmal and fibromyxoid elements. "Solid" variant of aneurysmal bone cyst. Cancer 51: 2278–2286.
2434. Sanfilippo R, Miceli R, Grosso F et al. (2011). Myxofibrosarcoma: prognostic factors and survival in a series of patients treated at a single institution. Ann Surg Oncol 18: 720–725.
2435. Sang DN, Albert DM (1982). Retinoblastoma: clinical and histopathologic features. Hum Pathol 13: 133–147.
2436. Sanjay BK, Sim FH, Unni KK et al. (1993). Giant-cell tumours of the spine. J Bone Joint Surg Br 75: 148–154.
2437. Sankar S, Lessnick SL (2011). Promiscuous partnerships in Ewing's sarcoma. Cancer Genet 204: 351–365.
2438. Santeusanio G, Bombonati A, Tarantino U et al. (2003). Multifocal epithelioid angiosarcoma of bone: a potential pitfall in the differential diagnosis with metastatic carcinoma. Appl Immunohistochem Mol Morphol 11: 359–363.
2439. Santonja C, Martin-Hita AM, Dotor A et al. (2001). Intimal angiosarcoma of the aorta with tumour embolisation causing mesenteric ischaemia. Report of a case diagnosed using CD31 immunohistochemistry in an intestinal resection specimen. Virchows Arch 438: 404–407.
2440. Sara AS, Evans HL, Benjamin RS (1990). Malignant melanoma of soft parts (clear cell sarcoma). A study of 17 cases, with emphasis on prognostic factors. Cancer 65: 367–374.
2441. Sari A, Tunakan M, Bolat B et al. (2007). Lipofibromatosis in a two-year-old girl: a case report. Turk J Pediatr 49: 319–321.
2442. Sartoris DJ, Mochizuki RM, Parker BR (1983). Lytic clavicular lesions in fibromatosis colli. Skeletal Radiol 10: 34–36.
2443. Sasaki D, Hatori M, Hosaka M et al. (2005). Lipofibromatosis arising in a pediatric forearm—a case report. Ups J Med Sci 110: 259–266.
2444. Sato K, Kubota T, Yoshida K et al. (1993). Intracranial extraskeletal myxoid chondrosarcoma with special reference to lamellar inclusions in the rough endoplasmic reticulum. Acta Neuropathol 86: 525–528.
2445. Savage SA, Mirabello L (2011). Using epidemiology and genomics to understand osteosarcoma etiology. Sarcoma 2011: 548151
2446. Sawada S, Florell S, Purandare SM et al. (1996). Identification of NF1 mutations in both alleles of a dermal neurofibroma. Nat Genet 14: 110–112.
2447. Sawada S, Honda M, Kamide R et al. (1995). Three cases of subungual glomus tumors with von Recklinghausen neurofibromatosis. J Am Acad Dermatol 32: 277–278.
2448. Sawyer JR, Sammartino G, Baker GF et al. (1994). Clonal chromosome aberrations in a case of nodular fasciitis. Cancer Genet Cytogenet 76: 154–156.
2449. Sawyer JR, Sammartino G, Gokden N et al. (2005). A clonal reciprocal t(2;7)(p13;p13) in plantar fibromatosis. Cancer Genet Cytogenet 158: 67–69.
2450. Sawyer JR, Swanson CM, Lukacs JL et al. (1998). Evidence of an association between 6q13-21 chromosome aberrations and locally aggressive behavior in patients with cartilage tumors. Cancer 82: 474–483.
2451. Sawyer JR, Tryka AF, Lewis JM (1992). A novel reciprocal chromosome translocation t(11;22)(p13;q12) in an intraabdominal desmoplastic small round-cell tumor. Am J Surg Pathol 16: 411–416.
2452. Schaffler G, Raith J, Ranner G et al. (1997). Radiographic appearance of an ossifying fibromyxoid tumor of soft parts. Skeletal Radiol 26: 615–618.
2453. Schaison F, Anract P, Coste F et al. (1999). [Chondrosarcoma secondary to multiple cartilage diseases. Study of 29 clinical cases and review of the literature]. Rev Chir Orthop Reparatrice Appar Mot 85: 834–845.
2454. Schajowicz F (1994) Giant-cell tumours (osteoclastoma). In: Schajowicz F ed, Tumours and tumour-like lesions of bone. Springer-Verlag: Berlin-Heidelberg-New York; 403–406; 540–551.
2455. Schajowicz F, Gallardo H (1970). Epiphysial chondroblastoma of bone. A clinicopathological study of sixty-nine cases. J Bone Joint Surg Br 52: 205–226.
2456. Schajowicz F, Santini Araujo E, Berenstein M (1983). Sarcoma complicating Paget's disease of bone. A clinicopathological study of 62 cases. J Bone Joint Surg Br 65: 299–307.
2457. Scheffel H, Stolzmann P, Plass A et al. (2008). Primary intimal pulmonary artery sarcoma: a diagnostic challenge. J Thorac Cardiovasc Surg 135: 949–950.
2458. Scheier M, Ramoni A, Alge A et al. (2008). Congenital fibrosarcoma as cause for fetal anemia: prenatal diagnosis and in utero treatment. Fetal Diagn Ther 24: 434–436.
2459. Scheipl S, Froehlich EV, Leithner A et al. (2012). Does insulin-like growth factor 1 receptor (IGF-1R) targeting provide new treatment options for chordomas? A retrospective clinical and immunohistochemical study. Histopathology 60: 999–1003.
2460. Scheithauer BW, Amrami KK, Folpe AL et al. (2011). Synovial sarcoma of nerve. Hum Pathol 42: 568–577.
2461. Scheithauer BW, Rubinstein LJ (1978). Meningeal mesenchymal chondrosarcoma: report of 8 cases with review of the literature. Cancer 42: 2744–2752.
2462. Scheithauer BW, Woodruff JM, Erlandson RA (1999). Miscellaneous benign neurogenic tumors. In: Atlas of Tumor Pathology, Tumors of the Peripheral Nervous System3 Edition. Rosai J, Sobin LH Armed Forces Institute of Pathology: Washington, DC: pp 219–282.
2463. Scheithauer BW, Woodruff JM, Erlandson RE. (1997). Tumors of the peripheral nervous system. Armed Forces Institute of Pathology: Washington.
2464. Schellenberg, Tetsuro M, Chang-En Yet al. (2012). Chapter 33: Werner Syndrome. The online Metabolic and Molecular Bases of Inherited disease :The McGraw-Hill Companies (http://www.ommbid.com/OMMBID/the_online_metabolic_and_molecular_bases_of_inherited_disease/b/abstract/part4/ch33). Accessed 24-2-2012.
2465. Schirosi L, Lantuejoul S, Cavazza A et al. (2008). Pleuro-pulmonary solitary fibrous tumors: a clinicopathologic, immunohistochemical, and molecular study of 88 cases confirming the prognostic value of de Perrot staging system and p53 expression, and evaluating the role of c-kit, BRAF, PDGFRs (alpha/beta), c-met, and EGFR. Am J Surg Pathol 32: 1627–1642.
2466. Schmale GA, Conrad EU, III, Raskind WH (1994). The natural history of hereditary multiple exostoses. J Bone Joint Surg Am 76: 986–992.
2467. Schmidt D, Harms D (1987). Epithelioid sarcoma in children and adolescents. An immunohistochemical study. Virchows Arch A Pathol Anat Histopathol 410: 423–431.
2468. Schmidt H, Bartel F, Kappler M et al. (2005). Gains of 13q are correlated with a poor prognosis in liposarcoma. Mod Pathol 18: 638–644.
2469. Schmidt H, Wurl P, Taubert H et al. (1999). Genomic imbalances of 7p and 17q in malignant peripheral nerve sheath tumors are clinically relevant. Genes Chromosomes Cancer 25: 205–211.
2470. Schneider-Stock R, Walter H, Radig K et al. (1998). MDM2 amplification and loss of heterozygosity at Rb and p53 genes: no simultaneous alterations in the oncogenesis of liposarcomas. J Cancer Res Clin Oncol 124: 532–540.
2471. Schneppenheim R, Fruhwald MC, Gesk S et al. (2010). Germline nonsense mutation and somatic inactivation of SMARCA4/BRG1 in a family with rhabdoid tumor predisposition syndrome. Am J Hum Genet 86: 279–284.
2472. Schober R, Reifenberger G, Kremer G et al. (1993). Symmetrical neurofibroma with Schwann cell predominance and focal formation of microneurinomas. Acta Neuropathol 85: 227–232.
2473. Schoenmakers EF, Wanschura S, Mols R et al. (1995). Recurrent rearrangements in the high mobility group protein gene, HMGI-C, in benign mesenchymal tumours. Nat Genet 10: 436–444.
2474. Schofield DE, Conrad EU, Liddell RM et al. (1995). An unusual round cell tumor of the tibia with granular cells. Am J Surg Pathol 19: 596–603.
2475. Schofield DE, Fletcher JA, Grier HE et al. (1994). Fibrosarcoma in infants and children. Application of new techniques. Am J Surg Pathol 18: 14–24.
2476. Schofield JB, Krausz T, Stamp GW et al. (1993). Ossifying fibromyxoid tumour of soft parts: immunohistochemical and ultrastructural analysis. Histopathology 22: 101–112.
2477. Schrage YM, Lam S, Jochemsen AG et al. (2009). Central chondrosarcoma progression is associated with pRb pathway alterations: CDK4 down-regulation and p16 overexpression inhibit cell growth in vitro. J Cell Mol Med 13: 2843–2852.
2478. Schuler PK, Weber A, Bode PK et al. (2009). MRI of intimal sarcoma of the pulmonary arteries. Circ Cardiovasc Imaging 2: e37–e39.
2479. Schwab JH, Antonescu CR, Athanasian EA et al. (2008). A comparison of intramedullary and juxtacortical low-grade osteogenic sarcoma. Clin Orthop Relat Res 466: 1318–1322.
2480. Schwartz ED, Hurst RW, Sinson G et al. (2002). Complete regression of intracranial arteriovenous malformations. Surg Neurol 58: 139–147.
2481. Schwartz HS, Dahir GA, Butler MG (1993). Telomere reduction in giant cell tumor of bone and with aging. Cancer Genet Cytogenet 71: 132–138.
2482. Schwartz HS, Unni KK, Pritchard DJ (1989). Pigmented villonodular synovitis. A retrospective review of affected large joints. Clin Orthop Relat Res 243–255.
2483. Schwartz HS, Walker R (1997). Recognizable magnetic resonance imaging characteristics of intramuscular myxoma. Orthopedics 20: 431–435.
2484. Schwartz HS, Zimmerman NB, Simon MA et al. (1987). The malignant potential of enchondromatosis. J Bone Joint Surg Am 69: 269–274.
2485. Schwartz RA, Dabski C, Dabska M (2000). The Dabska tumor: a thirty-year retrospect. Dermatology 201: 1–5.
2486. Schwartz RA, Janniger EJ (2011). On being a pathologist: Maria Dabska—the woman behind the eponym, a pioneer in pathology. Hum Pathol 42: 913–917.
2487. Schwindinger WF, Francomano CA, Levine MA (1992). Identification of a mutation in the gene encoding the alpha subunit of the stimulatory G protein of adenylyl cyclase in McCune-Albright syndrome. Proc Natl Acad Sci U S A 89: 5152–5156.
2488. Schwindinger WF, Levine MA (1993). McCune-Albright syndrome. Trends Endocrinol Metab 4: 238–242.
2489. Scinicariello F, Dolan MJ, Nedelcu I et al. (1994). Occurrence of human papillomavirus and p53 gene mutations in Kaposi's sarcoma. Virology 203: 153–157.
2490. Sciot R, Akerman M, Dal Cin P et al. (1997). Cytogenetic analysis of subcutaneous angiolipoma: further evidence supporting its difference from ordinary pure lipomas: a report of the CHAMP Study Group. Am J Surg Pathol 21: 441–444.
2491. Sciot R, Dal Cin P, De Vos R et al. (1993). Alveolar soft-part sarcoma: evidence for its myogenic origin and for the involvement of 17q25. Histopathology 23: 439–444.
2492. Sciot R, Dal Cin P, Fletcher C et al. (1995). t(9;22)(q22-31;q11-12) is a consistent marker of extraskeletal myxoid chondrosarcoma: evaluation of three cases. Mod Pathol 8: 765–768.
2493. Sciot R, Dal Cin P, Samson I et al. (1999). Clonal chromosomal changes in juxta-articular myxoma. Virchows Arch 434: 177–180.
2494. Sciot R, Dorfman H, Brys P et al. (2000). Cytogenetic-morphologic correlations in aneurysmal bone cyst, giant cell tumor of bone and combined lesions. A report from the CHAMP study group. Mod Pathol 13: 1206–1210.
2495. Sciot R, Rosai J, Dal Cin P et al. (1999). Analysis of 35 cases of localized and diffuse tenosynovial giant cell tumor: a report from the Chromosomes and Morphology (CHAMP) study group. Mod Pathol 12: 576–579.
2496. Sciot R, Samson I, Van den Berghe H et al. (1999). Collagenous fibroma (desmoplastic fibroblastoma): genetic link with fibroma of tendon sheath? Mod Pathol 12: 565–568.
2497. Scott SM, Reiman HM, Pritchard DJ et al. (1989). Soft tissue fibrosarcoma. A clinicopathologic study of 132 cases. Cancer 64: 925–931.
2498. Scotti C, Camnasio F, Rizzo N et al. (2008). Mammary-type myofibroblastoma of popliteal fossa. Skeletal Radiol 37: 549–553.
2499. Scrable HJ, Witte DP, Lampkin BC et al. (1987). Chromosomal localization of the human rhabdomyosarcoma locus by mitotic recombination mapping. Nature 329: 645–647.
2500. Sebenik M, Ricci A, Jr., DiPasquale B et al. (2005). Undifferentiated intimal sarcoma of large systemic blood vessels: report of 14 cases with immunohistochemical profile and review of the literature. Am J Surg Pathol 29: 1184–1193.
2501. Sebire NJ, Malone M (2003). Myogenin and MyoD1 expression in paediatric rhab-

domyosarcomas. J Clin Pathol 56: 412–416.
2502. Sebire NJ, Ramsay AD, Malone M et al. (2003). Extensive posttreatment ganglioneuromatous differentiation of rhabdomyosarcoma: malignant ectomesenchymoma in an infant. Pediatr Dev Pathol 6: 94–96.
2503. Seelig MH, Klingler PJ, Oldenburg WA et al. (1998). Angiosarcoma of the aorta: report of a case and review of the literature. J Vasc Surg 28: 732–737.
2504. Segal NH, Pavlidis P, Antonescu CR et al. (2003). Classification and subtype prediction of adult soft tissue sarcoma by functional genomics. Am J Pathol 163: 691–700.
2505. Seifert HW (1981). Ultrastructural investigation on cutaneous angioleiomyoma. Arch Dermatol Res 271: 91–99.
2506. Seijas R, Ares O, Sierra J et al. (2009). Oncogenic osteomalacia: two case reports with surprisingly different outcomes. Arch Orthop Trauma Surg 129: 533–539.
2507. Selvarajah S, Yoshimoto M, Ludkovski O et al. (2008). Genomic signatures of chromosomal instability and osteosarcoma progression detected by high resolution array CGH and interphase FISH. Cytogenet Genome Res 122: 5–15.
2508. Selvarajah S, Yoshimoto M, Prasad M et al. (2007). Characterization of trisomy 8 in pediatric undifferentiated sarcomas using advanced molecular cytogenetic techniques. Cancer Genet Cytogenet 174: 35–41.
2509. Semmelink HJ, Pruszczynski M, Wiersma-vanTilburg A et al. (1990). Cytokeratin expression in chondroblastomas. Histopathology 16: 257–263.
2510. Sencan A, Mir E, Sencan AB et al. (2000). Intrascrotal paratesticular rhabdomyoma: a case report. Acta Paediatr 89: 1020–1022.
2511. Senzaki H, Kiyozuka Y, Uemura Y et al. (1998). Juvenile hyaline fibromatosis: a report of two unrelated adult sibling cases and a literature review. Pathol Int 48: 230–236.
2512. Serra E, Puig S, Otero D et al. (1997). Confirmation of a double-hit model for the NF1 gene in benign neurofibromas. Am J Hum Genet 61: 512–519.
2513. Serra E, Rosenbaum T, Winner U et al. (2000). Schwann cells harbor the somatic NF1 mutation in neurofibromas: evidence of two different Schwann cell subpopulations. Hum Mol Genet 9: 3055–3064.
2514. Serrano-Egea A, Santos-Briz A, Garcia-Munoz H et al. (2001). Chest wall hamartoma. Report of two cases with secondary aneurysmal bone cysts. Pathol Res Pract 197: 835–839.
2515. Sestini R, Bacci C, Provenzano A et al. (2008). Evidence of a four-hit mechanism involving SMARCB1 and NF2 in schwannomatosis-associated schwannomas. Hum Mutat 29: 227–231.
2516. Sevenet N, Sheridan E, Amram D et al. (1999). Constitutional mutations of the hSNF5/INI1 gene predispose to a variety of cancers. Am J Hum Genet 65: 1342–1348.
2517. Shadan FF, Mascarello JT, Newbury RO et al. (2000). Supernumerary ring chromosomes derived from the long arm of chromosome 12 as the primary cytogenetic anomaly in a rare soft tissue chondroma. Cancer Genet Cytogenet 118: 144–147.
2518. Shaddix KK, Fakhre GP, Nields WW et al. (2008). Primary alveolar soft-part sarcoma of the liver: anomalous presentation of a rare disease. Am Surg 74: 43–46.
2519. Shaheen M, Deheshi BM, Riad S et al. (2006). Prognosis of radiation-induced bone sarcoma is similar to primary osteosarcoma. Clin Orthop Relat Res 450: 76–81.
2520. Shalaby A, Presneau N, Ye H et al. (2011). The role of epidermal growth factor receptor in chordoma pathogenesis: a potential therapeutic target. J Pathol 223: 336–346.
2521. Shannon P, Bedard Y, Bell R et al. (1997). Aneurysmal cyst of soft tissue: report of a case with serial magnetic resonance imaging and biopsy. Hum Pathol 28: 255–257.
2522. Shapeero LG, Vanel D, Couanet D et al. (1993). Extraskeletal mesenchymal chondrosarcoma. Radiology 186: 819–826.
2523. Shapiro F, Simon S, Glimcher MJ (1979). Hereditary multiple exostoses. Anthropometric, roentgenographic, and clinical aspects. J Bone Joint Surg Am 61: 815–824.
2524. Sharif S, Ferner R, Birch JM et al. (2006). Second primary tumors in neurofibromatosis 1 patients treated for optic glioma: substantial risks after radiotherapy. J Clin Oncol 24: 2570–2575.
2525. Shaughnessy JD, Jr., Zhan F, Burington BE et al. (2007). A validated gene expression model of high-risk multiple myeloma is defined by deregulated expression of genes mapping to chromosome 1. Blood 109: 2276–2284.
2526. Shaylor PJ, Peake D, Grimer RJ et al. (1999). Paget's osteosarcoma - no cure in sight. Sarcoma 3: 191–192.
2527. Shelekhova KV, Danilova AB, Michal M et al. (2008). Hybrid neurofibroma-perineurioma: an additional example of an extradigital tumor. Ann Diagn Pathol 12: 233–234.
2528. Shelekhova KV, Kazakov DV, Hes O et al. (2006). Phosphaturic mesenchymal tumor (mixed connective tissue variant): a case report with spectral analysis. Virchows Arch 448: 232–235.
2529. Sheng WQ, Hisaoka M, Okamoto S et al. (2001). Congenital-infantile fibrosarcoma. A clinicopathologic study of 10 cases and molecular detection of the ETV6-NTRK3 fusion transcripts using paraffin-embedded tissues. Am J Clin Pathol 115: 348–355.
2530. Shenker A, Weinstein LS, Sweet DE et al. (1994). An activating Gs alpha mutation is present in fibrous dysplasia of bone in the McCune-Albright syndrome. J Clin Endocrinol Metab 79: 750–755.
2531. Shete S, Amos CI, Hwang SJ et al. (2002). Individual-specific liability groups in genetic linkage, with applications to kindreds with Li-Fraumeni syndrome. Am J Hum Genet 70: 813–817.
2532. Sheth S, Li X, Binder S et al. (2011). Differential gene expression profiles of neurothekeomas and nerve sheath myxomas by microarray analysis. Mod Pathol 24: 343–354.
2533. Shields CL, Shields JA (2010). Retinoblastoma management: advances in enucleation, intravenous chemoreduction, and intra-arterial chemotherapy. Curr Opin Ophthalmol 21: 203–212.
2534. Shih LY, Dunn P, Leung WM et al. (1995). Localised plasmacytomas in Taiwan: comparison between extramedullary plasmacytoma and solitary plasmacytoma of bone. Br J Cancer 71: 128–133.
2535. Shim HS, Choi YD, Cho NH (2005). Malignant glomus tumor of the urinary bladder. Arch Pathol Lab Med 129: 940–942.
2536. Shima Y, Ikegami E, Takechi N et al. (2003). Congenital fibrosarcoma of the jejunum in a premature infant with meconium peritonitis. Eur J Pediatr Surg 13: 134–136.
2537. Shimada T, Mizutani S, Muto T et al. (2001). Cloning and characterization of FGF23 as a causative factor of tumor-induced osteomalacia. Proc Natl Acad Sci U S A 98: 6500–6505.
2538. Shimada T, Urakawa I, Yamazaki Y et al. (2004). FGF-23 transgenic mice demonstrate hypophosphatemic rickets with reduced expression of sodium phosphate cotransporter type IIa. Biochem Biophys Res Commun 314: 409–414.
2539. Shimizu S, Hashimoto H, Enjoji M (1984). Nodular fasciitis: an analysis of 250 patients. Pathology 16: 161–166.
2540. Shing DC, McMullan DJ, Roberts P et al. (2003). FUS/ERG gene fusions in Ewing's tumors. Cancer Res 63: 4568–4576.
2541. Shinohara N, Nonomura K, Ishikawa S et al. (2004). Medical management of recurrent aggressive angiomyxoma with gonadotropin-releasing hormone agonist. Int J Urol 11: 432–435.
2542. Shintaku M, Maeno K, Okabe H (2010). Chondroid chordoma of the skull base: immunohistochemical and ultrastructural study of two cases with special reference to microtubules within rough-surfaced endoplasmic reticulum. Med Mol Morphol 43: 241–245.
2543. Shlien A, Baskin B, Achatz MI et al. (2010). A common molecular mechanism underlies two phenotypically distinct 17p13.1 microdeletion syndromes. Am J Hum Genet 87: 631–642.
2544. Shlien A, Tabori U, Marshall CR et al. (2008). Excessive genomic DNA copy number variation in the Li-Fraumeni cancer predisposition syndrome. Proc Natl Acad Sci U S A 105: 11264–11269.
2545. Shmookler BM, Enzinger FM (1981). Pleomorphic lipoma: a benign tumor simulating liposarcoma. A clinicopathologic analysis of 48 cases. Cancer 47: 126–133.
2546. Shmookler BM, Enzinger FM, Weiss SW (1989). Giant cell fibroblastoma. A juvenile form of dermatofibrosarcoma protuberans. Cancer 64: 2154–2161.
2547. Shmookler BM, Lauer DH (1983). Retroperitoneal leiomyosarcoma. A clinicopathologic analysis of 36 cases. Am J Surg Pathol 7: 269–280.
2548. Shugart RR, Soule EH, Johnson EW (1963). Glomus tumor. Surg Gynecol Obstet 117: 334–334.
2549. Shukla N, Ameur N, Yilmaz I et al. (2012). Oncogene mutation profiling of pediatric solid tumors reveals significant subsets of embryonal rhabdomyosarcoma and neuroblastoma with mutated genes in growth signaling pathways. Clin Cancer Res 18: 748–757.
2550. Shuman C, Beckwith JB, Smith AC, Weksberg R. Beckwith- Wiedemann syndrome. In GeneReviews: Pagon RA, Bird TD, Dolan CR, Stephens K, Adam MP, editors. GeneReviews™ [http://genetest.org]. Seattle (WA): University of Washington, Seattle; 1993-.2000 Mar 03 [updated 2010 Dec 14].
2551. Side L, Taylor B, Cayouette M et al. (1997). Homozygous inactivation of the NF1 gene in bone marrow cells from children with neurofibromatosis type 1 and malignant myeloid disorders. N Engl J Med 336: 1713–1720.
2552. Sidwell RU, Rouse P, Owen RA et al. (2008). Granular cell tumor of the scrotum in a child with Noonan syndrome. Pediatr Dermatol 25: 341–343.
2553. Siebenrock KA, Unni KK, Rock MG (1998). Giant-cell tumour of bone metastasising to the lungs. A long-term follow-up. J Bone Joint Surg Br 80: 43–47.
2554. Siegal GP (1998). Primary tumors of bone. In: Pathology of Solid Tumors in Children. Stocker JT, Askin FB Chapman & Hall Medical: London: pp 183–212.
2555. Siegel HJ, Rock MG (2002). Occult phosphaturic mesenchymal tumor detected by Tc-99m sestamibi scan. Clin Nucl Med 27: 608–609.
2556. Sigel JE, Smith TA, Reith JD et al. (2001). Immunohistochemical analysis of anaplastic lymphoma kinase expression in deep soft tissue calcifying fibrous pseudotumor: evidence of a late sclerosing stage of inflammatory myofibroblastic tumor? Ann Diagn Pathol 5: 10–14.
2557. Siitonen HA, Sotkasiira J, Biervliet M et al. (2009). The mutation spectrum in RECQL4 diseases. Eur J Hum Genet 17: 151–158.
2558. Silverman TA, Enzinger FM (1985). Fibrolipomatous hamartoma of nerve. A clinicopathologic analysis of 26 cases. Am J Surg Pathol 9: 7–14.
2559. Simmons AD, Musy MM, Lopes CS et al. (1999). A direct interaction between EXT proteins and glycosyltransferases is defective in hereditary multiple exostoses. Hum Mol Genet 8: 2155–2164.
2560. Simon MP, Pedeutour F, Sirvent N et al. (1997). Deregulation of the platelet-derived growth factor B-chain gene via fusion with collagen gene COL1A1 in dermatofibrosarcoma protuberans and giant-cell fibroblastoma. Nat Genet 15: 95–98.
2561. Simons A, Schepens M, Jeuken J et al. (2000). Frequent loss of 9p21 (p16(INK4A)) and other genomic imbalances in human malignant fibrous histiocytoma. Cancer Genet Cytogenet 118: 89–98.
2562. Singer S, Antonescu CR, Riedel E et al. (2003). Histologic subtype and margin of resection predict pattern of recurrence and survival for retroperitoneal liposarcoma. Ann Surg 238: 358–370.
2563. Singer S, Corson JM, Demetri GD et al. (1995). Prognostic factors predictive of survival for truncal and retroperitoneal soft-tissue sarcoma. Ann Surg 221: 185–195.
2564. Singer S, Demetri GD, Baldini EH et al. (2000). Management of soft-tissue sarcomas: an overview and update. Lancet Oncol 1: 75–85.
2565. Singer S, Socci ND, Ambrosini G et al. (2007). Gene expression profiling of liposarcoma identifies distinct biological types/subtypes and potential therapeutic targets in well-differentiated and dedifferentiated liposarcoma. Cancer Res 67: 6626–6636.
2566. Singhi AD, Montgomery EA (2010). Colorectal granular cell tumor: a clinicopathologic study of 26 cases. Am J Surg Pathol 34: 1186–1192.
2567. Sirvent N, Coindre JM, Maire G et al. (2007). Detection of MDM2-CDK4 amplification by fluorescence in situ hybridization in 200 paraffin-embedded tumor samples: utility in diagnosing adipocytic lesions and comparison with immunohistochemistry and real-time PCR. Am J Surg Pathol 31: 1476–1489.
2568. Sirvent N, Forus A, Lescaut W et al. (2000). Characterization of centromere alterations in liposarcomas. Genes Chromosomes Cancer 29: 117–129.
2569. Sirvent N, Maire G, Pedeutour F (2003). Genetics of dermatofibrosarcoma protuberans family of tumors: from ring chromosomes to tyrosine kinase inhibitor treatment. Genes Chromosomes Cancer 37: 1–19.

2570. Sirvent N, Perrin C, Lacour JP et al. (2004). Monosomy 9q and trisomy 16q in a case of congenital solitary infantile myofibromatosis. Virchows Arch 445: 537–540.

2571. Sissons HA, Steiner GC, Dorfman HD (1993). Calcified spherules in fibro-osseous lesions of bone. Arch Pathol Lab Med 117: 284–290.

2572. Sjogren H, Meis-Kindblom J, Kindblom LG et al. (1999). Fusion of the EWS-related gene TAF2N to TEC in extraskeletal myxoid chondrosarcoma. Cancer Res 59: 5064–5067.

2573. Sjogren H, Meis-Kindblom JM, Orndal C et al. (2003). Studies on the molecular pathogenesis of extraskeletal myxoid chondrosarcoma-cytogenetic, molecular genetic, and cDNA microarray analyses. Am J Pathol 162: 781–792.

2574. Sjogren H, Orndal C, Tingby O et al. (2004). Cytogenetic and spectral karyotype analyses of benign and malignant cartilage tumours. Int J Oncol 24: 1385–1391.

2575. Sjogren H, Wedell B, Meis-Kindblom JM et al. (2000). Fusion of the NH2-terminal domain of the basic helix-loop-helix protein TCF12 to TEC in extraskeletal myxoid chondrosarcoma with translocation t(9;15)(q22;q21). Cancer Res 60: 6832–6835.

2576. Skalova A, Michal M, Husek K et al. (1993). Aggressive angiomyxoma of the pelvioperineal region. Immunohistological and ultrastructural study of seven cases. Am J Dermatopathol 15: 446–451.

2577. Skalova A, Vanecek T, Sima R et al. (2010). Mammary analogue secretory carcinoma of salivary glands, containing the ETV6-NTRK3 fusion gene: a hitherto undescribed salivary gland tumor entity. Am J Surg Pathol 34: 599–608.

2578. Skeletal Lesions Interobserver Correlation among Expert Diagnosticians (SLICED) Study Group (2007). Reliability of histopathologic and radiologic grading of cartilaginous neoplasms in long bones. J Bone Joint Surg Am 89: 2113–2123.

2579. Skuse GR, Kosciolek BA, Rowley PT (1991). The neurofibroma in von Recklinghausen neurofibromatosis has a unicellular origin. Am J Hum Genet 49: 600–607.

2580. Slater DN, Cotton DW, Azzopardi JG (1987). Oncocytic glomus tumour: a new variant. Histopathology 11: 523–531.

2581. Smida J, Baumhoer D, Rosemann M et al. (2010). Genomic alterations and allelic imbalances are strong prognostic predictors in osteosarcoma. Clin Cancer Res 16: 4256–4267.

2582. Smith A, Orchard D (2011). Infantile myofibromatosis: two families supporting autosomal dominant inheritance. Australas J Dermatol 52: 214–217.

2583. Smith AC, Squire JA, Thorner P et al. (2001). Association of alveolar rhabdomyosarcoma with the Beckwith-Wiedemann syndrome. Pediatr Dev Pathol 4: 550–558.

2584. Smith DM, Mahmoud HH, Jenkins JJ, III et al. (1995). Myofibrosarcoma of the head and neck in children. Pediatr Pathol Lab Med 15: 403–418.

2585. Smith GM, Johnson GD, Grimer RJ et al. (2011). Trends in presentation of bone and soft tissue sarcomas over 25 years: little evidence of earlier diagnosis. Ann R Coll Surg Engl 93: 542–547.

2586. Smith J, Botet JF, Yeh SD (1984). Bone sarcomas in Paget disease: a study of 85 patients. Radiology 152: 583–590.

2587. Smith ME, Fisher C, Weiss SW (1996). Pleomorphic hyalinizing angiectatic tumor of soft parts. A low-grade neoplasm resembling neurilemoma. Am J Surg Pathol 20: 21–29.

2588. Smith R, Owen LA, Trem DJ et al. (2006). Expression profiling of EWS/FLI identifies NKX2.2 as a critical target gene in Ewing's sarcoma. Cancer Cell 9: 405–416.

2589. Smith S, Fletcher CD, Smith MA et al. (1990). Cytogenetic analysis of a plexiform fibrohistiocytic tumor. Cancer Genet Cytogenet 48: 31–34.

2590. Smith-Zagone MJ, Prieto VG, Hayes RA et al. (2004). HMB-45 (gp103) and MART-1 expression within giant cells in an atypical fibroxanthoma: a case report. J Cutan Pathol 31: 284–286.

2591. Snyder EL, Sandstrom DJ, Law K et al. (2009). c-Jun amplification and overexpression are oncogenic in liposarcoma but not always sufficient to inhibit the adipocytic differentiation programme. J Pathol 218: 292–300.

2592. Sobreira NL, Cirulli ET, Avramopoulos D et al. (2010). Whole-genome sequencing of a single proband together with linkage analysis identifies a Mendelian disease gene. PLoS Genet 6: e1000991

2593. Soder S, Inwards C, Muller S et al. (2001). Cell biology and matrix biochemistry of chondromyxoid fibroma. Am J Clin Pathol 116: 271–277.

2594. Sola JB, Wright RW (1998). Arthroscopic treatment for lipoma arborescens of the knee: a case report. J Bone Joint Surg Am 80: 99–103.

2595. Solak O, Esme H, Sahin DA et al. (2007). Giant intraosseous lipoma of the rib. Thorac Cardiovasc Surg 55: 273–274.

2596. Soler JM, Piza G, Aliaga F (1997). Special characteristics of osteoid osteoma in the proximal phalanx. J Hand Surg Br 22: 793–797.

2597. Somerhausen NS, Fletcher CD (2000). Diffuse-type giant cell tumor: clinicopathologic and immunohistochemical analysis of 50 cases with extraarticular disease. Am J Surg Pathol 24: 479–492.

2598. Somers GR, Gupta AA, Doria AS et al. (2006). Pediatric undifferentiated sarcoma of the soft tissues: a clinicopathologic study. Pediatr Dev Pathol 9: 132–142.

2599. Somers GR, Tesoriero AA, Hartland E et al. (1998). Multiple leiomyosarcomas of both donor and recipient origin arising in a heart-lung transplant patient. Am J Surg Pathol 22: 1423–1428.

2600. Somers GR, Viero S, Nathan PC et al. (2005). Association of the t(12;22)(q13;q12) EWS/ATF1 rearrangement with polyphenotypic round cell sarcoma of bone: a case report. Am J Surg Pathol 29: 1673–1679.

2601. Song SE, Lee CH, Kim KA et al. (2010). Malignant glomus tumor of the stomach with multiorgan metastases: report of a case. Surg Today 40: 662–667.

2602. Sonobe H, Ro JY, Mackay et al. (1994). Primary pulmonary alveolar soft-part sarcoma: report of a case. Int J Surg Pathol 2: 57-61.

2603. Sontag LW, Pyle DI (1941). The appearance and nature of cyst-like areas in distal femoral metaphyses of children. Am J Roentgenol Radiat Ther 46: 185-188

2604. Sorensen PH, Lessnick SL, Lopez-Terrada D et al. (1994). A second Ewing's sarcoma translocation, t(21;22), fuses the EWS gene to another ETS-family transcription factor, ERG. Nat Genet 6: 146–151.

2605. Sorensen PH, Lynch JC, Qualman SJ et al. (2002). PAX3-FKHR and PAX7-FKHR gene fusions are prognostic indicators in alveolar rhabdomyosarcoma: a report from the children's oncology group. J Clin Oncol 20: 2672–2679.

2606. Sorensen PH, Shimada H, Liu XF et al. (1995). Biphenotypic sarcomas with myogenic and neural differentiation express the Ewing's sarcoma EWS/FLI1 fusion gene. Cancer Res 55: 1385–1392.

2607. Sotelo-Avila C, Bale PM (1994). Subdermal fibrous hamartoma of infancy: pathology of 40 cases and differential diagnosis. Pediatr Pathol 14: 39–52.

2608. Sotoda Y, Hirooka S, Kohi M et al. (2008). Intramuscular hemangioma in the right ventricle. Gen Thorac Cardiovasc Surg 56: 85–87.

2609. Souid AK, Ziemba MC, Dubansky AS et al. (1993). Inflammatory myofibroblastic tumor in children. Cancer 72: 2042–2048.

2610. Soule EH (1962). Proliferative (nodular) fasciitis. Arch Pathol 73: 437–444.

2611. Soule EH, Pritchard DJ (1977). Fibrosarcoma in infants and children: a review of 110 cases. Cancer 40: 1711–1721.

2612. Soussi T, Hamroun D, Hjortsberg L et al. (2010). MUT-TP53 2.0: a novel versatile matrix for statistical analysis of TP53 mutations in human cancer. Hum Mutat 31: 1020–1025.

2613. Soutar R, Lucraft H, Jackson G et al. (2004). Guidelines on the diagnosis and management of solitary plasmacytoma of bone and solitary extramedullary plasmacytoma. Br J Haematol 124: 717–726.

2614. Southgate J, Sarma U, Townend JV et al. (1998). Study of the cell biology and biochemistry of cherubism. J Clin Pathol 51: 831–837.

2615. Sovani V, Velagaleti GV, Filipowicz E et al. (2001). Ossifying fibromyxoid tumor of soft parts: report of a case with novel cytogenetic findings. Cancer Genet Cytogenet 127: 1–6.

2616. Sparkes RS, Sparkes MC, Wilson MG et al. (1980). Regional assignment of genes for human esterase D and retinoblastoma to chromosome band 13q14. Science 208: 1042–1044.

2617. Specht K, Haralambieva E, Bink K et al. (2004). Different mechanisms of cyclin D1 overexpression in multiple myeloma revealed by fluorescence in situ hybridization and quantitative analysis of mRNA levels. Blood 104: 1120–1126.

2618. Speer AL, Schofield DE, Wang KS et al. (2008). Contemporary management of lipoblastoma. J Pediatr Surg 43: 1295–1300.

2619. Spiegelberg BG, Sewell MD, Coltman T et al. (2009). Below-knee amputation through a joint-sparing proximal tibial replacement for recurrent tumour. J Bone Joint Surg Br 91: 815–819.

2620. Spillane AJ, Thomas JM, Fisher C (2000). Epithelioid sarcoma: the clinicopathological complexities of this rare soft tissue sarcoma. Ann Surg Oncol 7: 218–225.

2621. Spouge AR, Thain LM (2000). Osteoid osteoma: MR imaging revisited. Clin Imaging 24: 19–27.

2622. Springfield DS, Capanna R, Gherlinzoni F et al. (1985). Chondroblastoma. A review of seventy cases. J Bone Joint Surg Am 67: 748–755.

2623. Springfield DS, Rosenberg AE, Mankin HJ et al. (1994). Relationship between osteofibrous dysplasia and adamantinoma. Clin Orthop Relat Res 234–244.

2624. Spunt SL, Lobe TE, Pappo AS et al. (2000). Aggressive surgery is unwarranted for biliary tract rhabdomyosarcoma. J Pediatr Surg 35: 309–316.

2625. Squire J, Gallie BL, Phillips RA (1985). A detailed analysis of chromosomal changes in heritable and non-heritable retinoblastoma. Hum Genet 70: 291–301.

2626. Squire JA, Pei J, Marrano P et al. (2003). High-resolution mapping of amplifications and deletions in pediatric osteosarcoma by use of CGH analysis of cDNA microarrays. Genes Chromosomes Cancer 38: 215–225.

2627. Sraj SA, Lahoud LE, Musharafieh R et al. (2008). Nuchal-type fibroma of the ankle: a case report. J Foot Ankle Surg 47: 332–336.

2628. Sreekantaiah C, Karakousis CP, Leong SP et al. (1992). Cytogenetic findings in liposarcoma correlate with histopathologic subtypes. Cancer 69: 2484–2495.

2629. Sreekantaiah C, Leong SP, Davis JR et al. (1991). Cytogenetic and flow cytometric analysis of a clear cell chondrosarcoma. Cancer Genet Cytogenet 52: 193–199.

2630. Srigley JR, Ayala AG, Ordonez NG et al. (1985). Epithelioid hemangioma of the penis. A rare and distinctive vascular lesion. Arch Pathol Lab Med 109: 51–54.

2631. Staals EL, Bacchini P, Bertoni F (2006). Dedifferentiated central chondrosarcoma. Cancer 106: 2682–2691.

2632. Staals EL, Bacchini P, Bertoni F (2008). High-grade surface osteosarcoma: a review of 25 cases from the Rizzoli Institute. Cancer 112: 1592–1599.

2633. Staals EL, Bacchini P, Mercuri M et al. (2007). Dedifferentiated chondrosarcomas arising in preexisting osteochondromas. J Bone Joint Surg Am 89: 987–993.

2634. Stacchiotti S, Negri T, Palassini E et al. (2010). Sunitinib malate and figitumumab in solitary fibrous tumor: patterns and molecular bases of tumor response. Mol Cancer Ther 9: 1286–1297.

2635. Stacchiotti S, Palassini E, Sanfilippo R et al. (2012). Gemcitabine in advanced angiosarcoma: a retrospective case series analysis from the Italian Rare Cancer Network. Ann Oncol 23: 501–508.

2636. Stancheva-Ivanova MK, Wuyts W, van Hul E et al. (2011). Clinical and molecular studies of EXT1/EXT2 in Bulgaria. J Inherit Metab Dis 34: 917–921.

2637. Stanton RP, Abdel-Mota'al MM (1998). Growth arrest resulting from unicameral bone cyst. J Pediatr Orthop 18: 198–201.

2638. Stark B, Mor C, Jeison M et al. (1997). Additional chromosome 1q aberrations and der(16)t(1;16), correlation to the phenotypic expression and clinical behavior of the Ewing family of tumors. J Neurooncol 31: 3–8.

2639. Stark B, Zoubek A, Hattinger C et al. (1996). Metastatic extraosseous Ewing tumor. Association of the additional translocation der(16)t(1;16) with the variant EWS/ERG rearrangement in a case of cytogenetically inconspicuous chromosome 22. Cancer Genet Cytogenet 87: 161–166.

2640. Statz EM, Pochebit SM, Cooper A et al. (1989). Case report 525: Benign fibrous histiocytoma (BFH) of thumb. Skeletal Radiol 18: 299–302.

2641. Steelman C, Katzenstein H, Parham D et al. (2011). Unusual presentation of congenital infantile fibrosarcoma in seven infants with molecular-genetic analysis. Fetal Pediatr Pathol 30: 329–337.

2642. Steenman M, Westerveld A, Mannens M (2000). Genetics of Beckwith-Wiedemann syndrome-associated tumors: common genetic pathways. Genes Chromosomes Cancer 28:

1–13.
2643. Steeper TA, Rosai J (1983). Aggressive angiomyxoma of the female pelvis and perineum. Report of nine cases of a distinctive type of gynecologic soft-tissue neoplasm. Am J Surg Pathol 7: 463–475.
2644. Stefanato CM, Robson A, Calonje JE (2010). The histopathologic spectrum of regression in atypical fibroxanthoma. J Cutan Pathol 37: 310–315.
2645. Steigen SE, Schaeffer DF, West RB et al. (2009). Expression of insulin-like growth factor 2 in mesenchymal neoplasms. Mod Pathol 22: 914–921.
2646. Steiner GC (1979). Ultrastructure of benign cartilaginous tumors of intraosseous origin. Hum Pathol 10: 71–86.
2647. Stemmer-Rachamimov AO, Xu L, Gonzalez-Agosti C et al. (1997). Universal absence of merlin, but not other ERM family members, in schwannomas. Am J Pathol 151: 1649–1654.
2648. Stemmermann GN, Stout AP (1962). Elastofibroma dorsi. Am J Clin Pathol 37: 499–506.
2649. Stenman G, Andersson H, Mandahl N et al. (1995). Translocation t(9;22)(q22;q12) is a primary cytogenetic abnormality in extraskeletal myxoid chondrosarcoma. Int J Cancer 62: 398–402.
2650. Stenman G, Nadal N, Persson S et al. (1999). del(6)(q12q15) as the sole cytogenetic anomaly in a case of solitary infantile myofibromatosis. Oncol Rep 6: 1101–1104.
2651. Stephens PJ, Greenman CD, Fu B et al. (2011). Massive genomic rearrangement acquired in a single catastrophic event during cancer development. Cell 144: 27–40.
2652. Stevenson DA, Zhou H, Ashrafi S et al. (2006). Double inactivation of NF1 in tibial pseudarthrosis. Am J Hum Genet 79: 143–148.
2653. Stewart DR, Pemov A, Van Loo P et al. (2012). Mitotic recombination of chromosome arm 17q as a cause of loss of heterozygosity of NF1 in neurofibromatosis type 1-associated glomus tumors. Genes Chromosomes Cancer 51: 429–437.
2654. Stewart DR, Sloan JL, Yao L et al. (2010). Diagnosis, management, and complications of glomus tumours of the digits in neurofibromatosis type 1. J Med Genet 47: 525–532.
2655. Stickens D, Clines G, Burbee D et al. (1996). The EXT2 multiple exostoses gene defines a family of putative tumour suppressor genes. Nat Genet 14: 25–32.
2656. Stock C, Kager L, Fink FM et al. (2000). Chromosomal regions involved in the pathogenesis of osteosarcomas. Genes Chromosomes Cancer 28: 329–336.
2657. Stock N, Chibon F, Binh MB et al. (2009). Adult-type rhabdomyosarcoma: analysis of 57 cases with clinicopathologic description, identification of 3 morphologic patterns and prognosis. Am J Surg Pathol 33: 1850–1859.
2658. Stojadinovic A, Leung DH, Hoos A et al. (2002). Analysis of the prognostic significance of microscopic margins in 2,084 localized primary adult soft tissue sarcomas. Ann Surg 235: 424–434.
2659. Stone MD, Quincey C, Hosking DJ (1992). A neuroendocrine cause of oncogenic osteomalacia. J Pathol 167: 181–185.
2660. Storlazzi CT, Mertens F, Nascimento A et al. (2003). Fusion of the FUS and BBF2H7 genes in low grade fibromyxoid sarcoma. Hum Mol Genet 12: 2349–2358.
2661. Storlazzi CT, Wozniak A, Panagopoulos I et al. (2006). Rearrangement of the COL12A1 and COL4A5 genes in subungual exostosis: molecular cytogenetic delineation of the tumor-specific translocation t(X;6)(q13-14;q22). Int J Cancer 118: 1972–1976.
2662. Stout AP (1962). Fibrosarcoma in infants and children. Cancer 15: 1028–1040.
2663. Stout AP, HILL WT (1958). Leiomyosarcoma of the superficial soft tissues. Cancer 11: 844–854.
2664. Stratakis CA, Carney JA (2009). The triad of paragangliomas, gastric stromal tumours and pulmonary chondromas (Carney triad), and the dyad of paragangliomas and gastric stromal sarcomas (Carney-Stratakis syndrome): molecular genetics and clinical implications. J Intern Med 266: 43–52.
2665. Stratakis CA, Carney JA, Lin JP et al. (1996). Carney complex, a familial multiple neoplasia and lentiginosis syndrome. Analysis of 11 kindreds and linkage to the short arm of chromosome 2. J Clin Invest 97: 699–705.
2666. Stratakis CA, Kirschner LS, Carney JA (2001). Clinical and molecular features of the Carney complex: diagnostic criteria and recommendations for patient evaluation. J Clin Endocrinol Metab 86: 4041–4046.
2667. Stratton MR, Moss S, Warren W et al. (1990). Mutation of the p53 gene in human soft tissue sarcomas: association with abnormalities of the RB1 gene. Oncogene 5: 1297–1301.
2668. Strong LC, Riccardi VM, Ferrell RE et al. (1981). Familial retinoblastoma and chromosome 13 deletion transmitted via an insertional translocation. Science 213: 1501–1503.
2669. Strutton G, Weedon D (1987). Acro-angiodermatitis. A simulant of Kaposi's sarcoma. Am J Dermatopathol 9: 85–89.
2670. Stucky CC, Johnson KN, Gray RJ et al. (2011). Malignant peripheral nerve sheath tumors (MPNST): The Mayo Clinic Experience. Ann Surg Oncol 19:878-885.
2671. Su LD, Atayde-Perez A, Sheldon S et al. (1998). Inflammatory myofibroblastic tumor: cytogenetic evidence supporting clonal origin. Mod Pathol 11: 364–368.
2672. Suarez Vilela D, Gimenez Pizarro A, Rio Suarez M (1990). Vaginal rhabdomyoma and adenosis. Histopathology 16: 393–394.
2673. Suh JS, Cho J, Lee SH et al. (2000). Alveolar soft part sarcoma: MR and angiographic findings. Skeletal Radiol 29: 680–689.
2674. Sukov WR, Franco MF, Erickson-Johnson M et al. (2008). Frequency of USP6 rearrangements in myositis ossificans, brown tumor, and cherubism: molecular cytogenetic evidence that a subset of "myositis ossificans-like lesions" are the early phases in the formation of soft-tissue aneurysmal bone cyst. Skeletal Radiol 37: 321–327.
2675. Sultan I, Qaddoumi I, Yaser S et al. (2009). Comparing adult and pediatric rhabdomyosarcoma in the surveillance, epidemiology and end results program, 1973 to 2005: an analysis of 2,600 patients. J Clin Oncol 27: 3391–3397.
2676. Sultan I, Rodriguez-Galindo C, Saab R et al. (2009). Comparing children and adults with synovial sarcoma in the Surveillance, Epidemiology, and End Results program, 1983 to 2005: an analysis of 1268 patients. Cancer 115: 3537–3547.
2676A. Sumegi J, Nishio J, Nelson M et al. (2011). A novel t(4;22)(q31;q12) produces an EWSR1-SMARCA5 fusion in extraskeletal Ewing sarcoma/primitive neuroectodermal tumor. Mod Path 24:333-42.
2677. Sumegi J, Streblow R, Frayer RW et al. (2010). Recurrent t(2;2) and t(2;8) translocations in rhabdomyosarcoma without the canonical PAX-FOXO1 fuse PAX3 to members of the nuclear receptor transcriptional coactivator family. Genes Chromosomes Cancer 49: 224–236.
2678. Sumiyoshi K, Tsuneyoshi M, Enjoji M (1985). Myositis ossificans. A clinicopathologic study of 21 cases. Acta Pathol Jpn 35: 1109–1122.
2679. Sun R, Lin SF, Staskus K et al. (1999). Kinetics of Kaposi's sarcoma-associated herpesvirus gene expression. J Virol 73: 2232–2242.
2680. Sundaram M (2006). Imaging of Paget's disease and fibrous dysplasia of bone. J Bone Miner Res 21 Suppl 2: 28–30.
2681. Sundaram M, Akduman I, White LM et al. (1999). Primary leiomyosarcoma of bone. AJR Am J Roentgenol 172: 771–776.
2682. Surace C, Storlazzi CT, Engellau J et al. (2005). Molecular cytogenetic characterization of an ins(4;X) occurring as the sole abnormality in an aggressive, poorly differentiated soft tissue sarcoma. Virchows Arch 447: 869–874.
2683. Suster S, Fisher C (1997). Immunoreactivity for the human hematopoietic progenitor cell antigen (CD34) in lipomatous tumors. Am J Surg Pathol 21: 195–200.
2684. Suster S, Nascimento AG, Miettinen M et al. (1995). Solitary fibrous tumors of soft tissue. A clinicopathologic and immunohistochemical study of 12 cases. Am J Surg Pathol 19: 1257–1266.
2685. Suster S, Rosai J (1990). Hamartoma of the scalp with ectopic meningothelial elements. A distinctive benign soft tissue lesion that may simulate angiosarcoma. Am J Surg Pathol 14: 1–11.
2686. Suster S, Wong TY, Moran CA (1993). Sarcomas with combined features of liposarcoma and leiomyosarcoma. Study of two cases of an unusual soft-tissue tumor showing dual lineage differentiation. Am J Surg Pathol 17: 905–911.
2687. Swaby MG, Evans HL, Fletcher CD et al. (2011). Dermatofibrosarcoma protuberans with unusual sarcomatous transformation: a series of 4 cases with molecular confirmation. Am J Dermatopathol 33: 354–360.
2688. Swarts SJ, Neff JR, Johansson SL et al. (1996). Cytogenetic analysis of dedifferentiated chondrosarcoma. Cancer Genet Cytogenet 89: 49–51.
2689. Swarts SJ, Neff JR, Johansson SL et al. (1998). Significance of abnormalities of chromosomes 5 and 8 in chondroblastoma. Clin Orthop Relat Res 349:189–193.
2690. Sweet DE, Vinh TN, Devaney K (1992). Cortical osteofibrous dysplasia of long bone and its relationship to adamantinoma. A clinicopathologic study of 30 cases. Am J Surg Pathol 16: 282–290.
2691. Swelam WM, Cheng J, Ida-Yonemochi H et al. (2009). Oral solitary fibrous tumor: a cytogenetic analysis of tumor cells in culture with literature review. Cancer Genet Cytogenet 194: 75–81.
2692. Swensen JJ, Keyser J, Coffin CM et al. (2009). Familial occurrence of schwannomas and malignant rhabdoid tumour associated with a duplication in SMARCB1. J Med Genet 46: 68–72.
2693. Swift AC, Singh SD (1985). The presentation and management of the nasal glioma. Int J Pediatr Otorhinolaryngol 10: 253–261.
2694. Szudek J, Birch P, Riccardi VM et al. (2000). Associations of clinical features in neurofibromatosis 1 (NF1). Genet Epidemiol 19: 429–439.
2695. Szuhai K, Ijszenga M, de Jong D et al. (2009). The NFATc2 gene is involved in a novel cloned translocation in a Ewing sarcoma variant that couples its function in immunology to oncology. Clin Cancer Res 15: 2259–2268.
2696. Szuhai K, Ijszenga M, Knijnenburg J et al. (2007). Does parosteal liposarcoma differ from other atypical lipomatous tumors/well-differentiated liposarcomas? A molecular cytogenetic study using combined multicolor COBRA-FISH karyotyping and array-based comparative genomic hybridization. Cancer Genet Cytogenet 176: 115–120.
2697. Szuhai K, Jennes I, de Jong D et al. (2011). Tiling resolution array-CGH shows that somatic mosaic deletion of the EXT gene is causative in EXT gene mutation negative multiple osteochondromas patients. Hum Mutat 32: E2036–E2049.
2698. Szymanska J, Mandahl N, Mertens F et al. (1996). Ring chromosomes in parosteal osteosarcoma contain sequences from 12q13-15: a combined cytogenetic and comparative genomic hybridization study. Genes Chromosomes Cancer 16: 31–34.
2699. Szymanska J, Tarkkanen M, Wiklund T et al. (1996). Gains and losses of DNA sequences in liposarcomas evaluated by comparative genomic hybridization. Genes Chromosomes Cancer 15: 89–94.
2700. Tabori U, Nanda S, Druker H et al. (2007). Younger age of cancer initiation is associated with shorter telomere length in Li-Fraumeni syndrome. Cancer Res 67: 1415–1418.
2701. Taconis WK, Mulder JD (1984). Fibrosarcoma and malignant fibrous histiocytoma of long bones: radiographic features and grading. Skeletal Radiol 11: 237–245.
2702. Takahashi Y, Imamura T, Irie H et al. (2004). Myolipoma of the retroperitoneum. Pathol Int 54: 460–463.
2703. Takahashi Y, Oda Y, Kawaguchi K et al. (2004). Altered expression and molecular abnormalities of cell-cycle-regulatory proteins in rhabdomyosarcoma. Mod Pathol 17: 660–669.
2704. Takata H, Ikuta Y, Ishida O et al. (2001). Treatment of subungual glomus tumour. Hand Surg 6: 25–27.
2705. Takeuchi K, Soda M, Togashi Y et al. (2011). Pulmonary inflammatory myofibroblastic tumor expressing a novel fusion, PPFIBP1-ALK: reappraisal of anti-ALK immunohistochemistry as a tool for novel ALK fusion identification. Clin Cancer Res 17: 3341–3348.
2706. Takigawa K (1971). Chondroma of the bones of the hand. A review of 110 cases. J Bone Joint Surg Am 53: 1591–1600.
2707. Talbot C, Khan T, Smith M (2007). Infantile digital fibromatosis. J Pediatr Orthop B 16: 110–112.
2708. Tallini G, Dorfman H, Brys P et al. (2002). Correlation between clinicopathological features and karyotype in 100 cartilaginous and chordoid tumours. A report from the Chromosomes and Morphology (CHAMP) Collaborative Study Group. J Pathol 196: 194–203.
2709. Tamborini E, Casieri P, Miselli F et al. (2007). Analysis of potential receptor tyrosine kinase targets in intimal and mural sarcomas. J Pathol 212: 227–235.
2710. Tamborini E, Miselli F, Negri T et al. (2006). Molecular and biochemical analyses of platelet-derived growth factor receptor

(PDGFR) B, PDGFRA, and KIT receptors in chordomas. Clin Cancer Res 12: 6920–6928.

2711. Tan AY, Manley JL (2009). The TET family of proteins: functions and roles in disease. J Mol Cell Biol 1: 82–92.

2712. Tan D, Kraybill W, Cheney RT et al. (2005). Retiform hemangioendothelioma: a case report and review of the literature. J Cutan Pathol 32: 634–637.

2713. Tanaka H, Yasui N, Kuriskaki E et al. (1990). The Goltz syndrome associated with giant cell tumour of bone. A case report. Int Orthop 14: 179–181.

2714. Tanaka M, Kato K, Gomi K et al. (2009). Perivascular epithelioid cell tumor with SFPQ/PSF-TFE3 gene fusion in a patient with advanced neuroblastoma. Am J Surg Pathol 33: 1416–1420.

2715. Tanaka T, Kobayashi T, Iino M (2011). Transformation of benign fibrous histiocytoma into malignant fibrous histiocytoma in the mandible: case report. J Oral Maxillofac Surg 69: e285–e290.

2716. Tanas MR, Sboner A, Oliveira AM et al. (2011). Identification of a disease-defining gene fusion in epithelioid hemangioendothelioma. Sci Transl Med 3: 98ra82

2717. Tanda F, Rocca PC, Bosincu L et al. (1997). Rhabdomyoma of the tunica vaginalis of the testis: a histologic, immunohistochemical, and ultrastructural study. Mod Pathol 10: 608–611.

2718. Tang TT, Segura AD, Oechler HW et al. (1990). Inflammatory myofibrohistiocytic proliferation simulating sarcoma in children. Cancer 65: 1626–1634.

2719. Tantcheva-Poor I, Marathovouniotis N, Kutzner H et al. (2012). Vascular congenital dermatofibrosarcoma protuberans: a new histological variant of dermatofibrosarcoma protuberans. Am J Dermatopathol 34: e46–49.

2720. Tap WD, Eilber FC, Ginther C et al. (2011). Evaluation of well-differentiated/de-differentiated liposarcomas by high-resolution oligonucleotide array-based comparative genomic hybridization. Genes Chromosomes Cancer 50: 95–112.

2721. Tardio JC, Butron M, Martin-Fragueiro LM (2008). Superficial acral fibromyxoma: report of 4 cases with CD10 expression and lipomatous component, two previously underrecognized features. Am J Dermatopathol 30: 431–435.

2722. Tarkkanen M, Bohling T, Gamberi G et al. (1998). Comparative genomic hybridization of low-grade central osteosarcoma. Mod Pathol 11: 421–426.

2723. Tarkkanen M, Elomaa I, Blomqvist C et al. (1999). DNA sequence copy number increase at 8q: a potential new prognostic marker in high-grade osteosarcoma. Int J Cancer 84: 114–121.

2724. Tarkkanen M, Kaipainen A, Karaharju E et al. (1993). Cytogenetic study of 249 consecutive patients examined for a bone tumor. Cancer Genet Cytogenet 68: 1–21.

2725. Tarkkanen M, Larramendy ML, Bohling T et al. (2006). Malignant fibrous histiocytoma of bone: analysis of genomic imbalances by comparative genomic hybridisation and C-MYC expression by immunohistochemistry. Eur J Cancer 42: 1172–1180.

2726. Tarkkanen M, Nordling S, Bohling T et al. (1996). Comparison of cytogenetics, interphase cytogenetics, and DNA flow cytometry in bone tumors. Cytometry 26: 185–191.

2727. Tarkkanen M, Wiklund T, Virolainen M et al. (1994). Dedifferentiated chondrosarcoma

with t(9;22)(q34;q11-12). Genes Chromosomes Cancer 9: 136–140.

2728. Tarkkanen M, Wiklund TA, Virolainen MJ et al. (2001). Comparative genomic hybridization of postirradiation sarcomas. Cancer 92: 1992–1998.

2729. Tartaglia M, Zampino G, Gelb BD (2010). Noonan syndrome: clinical aspects and molecular pathogenesis. Mol Syndromol 1: 2–26.

2730. Tassano E, Nozza P, Tavella E et al. (2010). Cytogenetic characterization of a fibrous hamartoma of infancy with complex translocations. Cancer Genet Cytogenet 201: 66–69.

2731. Tassano E, Sementa AR, Tavella E et al. (2010). Trisomy 17 in congenital plexiform (multinodular) cellular schwannoma. Cancer Genet Cytogenet 203: 313–315.

2732. Taubert H, Berger D, Hinze R et al. (1998). How is the mutational status for tumor suppressors p53 and p16(INK4A) in MFH of the bone? Cancer Lett 123: 147–151.

2733. Taylor BS, Barretina J, Socci ND et al. (2008). Functional copy-number alterations in cancer. PLoS One 3: e3179

2734. Taylor JG, Cheuk AT, Tsang PS et al. (2009). Identification of FGFR4-activating mutations in human rhabdomyosarcomas that promote metastasis in xenotransplanted models. J Clin Invest 119: 3395–3407.

2735. Taylor MD, Mainprize TG, Rutka JT (2000). Molecular insight into medulloblastoma and central nervous system primitive neuroectodermal tumor biology from hereditary syndromes: a review. Neurosurgery 47: 888–901.

2736. Taylor R, Kashima TG, Knowles H et al. (2011). Osteoclast formation and function in pigmented villonodular synovitis. J Pathol 225: 151–156.

2737. Taylor RM, Kashima TG, Ferguson DJ et al. (2012). Analysis of stromal cells in osteofibrous dysplasia and adamantinoma of long bones. Mod Pathol 25: 56–64.

2738. Tazelaar HD, Batts KP, Srigley JR (2001). Primary extrapulmonary sugar tumor (PEST): a report of four cases. Mod Pathol 14: 615–622.

2739. Templeton SF, Solomon AR, Jr. (1996). Spindle cell lipoma is strongly CD34 positive. An immunohistochemical study. J Cutan Pathol 23: 546–550.

2740. Ten Heuvel SE, Hoekstra HJ, Bastiaannet E et al. (2009). The classic prognostic factors tumor stage, tumor size, and tumor grade are the strongest predictors of outcome in synovial sarcoma: no role for SSX fusion type or ezrin expression. Appl Immunohistochem Mol Morphol 17: 189–195.

2741. Ten Heuvel SE, Hoekstra HJ, Suurmeijer AJ (2008). Diagnostic accuracy of FISH and RT-PCR in 50 routinely processed synovial sarcomas. Appl Immunohistochem Mol Morphol 16: 246–250.

2742. Teo HE, Peh WC, Chan MY et al. (2005). Infantile lipofibromatosis of the upper limb. Skeletal Radiol 34: 799–802.

2743. Terada T, Fujimoto J, Shirakashi Y et al. (2011). Malignant glomus tumor of the palm: a case report. J Cutan Pathol 38: 381–384.

2744. Terrier-Lacombe MJ, Guillou L, Maire G et al. (2003). Dermatofibrosarcoma protuberans, giant cell fibroblastoma, and hybrid lesions in children: clinicopathologic comparative analysis of 28 cases with molecular data—a study from the French Federation of Cancer Centers Sarcoma Group. Am J Surg Pathol 27: 27–39.

2745. Terstappen LW, Johnsen S, Segers-Nolten IM et al. (1990). Identification and characterization of plasma cells in normal human bone marrow by high-resolution flow cytometry. Blood 76: 1739–1747.

2746. Terzis JK, Daniel RK, Williams HB et al. (1978). Benign fatty tumors of the peripheral nerves. Ann Plast Surg 1: 193–216.

2747. Tetzlaff MT, Liu P, O'Malley BW, Jr. et al. (2008). Report of a case of sinonasal undifferentiated carcinoma arising in a background of extensive nasal gliomatosis. Head Neck 30: 549–555.

2748. Theaker JM, Fletcher CD (1991). Heterotopic glial nodules: a light microscopic and immunohistochemical study. Histopathology 18: 255–260.

2749. Thomas D, Henshaw R, Skubitz K et al. (2010). Denosumab in patients with giant-cell tumour of bone: an open-label, phase 2 study. Lancet Oncol 11: 275–280.

2750. Thomas DM, Carty SA, Piscopo DM et al. (2001). The retinoblastoma protein acts as a transcriptional coactivator required for osteogenic differentiation. Mol Cell 8: 303–316.

2751. Thomas RM, Sobin LH (1995). Gastrointestinal cancer. Cancer 75: 154–170.

2752. Thompson J, Castillo M, Reddick RL et al. (1995). Nasopharyngeal nonossifying variant of ossifying fibromyxoid tumor: CT and MR findings. AJNR Am J Neuroradiol 16: 1132–1134.

2753. Thompson LD, Gyure KA (2000). Extracranial sinonasal tract meningiomas: a clinicopathologic study of 30 cases with a review of the literature. Am J Surg Pathol 24: 640–650.

2754. Thum C, Hollowood K, Birch J et al. (2011). Aberrant Melan-A expression in atypical fibroxanthoma and undifferentiated pleomorphic sarcoma of the skin. J Cutan Pathol 38: 954–960.

2755. Thurer RL, Thorsen A, Parker JA et al. (2000). FDG imaging of a pulmonary artery sarcoma. Ann Thorac Surg 70: 1414–1415.

2756. Thway K, Gibson S, Ramsay A et al. (2009). Beta-catenin expression in pediatric fibroblastic and myofibroblastic lesions: a study of 100 cases. Pediatr Dev Pathol 12: 292–296.

2757. Tiet TD, Hopyan S, Nadesan P et al. (2006). Constitutive hedgehog signaling in chondrosarcoma up-regulates tumor cell proliferation. Am J Pathol 168: 321–330.

2758. Timosca GC, Galesanu RM, Cotutiu C et al. (2000). Aggressive form of cherubism: report of a case. J Oral Maxillofac Surg 58: 336–344.

2759. Tinat J, Bougeard G, Baert-Desurmont S et al. (2009). 2009 version of the Chompret criteria for Li Fraumeni syndrome. J Clin Oncol 27: e108–e109.

2760. Tirabosco R, Mangham DC, Rosenberg AE et al. (2008). Brachyury expression in extra-axial skeletal and soft tissue chordomas: a marker that distinguishes chordoma from mixed tumor/myoepithelioma/parachordoma in soft tissue. Am J Surg Pathol 32: 572–580.

2761. Tirode F, Laud-Duval K, Prieur A et al. (2007). Mesenchymal stem cell features of Ewing tumors. Cancer Cell 11: 421–429.

2762. Tiziani V, Reichenberger E, Buzzo CL et al. (1999). The gene for cherubism maps to chromosome 4p16. Am J Hum Genet 65: 158–166.

2763. Tognon C, Garnett M, Kenward E et al. (2001). The chimeric protein tyrosine kinase ETV6-NTRK3 requires both Ras-Erk1/2 and PI3-kinase-Akt signaling for fibroblast transfor-

mation. Cancer Res 61: 8909–8916.

2764. Tognon C, Knezevich SR, Huntsman D et al. (2002). Expression of the ETV6-NTRK3 gene fusion as a primary event in human secretory breast carcinoma. Cancer Cell 2: 367–376.

2765. Togo T, Araki E, Ota M et al. (2007). Fibrous hamartoma of infancy in a patient with Williams syndrome. Br J Dermatol 156: 1052–1055.

2766. Tokano H, Sugimoto T, Noguchi Y et al. (2001). Sequential computed tomography images demonstrating characteristic changes in fibrous dysplasia. J Laryngol Otol 115: 757–759.

2767. Tomaszewski MM, Lupton GP (1997). Atypical fibroxanthoma. An unusual variant with osteoclast-like giant cells. Am J Surg Pathol 21: 213–218.

2768. Torabi A, Lele SM, DiMaio D et al. (2008). Lack of a common or characteristic cytogenetic anomaly in solitary fibrous tumor. Cancer Genet Cytogenet 181: 60–64.

2769. Torigoe T, Yazawa Y, Takagi T et al. (2007). Extraskeletal osteosarcoma in Japan: multiinstitutional study of 20 patients from the Japanese Musculoskeletal Oncology Group. J Orthop Sci 12: 424–429.

2770. Toro JR, Travis LB, Wu HJ et al. (2006). Incidence patterns of soft tissue sarcomas, regardless of primary site, in the surveillance, epidemiology and end results program, 1978-2001: An analysis of 26,758 cases. Int J Cancer 119: 2922–2930.

2771. Torres FX, Kyriakos M (1992). Bone infarct-associated osteosarcoma. Cancer 70: 2418–2430.

2772. Tosi P, Cintorino M, Toti P et al. (1989). Histopathological evaluation for the prognosis of retinoblastoma. Ophthalmic Paediatr Genet 10: 173–177.

2773. Tostar U, Malm CJ, Meis-Kindblom JM et al. (2006). Deregulation of the hedgehog signalling pathway: a possible role for the PTCH and SUFU genes in human rhabdomyoma and rhabdomyosarcoma development. J Pathol 208: 17–25.

2774. Toyosawa S, Tomita Y, Kishino M et al. (2004). Expression of dentin matrix protein 1 in tumors causing oncogenic osteomalacia. Mod Pathol 17: 573–578.

2775. Trassard M, Le Doussal V, Bui BN et al. (1996). Angiosarcoma arising in a solitary schwannoma (neurilemoma) of the sciatic nerve. Am J Surg Pathol 20: 1412–1417.

2776. Trattner A, Hodak E, David M et al. (1993). The appearance of Kaposi sarcoma during corticosteroid therapy. Cancer 72: 1779–1783.

2777. Trindade F, Tellechea O, Torrelo A et al. (2011). Wilms tumor 1 expression in vascular neoplasms and vascular malformations. Am J Dermatopathol 33: 569–572.

2778. Trkova M, Prochazkova K, Krutilkova V et al. (2007). Telomere length in peripheral blood cells of germline TP53 mutation carriers is shorter than that of normal individuals of corresponding age. Cancer 110: 694–702.

2779. Trofatter JA, MacCollin MM, Rutter JL et al. (1993). A novel moesin-, ezrin-, radixin-like gene is a candidate for the neurofibromatosis 2 tumor suppressor. Cell 72: 791–800.

2780. Trojani M, Contesso G, Coindre JM et al. (1984). Soft-tissue sarcomas of adults; study of pathological prognostic variables and definition of a histopathological grading system. Int J Cancer 33: 37–42.

2781. Trombetta D, Magnusson L, Von Steyern FV et al. (2011). Translocation t(7;19)(q22;q13)-a recurrent chromosome aberration in pseudomyogenic hemangioendothelioma? Cancer Genet 204: 211–215.

2782. Troum S, Dalton ML, Donner RS et al. (1996). Multifocal mesenchymal hamartoma of the chest wall in infancy. J Pediatr Surg 31: 713–715.

2783. Trovik CS, Bauer HC, Alvegard TA et al. (2000). Surgical margins, local recurrence and metastasis in soft tissue sarcomas: 559 surgically-treated patients from the Scandinavian Sarcoma Group Register. Eur J Cancer 36: 710–716.

2784. Tsai JC, Dalinka MK, Fallon MD et al. (1990). Fluid-fluid level: a nonspecific finding in tumors of bone and soft tissue. Radiology 175: 779–782.

2785. Tsai JW, Huang HY, Lee JC et al. (2011). Composite haemangioendothelioma: report of four cases with emphasis on atypical clinical presentation. Pathology 43: 176–180.

2786. Tsai JW, Tsou JH, Hung LY et al. (2010). Combined Erdheim-Chester disease and Langerhans cell histiocytosis of skin are both monoclonal: a rare case with human androgen-receptor gene analysis. J Am Acad Dermatol 63: 284–291.

2787. Tsang WY, Chan JK (1991). Kaposi-like infantile hemangioendothelioma. A distinctive vascular neoplasm of the retroperitoneum. Am J Surg Pathol 15: 982–989.

2788. Tsang WY, Chan JK (1992). Epithelioid variant of solitary circumscribed neuroma of the skin. Histopathology 20: 439–441.

2789. Tsang WY, Chan JK (1993). The family of epithelioid vascular tumors. Histol Histopathol 8: 187–212.

2790. Tsang WY, Chan JK, Chow LT et al. (1992). Perineurioma: an uncommon soft tissue neoplasm distinct from localized hypertrophic neuropathy and neurofibroma. Am J Surg Pathol 16: 756–763.

2791. Tsang WY, Chan JK, Lee KC et al. (1992). Aggressive angiomyxoma. A report of four cases occurring in men. Am J Surg Pathol 16: 1059–1065.

2792. Tsokos M, Webber BL, Parham DM et al. (1992). Rhabdomyosarcoma. A new classification scheme related to prognosis. Arch Pathol Lab Med 116: 847–855.

2793. Tsuchiya T, Sekine K, Hinohara S et al. (2000). Analysis of the p16INK4, p14ARF, p15, TP53, and MDM2 genes and their prognostic implications in osteosarcoma and Ewing sarcoma. Cancer Genet Cytogenet 120: 91–98.

2794. Tsuda M, Davis IJ, Argani P et al. (2007). TFE3 fusions activate MET signaling by transcriptional up-regulation, defining another class of tumors as candidates for therapeutic MET inhibition. Cancer Res 67: 919–929.

2795. Tsuji K, Ishikawa Y, Imamura T (2011). Technique for differentiating alveolar soft part sarcoma from other tumors in paraffin-embedded tissue: comparison of immunohistochemistry for TFE3 and CD147 and of reverse transcription polymerase chain reaction for ASP-SCR1-TFE3 fusion transcript. Hum Pathol 43: 356–363.

2796. Tsuji T, Yoshinaga M, Inomoto Y et al. (2007). Aggressive angiomyxoma of the vulva with a sole t(5;8)(p15;q22) chromosome change. Int J Gynecol Pathol 26: 494–496.

2797. Tsujimura T, Sakaguchi K, Aozasa K (1996). Phosphaturic mesenchymal tumor, mixed connective tissue variant (oncogenic osteomalacia). Pathol Int 46: 238–241.

2798. Tsuneyoshi M, Daimaru Y, Hashimoto H et al. (1985). Malignant soft tissue neoplasms with the histologic features of renal rhabdoid tumors: an ultrastructural and immunohistochemical study. Hum Pathol 16: 1235–1242.

2799. Tsuneyoshi M, Enjoji M, Iwasaki H et al. (1981). Extraskeletal myxoid chondrosarcoma—a clinicopathologic and electron microscopic study. Acta Pathol Jpn 31: 439–447.

2800. Tsuzuki T, Magi-Galluzzi C, Epstein JI (2004). ALK-1 expression in inflammatory myofibroblastic tumor of the urinary bladder. Am J Surg Pathol 28: 1609–1614.

2801. Tucker MA, D'Angio GJ, Boice JD, Jr. et al. (1987). Bone sarcomas linked to radiotherapy and chemotherapy in children. N Engl J Med 317: 588–593.

2802. Tucker T, Wolkenstein P, Revuz J et al. (2005). Association between benign and malignant peripheral nerve sheath tumors in NF1. Neurology 65: 205–211.

2803. Turc-Carel C, Aurias A, Mugneret F et al. (1988). Chromosomes in Ewing's sarcoma. I. An evaluation of 85 cases of remarkable consistency of t(11;22)(q24;q12). Cancer Genet Cytogenet 32: 229–238.

2804. Turc-Carel C, Limon J, Dal Cin P et al. (1986). Cytogenetic studies of adipose tissue tumors. II. Recurrent reciprocal translocation t(12;16)(q13;p11) in myxoid liposarcomas. Cancer Genet Cytogenet 23: 291–299.

2804A. Turc-Carel C, Philip I, Berger MP et al. (1984). Chromosome study of Ewing's sarcoma (ES) cell lines. Consistency of a reciprocal translocation t(11;22)(q24;q12). Cancer Genet. Cytogenet 12:1-19.

2805. Turcotte RE, Kurt AM, Sim FH et al. (1993). Chondroblastoma. Hum Pathol 24: 944–949.

2806. Tworek JA, Appelman HD, Singleton TP et al. (1997). Stromal tumors of the jejunum and ileum. Mod Pathol 10: 200–209.

2807. Tyler P, Saifuddin A (2010). The imaging of myositis ossificans. Semin Musculoskelet Radiol 14: 201–216.

2808. Tzellos TG, Dionyssopoulos A, Klagas I et al. (2009). Differential glycosaminoglycan expression and hyaluronan homeostasis in juvenile hyaline fibromatosis. J Am Acad Dermatol 61: 629–638.

2809. Ueda T, Aozasa K, Ohsawa M et al. (1989). Malignant lymphomas of bone in Japan. Cancer 64: 2387–2392.

2810. Ueda T, Araki N, Mano M et al. (2002). Frequent expression of smooth muscle markers in malignant fibrous histiocytoma of bone. J Clin Pathol 55: 853–858.

2811. Ueki Y, Lin CY, Senoo M et al. (2007). Increased myeloid cell responses to M-CSF and RANKL cause bone loss and inflammation in SH3BP2 "cherubism" mice. Cell 128: 71–83.

2812. Ueki Y, Tiziani V, Santanna C et al. (2001). Mutations in the gene encoding c-Abl-binding protein SH3BP2 cause cherubism. Nat Genet 28: 125–126.

2813. Uhrhammer NA, Lafarge L, Dos Santos L et al. (2006). Werner syndrome and mutations of the WRN and LMNA genes in France. Hum Mutat 27: 718–719.

2814. Ul-Hassan A, Sisley K, Hughes D et al. (2009). Common genetic changes in leiomyosarcoma and gastrointestinal stromal tumour: implication for ataxia telangiectasia mutated involvement. Int J Exp Pathol 90: 549–557.

2815. Unni KK, Inwards CY (2010) Dahlin's bone tumors: general aspects and data on 11 087 cases. Sixth edition. Lippincott Williams & Williams: Philadelphia; pp 179–183; 310–316.

2816. Unni KK (2005). Tumors of the bones and joints. Atlas of Tumor Pathology, Series IV. American Registry of Pathology in collaboration with the Armed Forces Institute of Pathology.

2817. Unni KK, Dahlin DC, McLeod RA et al. (1977). Intraosseous well-differentiated osteosarcoma. Cancer 40: 1337–1347.

2818. Unni KK, Inwards CY (2010). Dahlin's bone tumors: general aspects and data on 11 087 cases. Sixth edition. Lippincott Williams & Williams: Philadelphia.

2819. Upadhyaya M, Kluwe L, Spurlock G et al. (2008). Germline and somatic NF1 gene mutation spectrum in NF1-associated malignant peripheral nerve sheath tumors (MPNSTs). Hum Mutat 29: 74–82.

2820. Urabe A, Tsuneyoshi M, Enjoji M (1987). Epithelioid hemangioma versus Kimura's disease. A comparative clinicopathologic study. Am J Surg Pathol 11: 758–766.

2821. Uramoto N, Furukawa M, Yoshizaki T (2009). Malignant phosphaturic mesenchymal tumor, mixed connective tissue variant of the tongue. Auris Nasus Larynx 36: 104–105.

2822. Urano F, Umezawa A, Hong W et al. (1996). A novel chimera gene between EWS and E1A-F, encoding the adenovirus E1A enhancer-binding protein, in extraosseous Ewing's sarcoma. Biochem Biophys Res Commun 219: 608–612.

2823. Uriburu IJ, Levy VD (1998). Intraosseous growth of giant cell tumors of the tendon sheath (localized nodular tenosynovitis) of the digits: report of 15 cases. J Hand Surg Am 23: 732–736.

2824. Ushijima M, Hashimoto H, Tsuneyoshi M et al. (1986). Giant cell tumor of the tendon sheath (nodular tenosynovitis). A study of 207 cases to compare the large joint group with the common digit group. Cancer 57: 875–884.

2825. Ushijima M, Tsuneyoshi M, Enjoji M (1984). Dupuytren type fibromatoses. A clinicopathologic study of 62 cases. Acta Pathol Jpn 34: 991–1001.

2826. Vadgama B, Sebire NJ, Malone M et al. (2004). Sclerosing rhabdomyosarcoma in childhood: case report and review of the literature. Pediatr Dev Pathol 7: 391–396.

2827. Vaillo-Vinagre A, Ballestin-Carcavilla C, Madero-Garcia S et al. (2000). Primary angioleiomyoma of the iliac bone: clinical pathological study of one case with flow cytometric DNA content and S-phase fraction analysis. Skeletal Radiol 29: 181–185.

2828. Vakil-Adli A, Zandieh S, Hochreiter J et al. (2010). Synovial hemangioma of the knee joint in a 12-year-old boy: a case report. J Med Case Reports 4: 105

2829. Valdez TA, Desai U, Volk MS (2006). Recurrent fetal rhabdomyoma of the head and neck. Int J Pediatr Otorhinolaryngol 70: 1115–1118.

2830. Vallat-Decouvelaere AV, Dry SM, Fletcher CD (1998). Atypical and malignant solitary fibrous tumors in extrathoracic locations: evidence of their comparability to intrathoracic tumors. Am J Surg Pathol 22: 1501–1511.

2831. van Beerendonk HM, Rozeman LB, Taminiau AH et al. (2004). Molecular analysis of the INK4A/INK4A-ARF gene locus in conventional (central) chondrosarcomas and enchondromas: indication of an important gene for tumour progression. J Pathol 202: 359–366.

2832. van Capelle CI, Hogeman PH, van der Sijs-Bos CJ et al. (2007). Neurofibromatosis presenting with a cherubism phenotype. Eur J Pediatr 166: 905–909.

2833. van de Rijn M, Barr FG, Xiong QB et al. (1999). Poorly differentiated synovial sarcoma: an analysis of clinical, pathologic, and molecular genetic features. Am J Surg Pathol 23: 106–112.

2834. van den Berg E, Molenaar WM, Hoekstra HJ et al. (1992). DNA ploidy and karyotype in recurrent and metastatic soft tissue sarcomas. Mod Pathol 5: 505–514.

2835. van den Berg H, Kroon HM, Slaar A et al. (2008). Incidence of biopsy-proven bone tumors in children: a report based on the Dutch pathology registration "PALGA". J Pediatr Orthop 28: 29–35.

2836. van der Maten J, Blaauwgeers JL, Sutedja TG et al. (2003). Granular cell tumors of the tracheobronchial tree. J Thorac Cardiovasc Surg 126: 740–743.

2837. van der Woude HJ, Bloem JL, Holscher HC et al. (1994). Monitoring the effect of chemotherapy in Ewing's sarcoma of bone with MR imaging. Skeletal Radiol 23: 493–500.

2838. van der Woude HJ, Hazelbag HM, Bloem JL et al. (2004). MRI of adamantinoma of long bones in correlation with histopathology. AJR Am J Roentgenol 183: 1737–1744.

2839. van der Woude HJ, Verstraete KL, Hogendoorn PC et al. (1998). Musculoskeletal tumors: does fast dynamic contrast-enhanced subtraction MR imaging contribute to the characterization? Radiology 208: 821–828.

2840. van Doorninck JA, Ji L, Schaub B et al. (2010). Current treatment protocols have eliminated the prognostic advantage of type 1 fusions in Ewing sarcoma: a report from the Children's Oncology Group. J Clin Oncol 28: 1989–1994.

2841. Van Dorpe J, Ectors N, Geboes K et al. (1999). Is calcifying fibrous pseudotumor a late sclerosing stage of inflammatory myofibroblastic tumor? Am J Surg Pathol 23: 329–335.

2842. van Echten J, van den Berg E, van Baarlen J et al. (1995). An important role for chromosome 17, band q25, in the histogenesis of alveolar soft part sarcoma. Cancer Genet Cytogenet 82: 57–61.

2843. van Gaal JC, Flucke UE, Roeffen MH et al. (2012). Anaplastic lymphoma kinase aberrations in rhabdomyosarcoma: clinical and prognostic implications. J Clin Oncol 30: 308–315.

2844. Van Geertruyden J, Lorea P, Goldschmidt D et al. (1996). Glomus tumours of the hand. A retrospective study of 51 cases. J Hand Surg Br 21: 257–260.

2845. van Giffen NH, van Rhijn LW, van Ooij A et al. (2003). Benign fibrous histiocytoma of the posterior arch of C1 in a 6-year-old boy: a case report. Spine 28: E359–E363.

2846. van Hoeven KH, Factor SM, Kress Y et al. (1993). Visceral myogenic tumors. A manifestation of HIV infection in children. Am J Surg Pathol 17: 1176–1181.

2847. Van Hul W, Wuyts W, Hendrickx J et al. (1998). Identification of a third EXT-like gene (EXTL3) belonging to the EXT gene family. Genomics 47: 230–237.

2848. van Roggen JF, McMenamin ME, Fletcher CD (2001). Cellular myxoma of soft tissue: a clinicopathological study of 38 cases confirming indolent clinical behaviour. Histopathology 39: 287–297.

2849. van Unnik JA, Coindre JM, Contesso C et al. (1993). Grading of soft tissue sarcomas: experience of the EORTC Soft Tissue and Bone Sarcoma Group. Eur J Cancer 29A: 2089–2093.

2850. van Zelderen-Bhola SL, Bovee JV, Wessels HW et al. (1998). Ring chromosome 4 as the sole cytogenetic anomaly in a chondroblastoma: a case report and review of the literature. Cancer Genet Cytogenet 105: 109–112.

2851. Vanel D, De Paolis M, Monti C et al. (2001). Radiological features of 24 periosteal chondrosarcomas. Skeletal Radiol 30: 208–212.

2852. Vanel D, Shapeero LG, De Baere T et al. (1994). MR imaging in the follow-up of malignant and aggressive soft-tissue tumors: results of 511 examinations. Radiology 190: 263–268.

2853. Vang R, Kempson RL (2002). Perivascular epithelioid cell tumor ('PEComa') of the uterus: a subset of HMB-45-positive epithelioid mesenchymal neoplasms with an uncertain relationship to pure smooth muscle tumors. Am J Surg Pathol 26: 1–13.

2854. Vanni R, Marras S, Faa G et al. (1999). Chromosome instability in elastofibroma. Cancer Genet Cytogenet 111: 182–183.

2855. Varela-Duran J, Enzinger FM (1982). Calcifying synovial sarcoma. Cancer 50: 345–352.

2856. Varela-Duran J, Oliva H, Rosai J (1979). Vascular leiomyosarcoma: the malignant counterpart of vascular leiomyoma. Cancer 44: 1684–1691.

2857. Vargas SO, Perez-Atayde AR, Gonzalez-Crussi F et al. (2001). Giant cell angioblastoma: three additional occurrences of a distinct pathologic entity. Am J Surg Pathol 25: 185–196.

2858. Variend S, Bax NM, van Gorp J (1995). Are infantile myofibromatosis, congenital fibrosarcoma and congenital haemangiopericytoma histogenetically related? Histopathology 26: 57–62.

2859. Varikatt W, Soper J, Simmons G et al. (2008). Superficial acral fibromyxoma: a report of two cases with radiological findings. Skeletal Radiol 37: 499–503.

2860. Varley JM, Attwooll C, White G et al. (2001). Characterization of germline TP53 splicing mutations and their genetic and functional analysis. Oncogene 20: 2647–2654.

2861. Varras M, Akrivis C, Tsoukalos G et al. (2008). Tubal ectopic pregnancy associated with an extraskeletal chondroma of the fallopian tube: case report. Clin Exp Obstet Gynecol 35: 83–85.

2862. Vasconcelos C, Cunha TM, Felix A (2007). Lipoleiomyoma of the peritoneum. Acta Radiol 48: 10–12.

2863. Vayego SA, De Conti OJ, Varella-Garcia M (1996). Complex cytogenetic rearrangement in a case of unicameral bone cyst. Cancer Genet Cytogenet 86: 46–49.

2864. Vayego-Lourenco SA (2001). TP53 mutations in a recurrent unicameral bone cyst. Cancer Genet Cytogenet 124: 175–176.

2865. Velagaleti GV, Tapper JK, Panova NE et al. (2003). Cytogenetic findings in a case of nodular fasciitis of subclavicular region. Cancer Genet Cytogenet 141: 160–163.

2866. Vellios F, Baez J, Shumacker HB (1958). Lipoblastomatosis: a tumor of fetal fat different from hibernoma; report of a case, with observations on the embryogenesis of human adipose tissue. Am J Pathol 34: 1149–1159.

2867. Vencio EF, Reeve CM, Unni KK et al. (1998). Mesenchymal chondrosarcoma of the jaw bones: clinicopathologic study of 19 cases. Cancer 82: 2350–2355.

2868. Verbeke SL, Bertoni F, Bacchini P et al. (2011). Distinct histological features characterize primary angiosarcoma of bone. Histopathology 58: 254–264.

2869. Verbeke SL, Bovee JV (2011). Primary vascular tumors of bone: a spectrum of entities? Int J Clin Exp Pathol 4: 541–551.

2870. Verdegaal SH, Bovee JV, Pansuriya TC et al. (2011). Incidence, predictive factors, and prognosis of chondrosarcoma in patients with Ollier disease and Maffucci syndrome: an international multicenter study of 161 patients. Oncologist 16: 1771–1779.

2871. Verdijk RM, den Bakker MA, Dubbink HJ et al. (2010). TP53 mutation analysis of malignant peripheral nerve sheath tumors. J Neuropathol Exp Neurol 69: 16–26.

2872. Verelst SJ, Hans J, Hanselmann RG et al. (2004). Genetic instability in primary leiomyosarcoma of bone. Hum Pathol 35: 1404–1412.

2873. Vergel De Dios AM, Bond JR, Shives TC et al. (1992). Aneurysmal bone cyst. A clinicopathologic study of 238 cases. Cancer 69: 2921–2931.

2874. Vermaat M, Vanel D, Kroon HM et al. (2011). Vascular tumors of bone: imaging findings. Eur J Radiol 77: 13–18.

2875. Versini M, Jeandel PY, Fuzibet JG et al. (2010). [Erdheim-Chester disease: radiological findings]. Presse Med 39: e233–e237.

2876. Versteege I, Sevenet N, Lange J et al. (1998). Truncating mutations of hSNF5/INI1 in aggressive paediatric cancer. Nature 394: 203–206.

2877. Verstraete KL, De Deene Y, Roels H et al. (1994). Benign and malignant musculoskeletal lesions: dynamic contrast-enhanced MR imaging—parametric "first-pass" images depict tissue vascularization and perfusion. Radiology 192: 835–843.

2878. Avet-Loiseau H, Facon T, Grosbois B et al. (2002). Oncogenesis of multiple myeloma: 14q32 and 13q chromosomal abnormalities are not randomly distributed, but correlate with natural history, immunological features, and clinical presentation. Blood 99: 2185–2191.

2879. Veyssier-Belot C, Cacoub P, Caparros-Lefebvre D et al. (1996). Erdheim-Chester disease. Clinical and radiologic characteristics of 59 cases. Medicine (Baltimore) 75: 157–169.

2880. Viatour P, Sage J (2011). Newly identified aspects of tumor suppression by RB. Dis Model Mech 4: 581–585.

2881. Villani A, Tabori U, Schiffman J et al. (2011). Biochemical and imaging surveillance in germline TP53 mutation carriers with Li-Fraumeni syndrome: a prospective observational study. Lancet Oncol 12: 559–567.

2882. Viskochil D, Buchberg AM, Xu G et al. (1990). Deletions and a translocation interrupt a cloned gene at the neurofibromatosis type 1 locus. Cell 62: 187–192.

2883. Visuri T, Pulkkinen P, Paavolainen P (2006). Malignant tumors at the site of total hip prosthesis. Analytic review of 46 cases. J Arthroplasty 21: 311–323.

2884. Vogrincic GS, O'Connell JX, Gilks CB (1997). Giant cell tumor of tendon sheath is a polyclonal cellular proliferation. Hum Pathol 28: 815–819.

2885. von Hochstetter AR, Meyer VE, Grant JW et al. (1991). Epithelioid sarcoma mimicking angiosarcoma: the value of immunohistochemistry in the differential diagnosis. Virchows Arch A Pathol Anat Histopathol 418: 271–278.

2886. von Levetzow C, Jiang X, Gwye Y et al. (2011). Modeling initiation of Ewing sarcoma in human neural crest cells. PLoS One 6: e19305

2887. Voth H, Landsberg J, Hinz T et al. (2011). Management of dermatofibrosarcoma protuberans with fibrosarcomatous transformation: an evidence-based review of the literature.

J Eur Acad Dermatol Venereol 25: 1385–1391.

2888. Vujovic S, Henderson S, Presneau N et al. (2006). Brachyury, a crucial regulator of notochordal development, is a novel biomarker for chordomas. J Pathol 209: 157–165.

2889. Wachtel M, Dettling M, Koscielniak E et al. (2004). Gene expression signatures identify rhabdomyosarcoma subtypes and detect a novel t(2;2)(q35;p23) translocation fusing PAX3 to NCOA1. Cancer Res 64: 5539–5545.

2890. Walker PD, Rosai J, Dorfman RF (1981). The osseous manifestations of sinus histiocytosis with massive lymphadenopathy. Am J Clin Pathol 75: 131–139.

2891. Wallace MR, Marchuk DA, Andersen LB et al. (1990). Type 1 neurofibromatosis gene: identification of a large transcript disrupted in three NF1 patients. Science 249: 181–186.

2892. Walsh SN, Hurt MA (2008). Cutaneous fetal rhabdomyoma: a case report and historical review of the literature. Am J Surg Pathol 32: 485–491.

2893. Wang J, Zhu XZ, Zhang RY (2004). [Malignant granular cell tumor: a clinicopathologic analysis of 10 cases with review of literature]. Zhonghua Bing Li Xue Za Zhi 33: 497–502.

2894. Wang L, Bhargava R, Zheng T et al. (2007). Undifferentiated small round cell sarcomas with rare EWS gene fusions: identification of a novel EWS-SP3 fusion and of additional cases with the EWS-ETV1 and EWS-FEV fusions. J Mol Diagn 9: 498–509.

2895. Wang L, Motoi T, Khanin R et al. (2012). Identification of a novel, recurrent HEY1-NCOA2 fusion in mesenchymal chondrosarcoma based on a genome-wide screen of exon-level expression data. Genes Chromosomes Cancer 51: 127–139.

2896. Wang LL, Gannavarapu A, Kozinetz CA et al. (2003). Association between osteosarcoma and deleterious mutations in the RECQL4 gene in Rothmund-Thomson syndrome. J Natl Cancer Inst 95: 669–674.

2897. Wang LL, Levy ML, Lewis RA et al. (2001). Clinical manifestations in a cohort of 41 Rothmund-Thomson syndrome patients. Am J Med Genet 102: 11–17.

2898. Wang LL, Perlman EJ, Vujanic GM et al. (2007). Desmoplastic small round cell tumor of the kidney in childhood. Am J Surg Pathol 31: 576–584.

2899. Wang LL, Plon SE (1993). Rothmund-Thomson Syndrome.

2900. Wang NP, Marx J, McNutt MA et al. (1995). Expression of myogenic regulatory proteins (myogenin and MyoD1) in small blue round cell tumors of childhood. Am J Pathol 147: 1799–1810.

2901. Wang R, Lu YJ, Fisher C et al. (2001). Characterization of chromosome aberrations associated with soft-tissue leiomyosarcomas by twenty-four-color karyotyping and comparative genomic hybridization analysis. Genes Chromosomes Cancer 31: 54–64.

2902. Wang W-L, Evans HL, Meis JM et al. (2012). FUS rearrangements are rare in "pure" sclerosing epithelioid fibrosarcoma. Mod Pathol 25: 846–853.

2903. Wang WL, Bones-Valentin RA, Prieto VG et al. (2011). Sarcoma metastases to the skin: A clinicopathologic study of 65 patients. Cancer 118: 2900–2904.

2904. Wang WL, Mayordomo E, Zhang W et al. (2009). Detection and characterization of EWSR1/ATF1 and EWSR1/CREB1 chimeric transcripts in clear cell sarcoma (melanoma of soft parts). Mod Pathol 22: 1201–1209.

2905. Wang X, Asmann YW, Erickson-Johnson MR et al. (2011). High-resolution genomic mapping reveals consistent amplification of the fibroblast growth factor receptor substrate 2 gene in well-differentiated and dedifferentiated liposarcoma. Genes Chromosomes Cancer 50: 849–858.

2906. Wang X, Zamolyi RQ, Zhang H et al. (2010). Fusion of HMGA1 to the LPP/TPRG1 intergenic region in a lipoma identified by mapping paraffin-embedded tissues. Cancer Genet Cytogenet 196: 64–67.

2906A. Wasniewska M, De LF, Bertelloni S et al. (2004). Testicular microlithiasis: an unreported feature of McCune-Albright syndrome in males. J Pediatr 145: 670–672.

2907. Watanabe K, Suzuki T (2004). Epithelioid fibrosarcoma of the ovary. Virchows Arch 445: 410–413.

2908. Watanabe K, Tanaka M, Takashi K et al. (2008). Fibronexus in low-grade myofibrosarcoma: a case report. Ultrastruct Pathol 32: 97–100.

2909. Waters BL, Panagopoulos I, Allen EF (2000). Genetic characterization of angiomatoid fibrous histiocytoma identifies fusion of the FUS and ATF-1 genes induced by a chromosomal translocation involving bands 12q13 and 16p11. Cancer Genet Cytogenet 121: 109–116.

2910. Watts GD, Wymer J, Kovach MJ et al. (2004). Inclusion body myopathy associated with Paget disease of bone and frontotemporal dementia is caused by mutant valosin-containing protein. Nat Genet 36: 377–381.

2911. Weber-Hall S, Anderson J, McManus A et al. (1996). Gains, losses, and amplification of genomic material in rhabdomyosarcoma analyzed by comparative genomic hybridization. Cancer Res 56: 3220–3224.

2912. Wehrli BM, Huang W, de Crombrugghe B et al. (2003). Sox9, a master regulator of chondrogenesis, distinguishes mesenchymal chondrosarcoma from other small blue round cell tumors. Hum Pathol 34: 263–269.

2913. Wehrli BM, Weiss SW, Coffin CM (2001). Gardner syndrome. Am J Surg Pathol 25: 694–696.

2914. Wehrli BM, Weiss SW, Yandow S et al. (2001). Gardner-associated fibromas (GAF) in young patients: a distinct fibrous lesion that identifies unsuspected Gardner syndrome and risk for fibromatosis. Am J Surg Pathol 25: 645–651.

2915. Wei G, Antonescu CR, de Alava E et al. (2000). Prognostic impact of INK4A deletion in Ewing sarcoma. Cancer 89: 793–799.

2916. Wei Q, Zhu Y (2011). Collision tumor composed of mammary-type myofibroblastoma and eccrine adenocarcinoma of the vulva. Pathol Int 61: 138–142.

2917. Wei S, Pan Z, Siegal GP et al. (2012). Complex analysis of a recurrent pleomorphic hyalinizing angiectatic tumor of soft parts. Hum Pathol 43: 121–126.

2918. Weibolt VM, Buresh CJ, Roberts CA et al. (1998). Involvement of 3q21 in nodular fasciitis. Cancer Genet Cytogenet 106: 177–179.

2919. Weidner N, Santa Cruz D (1987). Phosphaturic mesenchymal tumors. A polymorphous group causing osteomalacia or rickets. Cancer 59: 1442–1454.

2920. Weinstein LS, Liu J, Sakamoto A et al. (2004). Minireview: GNAS: normal and abnormal functions. Endocrinology 145: 5459–5464.

2921. Weinstein LS, Shenker A, Gejman PV et al. (1991). Activating mutations of the stimulatory G protein in the McCune-Albright syndrome. N Engl J Med 325: 1688–1695.

2922. Weiss A, Khoury JD, Hoffer FA et al. (2007). Telangiectatic osteosarcoma: the St. Jude Children's Research Hospital's experience. Cancer 109: 1627–1637.
2923. Weiss RA, Whitby D, Talbot S et al. (1998). Human herpesvirus type 8 and Kaposi's sarcoma. J Natl Cancer Inst Monogr 51–54.
2924. Weiss SW. (1994). Histologic typing of soft tissue tumours. World Health Organization Histological Classification of Tumours. Springer: Berlin.
2925. Weiss SW, Dorfman HD (1977). Adamantinoma of long bone. An analysis of nine new cases with emphasis on metastasizing lesions and fibrous dysplasia-like changes. Hum Pathol 8: 141–153.
2926. Weiss SW, Enzinger FM (1977). Myxoid variant of malignant fibrous histiocytoma. Cancer 39: 1672–1685.
2927. Weiss SW, Enzinger FM (1982). Epithelioid hemangioendothelioma: a vascular tumor often mistaken for a carcinoma. Cancer 50: 970–981.
2928. Weiss SW, Goldblum JR (2001). Benign tumors and tumor-like lesions of synovial tissue. In: Enzinger and Weiss's Soft Tissue Tumours, 4th editionMosby-Harcourt: Philadelphia: pp 1037–1062.
2929. Weiss SW, Goldblum JR (2001). Enzinger and Weiss's soft tissue tumors, fourth edition. Mosby: St Louis.
2930. Weiss SW, Goldblum JR (2008). Enzinger & Weiss's soft tissue tumors, fifth edition. Mosby Elsevier: St Louis.
2931. Weiss SW, Ishak KG, Dail DH et al. (1986). Epithelioid hemangioendothelioma and related lesions. Semin Diagn Pathol 3: 259–287.
2932. Weiss SW, Langloss JM, Enzinger FM (1983). Value of S-100 protein in the diagnosis of soft tissue tumors with particular reference to benign and malignant Schwann cell tumors. Lab Invest 49: 299–308.
2933. Weiss SW, Rao VK (1992). Well-differentiated liposarcoma (atypical lipoma) of deep soft tissue of the extremities, retroperitoneum, and miscellaneous sites. A follow-up study of 92 cases with analysis of the incidence of "dedifferentiation". Am J Surg Pathol 16: 1051–1058.
2934. Weitzman S, Jaffe R (2005). Uncommon histiocytic disorders: the non-Langerhans cell histiocytoses. Pediatr Blood Cancer 45: 256–264.
2935. Weksberg R, Shuman C, Beckwith JB (2010). Beckwith-Wiedemann syndrome. Eur J Hum Genet 18: 8–14.
2936. Welborn J, Fenner S, Parks R (2010). Angioleiomyoma: a benign tumor with karyotypic aberrations. Cancer Genet Cytogenet 199: 147–148.
2937. Wells GC, Whimster IW (1969). Subcutaneous angiolymphoid hyperplasia with eosinophilia. Br J Dermatol 81: 1–14.
2938. Wenger DE, Wold LE (2000). Benign vascular lesions of bone: radiologic and pathologic features. Skeletal Radiol 29: 63–74.
2939. Wenger DE, Wold LE (2000). Malignant vascular lesions of bone: radiologic and pathologic features. Skeletal Radiol 29: 619–631.
2940. Wenig BM, Devaney K, Bisceglia M (1995). Inflammatory myofibroblastic tumor of the larynx. A clinicopathologic study of eight cases simulating a malignant spindle cell neoplasm. Cancer 76: 2217–2229.
2941. West RB, Harvell J, Linn SC et al. (2004). Apo D in soft tissue tumors: a novel marker for dermatofibrosarcoma protuberans. Am J Surg Pathol 28: 1063–1069.
2942. West RB, Rubin BP, Miller MA et al. (2006). A landscape effect in tenosynovial giant-cell tumor from activation of CSF1 expression by a translocation in a minority of tumor cells. Proc Natl Acad Sci U S A 103: 690–695.
2943. Wester SM, Beabout JW, Unni KK et al. (1982). Langerhans' cell granulomatosis (histiocytosis X) of bone in adults. Am J Surg Pathol 6: 413–426.
2944. Westermann FN, Langlois NE, Simpson JG (1997). Apoptosis in atypical fibroxanthoma and pleomorphic malignant fibrous histiocytoma. Am J Dermatopathol 19: 228–231.
2945. Wettach GR, Boyd LJ, Lawce HJ et al. (2008). Cytogenetic analysis of a hemosiderotic fibrolipomatous tumor. Cancer Genet Cytogenet 182: 140–143.
2946. Wexler LH, Ladanyi M (2010). Diagnosing alveolar rhabdomyosarcoma: morphology must be coupled with fusion confirmation. J Clin Oncol 28: 2126–2128.
2946A. Whang-Peng J, Triche TJ, Knutsen T et al. (1984). Chromosome translocation in peripheral neuroepithelioma. N Engl J Med 311, 584-5.
2947. Whibley C, Pharoah PD, Hollstein M (2009). p53 polymorphisms: cancer implications. Nat Rev Cancer 9: 95–107.
2948. Whitby D, Howard MR, Tenant-Flowers M et al. (1995). Detection of Kaposi sarcoma associated herpesvirus in peripheral blood of HIV-infected individuals and progression to Kaposi's sarcoma. Lancet 346: 799–802.
2949. White FV, Dehner LP, Belchis DA et al. (1999). Congenital disseminated malignant rhabdoid tumor: a distinct clinicopathologic entity demonstrating abnormalities of chromosome 22q11. Am J Surg Pathol 23: 249–256.
2950. White W, Shiu MH, Rosenblum MK et al. (1990). Cellular schwannoma. A clinicopathologic study of 57 patients and 58 tumors. Cancer 66: 1266–1275.
2951. Whitten RO, Benjamin DR (1987). Rhabdomyoma of the retroperitoneum. A report of a tumor with both adult and fetal characteristics: a study by light and electron microscopy, histochemistry, and immunochemistry. Cancer 59: 818–824.
2952. Whyte P, Buchkovich KJ, Horowitz JM et al. (1988). Association between an oncogene and an anti-oncogene: the adenovirus E1A proteins bind to the retinoblastoma gene product. Nature 334: 124–129.
2953. Wick MR, Siegal GP, Unni KK et al. (1981). Sarcomas of bone complicating osteitis deformans (Paget's disease): fifty years' experience. Am J Surg Pathol 5: 47–59.
2954. Wicking C, Shanley S, Smyth I et al. (1997). Most germ-line mutations in the nevoid basal cell carcinoma syndrome lead to a premature termination of the PATCHED protein, and no genotype-phenotype correlations are evident. Am J Hum Genet 60: 21–26.
2955. Wicklund CL, Pauli RM, Johnston D et al. (1995). Natural history study of hereditary multiple exostoses. Am J Med Genet 55: 43–46.
2956. Widemann BC (2009). Current status of sporadic and neurofibromatosis type 1-associated malignant peripheral nerve sheath tumors. Curr Oncol Rep 11: 322–328.
2957. Widhe B, Widhe T (2000). Initial symptoms and clinical features in osteosarcoma and Ewing sarcoma. J Bone Joint Surg Am 82: 667–674.
2958. Wiedemann HR (1964). Familial malformation complex with umbilical hernia and macroglossia - a "new syndrome"? J Genet Hum 13: 223–232.
2959. Wiegand S, Eivazi B, Barth PJ et al. (2008). Pathogenesis of lymphangiomas. Virchows Arch 453: 1–8.
2960. Wieland CN, Dyck R, Weenig RH et al. (2011). The role of CD10 in distinguishing atypical fibroxanthoma from sarcomatoid (spindle cell) squamous cell carcinoma. J Cutan Pathol 38: 884–888.
2961. Wiggs J, Nordenskjold M, Yandell D et al. (1988). Prediction of the risk of hereditary retinoblastoma, using DNA polymorphisms within the retinoblastoma gene. N Engl J Med 318: 151–157.
2962. Wiklund TA, Blomqvist CP, Raty J et al. (1991). Postirradiation sarcoma. Analysis of a nationwide cancer registry material. Cancer 68: 524–531.
2963. Wilder RB, Ha CS, Cox JD et al. (2002). Persistence of myeloma protein for more than one year after radiotherapy is an adverse prognostic factor in solitary plasmacytoma of bone. Cancer 94: 1532–1537.
2964. Wile AG, Evans HL, Romsdahl MM (1981). Leiomyosarcoma of soft tissue: a clinicopathologic study. Cancer 48: 1022–1032.
2965. Willems SM, Debiec-Rychter M, Szuhai K et al. (2006). Local recurrence of myxofibrosarcoma is associated with increase in tumour grade and cytogenetic aberrations, suggesting a multistep tumour progression model. Mod Pathol 19: 407–416.
2966. Willems SM, Mohseny AB, Balog C et al. (2009). Cellular/intramuscular myxoma and grade I myxofibrosarcoma are characterized by distinct genetic alterations and specific composition of their extracellular matrix. J Cell Mol Med 13: 1291–1301.
2967. Willems SM, Schrage YM, Baelde JJ et al. (2008). Myxoid tumours of soft tissue: the so-called myxoid extracellular matrix is heterogeneous in composition. Histopathology 52: 465–474.
2968. Williams A, Bartle G, Sumathi VP et al. (2011). Detection of ASPL/TFE3 fusion transcripts and the TFE3 antigen in formalin-fixed, paraffin-embedded tissue in a series of 18 cases of alveolar soft part sarcoma: useful diagnostic tools in cases with unusual histological features. Virchows Arch 458: 291–300.
2969. Williams J, Hodari A, Janevski P et al. (2010). Recurrence of giant cell tumors in the hand: a prospective study. J Hand Surg Am 35: 451–456.
2970. Williams K, Flanagan A, Folpe A et al. (2007). Lymphatic vessels are present in phosphaturic mesenchymal tumours. Virchows Arch 451: 871–875.
2971. Williams SB, Ellis GL, Meis JM et al. (1993). Ossifying fibromyxoid tumour (of soft parts) of the head and neck: a clinicopathological and immunohistochemical study of nine cases. J Laryngol Otol 107: 75–80.
2972. Williamson D, Missiaglia E, de Reynies A et al. (2010). Fusion gene-negative alveolar rhabdomyosarcoma is clinically and molecularly indistinguishable from embryonal rhabdomyosarcoma. J Clin Oncol 28: 2151–2158.
2973. Willman CL, Busque L, Griffith BB et al. (1994). Langerhans'-cell histiocytosis (histiocytosis X)—a clonal proliferative disease. N Engl J Med 331: 154–160.
2974. Wilson PR, Strutton GM, Stewart MR (1989). Atypical fibroxanthoma: two unusual variants. J Cutan Pathol 16: 93–98.
2975. Winik BC, Boente MC, Asial R (1998). Juvenile hyaline fibromatosis: ultrastructural study. Am J Dermatopathol 20: 373–378.
2976. Winter L, Langrehr J, Hanninen EL (2010). Primary angiosarcoma of the abdominal aorta: multi-row computed tomography. Abdom Imaging 35: 485–487.
2977. Wirman JA, Crissman JD, Aron BF (1979). Metastatic chondroblastoma: report of an unusual case treated with radiotherapy. Cancer 44: 87–93.
2978. Wise CA, Clines GA, Massa H et al. (1997). Identification and localization of the gene for EXTL, a third member of the multiple exostoses gene family. Genome Res 7: 10–16.
2979. Wittkop B, Davies AM, Mangham DC (2002). Primary synovial chondromatosis and synovial chondrosarcoma: a pictorial review. Eur Radiol 12: 2112–2119.
2980. Woertler K (2010). Tumors and tumor-like lesions of peripheral nerves. Semin Musculoskelet Radiol 14: 547–558.
2981. Wold LE, Dobyns JH, Swee RG et al. (1986). Giant cell reaction (giant cell reparative granuloma) of the small bones of the hands and feet. Am J Surg Pathol 10: 491–496.
2982. Wold LE, McLeod RA, Sim FH et al (1990). Atlas of orthopedic pathology. Saunders: Philadelphia-London.
2983. Wold LE, Unni KK, Beabout JW et al. (1982). Hemangioendothelial sarcoma of bone. Am J Surg Pathol 6: 59–70.
2984. Wold LE, Unni KK, Beabout JW et al. (1984). Dedifferentiated parosteal osteosarcoma. J Bone Joint Surg Am 66: 53–59.
2985. Wolf RE, Enneking WF (1996). The staging and surgery of musculoskeletal neoplasms. Orthop Clin North Am 27: 473–481.
2986. Wong NA, Young R, Malcomson RD et al. (2003). Prognostic indicators for gastrointestinal stromal tumours: a clinicopathological and immunohistochemical study of 108 resected cases of the stomach. Histopathology 43: 118–126.
2987. Woodruff JM, Christensen WN (1993). Glandular peripheral nerve sheath tumors. Cancer 72: 3618–3628.
2988. Woodruff JM, Godwin TA, Erlandson RA et al. (1981). Cellular schwannoma: a variety of schwannoma sometimes mistaken for a malignant tumor. Am J Surg Pathol 5: 733–744.
2989. Woodruff JM, Marshall ML, Godwin TA et al. (1983). Plexiform (multinodular) schwannoma. A tumor simulating the plexiform neurofibroma. Am J Surg Pathol 7: 691–697.
2990. Woodruff JM, Scheithauer BW, Kurtkaya-Yapicier O et al. (2003). Congenital and childhood plexiform (multinodular) cellular schwannoma: a troublesome mimic of malignant peripheral nerve sheath tumor. Am J Surg Pathol 27: 1321–1329.
2991. Woodruff JM, Selig AM, Crowley K et al. (1994). Schwannoma (neurilemoma) with malignant transformation. A rare, distinctive peripheral nerve tumor. Am J Surg Pathol 18: 882–895.
2992. Worrell JT, Ansari MQ, Ansari SJ et al. (1993). Atypical fibroxanthoma: DNA ploidy analysis of 14 cases with possible histogenetic implications. J Cutan Pathol 20: 211–215.
2993. Wu CC, Shete S, Amos CI et al. (2006). Joint effects of germ-line p53 mutation and sex on cancer risk in Li-Fraumeni syndrome. Cancer Res 66: 8287–8292.
2994. Wu CT, Inwards CY, O'Laughlin S et al. (1998). Chondromyxoid fibroma of bone: a clinicopathologic review of 278 cases. Hum Pathol 29: 438–446.
2995. Wu J, Brinker DA, Haas M et al. (2005).

Primary alveolar soft part sarcoma (ASPS) of the breast: report of a deceptive case with xanthomatous features confirmed by TFE3 immunohistochemistry and electron microscopy. Int J Surg Pathol 13: 81–85.

2996. Wu KL, Beverloo B, Lokhorst HM et al. (2007). Abnormalities of chromosome 1p/q are highly associated with chromosome 13/13q deletions and are an adverse prognostic factor for the outcome of high-dose chemotherapy in patients with multiple myeloma. Br J Haematol 136: 615–623.

2997. Wunder JS, Eppert K, Burrow SR et al. (1999). Co-amplification and overexpression of CDK4, SAS and MDM2 occurs frequently in human parosteal osteosarcomas. Oncogene 18: 783–788.

2998. Wurtz LD, Peabody TD, Simon MA (1999). Delay in the diagnosis and treatment of primary bone sarcoma of the pelvis. J Bone Joint Surg Am 81: 317–325.

2999. Wuyts W, Cleiren E, Homfray T et al. (2000). The ALX4 homeobox gene is mutated in patients with ossification defects of the skull (foramina parietalia permagna, OMIM 168500). J Med Genet 37: 916–920.

3000. Wuyts W, Van Hul W, Hendrickx J et al. (1997). Identification and characterization of a novel member of the EXT gene family, EXTL2. Eur J Hum Genet 5: 382–389.

3001. Wuyts W, Van Hul W, Wauters J et al. (1996). Positional cloning of a gene involved in hereditary multiple exostoses. Hum Mol Genet 5: 1547–1557.

3002. Wuyts W, Van Wesenbeeck L, Morales-Piga A et al. (2001). Evaluation of the role of RANK and OPG genes in Paget's disease of bone. Bone 28: 104–107.

3003. Xia L, Chen Y, Geng N et al. (2010). Multifocal myopericytoma in the maxillofacial region: a case report. Oral Surg Oral Med Oral Pathol Oral Radiol Endod 109: e59–e62.

3004. Xu GF, O'Connell P, Viskochil D et al. (1990). The neurofibromatosis type 1 gene encodes a protein related to GAP. Cell 62: 599–608.

3005. Xu W, Mulligan LM, Ponder MA et al. (1992). Loss of NF1 alleles in phaeochromocytomas from patients with type I neurofibromatosis. Genes Chromosomes Cancer 4: 337–342.

3006. Yamaguchi S, Yamazaki Y, Ishikawa Y et al. (2005). EWSR1 is fused to POU5F1 in a bone tumor with translocation t(6;22)(p21;q12). Genes Chromosomes Cancer 43: 217–222.

3007. Yamaguchi T, Dorfman HD (1998). Radiographic and histologic patterns of calcification in chondromyxoid fibroma. Skeletal Radiol 27: 559–564.

3008. Yamaguchi T, Dorfman HD (2001). Giant cell reparative granuloma: a comparative clinicopathologic study of lesions in gnathic and extragnathic sites. Int J Surg Pathol 9: 189–200.

3009. Yamaguchi T, Iwata J, Sugihara S et al. (2008). Distinguishing benign notochordal cell tumors from vertebral chordoma. Skeletal Radiol 37: 291–299.

3010. Yamaguchi T, Suzuki S, Ishiiwa H et al. (2004). Benign notochordal cell tumors. A comparative histological study of benign notochordal cell tumors, classic chordomas, and notochordal vestiges of fetal intervertebral discs. Am J Surg Pathol 28: 756–761.

3011. Yamaguchi T, Suzuki S, Ishiiwa H et al. (2004). Intraosseous benign notochordal cell tumours: overlooked precursors of classic chordomas? Histopathology 44: 597–602.

3012. Yamaguchi T, Watanabe-Ishiiwa H,

Suzuki S et al. (2005). Incipient chordoma: a report of two cases of early-stage chordoma arising from benign notochordal cell tumors. Mod Pathol 18: 1005–1010.

3013. Yamaguchi U, Hasegawa T, Hirose T et al. (2003). Sclerosing perineurioma: a clinicopathological study of five cases and diagnostic utility of immunohistochemical staining for GLUT1. Virchows Arch 443: 159–163.

3014. Yamamoto H, Kawana T (1988). Oral nerve sheath myxoma. Report of a case with findings of ultrastructural and immunohistochemical studies. Acta Pathol Jpn 38: 121–127.

3015. Yamamoto H, Yamaguchi H, Aishima S et al. (2009). Inflammatory myofibroblastic tumor versus IgG4-related sclerosing disease and inflammatory pseudotumor: a comparative clinicopathologic study. Am J Surg Pathol 33: 1330–1340.

3016. Yamashita K, Fletcher CD (2010). PEComa presenting in bone: clinicopathologic analysis of 6 cases and literature review. Am J Surg Pathol 34: 1622–1629.

3017. Yamazaki K (2007). An ultrastructural and immunohistochemical study of elastofibroma: CD 34, MEF-2, prominin 2 (CD133), and factor XIIIa-positive proliferating fibroblastic stromal cells connected by Cx43-type gap junctions. Ultrastruct Pathol 31: 209–219.

3018. Yandell DW, Campbell TA, Dayton SH et al. (1989). Oncogenic point mutations in the human retinoblastoma gene: their application to genetic counseling. N Engl J Med 321: 1689–1695.

3019. Yang BT, Wang YZ, Wang XY et al. (2011). Mesenchymal chondrosarcoma of the orbit: CT and MRI findings. Clin Radiol 67: 346–351.

3020. Yang J, Du X, Chen K et al. (2009). Genetic aberrations in soft tissue leiomyosarcoma. Cancer Lett 275: 1–8.

3021. Yang J, Yang D, Sun Y et al. (2011). Genetic amplification of the vascular endothelial growth factor (VEGF) pathway genes, including VEGFA, in human osteosarcoma. Cancer 117: 4925–4938.

3022. Yang J, Ylipaa A, Sun Y et al. (2011). Genomic and molecular characterization of malignant peripheral nerve sheath tumor identifies the IGF1R pathway as a primary target for treatment. Clin Cancer Res 17: 7563–7573.

3023. Yang JY, Kim JM (2009). Small cell extraskeletal osteosarcoma. Orthopedics 32: 217

3024. Yang P, Hirose T, Hasegawa T et al. (1994). Ossifying fibromyxoid tumor of soft parts: a morphological and immunohistochemical study. Pathol Int 44: 448–453.

3025. Yang XR, Ng D, Alcorta DA et al. (2009). T (brachyury) gene duplication confers major susceptibility to familial chordoma. Nat Genet 41: 1176–1178.

3026. Yarmish G, Klein MJ, Landa J et al. (2010). Imaging characteristics of primary osteosarcoma: nonconventional subtypes. Radiographics 30: 1653–1672.

3027. Yasuda T, Nishio J, Sumegi J et al. (2009). Aberrations of 6q13 mapped to the COL12A1 locus in chondromyxoid fibroma. Mod Pathol 22: 1499–1506.

3028. Yaziji H, Ranaldi R, Verdolini R et al. (2000). Primary alveolar soft part sarcoma of the stomach: a case report and review. Pathol Res Pract 196: 519–525.

3029. Ye C, Pan L, Huang Y et al. (2011). Somatic mutations in exon 17 of the TEK gene in vascular tumors and vascular malformations. J Vasc Surg 54: 1760–1768.

3030. Yen CC, Chen WM, Chen TH et al. (2009). Identification of chromosomal aberrations associated with disease progression and a novel 3q13.31 deletion involving LSAMP gene in osteosarcoma. Int J Oncol 35: 775–788.

3031. Yeoh GP, Bale PM, de Silva M (1989). Nasal cerebral heterotopia: the so-called nasal glioma or sequestered encephalocele and its variants. Pediatr Pathol 9: 531–549.

3032. Yi ES, Shmookler BM, Malawer MM et al. (1991). Well-differentiated extraskeletal osteosarcoma. A soft-tissue homologue of parosteal osteosarcoma. Arch Pathol Lab Med 115: 906–909.

3033. Yigit H, Turgut AT, Kosar P et al. (2009). Proliferative myositis presenting with a checkerboard-like pattern on CT. Diagn Interv Radiol 15: 139–142.

3034. Yokoyama R, Tsuneyoshi M, Enjoji M et al. (1993). Prognostic factors of malignant fibrous histiocytoma of bone. A clinical and histopathologic analysis of 34 cases. Cancer 72: 1902–1908.

3035. Yoo HJ, Choi JA, Chung JH et al. (2009). Angioleiomyoma in soft tissue of extremities: MRI findings. AJR Am J Roentgenol 192: W291–W294.

3036. Yoon TY, Kim JW (2006). Fibrous hamartoma of infancy manifesting as multiple nodules with hypertrichosis. J Dermatol 33: 427–429.

3037. Yoshida A, Ushiku T, Motoi T et al. (2010). Immunohistochemical analysis of MDM2 and CDK4 distinguishes low-grade osteosarcoma from benign mimics. Mod Pathol 23: 1279–1288.

3038. Yoshida A, Ushiku T, Motoi T et al. (2010). Well-differentiated liposarcoma with low-grade osteosarcomatous component: an underrecognized variant. Am J Surg Pathol 34: 1361–1366.

3039. Yoshimoto M, Graham C, Chilton-MacNeill S et al. (2009). Detailed cytogenetic and array analysis of pediatric primitive sarcomas reveals a recurrent CIC-DUX4 fusion gene event. Cancer Genet Cytogenet 195: 1–11.

3040. Younga J, Mott M, Hammoud ZT (2010). Venous hemangioma presenting as a superior sulcus tumor. Ann Thorac Surg 90: 2033–2035.

3041. Yu CE, Oshima J, Fu YH et al. (1996). Positional cloning of the Werner's syndrome gene. Science 272: 258–262.

3042. Yu J, Deshmukh H, Payton JE et al. (2011). Array-based comparative genomic hybridization identifies CDK4 and FOXM1 alterations as independent predictors of survival in malignant peripheral nerve sheath tumor. Clin Cancer Res 17: 1924–1934.

3043. Yu RC, Chu C, Buluwela L et al. (1994). Clonal proliferation of Langerhans cells in Langerhans cell histiocytosis. Lancet 343: 767–768.

3044. Yu Y, Demierre MF, Mahalingam M (2010). Anaplastic Kaposi's sarcoma: an uncommon histologic phenotype with an aggressive clinical course. J Cutan Pathol 37: 1088–1091.

3045. Zagars GK, Ballo MT, Pisters PW et al. (2003). Prognostic factors for patients with localized soft-tissue sarcoma treated with conservation surgery and radiation therapy: an analysis of 1225 patients. Cancer 97: 2530–2543.

3046. Zahm SH, Fraumeni JF, Jr. (1997). The epidemiology of soft tissue sarcoma. Semin Oncol 24: 504–514.

3047. Zalupski MM, Ensley JF, Ryan J et al.

(1990). A common cytogenetic abnormality and DNA content alterations in dedifferentiated chondrosarcoma. Cancer 66: 1176–1182.

3048. Zambrano E, Nose V, Perez-Atayde AR et al. (2004). Distinct chromosomal rearrangements in subungual (Dupuytren) exostosis and bizarre parosteal osteochondromatous proliferation (Nora lesion). Am J Surg Pathol 28: 1033–1039.

3049. Zambrano E, Perez-Atayde AR, Ahrens W et al. (2006). Pediatric sclerosing rhabdomyosarcoma. Int J Surg Pathol 14: 193–199.

3050. Zamecnik M, Dorociak F, Vesely L (1997). Calcifying fibrous pseudotumor after trauma. Pathol Int 47: 812

3051. Zamecnik M, Michal M (2001). Perineurial cell differentiation in neurofibromas. Report of eight cases including a case with composite perineurioma-neurofibroma features. Pathol Res Pract 197: 537–544.

3052. Zamecnik M, Michal M (2002). EMA+ cells in dermatofibrosarcoma protuberans. A study of 11 tumors suggesting perineurial cell differentiation. Cesk Patol 38: 55–62.

3053. Zamolyi RQ, Souza P, Nascimento AG et al. (2006). Intraabdominal myositis ossificans: a report of 9 new cases. Int J Surg Pathol 14: 37–41.

3054. Zand DJ, Huff D, Everman D et al. (2004). Autosomal dominant inheritance of infantile myofibromatosis. Am J Med Genet A 126A: 261–266.

3055. Zelger B, Weinlich G, Zelger B (2000). Perineuroma. A frequently unrecognized entity with emphasis on a plexiform variant. Adv Clin Path 4: 25–33.

3056. Zhan F, Barlogie B, Mulligan G et al. (2008). High-risk myeloma: a gene expression based risk-stratification model for newly diagnosed multiple myeloma treated with high-dose therapy is predictive of outcome in relapsed disease treated with single-agent bortezomib or high-dose dexamethasone. Blood 111: 968–969.

3057. Zhan RY, Pan XF, Wan S et al. (2011). Solitary intracerebral chondroma without meningeal attachment: a case report with review of the literature. J Int Med Res 39: 675–681.

3058. Zhang H, Erickson-Johnson M, Wang X et al. (2010). Molecular testing for lipomatous tumors: critical analysis and test recommendations based on the analysis of 405 extremity-based tumors. Am J Surg Pathol 34: 1304–1311.

3059. Zhang H, Macdonald WD, Erickson-Johnson M et al. (2007). Cytogenetic and molecular cytogenetic findings of intimal sarcoma. Cancer Genet Cytogenet 179: 146–149.

3060. Zhang J, Cheng K, Ding Y et al. (2011). Study of single voxel (1H MR spectroscopy of bone tumors: Differentiation of benign from malignant tumors. Eur J Radiol. In press.

3061. Zhang Q, Wang S, Divakaran J et al. (2010). Malignant glomus tumour of the lung. Pathology 42: 594–596.

3062. Zhang S, Bhalodia A, Swartz B et al. (2010). Fine needle aspiration of parapharyngeal space adult rhabdomyoma: a case report. Acta Cytol 54: 775–779.

3063. Zhang Y, Jorda M, Goldblum JR (2010). Perianal mammary-type myofibroblastoma. Ann Diagn Pathol 14: 358–360.

3064. Zhao C, Yamada T, Kuramochi S et al. (2000). Two cases of ectopic hamartomatous thymoma. Virchows Arch 437: 643–647.

3065. Zhao J, Roth J, Bode-Lesniewska B et al. (2002). Combined comparative genomic hybridization and genomic microarray for detection of gene amplifications in pulmonary artery intimal sarcomas and adrenocortical tumors. Genes Chromosomes Cancer 34: 48–57.

3066. Zheng MH, Robbins P, Xu J et al. (2001). The histogenesis of giant cell tumour of bone: a model of interaction between neoplastic cells and osteoclasts. Histol Histopathol 16: 297–307.

3067. Zhong M, De Angelo P, Osborne L et al. (2010). Dual-color, break-apart FISH assay on paraffin-embedded tissues as an adjunct to diagnosis of Xp11 translocation renal cell carcinoma and alveolar soft part sarcoma. Am J Surg Pathol 34: 757–766.

3068. Zhou P, Zhang H, Bu H et al. (2009). Paravertebral glomangiomatosis. Case report. J Neurosurg 111: 272–277.

3069. Zibat A, Missiaglia E, Rosenberger A et al. (2010). Activation of the hedgehog pathway confers a poor prognosis in embryonal and fusion gene-negative alveolar rhabdomyosarcoma. Oncogene 29: 6323–6330.

3070. Zielenska M, Marrano P, Thorner P et al. (2004). High-resolution cDNA microarray CGH mapping of genomic imbalances in osteosarcoma using formalin-fixed paraffin-embedded tissue. Cytogenet Genome Res 107: 77–82.

3071. Zillmer DA, Dorfman HD (1989). Chondromyxoid fibroma of bone: thirty-six cases with clinicopathologic correlation. Hum Pathol 20: 952–964.

3072. Zimmerman LE, Burns RP, Wankum G et al. (1982). Trilateral retinoblastoma: ectopic intracranial retinoblastoma associated with bilateral retinoblastoma. J Pediatr Ophthalmol Strabismus 19: 320–325.

3073. Zinzani PL, Carrillo G, Ascani S et al. (2003). Primary bone lymphoma: experience with 52 patients. Haematologica 88: 280–285.

3074. Zou C, Smith KD, Liu J et al. (2009). Clinical, pathological, and molecular variables predictive of malignant peripheral nerve sheath tumor outcome. Ann Surg 249: 1014–1022.

3075. Zucman J, Delattre O, Desmaze C et al. (1993). EWS and ATF-1 gene fusion induced by t(12;22) translocation in malignant melanoma of soft parts. Nat Genet 4: 341–345.

3076. Zukerberg LR, Nickoloff BJ, Weiss SW (1993). Kaposiform hemangioendothelioma of infancy and childhood. An aggressive neoplasm associated with Kasabach-Merritt syndrome and lymphangiomatosis. Am J Surg Pathol 17: 321–328.

3077. Zuntini M, Pedrini E, Parra A et al. (2010). Genetic models of osteochondroma onset and neoplastic progression: evidence for mechanisms alternative to EXT genes inactivation. Oncogene 29: 3827–3834.

3078. Zura RD, Minasi JS, Kahler DM (1999). Tumor-induced osteomalacia and symptomatic looser zones secondary to mesenchymal chondrosarcoma. J Surg Oncol 71: 58–62.

3079. Zurick AO, III, Lenge De Rosen V, Tan CD et al. (2011). Pulmonary artery intimal sarcoma masquerading as pulmonary embolism. Circulation 124: 1180–1181.

3080. Zustin J, Akpalo H, Gambarotti M et al. (2010). Phenotypic diversity in chondromyxoid fibroma reveals differentiation pattern of tumor mimicking fetal cartilage canals development: an immunohistochemical study. Am J Pathol 177: 1072–1078.

Subject index

List of abbreviations

aCGH	array comparative genomic hybridization
AFIP	Armed Forces Institute of Pathology
AIDS	acquired immunodeficiency syndrome
AJCC	American Joint Committee on Cancer
ALK	anaplastic lymphoma kinase
AP	anteroposterior
BAC	bacterial artificial chromosome
CGH	comparative genomic hybridization
CNS	central nervous system
CI	confidence interval
CRP	C-reactive protein
CT	computerized tomography
DAPI	4',6-diamidino-2-phenylindole
EBV	Epstein-Barr virus
EGFR	epidermal growth factor receptor
EMA	epithelial membrane antigen
ERG	ETS-related gene
ER	endoplasmic reticulum
ESR	erythrocyte sedimentation rate
FDG-PET	18F-fluorodeoxyglucose positron emission tomography
FISH	fluorescence in situ hybridization
FNCLCC	Fédération Nationale des Centres de Lutte Contre le Cancer
FS-MRI	fat-suppressed MRI
GFAP	glial-fibrillary acidic protein
H&E	haematoxylin and eosin
HHV8	human herpes virus 8
HIV	human immunodeficiency virus
HPF	high-power field
IGF1, IGF2	insulin-like growth factor 1, insulin-like growth factor 2
IHH	indian hedgehog
IRS	Intergroup Rhabdomyosarcoma Study
LDH	lactate dehydrogenase
LOH	loss of heterozygosity
MET	MET proto-oncogene (hepatocyte growth factor receptor)
MLPA	multiplex ligation-dependent probe amplification
MRI	magnetic resonance imaging
MSA	muscle specific actin
MITF	microphthalmia transcription factor
NCI	National Cancer Institute
NIH	National Institutes of Health
NOS	not otherwise specified
NSE	neuron-specific enolase
ORF	open reading frame
PAS	periodic acid-Schiff
PCR	polymerase chain reaction
PDGF	platelet derived growth factor

PEComa	perivascular epithelioid cell tumour
PET	positron emission tomography
RHG	reverse Giemsa banding
RT-PCR	reverse-transcriptase polymerase chain reaction
SEER	Surveillance Epidemiology and End Results
SHH	sonic hedgehog
SMA	smooth muscle actin
SNP	single nucleotide polymorphism
TFE3	transcription factor E3
TNM	tumour node metastasis
UICC	Union for International Cancer Control
UV	ultraviolet
VEGF3	vascular endothelial growth factor receptor 3